DATE OF RETURN
UNLESS RECALLED BY LIBRARY

30/9/2014	

PLEASE TAKE GOOD CARE OF THIS BOOK

Handbook of Headache

Paolo Martelletti, Timothy J. Steiner (Eds.)

Handbook of Headache
Practical Management

With 26 Figures and 91 Tables

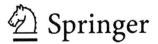 Springer

Lifting The Burden
in official relations with the World Health Organization
The Global Campaign against Headache

Editors
Paolo Martelletti
Department of Medical and Molecular Sciences
School of Health Sciences
Sapienza University of Rome
Rome
Italy

Timothy J. Steiner
Department of Neuroscience
Norwegian University of Science and Technology
Trondheim
Norway
and
Department of Neuroscience
Faculty of Medicine
Imperial College London
London
UK

ISBN 978-88-470-1699-6   e-ISBN 978-88-470-1700-9
Print and electronic bundle under ISBN 978-88-470-2009-2
DOI 10.1007/978-88-470-1700-9
Springer Milan Heidelberg Dordrecht London New York

Library of Congress Control Number: 2011928071

Springer is part of Springer Science+Business Media (www.springer.com)

Printed on acid-free paper

This volume is dedicated to all physicians tending
headache patients in their daily practice

Foreword

Headache is felt, at some time, by nearly everybody, and almost half the world's adults at any one time have recent personal experience of one or more headache disorders. In the Global Burden of Disease Study, updated in 2004, migraine on its own was found to account for 1.3% of all years of life lost to disability worldwide. While headache sometimes signals serious underlying illness, the public-health importance of headache disorders lies in their causal association with the personal and societal burdens of pain, disability, impaired quality of life and financial cost.

Despite the widespread occurrence and incapacitating nature of headache, headache disorders are under-recognized and under-treated everywhere. An important clinical barrier to effective headache management is lack of knowledge among health-care providers. Education is an important pillar to improve the management and thus reduce the burden of headache disorders. Most management of headache disorders lies in primary care, with non-specialists. Management by non-specialists in primary care can be made better by the provision of practical clinical management supports.

I am therefore pleased to note that the *Handbook of Headache* developed by *Lifting The Burden* includes information to support non-specialist primary health-care providers in identifying and managing headache disorders. The objectives of *Lifting the Burden,* a nongovernmental organization in official relations with World Health Organization, are not only to increase professional, public and political awareness of the global burden of headache but also to help in implementing effective and affordable local health-care solutions to it.

The *Handbook of Headache* is aimed at improving professional awareness and covers areas such as public-health importance of headache disorders and principles and details of good management. It also discusses the role of civil society in improving headache care. The *Handbook of Headache* is written and peer-reviewed by contributors from all over the world. I hope that the *Handbook of Headache* will be used by the global health community and civil society to improve headache care and services worldwide.

Dr. Ala Alwan
Assistant Director-General
NonCommunicable Diseases & Mental Health
World Health Organization
Geneva
Switzerland

Preface

Better access, without artificial barriers, to better headache services worldwide is the objective of *Lifting The Burden*: The Global Campaign Against Headache. Very large numbers of people have their lives affected by headache disorders, in particular migraine and tension-type headache, which collectively impose heavy individual and societal burdens and which are – or should be – public-health priorities. Because of these numbers, and also because specialist care is unnecessary in the great majority of cases, management of these disorders should lie very largely within the ambit of primary care. The *Handbook of Headache* is one of a range of management aids developed by *Lifting The Burden* specifically to support nonexpert primary health-care providers in this purpose. It supplements the others, offering all the basics of headache medicine together with detailed information on most aspects for the occasions when this may be required.

Clinicians confronted daily by headache disorders, and others who treat them less regularly or only occasionally, will find parts at least of the *Handbook of Headache* useful in their practice and, we hope, other parts to be of interest. The general approach of the *Handbook of Headache* favors practical management and application of current knowledge without discouraging innovative proposals and trends in basic and clinical research. In many cases, two levels of information, often under the headings "Established knowledge" and "Current research," go further than the practical and intellectual needs of the nonexpert in primary care and make useful offerings to a wider range of health-care professionals, to basic and clinical scientists in academia and industry whose interests lie in headache and related fields, to students and teachers of headache medicine, and to concerned laypeople.

The *Handbook of Headache* is, essentially, an educational project conceived by and published on behalf of *Lifting The Burden*: The Global Campaign Against Headache. Chapters cover the public-health importance of headache disorders (remarked upon above), the very major economic issues arising from such common and disabling ailments, the various causes of headache, the different clinical pictures of headache disorders, the basis of correct and timely diagnosis, the principles and detail of good management (including the challenges of difficult-to-treat headaches), the more common secondary headaches that must be recognized, troublesome facial pains, headache in children, adolescents and the elderly, the complex interactions between medication and headache, complementary and alternative approaches to headache care, and, finally, the present and future roles of nongovernmental organizations in better headache care. Along the way, other chapters clarify dilemmas such as surgical techniques proposed for the management of refractory chronic cluster headache, and discuss emerging therapies for chronic migraine. Comprehensive cross-referencing throughout, including hyperlinks in the online version, aims to facilitate navigation between related articles and, thereby, the practical usefulness of the *Handbook of Headache*. The multiple sections each have a subeditor and a subeditorial board. Renowned experts – scientists and physicians of all world regions, from developed and developing countries – have contributed. All chapters have been peer-reviewed by others from the panel of contributors. Coauthorship of most chapters has further ensured widely ranging content that is cross-culturally relevant, even in those parts of the world where headache management is still in its dawn. Chapters especially witnessing this global sensitivity include those on headache in the tropics and traditional treatments.

The *Handbook of Headache* is available in its entirety or in single constituent chapters. As an eReference it will be given hospitality on institutional platforms, and will be very easy to retrieve online, promoting wide dissemination of its content and achievement of its purpose: through education, the better practice of headache medicine everywhere, better headache services, the dismantling of barriers that restrict access to them and, ultimately, reduction in the burden of headache worldwide.

Paolo Martelletti
Chairman, *Lifting The Burden*
paolo.martelletti@uniroma1.it

Timothy J. Steiner
Director, *The Global Campaign Against Headache*
t.steiner@imperial.ac.uk

Editors-in-Chief

Paolo Martelletti
Department of Medical and Molecular
Sciences
School of Health Sciences
Sapienza University of Rome
Rome
Italy

Timothy J. Steiner
Department of Neuroscience
Norwegian University of Science
and Technology
Trondheim
Norway
and
Department of Neuroscience
Faculty of Medicine
Imperial College London
London
UK

Editorial Board

Messoud Ashina
Danish Headache Centre
Department of Neurology
Glostrup Hospital
University of Copenhagen
Glostrup, Copenhagen
Denmark
Part 7: *Cluster headache and other
trigeminal autonomic cephalalgias*

Rigmor Jensen
Danish Headache Centre
Department of Neurology
Glostrup Hospital
University of Copenhagen
Glostrup, Copenhagen
Denmark
Part 10: *Common or important secondary
headaches and facial pains*

Lars Bendtsen
Danish Headache Centre
Department of Neurology
Glostrup Hospital
University of Copenhagen
Glostrup, Copenhagen
Denmark
Part 6: *Tension-type headache*

Morris Levin
Department of Neurology
Dartmouth Headache Center
Dartmouth Hitchcock Medical Center
Lebanon, NH
USA
Part 4: *Correct and timely headache
diagnosis*

[†]Deceased

Table of Contents

Part 1   Overview of Headache Disorders

Part 2   Headache Disorders and Public Health

Part 3   The Causes of Headache

[†]Deceased

Part 15   Non-Governmental Organizations in Headache

List of Contributors

Mohammed Al Jumah
College of Medicine
KAIMRC, King Saud Ben Abdulaziz
University for Health Sciences
Riyadh
Saudi Arabia

Fabio Antonaci
University Consortium for Adaptive
Disorders and Head Pain (UCADH) and
Headache Science Centre
Pavia
Italy

Ichiro Arakawa
Faculty of Pharmaceutical Sciences
Teikyo Heisei University
Chiba
Japan

Messoud Ashina
Danish Headache Centre
Department of Neurology
Glostrup Hospital
University of Copenhagen
Glostrup, Copenhagen
Denmark

Sait Ashina
Department of Neurology
Albert Einstein College of Medicine
Montefiore Medical Center
Bronx, NY
USA

Sheena K. Aurora
Swedish Headache and Pain Center
Swedish Neurosciences Institute
Seattle, WA
USA

Thorsten Bartsch
Department of Neurology
University Hospital Schleswig-Holstein
University of Kiel
Kiel
Germany

Werner John Becker
University of Calgary and Alberta Health
Services
Calgary, AB
Canada

Lars Bendtsen
Danish Headache Centre
Department of Neurology
Glostrup Hospital
University of Copenhagen
Glostrup, Copenhagen
Denmark

David Bezov
Department of Neurology
Albert Einstein College of Medicine
Montefiore Medical Center
Bronx, NY
USA

Gretchen L. Birbeck
Department of Epidemiology & Neurology
Michigan State University
East Lansing, MI
USA
and
Chikankata Health Services
Mazabuka
Zambia

Carlos Alberto Bordini
Clínica Neurológica Batatais
Batatais, SP
Brazil

Susan W. Broner
The Headache Institute
St. Luke's-Roosevelt Hospital
New York, NY
USA

Dawn C. Buse
Department of Neurology
Albert Einstein College of Medicine of
Yeshiva University
Bronx, NY
USA
and
Ferkauf Graduate School of Psychology
of Yeshiva University
Montefiore Headache Center
Bronx, NY
USA

Maria Gabriella Buzzi
Post-Coma Unit and Headache Centre
IRCCS Fondazione Santa Lucia
Rome
Italy

Antonio Carolei
Department of Neurology
University of L'Aquila
L'Aquila
Italy

Donna Maria Coleston-Shields
Department of Neuropsychology
Neurosciences Unit
University Hospital
Coventry & Warwickshire
Coventry
UK

Giorgio Cruccu
Department of Neurological Sciences
Sapienza University of Rome
Rome
Italy

Boukje de Vries
Department of Human Genetics
Leiden University Medical Centre
Leiden
The Netherlands

David Dodick
Department of Neurology
Mayo Clinic Arizona
Phoenix, AZ
USA

Anne Ducros
Assistance Publique des Hôpitaux de Paris
Head and Neck Clinic
Hôpital Lariboisière
Paris
France

Lars Edvinsson
Department of Medicine
Lund University Hospital
Lund
Sweden

Stefan Evers
Department of Neurology
University of Münster
Münster
Germany

Ivano Farinelli
Department of Medical and Molecular
Sciences
School of Health Sciences
Sapienza University of Rome
Rome
Italy

Anna Ferrari
Headache and Drug Abuse Inter-Dep.
Research Centre
Division of Toxicology and Clinical
Pharmacology
University of Modena and Reggio Emilia
Modena
Italy

Lorenzo Gardella
Servicio of Neurology
Sanatorio Parque
Rosario, Santa Fe
Argentina

Astrid Gendolla
Regionales Schmerzzentrum Essen
Essen
Germany

Lara Gitto
CEIS Sanità (Centre for Health Economics
and Management – CHEM)
University Tor Vergata
Rome
Italy
and
University of Catania
Catania
Italy

Joost Haan
Department of Neurology
Rijnland Hospital
Leiderdorp
The Netherlands
and
Department of Neurology
Leiden University Medical Centre
Leiden
The Netherlands

Andrew D. Hershey
Division of Neurology
Department of Pediatrics
Headache Center
Cincinnati Children's Hospital Medical
Center
University of Cincinnati College of Medicine
Cincinnati, OH
USA

Valerie Hobbs
OUCH (UK) Organisation for the
Understanding of Cluster Headache
Tenby, Pembrokeshire
UK

Crispin Jenkinson
Health Services Research Unit
Department of Public Health and Primary
Care
University of Oxford
Oxford
UK

Rigmor Jensen
Danish Headache Centre
Department of Neurology
Glostrup Hospital
University of Copenhagen
Glostrup, Copenhagen
Denmark

Marielle A. Kabbouche
Division of Neurology
Department of Pediatrics
Headache Center
Cincinnati Children's Hospital Medical
Center
University of Cincinnati College of Medicine
Cincinnati, OH
USA

Regina N. M. Kamoga
Community Health And Information
Network (CHAIN)
Kampala
Uganda

Zaza Katsarava
Center for Neurology
University of Essen
Essen
Germany

Christian Lampl
Department of Neurology and Pain
Medicine
Headache Center
Konventhospital Barmherzige Brüder Linz
Linz
Austria

Morris Levin
Department of Neurology
Dartmouth Headache Center
Dartmouth Hitchcock Medical Center
Lebanon, NH
USA

Elizabeth W. Loder
Division of Headache and Pain
Department of Neurology
Brigham and Women's/Faulkner Hospitals
Boston, MA
USA

Antoinette Maassen van den Brink
Division of Vascular Medicine and
Pharmacology
Department of Internal Medicine
Erasmus University Medical Center
Rotterdam
The Netherlands

E. Anne MacGregor
The City of London Migraine Clinic
London
UK

Andrea Marcellusi
CEIS Sanità
(Centre for Health Economics and
Management – CHEM)
University Tor Vergata
Rome
Italy

Paolo Martelletti
Department of Medical and Molecular
Sciences
School of Health Sciences
Sapienza University of Rome
Rome
Italy

Isabel Pavão Martins
Unidade Neurológica de Investigação
Clínica
Instituto Medicina Molecular (IMM)
Lisbon Faculty of Medicine
Portugal Hospital de Sta Maria
Lisbon
Portugal

Ninan T. Mathew
Houston Headache Clinic
Houston, TX
USA

Alexander Mauskop
New York Headache Center
New York, NY
USA

Allison McLean
Alberta Health Services
Calgary, AB
Canada

Francesco Saverio Mennini
CEIS Sanità
(Centre for Health Economics and
Management – CHEM)
University Tor Vergata
Rome
Italy
and
Sapienza University of Rome
Rome
Italy

Dimos D. Mitsikostas
Neurology Department
Athens Naval Hospital
Athens
Greece

Jakob Møller Hansen
Danish Headache Centre
Department of Neurology
Glostrup Hospital
University of Copenhagen
Glostrup, Copenhagen
Denmark

Pasquale Montagna[†]
Department of Neurological Sciences
University of Bologna
Bologna
Italy

Andrea Negro
Department of Medical and Molecular
Sciences
School of Health Sciences
Sapienza University of Rome
Rome
Italy

Jes Olesen
Danish Headache Centre
Department of Neurology
Glostrup Hospital
University of Copenhagen
Glostrup, Copenhagen
Denmark

Vera Osipova
Department of Neurology and
Neurophysiology
Neurological Clinic
Sechenov Moskow Medical Academy
Moscow
Russian Federation

Koen Paemeleire
Department of Neurology
Ghent University Hospital
Ghent
Belgium

Juan A. Pareja
Department of Neurology
Hospital Quirón Madrid
Madrid
Spain

Suraj Perera
Ministry of Health Care & Nutrition
Colombo
Sri Lanka

Mario Fernando Prieto Peres
Universidade Federal de São Paulo
São Paulo
Brazil

Michele Peters
Health Services Research Unit
Department of Public Health and Primary
Care
University of Oxford
Oxford
UK

Sanjay Prakash
Department of Neurology
Medical College & SSG Hospital
Baroda, Gujarat
India

Luiz Paulo Queiroz
Department of Neurology
Universidade Federal de Santa Catarina
Florianópolis, SC
Brazil

Shireen Qureshi
Department of Internal Medicine
Saudi Aramco
Dhahran Health Center
Dhahran
Saudi Arabia

[†]Deceased

Alan Rapoport
The David Geffen School of Medicine
at UCLA
Los Angeles, CA
USA
and
The New England Center for Headache
Stamford, CT
USA

K. Ravishankar
The Headache and Migraine Clinic
Jaslok Hospital and Research Centre
Mumbai
India
and
The Headache and Migraine Clinic
Lilavati Hospital and Research Centre
Mumbai
India

Simona Sacco
Department of Neurology
University of L'Aquila
L'Aquila
Italy

Fumihiko Sakai
International Headache Center
Shinyurigaoka
Kitasato University Hospital
Asao Kawasaki, Kanagawa
Japan

Markus Schürks
Division of Preventive Medicine
Department of Medicine
Brigham and Women's Hospital
Harvard Medical School
Boston, MA
USA
and
Department of Neurology
University Hospital
Essen
Germany

Todd J. Schwedt
Washington University in St. Louis
School of Medicine
St. Louis, MO
USA

Henrik Winther Schytz
Danish Headache Center
Department of Neurology
Glostrup Hospital
University of Copenhagen
Glostrup, Copenhagen
Denmark

Timothy J. Steiner
Department of Neuroscience
Norwegian University of Science and
Technology
Trondheim
Norway
and
Department of Neuroscience
Faculty of Medicine
Imperial College London
London
UK

Lars Jacob Stovner
Department of Neuroscience
Norwegian National Headache Centre
Norwegian University of Science and
Technology
and
St. Olavs Hospital
Trondheim
Norway

Andreas Straube
Department of Neurology
University of Munich
Munich
Germany

Christina Sun-Edelstein
Department of Neurology
Centre for Clinical Neurosciences and
Neurological Research
St Vincent's Hospital
Melbourne
Australia

Cristina Tassorelli
Headache Science Centre
IRCCS "National Neurological Institute
C. Mondino" Foundation and University
Consortium for Adaptive Disorders and
Head Pain (UCADH)
University of Pavia
Pavia
Italy

Redda Tekle Haimanot
Department of Internal Medicine
Addis Ababa University
Addis Ababa
Ethiopia

Gisela M. Terwindt
Department of Neurology
Leiden University Medical Centre
Leiden
The Netherlands

Peer Carsten Tfelt-Hansen
Danish Headache Centre
Department of Neurology
Glostrup Hospital
University of Copenhagen
Glostrup, Copenhagen
Denmark

Andrea Truini
Department of Neurological Sciences
Sapienza University of Rome
Rome
Italy

Dominique Valade
Emergency Headache Center
Lariboisière Hospital
Assistance Publique des Hôpitaux de Paris
Paris
France

Sara Van Belle
Department of Public Health
Prince Leopold Institute of Tropical
Medicine
Antwerp
Belgium

Hans A. van Suijlekom
Department of Anesthesiology, ICU and
Pain Management
Catharina Ziekenhuis
Eindhoven
The Netherlands

Carlos M. Villalón
Departamento de Farmacobiología
Cinvestav-Coapa
México, DF
Mexico

Maurice B. Vincent
Hospital Universitário Clementino Fraga
Filho
Universidade Federal do Rio de Janeiro
Rio de Janeiro, RJ
Brazil

Shuu-Jiun Wang
Department of Neurology
Neurological Institute
Taipei Veterans General Hospital
Taipei
Taiwan
and
Department of Neurology
National Yang–Ming University School of
Medicine
Taipei
Taiwan

Tom Whitmarsh
Glasgow Homeopathic Hospital
Glasgow, Scotland
UK

Christian Wöber
Department of Neurology
Medical University of Vienna
Vienna
Austria

Çiçek Wöber-Bingöl
Department of Child and Adolescent
Psychiatry
Medical University of Vienna
Vienna
Austria

Lisa Yablon
New York Headache Center
New York, NY
USA

Sheng-Yuan Yu
Department of Neurology
Chinese PLA General Hospital
Beijing
People's Republic of China

Joanna M. Zakrzewska
Division of Diagnostic, Surgical and Medical
Sciences
Eastman Dental Hospital
UCLH NHS Foundation Trust
London
UK

Part 1

Overview of Headache Disorders

1 Overview of Common and Important Headache Disorders

Timothy J. Steiner[1,2] · *Paolo Martelletti*[3]
[1]Norwegian University of Science and Technology, Trondheim, Norway
[2]Faculty of Medicine, Imperial College London, London, UK
[3]School of Health Sciences, Sapienza University of Rome, Rome, Italy

Paolo Martelletti, Timothy J. Steiner (eds.), *Handbook of Headache*, DOI 10.1007/978-88-470-1700-9_1,
© Lifting The Burden 2011

Abstract: The purpose of this chapter is to provide a summary of headache disorders that are common or important in primary care. Later chapters cover all aspects in greater detail.

The key headache disorders are primary – migraine, tension-type headache, and cluster headache. A relatively small number of secondary headache disorders may be seen in primary care and are important because they are serious and need to be recognized.

Collectively, headache disorders are common and ubiquitous. They have a neurological basis, but headache rarely signals serious underlying illness. The huge public-health importance of headache arises from its causal association with personal and societal burdens of pain, disability, damaged quality of life, and financial cost.

Headache disorders have many types and subtypes, but a very small number of them impose almost all of these burdens. Most of these can be effectively treated. They are diagnosed clinically, requiring no special investigations. Their management belongs in primary care.

Mismanagement and overuse of medications to treat acute headache are major risk factors for disease aggravation.

Headache

Headache is a painful feature of a relatively small number of primary headache disorders that in many cases are lifelong conditions. Headache also occurs as a characteristic symptom of many other conditions; these are termed secondary headache disorders. Although the International Headache Society classifies almost 200 distinct headache disorders – under 14 headings, the first four of which cover the primary headache disorders (❷ *Table 1.1*) – most are not of significance in primary care. A few are, and must be recognized, because they are serious.

There are regional variations, but headache disorders are highly prevalent throughout the world. Collectively, they are among the most common disorders of the nervous system. They affect people of all ages, races, income levels, and geographical areas. Furthermore, some of them cause substantial disability, which is imposed on all populations along with a very considerable socioeconomic burden.

Despite this, headache is underestimated in scope and scale, and headache disorders remain under-recognized and undertreated everywhere.

Migraine

Migraine is a primary headache disorder, probably with a genetic basis. Activation of a mechanism deep in the brain causes release of pain-producing inflammatory substances around the nerves and blood vessels of the head. Why this happens periodically and what brings the process to an end in spontaneous resolution of attacks are uncertain.

Usually starting at puberty, migraine is recurrent throughout life in many cases. Adults with migraine describe episodic attacks with specific features (❷ *Table 1.2*), of which headache and nausea are the most characteristic. In children, attacks tend to be shorter-lasting and abdominal symptoms more prominent. Attack frequency is typically once or twice a month but can be anywhere between once a year and once a week, often subject to lifestyle and environmental factors.

◘ Table 1.1

The international classification of headache disorders (International Headache Society Classification Subcommittee 2004)

Primary headaches	1. Migraine, *including*: 1.1 Migraine without aura 1.2 Migraine with aura
	2. Tension-type headache, *including*: 2.1 Infrequent episodic tension-type headache 2.2 Frequent episodic tension-type headache 2.3 Chronic tension-type headache
	3. Cluster headache and other trigeminal autonomic cephalalgias, *including*: 3.1 Cluster headache
	4. Other primary headaches
Secondary headaches	5. Headache attributed to head and/or neck trauma, *including*: 5.2 Chronic posttraumatic headache
	6. Headache attributed to cranial or cervical vascular disorder, *including*: 6.2.2 Headache attributed to subarachnoid hemorrhage 6.4.1 Headache attributed to giant cell arteritis
	7. Headache attributed to nonvascular intracranial disorder, *including*: 7.1.1 Headache attributed to idiopathic intracranial hypertension 7.4 Headache attributed to intracranial neoplasm
	8. Headache attributed to a substance or its withdrawal, *including*: 8.1.3 Carbon monoxide-induced headache 8.1.4 Alcohol-induced headache 8.2 Medication-overuse headache 8.2.1 Ergotamine-overuse headache 8.2.2 Triptan-overuse headache 8.2.3 Analgesic-overuse headache
	9. Headache attributed to infection, *including*: 9.1 Headache attributed to intracranial infection
	10. Headache attributed to disorder of homoeostasis
	11. Headache or facial pain attributed to disorder of cranium, neck, eyes, ears, nose, sinuses, teeth, mouth, or other facial or cranial structures, *including*: 11.2.1 Cervicogenic headache 11.3.1 Headache attributed to acute glaucoma
	12. Headache attributed to psychiatric disorder
Neuralgias and other headaches	13. Cranial neuralgias, central and primary facial pain and other headaches, *including*: 13.1 Trigeminal neuralgia
	14. Other headache, cranial neuralgia, central or primary facial pain

◨ Table 1.2

Typical features of adult migraine headache

Headache	Moderate or severe in intensity One-sided and/or pulsating Aggravated by routine physical activity
Duration	Hours to 2–3 days
Accompanying symptoms	Nausea and sometimes vomiting and/or dislike or intolerance of normal levels of light and sound

Migraine is most disabling to those aged 35–45 years, but it can trouble much younger people, including children. In Europe and the USA, migraine affects 6–8% of men and 15–18% of women. The higher rates in women are hormonally driven. Similar patterns probably exist in Central and South America, with prevalences only slightly lower. In India, migraine is likely to be common: high temperatures and light levels for more than 8 months of the year, the heavy noise pollution and the Indian habits of omitting breakfast, frequent fasting, and eating rich, spicy, and fermented food are thought to be common triggers. Migraine appears less prevalent, but still common, elsewhere in Asia (around 8–10%) and in Africa (3–7%). In these areas, population-based studies are now being performed.

Tension-Type Headache

The mechanism of tension-type headache is poorly understood although it has long been regarded as a headache with muscular origins. It may be stress-related or associated with musculoskeletal problems in the neck.

Tension-type headache has distinct subtypes. Episodic tension-type headache, like migraine, occurs in attack-like episodes. These usually last no more than a few hours but can persist for several days. Chronic tension-type headache, one of the chronic daily headache syndromes, is present most of the time and can be unremitting over long periods. It is less common, but much more disabling to those affected.

Headache in either case is usually mild or moderate and generalized, though it can be one-sided. It is described as pressure or tightness, like a band around the head, sometimes spreading into or from the neck. It lacks the specific features and associated symptoms of migraine.

Tension-type headache pursues a highly variable course, often beginning during the teenage years and reaching peak levels in the 30s. It affects three women to every two men. Episodic tension-type headache is the most common headache disorder, reported by over 70% of some populations although its prevalence appears to vary greatly worldwide. In Japan, for example, 22% of the population report this disorder, while a prevalence of only 3% has been recorded in a rural population of Saudi Arabia. Lack of reporting and underdiagnosis are likely factors here, and cultural attitudes to reporting a relatively minor complaint may explain at least part of the variation elsewhere. Chronic tension-type headache affects 1–3% of adults.

Cluster Headache

Cluster headache is one of a group of primary headache disorders (trigeminal autonomic cephalalgias) of uncertain mechanism that are characterized by frequently recurring, short-lasting but extremely severe headache.

Cluster headache also has episodic and chronic forms. Episodic cluster headache occurs in bouts (clusters), typically of 6–12 weeks' duration once a year or 2 years and at the same time of the year. Strictly one-sided intense pain develops around the eye once or more times daily, mostly at night. Unable to stay in bed, the affected person agitatedly paces the room, even going outdoors, until the pain diminishes after 30–60 min. The eye is red and waters, the nose runs or is blocked on the affected side, and the eyelid may droop. In the less common chronic cluster headache, there are no remissions between clusters. The episodic form can become chronic, and vice versa.

Though relatively uncommon, affecting no more than 3 per 1,000 adults, cluster headache is highly recognizable. It is unusual among primary headache disorders in affecting six men to each woman. Most people developing cluster headache are in their 20s or older. Once present, the condition may persist intermittently for 40 years or more.

Medication-Overuse Headache

Chronic excessive use of medication to treat headache is the cause of medication-overuse headache, another of the chronic daily headache syndromes.

Medication-overuse headache is oppressive, persistent, and often at its worst on awakening in the morning. A typical history begins with episodic headache – migraine or tension-type headache – treated with an analgesic or other medication for each attack. Over time, headache episodes become more frequent, as does medication intake. In the end stage, which not all patients reach, headache persists all day, fluctuating with medication use repeated every few hours. This evolution occurs over a few weeks or much, much longer. A common and probably key factor at some stage in the development of medication-overuse headache is a switch to preemptive use of medication, in anticipation of the headache.

All medications for the acute or symptomatic treatment of headache, in overuse, are associated with this problem, but what constitutes overuse is not clear in individual cases. Suggested limits are the regular intake of simple analgesics on 15 or more days per month or of codeine- or barbiturate-containing combination analgesics, ergotamine or triptans, or any combination of these, on more than 10 days a month. Frequency of use is important: even when the total quantities are similar, low daily doses carry greater risk than larger weekly doses.

In terms of prevalence, medication-overuse headache far outweighs all other secondary headaches. It affects more than 1% of some populations, women more than men, and children also.

Serious Secondary Headaches (Headaches to Worry About)

Some headaches signal serious underlying disorders. These may demand immediate intervention. Although relatively uncommon, they worry nonspecialists because they are in the differential diagnosis of primary headache disorders. The reality is that intracranial lesions give rise to histories and physical signs that should bring them to mind.

A history indicative of raised intracranial pressure should first suggest *intracranial neoplasm*. Intracranial tumors rarely produce headache until quite large, when raised intracranial pressure is apparent in the history and, in all likelihood, focal neurological signs are present. Because of their infrequency, brain scanning is not justified as a routine investigation in patients with headache.

Meningitis and its associated headache occur in an obviously ill patient. The signs of fever and neck stiffness, later accompanied by nausea and disturbed consciousness, reveal the cause.

Subarachnoid hemorrhage is by far the most common cause of incapacitating headache of abrupt onset, often described as the worst headache ever. It is usually unilateral at onset and accompanied by nausea, vomiting, and impaired consciousness, but may be less severe and without associated signs. Neck stiffness may take some hours to develop. Subarachnoid hemorrhage is very serious (50% of patients die, often before arriving at hospital, and 50% of survivors are left disabled). Unless there is a clear history of similar uncomplicated episodes, headache with these characteristics demands urgent investigation.

New headache in any patient over 50 years of age should raise the suspicion of *giant cell (temporal) arteritis*. This condition is conspicuously associated with headache, which can be severe. The patient, who does not feel entirely well, may also complain of marked scalp tenderness. Jaw claudication is highly suggestive. This disorder must be recognized: there is major risk of blindness, preventable by immediate steroid treatment.

Primary angle-closure glaucoma, rare before middle age, may present dramatically with acute ocular hypertension, a painful red eye with the pupil mid-dilated and fixed, and, essentially, impaired vision. In other cases, headache or eye pain may be episodic and mild.

Idiopathic intracranial hypertension is a rare cause of headache not readily diagnosed on the history alone. Papilledema indicates the diagnosis in adults, but is not seen invariably in children with the condition.

More commonly encountered in the tropics are the acute infections, *viral encephalitis*, *malaria*, and *Dengue fever*, all of which can present with sudden severe headache with or without a neurological deficit. These conditions should be kept in mind wherever they are likely to occur.

Other disorders seen more in the tropics that may present with subacute or chronic headache are *tuberculosis*, *neurocysticercosis*, *neurosarcoidosis*, and *HIV-related infections*. These are often diagnosed only on imaging.

Other Headaches Common in Primary Care

Only a small number of other headache disorders are likely to be seen in primary care. Guidance on their diagnosis is given elsewhere in this Handbook.

Chronic posttraumatic headache, usually secondary to moderate or severe head injury, has no specific features but often occurs as part of the posttraumatic syndrome. This includes symptoms such as equilibrium disturbance, poor concentration, decreased work ability, irritability, depressive mood, and sleep disturbances.

Headache attributed to low cerebrospinal fluid (CSF) pressure has three subtypes, presenting similarly but distinguished by etiology. This headache may develop up to 5 days after lumbar puncture (often resolving spontaneously within a week). Persistent CSF leakage may be caused by another clinical procedure, or by trauma. Low CSF pressure may also develop spontaneously, often with a history of trivial increase in intracranial pressure, such as occurs on vigorous coughing, or after a sudden drop in atmospheric pressure.

Classical trigeminal neuralgia is characterized by unilateral brief electric shock-like pains, abrupt in onset and termination, limited to the distribution of one or more divisions of the trigeminal nerve (usually the second or third). These occur spontaneously, or are evoked by trivial stimuli such as washing, shaving, brushing the teeth, smoking, or talking. They commonly cause facial muscle spasm on the affected side (*tic douloureux*). Between paroxysms there may be no symptoms, or a dull background pain may persist.

Persistent idiopathic facial pain (formerly known as atypical facial pain) is deep and poorly localized, confined at onset to a limited area on one side of the face, and present daily for all or most of the day. It lacks the characteristics of a cranial neuralgia and is not attributable to another disorder (pain may be initiated by surgery or injury to the face, teeth or gums, but persists without any demonstrable local cause).

Over-Diagnosed Headaches

Headache should not be attributed to sinus disease in the absence of other symptoms indicative of it. Errors of refraction are overestimated as a cause of headache. Dental problems may cause jaw or facial pain but rarely headache.

Management and Prevention of Headache Disorders

Health-Care Policy

The volume of headache referrals to neurologists seen in better-resourced countries is difficult to justify (see ❷ Chap. 5), and should not be repeated in countries where headache-related health services are being developed. The common headache disorders require no special investigation: they are diagnosed and managed with skills generally available to physicians. Management of headache therefore belongs in primary care for all but a very small minority of patients. Models of health care vary but, in most countries, primary care has an acknowledged and important role. It is a role founded on recognition that decisions in primary care take account of important patient-related factors such as family medical history and patients' individual expectations and values. The continuity and long-term relationships of primary care generate awareness of these, while promoting trust and satisfaction among patients.

Even in primary care, however, the needs of the headache patient are not met in the time usually allocated to a consultation in many health systems. Nurses and pharmacists can complement the delivery of health care by primary care physicians.

Successful management of headache disorders follows five essential steps:

- The affected person must seek medical treatment.
- A correct diagnosis should be made.

- The treatment offered must be appropriate to the diagnosis.
- The treatment should be taken as directed.
- The patient should be followed up to assess the outcome of treatment, which should be changed if necessary.

Headache Diagnosis

The key to getting the diagnosis right is sufficient time committed to a systematic history. This must highlight or elicit description of the characteristic features of the important headache disorders described above (❍ *Table 1.3*). Different headache types are not mutually exclusive: patients are often aware of more than one headache type, and a separate history should be taken for each.

The correct diagnosis is not always evident initially, especially when more than one headache disorder is present, but the history should awaken suspicion of the important secondary headaches. Once it is established that there is no serious underlying disorder, a diary kept for a few weeks to record the pattern of attacks, symptoms, and medication use will usually clarify the diagnosis.

Physical examination rarely reveals unexpected signs after an adequately taken history, but should include blood pressure measurement and a brief but comprehensive neurological examination including the optic fundi: more is not required unless the history

◘ **Table 1.3**

An approach to the headache history

1. How many different headache types does the patient experience? Separate histories are necessary for each. It is reasonable to concentrate on the most bothersome to the patient but others should always attract some enquiry in case they are clinically important.	
2. *Time questions*	(a) Why consulting now? (b) How recent in onset? (c) How frequent, and what temporal pattern (especially distinguishing between episodic and daily or unremitting)? (d) How long lasting?
3. *Character questions*	(a) Intensity of pain (b) Nature and quality of pain (c) Site and spread of pain (d) Associated symptoms
4. *Cause questions*	(a) Predisposing and/or trigger factors (b) Aggravating and/or relieving factors (c) Family history of similar headache
5. *Response questions*	(a) What does the patient do during the headache? (b) How much is activity (function) limited or prevented? (c) What medication has been and is used, and in what manner?
6. *State of health between attacks*	(a) Completely well, or residual or persisting symptoms? (b) Concerns, anxieties, fears about recurrent attacks, and/or their cause

is suggestive. Examination of the head and neck may find muscle tenderness, limited range of movement or crepitation, which suggest a need for physical forms of treatment but not necessarily headache causation.

Investigations, including neuroimaging, rarely contribute to the diagnosis of headache when the history and examination have not suggested an underlying cause.

Realistic Objectives

There are few patients troubled by headache whose lives cannot be improved by the right management, with the objective of minimizing impairment of life and lifestyle (❯ *Table 1.4*). Cure is rarely a realistic aim in primary headache disorders, but people disabled by headache should not have unduly low expectations of what is achievable through optimum management. Medication-overuse headache and other secondary headaches are, at least in theory, resolved through treatment of the underlying cause.

Predisposing and Trigger Factors

Migraine in particular is subject to certain physiological and external environmental factors. While predisposing factors increase susceptibility to attacks, trigger factors may initiate them. The two may combine.

Attempts to control migraine by managing these factors are often disappointing. A few predisposing factors (stress, depression, anxiety, menopause, head or neck trauma) are well recognized but not always avoidable or treatable. Trigger factors are important and their influence real in some patients, although dietary sensitivities affect, at most, 20% of people with migraine. Other lifestyle and environmental trigger factors suggest people with migraine react adversely to change in routine. Many attacks have no obvious triggers and, again, those that are identified are not always avoidable. Diaries may be useful in detecting triggers but the process is complicated as triggers appear to be cumulative, jointly overflowing the "threshold" above which attacks are initiated. Too much effort in seeking triggers causes introspection and

◻ Table 1.4

Seven elements of good headache management

1. Evident interest and investment of time to inform, explain, reassure, and educate
2. Correct and timely diagnosis
3. Agreed high but realistic objectives
4. Identification of predisposing and/or trigger factors and their avoidance through appropriate lifestyle modifications
5. Intervention (optimal management of most primary headaches combines adequate but not excessive use of effective and cost-effective pharmaceutical remedies with non-pharmacological approaches; secondary headaches generally require treatment of the underlying cause)
6. Follow-up to ensure optimum treatment has been established
7. Referral to specialist care when these measures fail

can be counterproductive. Enforced lifestyle change to avoid triggers can itself adversely affect quality of life.

In tension-type headache, stress may be obvious and likely to be etiologically implicated. Musculoskeletal involvement may be evident in the history or on examination. Sometimes, neither of these is apparent. In the Muslim world, a marked rise in tension-type headache incidence on the first day of fasting is observed in people ordinarily susceptible to headache.

Cluster headache is usually but not always a disease of smokers, many of them heavy. However, patients with cluster headache who still smoke cannot be promised that giving up will end or even improve their headaches. Alcohol potently triggers cluster headache and most patients have learnt to avoid it during clusters.

Patient Information

Patients who are informed about and understand their disorder, and the purpose, nature, and expected effects of treatments for it, can be expected generally to adhere better to recommendations and have better outcomes. In this Handbook, each of the sections on the major headache disorders concludes with suggested information to patients.

Therapeutic Intervention

The purpose of pharmacotherapy of primary headache, once nondrug measures have been fully exploited, is to control symptoms so that the impact of the disorder on each individual patient's life and lifestyle is minimized. This requires a therapeutic plan tailored for each patient, and patients with two or more coexisting headache disorders are likely to require separate plans for each disorder.

Use of drugs for headache should, where possible, follow local guidelines that take account of local resources. The following are general guidelines.

No details of treatment are included in this overview: later chapters cover these for each headache type. The following observations are worth making here.

Migraine

Most people with migraine require drugs for the acute attack. Large numbers manage themselves, with no more than symptomatic over-the-counter remedies, and for many this appears adequate. Advice on correct usage (formulation, timing, dosage) may improve outcomes.

For the remainder, the great majority should be perfectly well manageable in primary care. The goal of acute therapy – resolution of symptoms and full return of function within 2 h – is not attainable by everyone with drugs currently available. When symptom control with best acute therapy is inadequate, it can be supplemented with prophylactic medication aiming to reduce the number of attacks. Drugs in a range of pharmacological classes have limited but often useful prophylactic efficacy against migraine. The choice of agent is guided by local availability, but otherwise by comorbidities and contraindications. Because poor compliance is a major factor impairing effectiveness, drugs given once daily are preferable, all else being equal.

Tension-Type Headache

Reassurance and over-the-counter analgesics are usually sufficient for infrequent episodic tension-type headache. Most people with this condition manage themselves: it is self-limiting and, although it may be temporarily disabling, it rarely raises anxieties.

People consult doctors because of episodic tension-type headache when it is becoming frequent and, in all likelihood, no longer responding to painkillers. Symptomatic medication is contraindicated for tension-type headache occurring on more than 2 days/week: when it is already being taken at high frequency, a diagnosis of chronic tension-type headache rather than medication-overuse headache cannot be made with confidence.

Cluster Headache

Because of its relative rarity, cluster headache has a tendency to be misdiagnosed, sometimes for years. It is the one primary headache that may not be best managed in primary care, but the primary care physician has an important role not only in recognizing it at once but also in discouraging inappropriate "treatments" (tooth extraction is not infrequent).

Medication-Overuse Headache

Prevention is the ideal management of medication-overuse headache, with education the key factor: many patients with medication-overuse headache are otherwise unaware of it as a medical condition. Once this disorder has developed, early intervention is important since the long-term prognosis depends on the duration of medication overuse. Treatment is withdrawal of the suspected medication(s). Despite initial worsening, within 2 weeks usually, the headache shows signs of improvement, which continues for weeks to months; 50–75% of patients revert to their original episodic headache type.

Other Headaches

All of the serious secondary headaches described above require specialist referral. In most cases, this should be immediate or urgent.

Headache attributed to low CSF pressure is likely to require specialist intervention whatever its etiology if it persists beyond a week.

Chronic posttraumatic headache and persistent idiopathic facial pain may be difficult to manage, and generally require specialist care. This is true also of classical trigeminal neuralgia. Many, possibly most, patients with this condition have compression of the trigeminal root by tortuous or aberrant vessels for which surgery may be appropriate. Rarely this disorder occurs bilaterally, in which case a central cause such as multiple sclerosis must be considered.

Follow-Up, and Referral

Neither the first diagnosis, nor the first-proposed treatment plan, may be correct. Follow-up is essential.

For migraine and episodic tension-type headache, the interval to follow-up is usually determined by attack frequency. Acute treatment may need several trials before its effect can be judged. Prophylaxis generally achieves observable benefit only after 3–4 weeks (although adverse effects may occur sooner).

For chronic tension-type headache, follow-up provides often-needed psychological support while recovery is slow.

In medication-overuse headache, early review is essential once withdrawal from medication has begun in order to check that it is being achieved: Nothing is less helpful than discovering, 3 months later, that the patient ran into difficulties and gave up the attempt. During later follow-up, the underlying primary headache condition is likely to reemerge and require reevaluation and a new therapeutic plan. Most patients with medication-overuse headache require extended support: the relapse rate is around 40% within 5 years.

Urgent referral for specialist management is recommended at each onset of cluster headache. Weekly review is unlikely to be too frequent, and allows dosage incrementation of potentially toxic drugs to be as rapid as possible.

In all other cases, specialist referral is appropriate when the diagnosis remains (or becomes) unclear or these standard management options fail.

Acknowledgment

The text of this chapter is closely based on educational materials developed for primary-care physicians by *Lifting The Burden: the Global Campaign Against Headache.*

References

International Headache Society Classification Subcommittee (2004) The international classification of headache disorders, 2nd edn. Cephalalgia 24(Suppl 1):S1–S160

Part 2

Headache Disorders and Public Health

2 Epidemiology of Common Headache Disorders

Lars Jacob Stovner[1] · *Redda Tekle Haimanot*[2]
[1]Norwegian National Headache Centre, Norwegian University of Science and Technology and St. Olavs Hospital, Trondheim, Norway
[2]Addis Ababa University, Addis Ababa, Ethiopia

Paolo Martelletti, Timothy J. Steiner (eds.), *Handbook of Headache*, DOI 10.1007/978-88-470-1700-9_2,
© Lifting The Burden 2011

Abstract: This chapter starts with a brief discussion of some main methodological issues related to headache epidemiology, such as case definitions, method of data collection, time frame of the headache, and representativeness of the source population. It then presents the results of all major studies of adequate methodology, demonstrating that the 1-year prevalence of headache is around 50%, of migraine 11%, of tension-type headache (TTH) almost 40%, and of chronic daily headache (CDH) 3%. Cluster headache has a lifetime prevalence of 0.2%. Most headaches affect women more than men, and migraine is particularly prevalent among young and middle-aged adult women. Migraine often starts in childhood in men, but often at a later age in women. The disease varies considerably through life, but it tends to be a lifelong disorder in the majority. Headaches are more prevalent among those of lower socioeconomic status, and there may also be geographical and racial variations in the prevalence.

Many associations between headaches and potential risk factors and comorbid diseases have been found, but the degree to which these associations represent causal connections is largely unknown. For disorders like anxiety, depression, epilepsy, and others, the comorbidity with migraine may be due to common pathophysiological mechanisms. Migraine with aura seems to be a risk factor for cerebrovascular ischemic events among younger women. A most important task for headache epidemiological research in the future will be to identify preventable risk factors for and consequences of headache.

Introduction

Epidemiology has been defined as "the study of distribution and determinants of disease frequency" (Hennekens and Buring 1987). In the headache science, epidemiology has till now mostly been concerned with describing how the different headaches are distributed among men and women, in different age, race, and socioeconomic groups, in urban and rural settings, and in different countries. Such descriptive epidemiology has been important for describing prevalences of headache, and combined with other information, to assess the economical, societal, and psychological burden of headache. This part of epidemiology is important for informing health-care providers and health authorities with the necessary knowledge to assign resources to headache that are proportional to the size of the problem.

Increasingly, however, headache epidemiology is a basic science involved in the mapping of headache determinants, i.e., causes and mechanisms that may lead to better treatment and preferably prevention. One hopes that this so-called analytical headache epidemiology may contribute as much to the understanding and control of headache as it has done for some cancer types and cardiovascular diseases.

Regardless of whether the aim of epidemiology is descriptive or analytical, there are certain methodological issues that should be addressed. Certain problems are relatively specific to headache epidemiology, and an understanding of these problems is necessary for interpreting the results of published studies, and for performing headache epidemiological studies (Stovner 2006).

Methodological Issues in Headache Epidemiology

Case definition, or how to define who has a certain headache (is a case) and who has not, is a problem since headache diagnoses usually are made on the basis of subjective experiences without any objective signs or markers. In many studies, a screening question is used to define subpopulations with and without headache. Significantly higher headache prevalences will be found if the screening question is a neutral one ("do you have headache?") than if it specifies or implies some degree of headache (e.g., "do you *suffer* from headache?," "do you have recurrent headaches" or "do you have severe headache?") (Stovner et al. 2006). Headache diagnoses are ultimately dependent on self-report, and recall problems are probably a bigger problem if one asks about headache in a relatively distant past. In addition, cultural differences related to the threshold for reporting pain may contribute to variation in headache prevalence in different regions or over time. The effect of this factor is largely unknown.

For diagnosing one of the headache subtypes, epidemiological studies should use the criteria of the International Headache Society from 1988 or, in recent years, the revision from 2004 (International Classification of Headache Disorders, 2nd edition (IHCD-2)). However, these criteria are often difficult to apply stringently in many studies, and hence they are often used with some modifications. The way this may influence the results is not well known. Also, one should be aware of the importance of the number of diagnoses used. Studies from the USA (Patel et al. 2004) and France (Lanteri-Minet et al. 2005) indicate that the migraine prevalence will almost double if not only strict migraine (ICHD-2, 1.1 and 1.2) but also probable migraine (ICHD-2, 1.6) are counted as migraine.

In most headache epidemiological studies, the fact that multiple headache types often coexist in the same individuals can be a significant problem. The extent to which multiple headaches can be diagnosed is highly dependent on the *method of data collection*. To make reliable diagnoses of several coexisting headaches, including the rare primary or secondary headaches, it is necessary that *personal interview and examination* is performed by a neurologist using the diagnostic criteria (the "gold-standard" method). This approach is expensive and has been used in a limited number of population studies (❷ *Table 2.1*). However, multiple headache types are of less importance when the study aim is to identify only migraine or TTH sufferers. In *questionnaire studies*, it is usually not possible to diagnose more than one headache type, so the participants may be asked to answer based on their overall most distressing headache.

In all headache epidemiological studies, it is important to define the *time frame* for the headache. Asking participants if they have ever had a headache will give the *lifetime prevalence*. At least in elderly, this may be imprecise due to recall bias. Most commonly, 1-*year prevalence* is used since it is considered reasonably reliable. Also, it defines the proportion of the population that has an active disease, therefore being relevant for assessing the burden of headache in society. The 6- *or 3-month prevalences* will give similar information, and probably also studies not specifying a time frame, only asking a question like "do you suffer from headache?." In general, it is highly advisable to specify a time frame, and most studies to date have been done with the 1-year prevalence (❷ *Table 2.1*).

In all studies not using the gold-standard method, there should be a validation of the diagnostic method to estimate the degree of diagnostic accuracy (sensitivity, specificity, positive, and negative predictive values) between the method applied and the gold-standard method in a random sample of participants.

In all epidemiological studies, it is of vital importance to know the *source population*, i.e., the population from which study participants are drawn. Samples from a country, region, city, or smaller community may be representative for the whole population, and primary school students for their age group, whereas university students, or company employees are probably not representative since they are likely to be more healthy, and patients less healthy than the average. To ensure representativeness of the sample, the participation rate is important. If certain age or socioeconomic groups have a higher nonparticipation rate than the average, this

□ Table 2.1

Studies reporting 1-year prevalence of headache in general, migraine, TTH and "chronic daily headache" (CDH)

Country (year)	Reference	Method	N	Age range (years)	Headache M	Headache F	Headache Tot.	Migraine M	Migraine F	Migraine Tot.	TTH M	TTH F	TTH Tot.	CDH M	CDH F	CDH Tot.
Africa																
Ethiopia 1995	Tekle Haimanot et al. (1995)	P.i.	15,000	≥20				1.7	4.2	3.0				1.0	2.3	1.7
Tanzania 2004	Dent et al. (2004)	P.i.	3,351	≥11	18.8	26.4	23.1	2.5	7.0	5.0						
Tanzania 2009	Winkler et al. (2009a, b)	P.i.	7,412	All			12	2.2	6.4	4.3	5.3	8.8	7.0			
Zimbabwe 1983	Levy 1983	P.i.	5,028	5–70	17.5	27.1	20.0									
Africa (Mean)					18.2	26.8	18.4	2.1	5.9	4.1	5.3	8.8	7.0	1.0	2.3	1.7
Asia																
Japan 1997	Sakai (2008)	T.i.	4,029	≥15			55.6	3.6	13.0	8.4						
Japan 2004	Takeshima et al. (2004)	Q	4,795	≥15	19.1	36.6	28.5	2.3	9.1	6.0	16.2	26.4	21.7	1.5	2.7	2.1
Korea 1998	Roh et al. (1998)	T.i.	5,556	≥15		68		20.2	24.3	22.3						
Malaysia 1996	Alders et al. (1996)	Q	561	≥5				6.7	11.3	9	23.3	29.6	26.5			
Oman 2002	Deleu et al. (2002)	Q	1,158	≥10			78.8			10.1						
Taiwan 2000	Wang et al. (2000)	Q	3,377	≥15	50	72	62	3.4	11.2	7.7						
Taiwan 2001	Lu et al. (2001)	Q	3,377	≥15										1.9	4.3	3.2
Asia (Mean)					34.6	54.3	58.6	7.2	13.8	10.6	19.8	28.0	24.1	1.5	2.7	2.1
Australia/Oceania																
New Zealand 1985	Paulin et al. (1985)	Q	1,139	≥16	39	60	50									
Europe																
Austria 2003	Lampl et al. (2003)	P.i.	997	≥15	43.6	54.6	49.4	6.1	13.8	10.2						
Croatia 2001	Zivadinov et al. (2001)	P.i.	3,794	15–65				13	20.2	16.7						
Denmark 1991	Rasmussen et al. (1991)	P.i.	740	25–64				6	15	10	63	86	74			3

Study	Reference		N	Age												
Denmark 2005	Lyngberg et al. (2005)	P.i.	207	25–36				5.4	23.5	15.5	81.5	90.4	86.5			
Finland 1981	Nikiforow (1981)	P.i.	200	>15	69	83	77									
Georgia 2009	Katsarava et al. (2009b)	P.i.	1,145	≥16			74.5	10.8	18.8	15.6	29	42.8	37.3	5.1	9.3	7.6
Greece 1996	Mitsikostas et al. (1996)	Q	3,501	15–75	19.0	40.0	29							2.1	6.8	4.5
Hungary 2000	Bank and Marton (2000)	Q	813	15–80				2.7	6.9	9.6						
Italy 1988	D'Alessandro et al. (1988)	Q	1,154	>7	35.3	46.2	46									
Netherlands 1999	Launer et al. (1999)	Q	6,491	20–65				7.5	25	16.3						
Norway 2000	Hagen et al. (2000)	Q	51,383	≥20	29.6	45.7	37.7	7.5	15.6	11.6				1.7	2.8	2.4
Norway 2008	Grande et al. (2008)	Q	20,598	30–44												2.9
Spain 1999	Castillo et al. (1999)	Q	2,253	>14										1.0	8.7	4.7
Sweden 2000	Mattsson et al. (2000)	Q	728	40–74					18							
Sweden 2001	Dahlof and Linde (2001)	Q	1,668	18–74	50	76	63	9.5	16.7	13.2						
Switzerland 1994	Merikangas et al. (1994)	P.i.	379	29–30						24.6						
Turkey 2003	Koseoglu et al. (2003)	P.i.	1,146	45–64								18.8				
UK 1975	Waters and O'Connor (1975)	Q	1,718	>21	63.5	78.4										
UK 2003	Steiner et al. (2003)	T.i.	4,007	16–65				7.6	18.3	14.3						
UK 2005	Boardman et al. (2003)	Q	1,589	18–90			76									
Europe (mean)					*44.3*	*60.6*	*56.6*	*7.6*	*17.4*	*14.3*	*57.8*	*59.5*	*65.9*	*2.5*	*6.9*	*4.2*
North America																
Canada 1994	O'Brien et al. (1994)	T.i.	2,922	>18	83.9	90.6		7.4	21.9							
USA 1992	Stewart et al. (1992)	Q	20,468	12–80				5.7	17.6							
USA 1994	Kryst and Scherl (1994)	T.i.	653	>20			13.4	4.5	9.8	8.5						
USA 1996	Stewart et al. (1996)	T.i.	12,328	18–65				8.9	19.0							
USA 1997	Schwartz et al. (1997)	T.i.	13,343	18–65		59.7				13.3						

▢ Table 2.1 (Continued)

Country (year)	Reference	Method	N	Age range (years)	Headache			Migraine			TTH			CDH		
					M	F	Tot.	M	F	Tot.	M	F	Tot.	M	F	Tot.
USA 1998	Schwartz et al. (1998a)	T.i.	13,345	18–65							37.7	44.8	40.3	1.4	2.8	2.2
USA 2001	Lipton et al. (2001)	Q	29,727	>12				6.2	18.2							
USA 2002	Lipton et al. (2002)	T.i.	4,804	18–65				6.0	17.2							
USA 2004	Patel et al. (2004)	T.i.	8,579	18–55				6.6	19.2	14.7						
USA 2006	Bigal et al. (2006a)	T.i.	145,335	≥18				8.4	18.4	15.0						
N. America (mean)					83.9	90.6	36.6	6.7	17.7	12.9	37.7	44.8	40.3	1.4	2.8	2.2
Central/South America																
Argentina 2005	Morillo et al. (2005)	Q	>500	≥15				3.8	6.1	5.0						
Brazil 2002	Wiehe et al. (2002)	P.i.	1,174	≥18	54.4	71.8	63.1									
Brazil 2005	Morillo et al. (2005)	Q	>500	≥5				7.8	17.4	12.6				5,2	9,3	7,3
Brazuil 2008	Queiroz et al. (2008a, b, 2009)	Q	4,075	18–79			72.2	9.3	20.9	15.2	15.4	9.5	13.0	4.0	9.5	6.9
Chile 1997	Lavados and Tenhamm (1997)	Q	1,385	≥15				2.0	11.9	7.3						
Chile 1998	Lavados and Tenhamm (1998)	Q	1,385	≥15							18.1	35.2	26.9	1,1	3,9	2,6
Colombia 2005	Morillo et al. (2005)	Q	>500	≥15				4.8	13.8	9.3						
Ecuador 2005	Morillo et al. (2005)	Q	>500	≥15				2.9	13.5	8.2						
Mexico 2005	Morillo et al. (2005)	Q	>500	≥15				3.9	12.1	10.0						
Peru 1997	Jaillard et al. (1997)	P.i.	3,246	≥15	17.5	38.2	28.7	2.3	7.8	5.3						
Puerto Rico 2003	Miranda (94)	T.i.	1,610	All ages	27.0	40.0	35.9	6.0	16.7	13.5						
Venezuela 2005	Morillo et al. (2005)	Q	>500	≥15				4.7	12.2	8.5						
C/S Am. (mean)					33.0	50.0	50.0	4.8	13.2	9.5	16.8	22.4	20.0	4.0	9.5	6.9
Global mean					39.8	55.4	48.9	6.1	14.9	11.2	32.2	39.2	37.0	2.2	5.6	3.8

Asia	Children and youth															
Taiwan 2005	Wang et al. (2005)	Q	13,426	13–15				4.9	8.9	6.8						
China 2001	Kong et al. (2001)	Q	2,120	5–16			2.8			0.5						
Taiwan 2006	Wang et al. (2006)	Q	7,900	12–14										0.8	2.4	1.5
UAE 1998	Bener et al. (1998)	Q	1,159	6–14			36.9			3.8						
Iran 2006	Ayatollahi and Khosravi (2006)	P.i.	2,226	6–13			31.0	1.4	2.1	1.7	4.3	6.8	5.5			
Asia (mean)							*23.6*	*3.2*	*5.5*	*3.2*	*4.3*	*6.8*	*5.5*	*0.8*	*2.4*	*1.5*
Australia/Oceania																
Australia 1994	Wilkinson et al. (1994)	Q	851	5–12			22									
Europe																
Finland 1983	Sillanpää (1983)	Q	3,784	13	79.8	84.2	82.0									
Finland 1994	Metsähonkala and Sillanpää (1994)	Q	3,580	8–9			36.5	3	2.3	2.7						
Finland 1991	Sillanpaa et al. (1991)	Q	4,405	5			19.5									
Greece 1999	Mavromichalis et al. (1999)	Q	3,509	4–15				5.2	7.3	6.2						
Italy 1995	Raieli et al. (1995)	P.i.	1,445	11–14	19.9	28.1	23.9	2.7	3.3	3						
Norway 2004	Zwart et al. (2004)	Q	8,255	13–19	69.4	84.2	76.8	4.8	9.1	7.0	12.5	23.2	18.0	0.2	0.8	0.5
Sweden 2004	Laurell et al. (2004)	Q	1,850	7–15	39.3	50.3	44.8	9.8	12.2	11.0	7.9	11.8	9.8			
Turkey 2006	Karli et al. (2006)	Q	2,387	12–17	45.1	59.8	52.2			14.5						
UK 1977	Deubner (1977)	Q	600	10–20	74.4	81.5										
UK 1994	Abu-Arefeh and Russell (1994)	Q	2,165	5–15			66	9.7	11.5	10.6						
Europe (mean)					*54.7*	*64.7*	*50.2*	*5.9*	*7.6*	*7.9*	*10.2*	*17.5*	*13.9*	*0.2*	*0.8*	*0.5*
North America																
USA 2000	Rhee (2001)	P.i.	4,591	11–21			91									
USA 2007	Bigal et al. (2007)	Q	18,714	12–19				5.0	7.7	6.3						

◘ Table 2.1 (Continued)

Country (year)	Reference	Method	N	Age range (years)	Headache			Migraine			TTH			CDH		
					M	F	Tot.	M	F	Tot.	M	F	Tot.	M	F	Tot.
Central/South America																
Brazil 1998	Antoniuk et al. (1998)	Q	460	10–14	86.0	92.7	90.0									
Brazil 1996	Barea (118)	P.i.	538	10–18	77.9	87.9	82.9	9.6	10.3	9.9	68.3	76.7	72.3			
C/S Am. (mean)					81.95	90.3	86.45	9.6	10.3	9.9	68.3	76.7	72.3			
Asia																
Elderly																
Taiwan 1997	Wang et al. (1997)	P.i.	1,533	≥65	22	51	38	0.7	4.7	3				1.8	5.6	3.9
Thailand 1991	Srikiatkhachorn (1991)	P.i.	241	≥61	27.8	59.5	54.8									
Asia (mean)					24.9	55.3	46.4	0.7	4.7	3.0				1.8	5.6	3.9
Europe																
Italy 2001	Prencipe et al. (2001)	P.i.	833	≥65	36.6	62.1	51	7.4	13.8	11				2.5	6	4.4
Italy 2003	Camarda and Monastero (2003)	P.i.	1,031	≥65	16.5	26.3	21.8	2.3	6.4	4.6						
Europe (mean)					26.6	44.2	36.4	4.9	10.1	7.8				2.5	6	4.4
North America																
USA 1989	Cook (123)	P.i.		≥65	36	53	45									
South America																
Brazil 2008	Bensenor et al. (2008)	P.i.	2,072	>65	33.7	53.1	45.6	5.1	14.1	10.6	28.1	36.3	33.1			

CDH: Chronic daily headache, TTH: Tension-type headache, M: Males, F :Females, Tot.: Total, N: number, P.i.: Personal interview, T.i.: Telephone interview, Q: Questionnaire

may distort the results. If headache is the main object of the study, individuals suffering from headache may be more likely to participate than non-headache sufferers, and the headache prevalence may be overrated. If participation is found to vary substantially by demographic characteristics, prevalence rates are often adjusted to compensate for differential participation.

Prevalences of Various Headaches

Due to the large variations in the method of different studies, it is not surprising the prevalences vary considerably from one study to another, and from country to country. A review of most prevalence studies has been published (Stovner et al. 2007). In the tables, we have reported the studies giving 1-year prevalence of headache in general, migraine, and tension-type headache (TTH). Also, we have included "chronic daily headache" (CDH), which is not a formal diagnosis, but which is often reported in studies. This term is used if the headache occurs on more days than not ($\geq$15 days per month, or $\geq$180 days per year, or "daily").

As can be seen from the ❷ *Table 2.1*, there are relatively large differences in the prevalences from country to country, and between the continents. The amount of available data for the various continents varies considerably. The global mean of all these studies for headache during the last year among adults is 48.9%. For migraine it is 11.2%, for TTH 37%, and for CDH 3.8%. For all headache categories, the figures are higher for women than for men. Among children and youth the prevalence of headache seems to be similar (50.5%), but the figures are lower for all the headache subcategories (migraine 6.5%, TTH 26.4%, and CDH 1%). Among elderly, there seems to be somewhat less headache in general (41.8%) and migraine (7.4%), whereas figures for TTH (33.1%) and CDH (4.2%) are quite high. Previous comparisons of headache prevalence among different age groups have shown similar trends, that headache in general is high from youth and then declines markedly after 60 years of age (❷ *Fig. 2.1*), whereas migraine prevalence has a marked peak in young and middle-aged adults, particularly among women (❷ *Fig. 2.2*). There seems to be somewhat lower prevalences in Africa, but data from this and some other continents are scarce, and in general, it is not known whether these differences are real or due to variations in methodology.

The criteria for migraine with aura are not easy to apply correctly in epidemiological studies, and usually, it is demanded that the diagnosis should be made by personal interview by a neurologist. In several studies from Europe, North America, and Japan, it has been found that 30–40% of all migraineurs have migraine with aura (Lampl et al. 2003; Lipton et al. 2002; Sakai and Igarashi 1997; Zivadinov et al. 2001). The proportion with aura seems to increase with increasing age (Bigal et al. 2006a).

Chronic migraine is a relatively new and somewhat disputed condition. Based on the original strict criteria, one study has found a prevalence of 0.01% among young adults (30–44 years of age) (Grande et al. 2008). The revised criteria require at least 8 days with migraine and 15 days with headache per month for at least 3 months (Olesen et al. 2006). No epidemiological studies have applied these criteria, but a recent review has estimated that the prevalence is less than 1% if relatively strict criteria are applied (Natoli et al. 2009).

Medication overuse headache can be considered a complication of one of the primary headaches, usually occurring among patients with either migraine or TTH. The original ICHD 2 criteria required that the diagnosis should be made only after successful treatment of the condition ("The International Classification of Headache Disorders. 2nd Edition" 2004; Olesen et al. 2006), which is feasible in the clinic, but not in epidemiological studies. In the

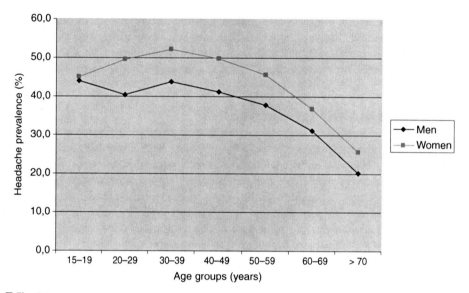

□ Fig. 2.1
Headache prevalence related to age in men and women (Reproduced from Stovner et al. 2006 by courtesy of Cephalalgia)

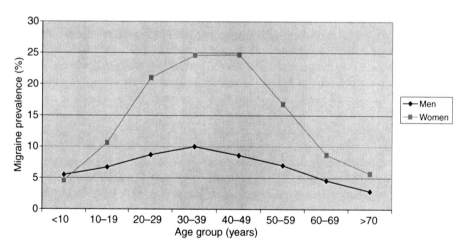

□ Fig. 2.2
Migraine prevalence related to age in men and women (Reproduced from Stovner et al. 2006 by courtesy of Cephalalgia)

revised criteria, the diagnosis can be made based on headache frequency and medication intake alone (Olesen et al. 2006). Among those with chronic headache, medication overuse is frequent, and possible medication overuse headache (i.e., headache and use of medication ≥15 days per month ≥3 months) was found to affect 0.9% in Georgia (Katsarava et al. 2009b) and 1% of adults in Spain (Castillo et al. 1999; Colas et al. 2004). In the HUNT studies in Norway from the 1990s, the prevalence was 1% in adults (Zwart et al. 2003b) and 0.5% in adolescents (Dyb et al. 2006), whereas a more recent study in the same country showed 1.7% in young adults (Aaseth et al. 2008). In Germany, a recent study demonstrated a prevalence of 2% (Katsarava and Diener 2008).

Cluster headache should be diagnosed on the basis of personal interview and examination by a neurologist, and since the condition is quite rare, this must be performed in a relatively large population to detect any cases at all. Till now, only lifetime prevalences have been reported. In a study in which the diagnosis was made by face-to-face interview by a headache expert among more than 1,800 inhabitants of a Norwegian rural community, a lifetime prevalence of 0.326% was found (Sjaastad and Bakketeig 2003). One study in an Italian town among >10,000 patients registered in the lists of general practitioners found cluster headache among 0.279%. The sample was said to be representative of the general population (Torelli et al. 2005). Questionnaires or telephone interviews were used to screen the population, and suspected cases were interviewed by a headache specialist to confirm the diagnosis. These prevalences are similar to that of a Swedish twin registry study giving a lifetime prevalence of around 0.2% (Ekbom et al. 2006). In Germany, suspected cluster headache cases detected by a questionnaire and interviewed by a neurologist in a population-based study revealed a prevalence of 0.12% (Katsarava et al. 2007). In Georgia, one case was found in door-to-door survey among 1,145 individuals, which corresponds to 0.09% (Katsarava et al. 2009a). In Ethiopia, five patients among 15,000 subjects were found, corresponding to 0.03% of the population (Tekle Haimanot et al. 1995). In most studies on cluster headache, there is a marked male dominance, from 57% to 85% in the studies mentioned above.

Headache Incidence and Headache Course

Incidence refers to the number of new cases with a disorder in a defined population at risk during a given period of time. There are relatively few studies on incidence of headache.

In one study (Stewart et al. 1991), participants aged 12–29 were asked about the first occurrence of their migraine headache. It appeared that in both sexes, migraine with aura tended to start earlier than migraine without aura, but the peak incidence came at a younger age in boys. Incidence of migraine with aura peaked at 5 years in boys, and at 12–13 years in girls. Migraine without aura reached the highest incidence between 10 and 11 years in boys, and between 14 and 17 years in girls. New cases of migraine after the age of 20 were rare in men, but quite common among women.

In one important study on the course of migraine, 9,000 Swedish schoolchildren between 7 and 15 years were screened for migraine. It was found that 3.9% had migraine with an average age of onset of 6 years and 73% of these were followed for 40 years (Bille 1997). During puberty, only 40% of these still had migraine, but at around 30 years of age, 60% had migraine, and at 50 years, there were still more than 50%. This indicates that for most children with migraine, the disease will be a near lifelong affliction.

In one study from the UK, randomly selected adults were asked about recent headache and headache during their life time at baseline and 1 year later (Boardman et al. 2005). Among those who at baseline had not had headache within the last 3 months, 33% had such headache 1 year later. The incidence of headache among those who had never had a headache was 8%. Among those who had had recent headache at baseline, 94% had recent headache after 1 year, showing that headache is relatively stable over time, although most (85%) had had one or more changes in their headache characteristics.

Risk Factors and Comorbid Conditions

Apart from age and sex, headache epidemiological studies have indicated several factors that are associated with high headache prevalence and incidences, but for most factors, it is not known whether these associations represent causal connections.

The relation between headache and socioeconomic status has been addressed in some studies. Both migraine and headache in general were associated with low socioeconomic status in a large Norwegian study (Hagen et al. 2002c), and this has also been found in North America (Breslau et al. 1991; Scher et al. 2003; Stewart et al. 1992) but not in some smaller European studies (Gobel et al. 1994; Launer et al. 1999; Linde and Dahlöf 2004; Rasmussen 1992; Steiner et al. 2003). It is not known why low socioeconomic status is associated with high headache prevalence, but higher levels of stress and worries in daily life, unhealthy diets and lifestyle, poor health in general, or less access to health care may be possible explanations. One may also speculate that low socioeconomic status may, at least partly, be caused by headache. In one Swedish study, half of the patients reported a negative influence of migraine on their ability to pursue studies and one-third a negative influence on their finances (Linde and Dahlöf 2004). In the USA, headache patients have been found to have somewhat reduced labor force participation (Stang et al. 1998). However, in some European studies, employment status has not been found to be related to headache (Boardman et al. 2003; Rasmussen 1992).

Some studies have also addressed the influence of race on headache prevalence. It is notable that headache prevalences seem to be lower in Africa (See ❷ *Table 2.1*) than on the other continents. In the USA, higher prevalences of both migraine and TTH have been found among whites (Caucasians) than among other racial groups (African and Asian Americans) (Carson et al. 2004; Schwartz et al. 1998a; Stewart et al. 1996). In Singapore, Non-Chinese were more likely to suffer from migraine and severe headaches than the Chinese (Ho and Ong 2001). Most of these studies have tried to adjust for differences in socioeconomic status, and it is speculated that racial variations may reflect differences in the genetical susceptibility to headache (Stewart et al. 1996).

Cardiovascular risk factors, including smoking and obesity may be important also for headache prevalence (Bigal et al. 2006b; Scher et al. 2003; Aamodt et al. 2006). Among dietary factors, caffeine seems to be associated with moderate increase in headache prevalence, and be a risk factor for transforming migraine to a chronic headache (Hagen et al. 2009; Scher et al. 2004). Use of estrogen-containing oral contraceptives and hormone replacement therapy are also related to headache prevalence in women (Aegidius et al. 2006, 2007). For many of these factors, it cannot be known for certain whether patients develop headache because of the use, or whether the use is a consequence of the headache. For example, many women use estrogen-containing pills to alleviate certain complaints related to menstruation or climacterium, and headache may be part of these complaints. Also, cigarette smoking may for some be a way to relieve stress and pain. At least one study has found that low alcohol consumption is associated with high headache prevalence (Aamodt et al. 2006). This is most certainly because people with headache tend to avoid alcohol because of its headache-inducing properties.

Many disorders have been found to be comorbid with migraine, and also headaches in general. Comorbidity is generally understood as the greater than coincidental association between two disorders (Scher et al. 2005a). Several studies have concerned psychiatric disease, like anxiety and depression, which have proved to be strongly associated not only with migraine (Breslau et al. 2001, 2003; Kececi et al. 2003; Merikangas and Stevens 1997; Molgat and Patten 2005; Torelli and D'Amico 2004), but also with headache in general (Zwart et al. 2003a). The strength of the association may be more dependent on headache frequency than on headache type (Zwart et al. 2003a). It is discussed whether headache causes depression and worries or vice versa. At least with regard to the relation between migraine and major depression, it has been found to be bidirectional, i.e., migraine seems to be a risk factor for depression, and depression for migraine. This observation may indicate that the two disorders share some etiological factors (Breslau et al. 2003).

It is also well documented that patients with headache not only suffer from pain in the head, but also in other parts of the body. This has been shown both in children (Anttila et al. 2001; Borge et al. 1994; Santalahti et al. 2005) and in adults (10, 11). In the large HUNT study from Norway, both patients with migraine and patients with other headaches had 15–20% increased chance of having chronic musculoskeletal pain compared to those without head-aches. This was true for all age groups, and it was true for all parts of the body (Hagen et al. 2002a). A likely explanation for this is that migraine to some degree is a disorder of altered pain perception that is not limited to the head.

A few studies have also focused on gastrointestinal complaints. In population-based studies, an association has been found not only between migraine and abdominal pain (Stordal et al. 2005), but also to painful disorders like heartburn, dyspepsia, and peptic ulcer (Bingefors and Isacson 2004; Aamodt et al. 2008). This comorbidity may, at least partly, be explained by medication, as many headache drugs (Acetyl salicylic acid, nonsteroidal anti-inflammatory drugs (NSAIDS)) may cause many of these symptoms. Also, there may be an underlying dysregulation of the autonomic nervous system and pain perception that causes both migraine and gastrointestinal complaints (Aamodt et al. 2008).

Migraine and epilepsy are both brain disorders occurring in attacks, and which both may involve an aura phase. In a large American study of almost 2,000 epilepsy patients, migraine was almost twice as frequent among those with epilepsy as in those without it. In a Norwegian population-based study among 1,800 residents in a community, active epilepsy occurred twice as often among migraine patients, and the association was even stronger in migraine with aura. However, if one also included those who had previously suffered from epilepsy, there was no association between the diseases (Brodtkorb et al. 2008). The cause of the association is not well understood. In a few patients, migraine may precipitate seizures, the so-called migralepsy. It is probably more common that seizures are accompanied by headache, often of migraineous type. Also, the fact that migraine is more common among relatives of epilepsy patients (Ottman and Lipton 1994), is taken as evidence that some genes may dispose for both disorders (Ottman and Lipton 1994).

Some studies have demonstrated that asthma is comorbid with migraine and other headaches (Terwindt et al. 2000; Aamodt et al. 2007a). This is also true for other lung disorders like chronic bronchitis. For asthma, there may be several explanations for the relation to migraine. Beta-blockers for migraine prophylaxis may precipitate asthma, and so may some painkillers like acetylic salicylic acid and NSAIDS. Also, one may speculate in common pathogenetic factors related to autonomic instability. A psychological explanation is that the stress connected with having one attackwise and unpredictable disorder will increase the likelihood of eliciting another such disorder.

Migraine is often referred to as a vascular headache, and the relation to other vascular disorders has been subject to much scrutiny. In particular, the association to cerebrovascular events has been studied, since the migraine aura may resemble transitory ischemic attacks, and also since some aura attacks may give rise to a stroke ("migrainous infarction"). In short, there are now several studies that link migraine, and in particular migraine with aura, to stroke in women below 45 years of age (Kruit et al. 2004; Kurth et al. 2006; Merikangas et al. 1997;

Tzourio et al. 1993, 1995). The risk is manifold higher in women who also smoke and use oral contraceptives. An increase in subclinical brain lesions has been found in women with migraine, both with and without aura (Kruit et al. 2004). There are several explanation for this comorbidity, like cerebral oligoemia of the aura phase, and also prothrombotic and endothelial factors (Kurth et al. 2006). Younger women with migraine and aura should be advised about the dangers related to using oral contraceptives, and smoking should be strongly discouraged.

As to cardiac infarctions, no definite associations have been found neither to migraine with or without aura, at least not for individuals older than 40 (Cook et al. 2002; Rose et al. 2003). This is surprising, considering that migraineurs as a group tend to have some risk factors for cardiovascular disease (Scher et al. 2005b). On the other hand, diabetes may be less prevalent among migraineurs than among others (Aamodt et al. 2007b). It is also most interesting that migraine tends to be associated with normal or low blood pressure (Hagen et al. 2002b), particularly low pulse pressure (Gudmundsson et al. 2006; Tronvik et al. 2008; Tzourio et al. 2003). This has also been found for other chronic pains (Hagen et al. 2005), and it may be explained by a neurophysiological mechanism called "hypertension-associated hypalgesia," describing a common regulation of blood pressure and pain perception at the brainstem level (Tronvik et al. 2008).

Conclusions

Globally, the 1-year prevalence of headache is around 50%, of migraine 11%, of TTH almost 40%, and of CDH 3%. Cluster headache has a lifetime prevalence of 0.2%. Most headaches affect women more than men, and migraine is particularly prevalent among young and middle-aged adult women. Migraine often starts in childhood in men, but often at a later age in women. The disease varies considerably through life, but it tends to be a lifelong disorder in the majority. Headaches are more prevalent among those of lower socioeconomic status, and there may also be geographical and racial variations in the prevalence.Many associations between headaches and potential risk factors and comorbid diseases have been found, but the degree to which these associations represent causal connections is largely unknown. For disorders like anxiety, depression, epilepsy, and others, the comorbidity with migraine may be due to common pathophysiological mechanisms. Migraine with aura seems to be a risk factor for cerebrovascular ischemic events among younger women. A most important task for headache epidemiological research in the future will be to identify preventable risk factors for and consequences of headache.

References

Aamodt AH, Stovner LJ, Hagen K, Brathen G, Zwart J (2006) Headache prevalence related to smoking and alcohol use. The Head-HUNT study. Eur J Neurol 13(11):1233–1238

Aamodt AH, Stovner LJ, Langhammer A, Hagen K, Zwart JA (2007a) Is headache related to asthma, hay fever, and chronic bronchitis? The Head-HUNT study. Headache 47(2):204–212

Aamodt AH, Stovner LJ, Midthjell K, Hagen K, Zwart JA (2007b) Headache prevalence related to diabetes mellitus. The Head-HUNT study. Eur J Neurol 14(7):738–744

Aamodt AH, Stovner LJ, Hagen K, Zwart JA (2008) Comorbidity of headache and gastrointestinal complaints. The Head-HUNT study. Cephalalgia 28(2):144–151

Aaseth K, Grande RB, Kvaerner KJ, Gulbrandsen P, Lundqvist C, Russell MB (2008) Prevalence of secondary chronic headaches in a population-based sample of 30–44-year-old persons. The Akershus study of chronic headache. Cephalalgia 28(7):705–713

Abu-Arefeh I, Russell G (1994) Prevalence of headache and migraine in schoolchildren. BMJ 309(6957):765–769

Aegidius K, Zwart JA, Hagen K, Schei B, Stovner LJ (2006) Oral contraceptives and increased headache prevalence: the Head-HUNT study. Neurology 66(3):349–353

Aegidius KL, Zwart JA, Hagen K, Schei B, Stovner LJ (2007) Hormone replacement therapy and headache prevalence in postmenopausal women. The Head-HUNT study. Eur J Neurol 14(1):73–78

Alders EE, Hentzen A, Tan CT (1996) A community-based prevalence study on headache in Malaysia. Headache 36(6):379–384

Antoniuk S, Kozak MF, Michelon L, Montemór Netto MR (1998) Prevalence of headache in children of a school from Curitiba, Brazil, comparing data obtained from children and parents. Arq Neuropsiquiatr 56(4):726–733

Anttila P, Metsahonkala L, Mikkelsson M, Helenius H, Sillanpaa M (2001) Comorbidity of other pains in schoolchildren with migraine or nonmigrainous headache. J Pediatr 138(2):176–180

Ayatollahi SM, Khosravi A (2006) Prevalence of migraine and tension-type headache in primary-school children in Shiraz. East Mediterr Health J 12(6):809–817

Bank J, Marton S (2000) Hungarian migraine epidemiology. Headache 40:164–169

Bener A, Swadi H, Qassimi EMA, Uduman S (1998) Prevalence of headache and migraine in schoolchildren in the United Arab Emirates. Ann Saudi Med 18(6):522–524

Bensenor IM, Lotufo PA, Goulart AC, Menezes PR, Scazufca M (2008) The prevalence of headache among elderly in a low-income area of Sao Paulo, Brazil. Cephalalgia 28(4):329–333

Bigal ME, Liberman JN, Lipton RB (2006a) Age-dependent prevalence and clinical features of migraine. Neurology 67(2):246–251

Bigal ME, Liberman JN, Lipton RB (2006b) Obesity and migraine: a population study. Neurology 66(4):545–550

Bigal ME, Lipton RB, Winner P, Reed ML, Diamond S, Stewart WF (2007) Migraine in adolescents: association with socioeconomic status and family history. Neurology 69(1):16–25

Bille B (1997) A 40-year follow-up of school children with migraine. Cephalalgia 17(4):488–491

Bingefors K, Isacson D (2004) Epidemiology, co-morbidity, and impact on health-related quality of life of self-reported headache and musculoskeletal pain–a gender perspective. Eur J Pain 8(5):435–450

Boardman HF, Thomas E, Croft PR, Millson DS (2003) Epidemiology of headache in an English district. Cephalalgia 23(2):129–137

Boardman HF, Thomas E, Millson DS, Croft PR (2005) One-year follow-up of headache in an adult general population. Headache 45(4):337–345

Borge AI, Nordhagen R, Moe B, Botten G, Bakketeig LS (1994) Prevalence and persistence of stomach ache and headache among children. Follow-up of a cohort of Norwegian children from 4 to 10 years of age. Acta Paediatr 83(4):433–437

Breslau N, Davis GC, Andreski P (1991) Migraine, psychiatric disorders, and suicide attempts: an epidemiologic study of young adults. Psychiatry Res 37(1):11–23

Breslau N, Schultz LR, Stewart WF, Lipton R, Welch KM (2001) Headache types and panic disorder: directionality and specificity. Neurology 56(3):350–354

Breslau N, Lipton RB, Stewart WF, Schultz LR, Welch KM (2003) Comorbidity of migraine and depression: investigating potential etiology and prognosis. Neurology 60(8):1308–1312

Brodtkorb E, Bakken IJ, Sjaastad O (2008) Comorbidity of migraine and epilepsy in a Norwegian community. Eur J Neurol 15(12):1421–1423

Camarda R, Monastero R (2003) Prevalence of primary headaches in Italian elderly: preliminary data from the Zabut aging project. Neurol Sci 24(Suppl 2): S122–S124

Carson AL, Rose KM, Sanford CP, Ephross SA, Stang PE, Hunt KJ et al (2004) Lifetime prevalence of migraine and other headaches lasting 4 or more hours: the Atherosclerosis Risk in Communities (ARIC) study. Headache 44(1):20–28

Castillo J, Munoz P, Guitera V, Pascual J (1999) Epidemiology of chronic daily headache in the general population. Headache 39:190–196

Colas R, Munoz P, Temprano R, Gomez C, Pascual J (2004) Chronic daily headache with analgesic overuse: epidemiology and impact on quality of life. Neurology 62(8):1338–1342

Cook NR, Bensenor IM, Lotufo PA, Lee IM, Skerrett PJ, Chown MJ et al (2002) Migraine and coronary heart disease in women and men. Headache 42(8):715–727

Dahlof C, Linde M (2001) One-year prevalence of migraine in Sweden: a population-based study in adults. Cephalalgia 21(6):664–671

D'Alessandro R, Benassi G, Lenzi PL, Gamberini G, Sacquegna T, De Carolis P et al (1988) Epidemiology of headache in the republic of San Marino. J Neurol Neurosurg Psychiatry 51(1):21–27

Deleu D, Khan MA, Al Shehab TA (2002) Prevalence and clinical characteristics of headache in a rural community in oman. Headache 42(10):963–973

Dent W, Spiss H, Helbok R, Matuja W, Scheunemann S, Schmutzhard E (2004) Prevalence of migraine in a rural area in South Tanzania: a door-to-door survey. Cephalalgia 24(11):960–966

Deubner DC (1977) An epidemiologic study of migraine and headache in 10-20 year olds. Headache 17(4):173–180

Dyb G, Holmen TL, Zwart JA (2006) Analgesic overuse among adolescents with headache: the Head-HUNT-youth study. Neurology 66(2):198–201

Ekbom K, Svensson DA, Pedersen NL, Waldenlind E (2006) Lifetime prevalence and concordance risk of cluster headache in the Swedish twin population. Neurology 67(5):798–803

Gobel H, Petersen-Braun M, Soyka D (1994) The epidemiology of headache in Germany: a nationwide survey of a representative sample on the basis of the headache classification of the International Headache Society. Cephalalgia 14(2):97–106

Grande RB, Aaseth K, Gulbrandsen P, Lundqvist C, Russell MB (2008) Prevalence of primary chronic headache in a population-based sample of 30- to 44-year-old persons. The Akershus study of chronic headache. Neuroepidemiology 30(2):76–83

Gudmundsson LS, Thorgeirsson G, Sigfusson N, Sigvaldason H, Johannsson M (2006) Migraine patients have lower systolic but higher diastolic blood pressure compared with controls in a population-based study of 21,537 subjects. The Reykjavik study. Cephalalgia 26(4):436–444

Hagen K, Zwart JA, Vatten L, Stovner LJ, Bovim G (2000) Prevalence of migraine and non-migrainous headache–head-HUNT, a large population-based study. Cephalalgia 20(10):900–906

Hagen K, Einarsen C, Zwart JA, Svebak S, Bovim G (2002a) The co-occurrence of headache and musculoskeletal symptoms amongst 51 050 adults in Norway. Eur J Neurol 9(5):527–533

Hagen K, Stovner LJ, Vatten L, Holmen J, Zwart JA, Bovim G (2002b) Blood pressure and risk of headache: a prospective study of 22 685 adults in Norway. J Neurol Neurosurg Psychiatry 72(4):463–466

Hagen K, Vatten L, Stovner LJ, Zwart JA, Krokstad S, Bovim G (2002c) Low socio-economic status is associated with increased risk of frequent headache: a prospective study of 22718 adults in Norway. Cephalalgia 22(8):672–679

Hagen K, Zwart JA, Holmen J, Svebak S, Bovim G, Stovner LJ (2005) Does hypertension protect against chronic musculoskeletal complaints? The Nord-Trondelag health study. Arch Intern Med 165(8):916–922

Hagen K, Thoresen K, Stovner LJ, Zwart JA (2009) High dietary caffeine consumption is associated with a modest increase in headache prevalence: results from the Head-HUNT study. J Headache Pain 10(3):153–159

Hennekens CH, Buring J (1987) Epidemiology in medicine. Little, Brown & Company, Boston

Ho KH, Ong BK (2001) Headache characteristics and race in Singapore: results of a randomized national survey. Headache 41(3):279–284

International Headache Society (2004) The international classification of headache disorders, 2nd edn. Cephalalgia 24(Suppl 1):1–160

Jaillard AS, Mazetti P, Kala E (1997) Prevalence of migraine and headache in a high-altitude town of Peru: a population-based study. Headache 37(2):95–101

Karli N, Akis N, Zarifoglu M, Akgoz S, Irgil E, Ayvacioglu U et al (2006) Headache prevalence in adolescents aged 12–17: a student-based epidemiological study in Bursa. Headache 46(4):649–655

Katsarava Z, Diener HC (2008) Medication overuse headache in Germany. Cephalalgia 28(11):1221–1222

Katsarava Z, Obermann M, Yoon MS, Dommes P, Kuznetsova J, Weimar C et al (2007) Prevalence of cluster headache in a population-based sample in Germany. Cephalalgia 27(9):1014–1019

Katsarava Z, Dzagnidze A, Kukava M, Mirvelashvili E, Djibuti M, Janelidze M et al (2009a) Prevalence of cluster headache in the republic of Georgia: results of a population-based study and methodological considerations. Cephalalgia 29(9):949–952

Katsarava Z, Dzagnidze A, Kukava M, Mirvelashvili E, Djibuti M, Janelidze M et al (2009b) Primary headache disorders in the republic of Georgia: prevalence and risk factors. Neurology 73(21):1796–1803

Kececi H, Dener S, Analan E (2003) Co-morbidity of migraine and major depression in the Turkish population. Cephalalgia 23(4):271–275

Kong CK, Cheng WW, Wong LY (2001) Epidemiology of headache in Hong Kong primary-level schoolchildren: questionnaire study. Hong Kong Med J 7(1):29–33

Koseoglu E, Nacar M, Talaslioglu A, Cetinkaya F (2003) Epidemiological and clinical characteristics of migraine and tension type headache in 1146 females in Kayseri, Turkey. Cephalalgia 23(5):381–388

Kruit MC, van Buchem MA, Hofman PA, Bakkers JT, Terwindt GM, Ferrari MD et al (2004) Migraine as a risk factor for subclinical brain lesions. JAMA 291(4):427–434

Kryst S, Scherl E (1994) A population-based survey of the social and personal impact of headache. Headache 34(6):344–350

Kurth T, Gaziano JM, Cook NR, Logroscino G, Diener HC, Buring JE (2006) Migraine and risk of cardiovascular disease in women. JAMA 296(3):283–291

Lampl C, Buzath A, Baumhackl U, Klingler D (2003) One-year prevalence of migraine in Austria: a nation-wide survey. Cephalalgia 23(4):280–286

Lanteri-Minet M, Valade D, Geraud G, Chautard MH, Lucas C (2005) Migraine and probable migraine–results of FRAMIG 3, a French nationwide survey carried out according to the 2004 IHS classification. Cephalalgia 25(12):1146–1158

Launer LJ, Terwindt GM, Ferrari MD (1999) The prevalence and characteristics of migraine in a population-based cohort: the GEM study. Neurology 53(3):537–542

Laurell K, Larsson B, Eeg-Olofsson O (2004) Prevalence of headache in Swedish schoolchildren, with a focus on tension-type headache. Cephalalgia 24(5):380–388

Lavados PM, Tenhamm E (1997) Epidemiology of migraine headache in Santiago, Chile: a prevalence study. Cephalalgia 17(7):770–777

Lavados PM, Tenhamm E (1998) Epidemiology of tension-type headache in Santiago, Chile: a prevalence study. Cephalalgia 18(8):552–558

Levy LM (1983) An epidemiological study of headache in an urban population in Zimbabwe. Headache 23(1):2–9

Linde M, Dahlöf C (2004) Attitudes and burden of disease among self-considered migraineurs–a nation-wide population-based survey in Sweden. Cephalalgia 24(6):455–465

Lipton RB, Stewart WF, Diamond S, Diamond ML, Reed M (2001) Prevalence and burden of migraine in the United States: data from the American Migraine study II. Headache 41(7):646–657

Lipton RB, Scher AI, Kolodner K, Liberman J, Steiner TJ, Stewart WF (2002) Migraine in the United States: epidemiology and patterns of health care use. Neurology 58(6):885–894

Lu SR, Fuh JL, Chen WT, Juang KD, Wang SJ (2001) Chronic daily headache in Taipei, Taiwan: prevalence, follow-up and outcome predictors. Cephalalgia 21(10):980–986

Lyngberg AC, Rasmussen BK, Jorgensen T, Jensen R (2005) Has the prevalence of migraine and tension-type headache changed over a 12-year period? A Danish population survey. Eur J Epidemiol 20(3):243–249

Mattsson P, Svardsudd K, Lundberg PO, Westerberg CE (2000) The prevalence of migraine in women aged 40–74 years: a population-based study. Cephalalgia 20(10):893–899

Mavromichalis I, Anagnostopoulos D, Metaxas N, Papanastassiou E (1999) Prevalence of migraine in schoolchildren and some clinical comparisons between migraine with and without aura. Headache 39(10):728–736

Merikangas KR, Stevens DE (1997) Comorbidity of migraine and psychiatric disorders. Neurol Clin 15(1):115–123

Merikangas KR, Whitaker AE, Isler H, Angst J (1994) The Zurich Study: XXIII. Epidemiology of headache syndromes in the Zurich cohort study of young adults. Eur Arch Psychiatry Clin Neurosci 244(3):145–152

Merikangas KR, Fenton BT, Cheng SH, Stolar MJ, Risch N (1997) Association between migraine and stroke in a large-scale epidemiological study of the United States. Arch Neurol 54(4):362–368

Metsähonkala L, Sillanpää M (1994) Migraine in children–an evaluation of the IHS criteria. Cephalalgia 14(4):285–290

Mitsikostas DD, Tsaklakidou D, Athanasiadis N, Thomas A (1996) The prevalence of headache in Greece: correlations to latitude and climatological factors. Headache 36(3):168–173

Molgat CV, Patten SB (2005) Comorbidity of major depression and migraine–a Canadian population-based study. Can J Psychiatry 50(13):832–837

Morillo LE, Alarcon F, Aranaga N, Aulet S, Chapman E, Conterno L et al (2005) Prevalence of migraine in Latin America. Headache 45(2):106–117

Natoli J, Manack A, Dean B, Butler Q, Turkel C, Stovner L et al (2009) Global prevalence of chronic migraine: a systematic review. Cephalalgia 30(5):599–609

Nikiforow R (1981) Headache in a random sample of 200 persons: a clinical study of a population in northern Finland. Cephalalgia 1(2):99–107

O'Brien B, Goeree R, Streiner D (1994) Prevalence of migraine headache in Canada: a population-based survey. Int J Epidemiol 23(5):1020–1026

Olesen J, Bousser MG, Diener HC, Dodick D, First M, Goadsby PJ et al (2006) New appendix criteria open for a broader concept of chronic migraine. Cephalalgia 26(6):742–746

Ottman R, Lipton RB (1994) Comorbidity of migraine and epilepsy. Neurology 44(11):2105–2110

Patel NV, Bigal ME, Kolodner KB, Leotta C, Lafata JE, Lipton RB (2004) Prevalence and impact of migraine and probable migraine in a health plan. Neurology 63(8):1432–1438

Paulin JM, Waal-Manning HJ, Simpson FO, Knight RG (1985) The prevalence of headache in a small New Zealand town. Headache 25(3):147–151

Prencipe M, Casini AR, Ferretti C, Santini M, Pezzella F, Scaldaferri N et al (2001) Prevalence of headache in an elderly population: attack frequency, disability, and use of medication. J Neurol Neurosurg Psychiatry 70(3):377–381

Queiroz L, Peres M, Kowacs F, Piovesan E, Ciciarelli M, Souza J et al (2008a) Chronic daily headache in Brazil: a nationwide population-based study. Cephalalgia 28:1264–1269

Queiroz LP, Peres MF, Piovesan EJ, Kowacs F, Ciciarelli MC, Souza JA et al (2008b) A nationwide population-based study of tension-type headache in Brazil. Headache 49(1):71–78

Queiroz LP, Peres MF, Piovesan EJ, Kowacs F, Ciciarelli MC, Souza JA et al (2009) A nationwide population-based study of migraine in Brazil. Cephalalgia 29(6):642–649

Raieli V, Raimondo D, Cammalleri R, Camarda R (1995) Migraine headaches in adolescents: a student population-based study in Monreale. Cephalalgia 15(1):5–12

Rasmussen BK (1992) Migraine and tension-type headache in a general population: psychosocial factors. Int J Epidemiol 12(6):1138–1143

Rasmussen BK, Jensen R, Schroll M, Olesen J (1991) Epidemiology of headache in a general population–a prevalence study. J Clin Epidemiol 44(11):1147–1157

Rhee H (2001) Additional thoughts about racial differences in the prevalence of headaches in US adolescents. Headache 41(4):419–420

Roh JK, Kim JS, Ahn YO (1998) Epidemiologic and clinical characteristics of migraine and tension-type headache in Korea. Headache 38(5):356–365

Rose KM, Perry AL, Brown CA, Folsom AR, Sanford CP, Stang PE et al (2003) Migraine and other headaches with and without aura and coronary heart disease: findings from the ARIC study. Circulation 107(7):P13

Sakai F (2008) Migrainology learned from patients. Rinsho Shinkeigaku 48(11):785–791

Sakai F, Igarashi H (1997) Prevalence of migraine in Japan: a nationwide survey. Cephalalgia 17(1):15–22

Santalahti P, Aromaa M, Sourander A, Helenius H, Piha J (2005) Have there been changes in children's psychosomatic symptoms? A 10-year comparison from Finland. Pediatrics 115(4):e434–e442

Scher AI, Stewart WF, Ricci JA, Lipton RB (2003) Factors associated with the onset and remission of chronic daily headache in a population-based study. Pain 106(1–2):81–89

Scher AI, Stewart WF, Lipton RB (2004) Caffeine as a risk factor for chronic daily headache: a population-based study. Neurology 63(11):2022–2027

Scher AI, Bigal ME, Lipton RB (2005a) Comorbidity of migraine. Curr Opin Neurol 18(3):305–310

Scher AI, Terwindt GM, Picavet HS, Verschuren WM, Ferrari MD, Launer LJ (2005b) Cardiovascular risk factors and migraine: the GEM population-based study. Neurology 64(4):614–620

Schwartz BS, Stewart WF, Lipton RB (1997) Lost workdays and decreased work effectiveness associated with headache in the workplace. J Occup Environ Med 39(4):320–327

Schwartz BS, Stewart WF, Simon D, Lipton RB (1998a) Epidemiology of tension-type headache. JAMA 279(5):381–383

Sillanpää M (1983) Prevalence of headache in prepuberty. Headache 23(1):10–14

Sillanpaa M, Piekkala P, Kero P (1991) Prevalence of headache at preschool age in an unselected child population. Cephalalgia 11(5):239–242

Sjaastad O, Bakketeig LS (2003) Cluster headache prevalence. Vaga study headache epidemiology. Cephalalgia 23(7):528–533

Srikiatkhachorn A (1991) Epidemiology of headache in the Thai elderly: a study in the Bangkae home for the aged. Headache 31(10):677–681

Stang P, Von Korff M, Galer BS (1998) Reduced labor force participation among primary care patients with headache. J Gen Intern Med 13(5):296–302

Steiner TJ, Scher AI, Stewart WF, Kolodner K, Liberman J, Lipton RB (2003) The prevalence and disability burden of adult migraine in England and their relationships to age, gender and ethnicity. Cephalalgia 23(7):519–527

Stewart WF, Linet MS, Celentano DD, Van Natta M, Ziegler D (1991) Age- and sex-specific incidence rates of migraine with and without visual aura. Am J Epidemiol 134(10):1111–1120

Stewart WF, Lipton RB, Celentano DD, Reed ML (1992) Prevalence of migraine headache in the United States. Relation to age, income, race, and other sociodemographic factors. JAMA 267(1):64–69

Stewart WF, Lipton RB, Liberman J (1996) Variation in migraine prevalence by race. Neurology 47(1):52–59

Stordal K, Nygaard EA, Bentsen BS (2005) Recurrent abdominal pain: a five-year follow-up study. Acta Paediatr 94(2):234–236

Stovner LJ (2006) Headache epidemiology: how and why? J Headache Pain 7(3):141–144

Stovner LJ, Zwart JA, Hagen K, Terwindt G, Pascual J (2006) Epidemiology of headache in Europe. Eur J Neurol 13(4):333–345

Stovner LJ, Hagen K, Jensen R, Katsarava Z, Lipton R, Scher A et al (2007) The global burden of headache: a documentation of headache prevalence and disability worldwide. Cephalalgia 27(3):193–210

Takeshima T, Ishizaki K, Fukuhara Y, Ijiri T, Kusumi M, Wakutani Y et al (2004) Population-based door-to-door survey of migraine in Japan: the Daisen study. Headache 44(1):8–19

Tekle Haimanot R, Seraw B, Forsgren L, Ekbom K, Ekstedt J (1995) Migraine, chronic tension-type headache, and cluster headache in an Ethiopian rural community. Cephalalgia 15(6):482–488

Terwindt GM, Ferrari MD, Tijhuis M, Groenen SM, Picavet HS, Launer LJ (2000) The impact of migraine on quality of life in the general population: the GEM study. Neurology 55(5):624–629

Torelli P, D'Amico D (2004) An updated review of migraine and co-morbid psychiatric disorders. Neurol Sci 25(Suppl 3):S234–S235

Torelli P, Beghi E, Manzoni GC (2005) Cluster headache prevalence in the Italian general population. Neurology 64(3):469–474

Tronvik E, Stovner LJ, Hagen K, Holmen J, Zwart JA (2008) High pulse pressure protects against headache: prospective and cross-sectional data (HUNT study). Neurology 70(16):1329–1336

Tzourio C, Iglesias S, Hubert JB, Visy JM, Alpérovitch A, Tehindrazanarivelo A et al (1993) Migraine and risk of ischaemic stroke: a case-control study. BMJ 307(6899):289–292

Tzourio C, Tehindrazanarivelo A, Iglésias S, Alpérovitch A, Chedru F, d'Anglejan-Chatillon J et al (1995) Case-control study of migraine and risk of ischaemic stroke in young women. BMJ 310(6983):830–833

Tzourio C, Gagniere B, El Amrani M, Alperovitch A, Bousser MG (2003) Relationship between migraine, blood pressure and carotid thickness. A population-based study in the elderly. Cephalalgia 23(9):914–920

Wang SJ, Liu HC, Fuh JL, Liu CY, Lin KP, Chen HM et al (1997) Prevalence of headaches in a Chinese elderly population in Kinmen: age and gender effect and cross-cultural comparisons. Neurology 49(1):195–200

Wang SJ, Fuh JL, Young YH, Lu SR, Shia BC (2000) Prevalence of migraine in Taipei, Taiwan: a population-based survey. Cephalalgia 20(6):566–572

Wang SJ, Fuh JL, Juang KD, Lu SR (2005) Rising prevalence of migraine in Taiwanese adolescents aged 13–15 years. Cephalalgia 25(6):433–438

Wang SJ, Fuh JL, Lu SR, Juang KD (2006) Chronic daily headache in adolescents: prevalence, impact, and medication overuse. Neurology 66(2):193–197

Waters WE, O'Connor PJ (1975) Prevalence of migraine. J Neurol Neurosurg Psychiatry 38(6):613–616

Wiehe M, Fuchs SC, Moreira LB, Moraes RS, Fuchs FD (2002) Migraine is more frequent in individuals with optimal and normal blood pressure: a population-based study. J Hypertens 20(7):1303–1306

Wilkinson IA, Halliday JA, Henry RL, Hankin RG, Hensley MJ (1994) Headache and asthma. J Paediatr Child Health 30(3):253–256

Winkler A, Dent W, Stelzhammer B, Kerschbaumsteiner K, Meindl M, Kaaya J et al (2009a) Prevalence of migraine headache in a rural area of northern Tanzania: a community-based door-to-door survey. Cephalalgia 30(5):582–592

Winkler A, Stelzhammer B, Kerschbaumsteiner K, Meindl M, Dent W, Kaaya J et al (2009b) The prevalence of headache with emphasis on tension-type headache in rural Tanzania: a community-based study. Cephalalgia 29(12):1317–1325

Zivadinov R, Willheim K, Jurjevic A, Sepic-Grahovac D, Bucuk M, Zorzon M (2001) Prevalence of migraine in Croatia: a population-based survey. Headache 41(8):805–812

Zwart JA, Dyb G, Hagen K, Odegard KJ, Dahl AA, Bovim G et al (2003a) Depression and anxiety disorders associated with headache frequency. The Nord-Trondelag health study. Eur J Neurol 20(10):147–152

Zwart JA, Dyb G, Hagen K, Svebak S, Holmen J (2003b) Analgesic use: a predictor of chronic pain and medication overuse headache: the Head-HUNT Study. Neurology 61(2):160–164

Zwart JA, Dyb G, Holmen TL, Stovner LJ, Sand T (2004) The prevalence of migraine and tension-type headaches among adolescents in Norway. The Nord-Trondelag health study (Head-HUNT-youth), a large population-based epidemiological study. Cephalalgia 24(5):373–379

3 The Burden of Headache

Lars Jacob Stovner[1] · *Luiz Paulo Queiroz*[2]
[1]Norwegian National Headache Centre, Norwegian University of Science and Technology and St. Olavs Hospital, Trondheim, Norway
[2]Universidade Federal de Santa Catarina, Florianópolis, SC, Brazil

Paolo Martelletti, Timothy J. Steiner (eds.), *Handbook of Headache*, DOI 10.1007/978-88-470-1700-9_3,
© Lifting The Burden 2011

Abstract: Studies on headache burden are mostly performed to show the size of the public health problem. This chapter, dealing with the noneconomic aspects of headache burden, describes the methods and validated instruments to measure disability and reduction in the quality of life due to headache and refers some interesting results from such studies. Most studies until now have dealt with migraine, but there are also some studies on headache in general and cluster headache in particular. According to disease burden assessments by the World Health Organization, migraine alone may be among the 20 most disabling conditions worldwide. For tension-type headache, there are not sufficient data yet. Some data indicate that this headache type, due to its high prevalence, may entail a higher burden than migraine. Part of the headache burden may be due to psychiatric comorbidities of headache. A few studies indicate that headaches may lead to reductions in quality of life that are higher than in many other chronic disorders. The interictal burden of, e.g., migraine and cluster headache is probably mostly related to worry for later attacks and restrictions in lifestyle to avoid attacks, but some people also fail to recover completely. It has also been shown that migraine, in several ways, influences the lives of partners and children.

Introduction

For most people, having a headache from time to time is a nuisance, but it is not a serious health problem. However, there is a sizeable proportion of humankind for whom this is not true, and for seriously affected patients, the general lack of understanding of headache as a potentially disabling condition is a problem in addition to the pain and suffering. The trivialization of headache as a public health problem has far-reaching implications, such as inadequate resources to headache treatment and prevention, little attention in the curricula of medical schools, low funding of headache research, and lack of understanding for headache among relatives, employers, teachers, and colleagues. For this reason, headache patients and headache experts have in recent years tried to measure in different ways the disease burden that headache patients carry, and to compare it with that of other disorders. Headache burden can be measured along many dimensions, namely, the economic burden, the loss of function, the missed opportunities, the suffering itself, and the reduction in quality of life.

One of the main aims of the burden of headache studies is to get a clear picture of the way headache influences public health so that appropriate measures can be implemented to alleviate the different burdens. Part of the effort has a clear political objective, i.e., trying to convince relevant decision makers that headache is one of the major public health problems.

In this chapter, we consider the noneconomic impact of headache, whereas the economic consequences are treated in ❷ Chap. 2. We believe that the pain, suffering, and disability caused by headaches are as important as the economic consequences, from both a purely humanitarian and a public health perspective. Most of the literature is on migraine, but there are also some studies on tension-type headache (TTH) and cluster headache.

Disability Related to Headache Disorders

In a study performed in young women in nine Western European countries, 86% of migraineurs stated that their life would have been better if they did not suffer from migraine (Dueland et al. 2004). An even more dramatic evidence of the impact of headache on the public health is the finding that 300,000 persons in the USA stay in bed each day (24 h) due to headaches, according to a calculation based on data from a large population-based survey (Hu et al. 1999). A German study has shown that, on average, patients with migraine or TTH had around 1 month every year affected by headaches (Gobel et al. 1994). However, the main burden of headache is carried by a minority of sufferers. A Swedish study has shown that 27% of migraine patients had 68% of all attacks (Linde and Dahlöf 2004). Three to 4% of the European population have headache half of the days or more per month (Stovner et al. 2007).

Several instruments have been developed to measure the disability related to headache. Perhaps the most widely used is the Migraine Disability Assessment Scale (MIDAS) (Lipton et al. 2001) whose validity has been well documented (Stewart et al. 2000). The scale can be accessed on the webpage of the American Migraine Society (http://www.achenet.org/tools/migraine/index.asp). Originally developed for migraine, it is now also used for other headache types. With this instrument, days with absence from work (job or household chores), days with ≥50% reduction in productivity and days with inability to participate in social activities, are counted during a 3 months' period. The score can be used to classify patients into four grades: where 1 (0–5 days) is minimal; 2 (6–10 days) is mild, 3 (11–20) is moderate, and >20 is severe disability.

In France, among those with active migraine, 22% had grades 3 or 4, implying that 1.5% of the whole French population has 11 days or more during the last 3 months' period when headache affected work/household chores or leisure activities (Lucas et al. 2005). MIDAS grades 3 or 4 were even more common among migraineurs in a US (Hamelsky et al. 2005) and a multinational Latin American study, (Morillo et al. 2005) 54 and 50%, respectively.

In the UK, among patients with headache in general (both migraine and non-migraine headache) comprising 70% of the study population, 10.3% (7.2% of the total population) had MIDAS grade 3 or 4 (Boardman et al. 2003).

Comparing the percentage of the general population with MIDAS disability grade 3–4 due to migraine in France (1.5%) (Lucas et al. 2005) with the percentage with same disability due to headache in general in England (7.2%) (Boardman et al. 2003), it seems that non-migraine headache causes more disability in the population than migraine.

The PedMIDAS is a similar instrument used in children and adolescents to measure primarily whole or partial loss of days for school, homework, and play/sport activities during the last 3 months (Hershey et al. 2001). In a study from Turkey, among 7,700 students from 9 to 17 years of age, 83% had had headache, and among these, the average PedMIDAS score was almost 10 days in boys and 11.5 days in girls (Hershey et al. 2001). This instrument has also been used among 1,500 German children 11–14 years of age (Kroner-Herwig et al. 2010). Among the 67% who had had at least 1 day of headache during the last 3 months, 11.9% had PedMIDAS grade 2 (mild), 1.6% grade 3 (moderate), and 1.1% grade 4 (severe). A number of implausible answers indicate that some of the questions may have low reliability in this age group.

The HALT (Headache-Attributed Lost Time) index is a close derivative of MIDAS to be used for headache burden studies, which will be conducted by *Lifting The Burden*: the Global Campaign against Headache (Steiner 2005).

Another well-known scale is the Headache Impact Test (HIT). The HIT-6 is a paper-based short form tool, derived from the 54-item HIT, which is an Internet-based one, to assess the burden in the previous month (Kosinski et al. 2003). It is used both in clinical practice and research. The HIT-6 consists of six items: pain, social functioning, role functioning, vitality, cognitive functioning, and psychological distress. Questions are answered by "never," "rarely," "sometimes," "very often," and "always." The responses can be summed to scores ranging from 36 to 78. A higher score indicates a greater impact of headache on the respondent's daily life (Shin et al. 2008). The scores can be stratified in four levels of impact. The HIT-6 scale correlates with both headache severity and with QoL (Quality of Life), across different diagnostic groups of headache (Nachit-Ouinekh et al. 2005), and it has been used to identify patients in a GP population that are suitable for migraine treatment (De Diego and Lanteri-Minet 2005). The scores on HIT-6 and MIDAS are highly correlated, but the MIDAS seems to be more influenced by headache frequency and HIT-6 is more influenced by headache intensity (Sauro et al. 2010).

In the World Health Organization (WHO), the preferred measure of disease burden is "Disability Adjusted Life Years" (DALYs), which is a sum of the years of life lost (YLL) and the years lived with disability (YLDs). The YLDs are determined by the incidence and duration of the disorder and by a disability weight ranging between 0 and 1 (Leonardi et al. 2005). Although migraine entails no increased mortality (i.e., YLL = 0), migraine was number 19 of the leading causes of DALYs among women aged 15–44 and with regard to YLDs, it was number 19 for both sexes and number 12 for women, irrespective of age. Using the WHO data for a calculation of the burden of "brain disorders" (i.e., the psychiatric and neurological disorders) in Europe, the weight of migraine was lower than that of the major psychiatric disorders, dementia, stroke, and injuries, but higher than that of epilepsy, multiple sclerosis, and Parkinson's disease (Olesen and Leonardi 2003).

In a recent report on the global prevalence and burden of headache disorders, the burden of migraine and TTH was measured in a similar way as the DALYs by combining data on prevalence, mean number and duration of headache attacks and headache intensity from studies containing such information. For the world as a whole, it was demonstrated that TTH resulted in a higher population burden than migraine, each accounting for approximately 55% and 45% of the total burden. The data for Europe indicated an even higher burden due to TTH compared to migraine (Stovner et al. 2007). If one uses the European data from this study, it can be calculated that the hours with migraine headache would add up to between 34 and 100 h per year, if distributed on each adult individual in the population. The data on TTH are too scarce to use for similar calculations.

Studies Using Validated QoL-Instruments

To evaluate QoL in patients with headache, the most commonly used tools are the Medical Outcomes Study 36-Item Short Form (SF-36), the Migraine-Specific QoL Questionnaire (MSQ), and the Qualité de Vie et Migraine (QVM) (Nachit-Ouinekh et al. 2005).

Several studies have used the SF-36 instrument. This questionnaire, which is not a headache-specific tool, measures eight domains of QoL: physical and social functioning, role limitations because of physical or emotional problems, mental health, energy/vitality, pain, and general health perception (Brandes 2008). The scores range from 0 (lowest level of functioning) to 100 (highest level).

In a study from Taiwan, SF-36 scores differed among headache diagnoses, being lower in patients with chronic headaches than in those with episodic headaches, and they were significantly influenced by psychological distress (Wang et al. 2001). In a US study (Osterhaus et al. 1994) recruiting migraine patients from a medication trial, it was demonstrated that migraineurs had lower QoL than the general US population, most marked for bodily pain, physical role limitations, and social functioning. A Dutch population-based study using the same instrument found that migraine had a negative influence on all dimensions compared to controls. The negative influence on QoL was larger than that of for example asthma, and it increased with increasing headache frequency (Terwindt et al. 2000).

Two population-based studies from Spain among chronic daily headache sufferers showed a marked negative influence, most marked for those with medication overuse, but similar for those with a headache of a migraine or a tension type (Guitera et al. 2002). One of these studies showed that the headache frequency may have a greater impact than headache intensity on QoL (Guitera et al. 2002) and the other study showed that chronic headache with medication overuse was associated with a decrease in all QoL aspects studied with SF-36, most marked for role physical and bodily pain (Colás et al. 2004). A study from UK showed that migraineurs with high or moderate disability had a marked reduction on all dimensions on the SF-36 (Lipton et al. 2003b). A Swedish study compared SF-36 results in the two sexes and in participants with different pain conditions. For headache, there was a gender difference. In men, it influenced mostly physical function, physical role, and bodily pain, whereas in women it affected vitality, social functioning, emotional functioning, and mental health (Bingefors and Isacson 2004).

In a French study, migraineurs had significantly lower scores than headache-free controls on all SF-36 dimensions and lower scores on the pain dimension than those with other headaches or with TTH (Michel et al. 1997). The SF-36 has also been used to demonstrate that QoL can be significantly improved by effective treatment of the headache disorders (D'Amico et al. 2006).

One study comparing migraineurs in the USA and the UK used a shorter QoL instrument, the SF-12, which contains a physical and a mental component (Lipton et al. 2000b). In both countries, migraineurs had lower scores than controls on both components even after adjusting for socioeconomic status and for depression. However, in those with both migraine and depression, the QoL was significantly reduced in comparison to those who were not depressed.

Qualité de vie et migraine (QVM) is a disease-specific QoL instrument. In a French study that used this, the QoL was found to be lowest among those with chronic headache, intermediate among migraineurs, and highest among subjects with other forms of episodic headache (Duru et al. 2004).

The MSQ is a migraine-specific instrument to assess QoL (Martin et al. 2000). It is nowadays in the version 2.1, which is a 13-item questionnaire, divided in three domains: role restrictive, role preventive, and emotional functioning. Scores are summed without weights (Cole et al. 2007). It has been used to demonstrate that migraine education improves quality of life, especially among those with a high degree of anxiety connected with their headache (Smith et al. 2010).

The total burden of headache may not only be related to the headache per se, but also to comorbid conditions (see ❷ Chap. 10 Comorbidities of Headache Disorders). European population-based studies have demonstrated that depression and/or anxiety occur two to three times more often among migraineurs than in the general population (Kececi et al. 2003; Lipton et al. 2000a). Depression adds to the reduction in QoL in migraine (Lipton et al. 2000b). This comorbidity may be as important for non-migraine headache (Zwart et al. 2003), but it is not known how this comorbidity influences the QoL in other headaches. In addition, it has been found that headache is comorbid with other bodily pain, both in Finnish children (Anttila et al. 2001) and in Norwegian adults (Hagen et al. 2002).

Family Impact

Headaches may also affect the patients' spouses and children. In a population-based Swedish study (Linde and Dahlöf 2004), the percentage of migraine sufferers who reported a negative impact of migraine was 76% for attendance to work, 67% for family situation, 59% for leisure time, 48% for pursuing studies, 46% for sexual life, 37% for their social position, 31% for love, 30% for their financial situation, 27% for making a career, and 11% for making friends.

One study has measured the impact of migraine on the family of two population samples in the USA and the UK (Lipton et al. 2003a). The results were very similar in both countries. More than 60% of patients reported a marked impact on the ability to do household chores because of their migraine during the past 3 months and it was markedly reduced in 20% of the patients' partners. Almost 46% of patients and 24% of the partners had missed days of family or social activities due to the proband's migraine, and 16% of the patients and 12% of the partners had avoided making plans for family or social activities due to proband's migraine. More than 60% stated that it had a moderate to marked influence on the relation with their children, 40% stated that they would have been a better guardian or parent without migraine; more than 10% stated that their children had missed school and 10% said that their children had been late to school because of their headache. Forty-six percent stated that they would have been a better partner without headaches, and 5% stated that they had had fewer children because of headache, 0.4% that they had avoided having children, and 15% that they had avoided oral contraception. Compared with a control group, the partners of migraine patients were significantly more dissatisfied with the demands, responsibility, and duties placed upon them and with their ability to perform.

The Burden of Cluster Headache

Few studies have addressed this headache type in particular. In a Danish study in which 85 such patients were compared with a matched control group, 75% reported restrictions in their daily living during cluster periods, and 13% outside the periods (Jensen et al. 2007). During the periods, 25% of the patients had to reduce their participation in social activities, family life and housework to less than one-third of the normal. In 96% of the patients, the disease had caused lifestyle changes within the last decade, most often in their sleeping habits and their alcohol consumption. More than 90% worked through a cluster period, but over 80% reported decreased working ability.

Interictal Burden

This refers to the complaints and limitations headache sufferers have when they do not have head pain (for review, cf. Brandes 2008). An important aspect of attackwise headaches is their unpredictability. This confers serious limitation on the ability to plan and take on responsibilities for many patients. In addition, many patients live in a constant worry about the next attack (Dueland et al. 2004; Linde and Dahlöf 2004). Also, there may in some patients be headache features that last longer than the pain. Indeed, a Swedish study has shown that the disability is not only related to the attacks since many migraine patients feel an impairment also between attacks (Dahlöf and Dimenäs 1995). Nine percent of the patients report that they have some residual disability since they do not recover completely between attacks. It is difficult to measure the interictal burden, but in a small proportion of patients, it is probably considerable.

References

Anttila P, Metsahonkala L, Mikkelsson M, Helenius H, Sillanpaa M (2001) Comorbidity of other pains in schoolchildren with migraine or nonmigrainous headache. J Pediatr 138(2):176–180

Bingefors K, Isacson D (2004) Epidemiology, co-morbidity, and impact on health-related quality of life of self-reported headache and musculoskeletal pain – a gender perspective. Eur J Pain 8(5):435–450

Boardman HF, Thomas E, Croft PR, Millson DS (2003) Epidemiology of headache in an English district. Cephalalgia 23(2):129–137

Brandes JL (2008) The migraine cycle: patient burden of migraine during and between migraine attacks. Headache 48(3):430–441

Colás R, Muñoz P, Temprano R, Gómez C, Pascual J (2004) Chronic daily headache with analgesic overuse: epidemiology and impact on quality of life. Neurology 62(8):1338–1342

Cole JC, Lin P, Rupnow MF (2007) Validation of the migraine-specific quality of life questionnaire version 2.1 (MSQ v. 2.1) for patients undergoing prophylactic migraine treatment. Qual Life Res 16(7):1231–1237

D'Amico D, Solari A, Usai S, Santoro P, Bernardoni P, Frediani F et al (2006) Improvement in quality of life and activity limitations in migraine patients after prophylaxis. A prospective longitudinal multicentre study. Cephalalgia 26(6):691–696

Dahlöf CG, Dimenäs E (1995) Migraine patients experience poorer subjective well-being/quality of life even between attacks. Cephalalgia 15(1):31–36

De Diego EV, Lanteri-Minet M (2005) Recognition and management of migraine in primary care: influence of functional impact measured by the headache impact test (HIT). Cephalalgia 25(3):184–190

Dueland AN, Leira R, Burke TA, Hillyer EV, Bolge S (2004) The impact of migraine on work, family, and leisure among young women – a multinational study. Curr Med Res Opin 20(10):1595–1604

Duru G, Auray JP, Gaudin AF, Dartigues JF, Henry P, Lantéri-Minet M et al (2004) Impact of headache on quality of life in a general population survey in France (GRIM2000 Study). Headache 44(6):571–580

Gobel H, Petersen-Braun M, Soyka D (1994) The epidemiology of headache in Germany: a nationwide survey of a representative sample on the basis of the headache classification of the International Headache Society. Cephalalgia 14(2):97–106

Guitera V, Muñoz P, Castillo J, Pascual J (2002) Quality of life in chronic daily headache: a study in a general population. Neurology 58(7):1062–1065

Hagen K, Einarsen C, Zwart JA, Svebak S, Bovim G (2002) The co-occurrence of headache and musculoskeletal symptoms amongst 51 050 adults in Norway. Eur J Neurol 9(5):527–533

Hamelsky SW, Lipton RB, Stewart WF (2005) An assessment of the burden of migraine using the willingness to pay model. Cephalalgia 25(2):87–100

Hershey AD, Powers SW, Vockell AL, LeCates S, Kabbouche MA, Maynard MK (2001) PedMIDAS: development of a questionnaire to assess disability of migraines in children. Neurology 57(11):2034–2039

Hu XH, Markson LE, Lipton RB, Stewart WF, Berger ML (1999) Burden of migraine in the United States: disability and economic costs. Arch Intern Med 159(8):813–818

Jensen RM, Lyngberg A, Jensen RH (2007) Burden of cluster headache. Cephalalgia 27(6):535–541

Kececi H, Dener S, Analan E (2003) Co-morbidity of migraine and major depression in the Turkish population. Cephalalgia 23(4):271–275

Kosinski M, Bayliss MS, Bjorner JB, Ware JE Jr, Garber WH, Batenhorst A et al (2003) A six-item short-form survey for measuring headache impact: the HIT-6. Qual Life Res 12(8):963–974

Kroner-Herwig B, Heinrich M, Vath N (2010) The assessment of disability in children and adolescents with headache: adopting PedMIDAS in an epidemiological study. Eur J Pain 14(9):951–958

Leonardi M, Steiner TJ, Scher AT, Lipton RB (2005) The global burden of migraine: measuring disability in headache disorders with WHO's classification of functioning, disability and health (ICF). J Headache Pain 6(6):429–440

Linde M, Dahlöf C (2004) Attitudes and burden of disease among self-considered migraineurs – a nationwide population-based survey in Sweden. Cephalalgia 24(6):455–465

Lipton RB, Hamelsky SW, Kolodner KB, Steiner TJ, Stewart WF (2000a) Migraine, quality of life, and depression: a population-based case-control study. Neurology 55(5):629–635

Lipton RB, Hamelsky SW, Kolodner KB, Steiner TJ, Stewart WF (2000b) Migraine, quality of life, and depression: a population-based case-control study. Neurology 55(5):629–635

Lipton RB, Stewart WF, Sawyer J, Edmeads JG (2001) Clinical utility of an instrument assessing migraine disability: the migraine disability assessment (MIDAS) questionnaire. Headache 41(9): 854–861

Lipton RB, Bigal ME, Kolodner K, Stewart WF, Liberman JN, Steiner TJ (2003a) The family impact of migraine: population-based studies in the USA and UK. Cephalalgia 23(6):429–440

Lipton RB, Liberman JN, Kolodner KB, Bigal ME, Dowson A, Stewart WF (2003b) Migraine headache disability and health-related quality-of-life: a population-based case-control study from England. Cephalalgia 23(6):441–450

Lucas C, Chaffaut C, Artaz MA, Lantéri-Minet M (2005) FRAMIG 2000: medical and therapeutic management of migraine in France. Cephalalgia 25(4):267–279

Martin BC, Pathak DS, Sharfman MI, Adelman JU, Taylor F, Kwong WJ et al (2000) Validity and reliability of the migraine-specific quality of life questionnaire (MSQ Version 2.1). Headache 40(3): 204–215

Michel P, Dartigues JF, Lindoulsi A, Henry P (1997) Loss of productivity and quality of life in migraine sufferers among French workers: results from the GAZEL cohort. Headache 37(2):71–78

Morillo LE, Alarcon F, Aranaga N, Aulet S, Chapman E, Conterno L et al (2005) Prevalence of migraine in Latin America. Headache 45(2):106–117

Nachit-Ouinekh F, Dartigues JF, Henry P, Becg JP, Chastan G, Lemaire N et al (2005) Use of the headache impact test (HIT-6) in general practice: relationship with quality of life and severity. Eur J Neurol 12(3):189–193

Olesen J, Leonardi M (2003) The burden of brain diseases in Europe. Eur J Neurol 10(5):471–477

Osterhaus JT, Townsend RJ, Gandek B, Ware JE (1994) Measuring the functional status and well-being of patients with migraine headache. Headache 34(6): 337–343

Sauro KM, Rose MS, Becker WJ, Christie SN, Giammarco R, Mackie GF et al (2010) HIT-6 and MIDAS as measures of headache disability in a headache referral population. Headache 50:383–395

Shin HE, Park JW, Kim YI, Lee KS (2008) Headache impact test-6 (HIT-6) scores for migraine patients: their relation to disability as measured from a headache diary. J Clin Neurol 4(4):158–163

Smith TR, Nicholson RA, Banks JW (2010) Migraine education improves quality of life in a primary care setting. Headache 50(4):600–612

Steiner TJ (2005) Lifting the burden: the global campaign to reduce the burden of headache worldwide. J Headache Pain 6(5):373–377

Stewart WF, Lipton RB, Kolodner KB, Sawyer J, Lee C, Liberman JN (2000) Validity of the migraine disability assessment (MIDAS) score in comparison to a diary-based measure in a population sample of migraine sufferers. Pain 88(1):41–52

Stovner L, Hagen K, Jensen R, Katsarava Z, Lipton R, Scher A et al (2007) The global burden of headache: a documentation of headache prevalence and disability worldwide. Cephalalgia 27(3):193–210

Terwindt GM, Ferrari MD, Tijhuis M, Groenen SM, Picavet HS, Launer LJ (2000) The impact of migraine on quality of life in the general population: the GEM study. Neurology 55(5):624–629

Wang SJ, Fuh JL, Lu SR, Juang KD (2001) Quality of life differs among headache diagnoses: analysis of SF-36 survey in 901 headache patients. Pain 89(2–3): 285–292

Zwart JA, Dyb G, Hagen K, Odegard KJ, Dahl AA, Bovim G et al (2003) Depression and anxiety disorders associated with headache frequency. The Nord-Trondelag Health Study. Eur J Neurol 20(10):147–152

4 Economics of Headache

Francesco Saverio Mennini[1,2] · *Lara Gitto*[1,3] · *Andrea Marcellusi*[1] ·
Fumihiko Sakai[4] · *Ichiro Arakawa*[5]
[1]University Tor Vergata, Rome, Italy
[2]Sapienza University of Rome, Rome, Italy
[3]University of Catania, Catania, Italy
[4]Kitasato University Hospital, Asao Kawasaki, Kanagawa, Japan
[5]Faculty of Pharmaceutical Sciences, Teikyo Heisei University,
Chiba, Japan

Paolo Martelletti, Timothy J. Steiner (eds.), *Handbook of Headache*, DOI 10.1007/978-88-470-1700-9_4,
⸳ Lifting The Burden 2011

Abstract: On the World Health Organization's ranking of causes of disability, headache disorders are among the ten most disabling conditions, and among the five most disabling for women.

Hence, the impact of headache disorders is a problem of enormous proportions, both for individual and society. Health economic literature tried to assess the effects on individuals by examining the socioeconomic burden of headache disorders and identifying direct and indirect cost related to headache.

Migraine has a considerable impact on functional capacity, resulting in disrupted work and social activities. Indirect costs associated with reduced productivity represent a substantial proportion of the total cost of migraine as well. It is not surprising that chronic headache is one of modern society's most costly illnesses.

Headache is well far behind other pathologies, where there is a greater knowledge of the economic aspects of both the pathology-related costs and the likely benefits resulting from different therapeutic approaches.

Notwithstanding the disease costing problems, it is important for the economic analysis to gain ground since there is a growing need to keep account of the available resources and the results attainable in the health care policies, from the central to the peripheral levels, where the evaluation tools referred to above prove even more expedient.

Given the social relevance of migraine, it is important to increase the knowledge related to the economic consequences of prevention through an increase of availability of health service.

From the analysis of prevalence, incidence, morbidity, and consequence of the state of health caused by headache and by looking at the Asian experience as well, it seems important to warn the scientific community and policy makers to implement specific "observatories." For this reason, it is useful to increase economic evaluation studies to be able to estimate economic and financial costs of headache and its prevention (as in The Global Campaign to Reduce the Burden of Headache Worldwide – WHO).

Introduction

Migraine is a very common disorder, affecting about 11% of adult populations in Western countries, and it belongs to the primary headache. Migraine is sometimes a progressive disease with cardiovascular, cerebrovascular, and long-term neurologic effects (Hazard et al. 2009).

On the World Health Organization's ranking of causes of disability, headache disorders are among the ten most disabling conditions, and among the five most disabling for women. In all studies, regardless of nationality, women stay away from work more often than men. Moreover, women tended to lose more workdays than men, even if indirect costs were similar due to lower salaries and labor force participation among women (Stovner and Andrée 2008). Hence, the impact of headache disorders is a problem of enormous proportions, both for individual and society. Health economic literature tried to assess the effects on individuals by examining the socioeconomic burden of headache disorders (Clarke et al. 1996; Rasmussen 1999; Lanteri-Minet et al. 2003) and identifying direct and indirect cost related to headache.

Direct costs concern mainly expenses for drugs, which are not often assumed in an appropriate way. The most of the people suffering from migraine, in fact, manage headache without conventional medical advice and generally treat their attacks with over-the-counter medication. They neither seek medical attention nor are accurately diagnosed by a physician. This gives often rise to a high percentage of visits to different health professionals and, once the disease has become chronic, to a large number of prescriptions for medication, which in turn produces an increase in costs (Volcy-Gomez 2006).

Migraine has a considerable impact on functional capacity, resulting in disrupted work and social activities (Solomon and Price 1997). Indirect costs associated with reduced productivity represent a substantial proportion of the total cost of migraine as well. Hence, migraine has a major impact on the working sector of the population (prevalence of migraine is the highest during the peak productive years – between the ages of 25 and 55), therefore determining that indirect costs outweigh the direct costs.

It is not surprising that chronic headache is one of the modern society's most costly illnesses (Lanteri-Minet et al. 2003). In EU countries, the working days lost as a result of migraine vary from 1.9 to 3.2 days/patient/year. The overall cost of migraine has been estimated to be €27 billion in the EU countries; adding the cost for other types of headache (tension-type headache and chronic headache), the impact is much greater (Stovner and Andrée 2008).

During the last years several studies on chronic headaches have gone further the analysis of costs, stressing the negative influence of headache on quality of life parameters (Blumenfeld 2003).

Since standardized measures to evaluate losses of utility due to migraine have not been properly developed so far, the issue of costs is still the most relevant: the approach of cost of illness is particularly well suited to analyze the burden of headache (Donia Sofio et al. 2003).

The chapter is organized as follows: the next section will discuss the issue of costs, both direct and indirect, describing as well some indicators developed in the medical and economic literature on headache and related to the severity of headache (and, consequently, to the level of costs that will arise for treating the symptoms). ❷ Section "Migraine and Quality of Life" will illustrate the new perspectives of economics of headache: studies are now focusing on the issue of quality of life, so that cost-utility analyses are becoming more common in the literature. ❷ Section "Treatment of Migraine with New Drugs and Improvements in Terms of Cost Savings and Quality of Life" will look, instead, at the newest therapeutic opportunities for headache, mentioning the consequences in terms of cost savings. ❷ Section "Economics of Headache in Asia and Japan" will offer an overview of the management of headache in Asia and Japan. Some final remarks will conclude the chapter.

Direct and Indirect Costs of Migraine

The financial burden of migraine has constituted the main issue of many analyses.

Economic analyses make a distinction among direct and indirect costs. Direct costs include all the healthcare costs caused by a disease, from its diagnosis to the patient's treatment and rehabilitation. Among the resources employed for the treatment of headache there are the clinical and instrumental analyses called for by a diagnosis, drugs, and other therapeutic measures. The resources include as well the services provided by the health personnel (physicians, nurses, and other workers) and that part of overhead costs imputable to the disease. Hospital costs represent only a very small portion of total migraine management costs (Hu et al. 1999): the rate of hospitalization is less than 10% and varies from 2% in Denmark to 7% in the USA.

Although indirect costs appear to be the most difficult to be estimated, even direct costs may have been underestimated. This conclusion derives by considering that medical claims do not capture all migraine-related treatment costs, because the disease is often not treated with specific therapies; moreover, it is quite complicated to measure all the over-the-counter or preventive medications as well as nondrug-related interventions.

There is a general agreement on the circumstance that a high percentage of people suffering from migraine never consult a physician for their illness – between 19% and 44% as reported by various studies – and that only a small percentage – from 16% to 36% – regularly consult a physician (Edmeads et al. 1993).

Direct costs may be differentiated depending on who provides the resources: health service, regardless of the type of system existing in the various countries (national healthcare service, panel-based healthcare system, or health insurance), or the patients themselves and their relatives.

Comparing direct costs for people suffering from migraine (including episodic migraine) versus people who do not, the former use more medical care (on average 2.3 more physician office visits) and incur on average $697 more in medical care costs per year. The need for medical consultation increases with the severity of symptoms: those with a claims-based diagnosis of migraine tend to use more care compared to those without such a diagnosis (5.1 more visits) (Lafata et al. 2004).

Indirect costs have been estimated to be due mainly to losses of productivity and absenteeism: some studies (Stewart et al. 2003; Hu et al. 1999) provided an estimation for headache costs of more of $14.5 billion (of which $7.9 billion were due to absenteeism, $5.4 billion to diminished productivity, and only $1.2 billion to medical costs).

Severe migraine can lead to disruption of work, family, and social life: hence, the direct costs of migraine, due to medical care, are small compared with the indirect costs caused by absence from work and reduced productivity (Lipton et al. 1994, 1997, 2001).

A significant increase in the economic burden of migraine occurs when the latter is comorbid with anxiety and depression (Pesa and Lage 1994).

Studies already existing in literature, in fact, reveal that migraine is currently underdiagnosed and undertreated. The development of suitable measures of severity may be useful in assessing the need for patient care and treatment and helps in targeting those that are more disabled by migraine. The identification of patients who need more care should reduce the impact of migraine on the individual and the burden of migraine on society. Measures of severity may be seen as predictors of disability and healthcare use.

Among the indicators developed in the economic literature and reported by some studies (i.e., Hu et al. 1999) it is possible to mention:

– *Bedridden days per year.* Total number of bedridden days per year (BDY) was calculated as follows:

$$BDY = NMS \times FAY \times PAB \times ABH/24$$

where NMS is the number of migraine sufferers in an age and sex stratum; FAY, the frequency of migraine attacks per year; PAB is the average percentage of attacks for which patients need bed rest; ABH, the average bedridden hours when lying down with a migraine attack (by dividing by 24, bedridden hours were converted into bedridden days).

Migraine-related disability is calculated as a function of the number of bedridden days in patients aged 20–64 years based on results of a previous American study (the Baltimore County Migraine Study). Subjects reported how often they needed bed rest when experiencing a migraine attack; response options were: never, rarely, less than 50% of the time, and more than 50% of the time; for calculations, these were translated into rates of 0%, 10%, 25%, and 75%.

– *Healthcare resource use*. The costs of healthcare resource utilization associated with migraine included both inpatient, outpatient, and prescription drug claims for employees from 40 large firms in the United States (data of 1994). Migraine-related drug costs were estimated only for those patients who had at least one migraine-related medical encounter.

– *Economic losses due to missed workdays*. The total number of migraine-related missed workdays (TMWD) per year may be calculated for each age- and gender-specific stratum as follows:

$$TMWD = NMS \times MWD \times PWP \times WHW/40$$

where MWD is average migraine-related missed workdays per year; PWP is the percentage of the population working for pay, estimated at 73% for males and 57% for females; WHW is the average working hours per week, most recently reported as 35 working hours for both sexes (by dividing by 40, working hours have been converted into the standard full-time level – 8 working hours per day).

Missed workdays and impaired work performance were combined with data from the Bureau of Labor Statistics with respect to percentage of population working for pay and average working hours per week.

– *Impaired work performance* is a function of the number of workdays with migraine (NWDM) and reduced work efficiency during the attacks.

The NWDM may be estimated as follows:

$$NWDM = NMS \times WDM \times PWP \times WHW/40.$$

The average number of workdays with migraine (WDM) per year can be estimated based on patient self-reporting.

– *Lost workday equivalent (LWDE)*. LWDE due to impaired work performance was calculated as follows:

$$LWDE = NWDM \times (1 - EWM)$$

where EWM is the average effectiveness at work with migraine, estimated at 42% for men and 34% for women.

– *Economic loss due to reduced productivity*. The total employment lost due to migraine (TELM) in dollar terms, assuming 8 h for each working day, is:

$$TELM = (TMWD + LWDE) \times \text{hourly salary} \times 8.$$

Such indicators put in evidence what extent patients with migraine are frequently disabled during their acute attacks.

Although migraine-related disability can be reflected by both bedridden days and restricted activities, bedridden days have been more emphasized because of the ease in reporting and quantifying them. In fact, about one third of migraine sufferers experienced severe disability or the need for bed rest following attacks, and an additional 50% reported mild or moderate disability.

Other indicators have been developed in other studies. In Hawkins et al. (2007), the authors compared the average annual indirect expenditures of a group of employees with migraine with a matched group of employees without migraine: the burden of illness of migraine was defined as the difference in average indirect expenditures per person between migraine and control cohorts. Indirect cost components were workplace absence, short-term disability, and workers' compensation claims. In this study, controls were matched to the migraine cohort according to the predicted probability of having a migraine; this probability was estimated for each patient on the basis of a logistic regression analysis of having a migraine that controlled for demographics (age, gender, region, location, year, and type of insurance) and overall comorbidities. A second-stage regression was used to estimate the indirect burden of migraine. Specifically, the second-stage regression used total indirect expenditures as the dependent variable and the same independent variables used in the propensity score matching, plus a dummy indicator to denote migraine patients. The second-stage regression estimated by applying a generalized linear model (GLM), controlled for any remaining differences between the cohorts after matching.

It was estimated that employees with migraine cost approximately $12 billion per year due to absenteeism, short-term disability, and/or workers' compensation claims. Most of the indirect migraine expenditures were driven by absenteeism. In a cross-study comparison, the estimated per-employee absenteeism plus short-term disability expenditures for migraine were shown to be greater than those of other common conditions such as chronic obstructive pulmonary disorder, heart disease, depression, chronic renal failure, diabetes, and asthma.

Compared with the study by Hu et al., which found absenteeism costs to be about $8 billion ($10.1 billion – data of 2004), the estimate of absence costs from Hawkins et al.'s study is of $9 billion: the difference is due to the use of different sets of indirect cost components (in their study, Hu et al. did not include short-term disability and workers' claims).

Loss of production capacity (so-called debility) might occur as well when an ill individual goes to work – "presenteeism": it is easy to understand how an individual suffering from migraine will not have the same level of productivity as a non suffering individual. Although evaluation of loss of productivity due to migraine is extremely subjective, the residual level of effectiveness calculated in the various studies is fairly similar, between 56% and 72% (Cerbo et al. 2001).

Presenteeism has been estimated among the most important drivers of overall costs: its impact accounts for 89% of the total cost burden (Goetzel et al. 2004).

Other international studies (Bigal et al. 2003) have estimated the burden of migraine giving some insights about possible indicators to apply (e.g., ❷ Sect. "Economics of Headache in Asia and Japan" of this chapter, reporting the Asian experience).

The results, related to different levels of care, showed how the estimated cost of a consultation for migraine on the primary care level was US $11.53; on the secondary care level, US $22.18; in the emergency department, $34.82; and for hospitalization, US $217.93.

A study aimed at estimating the burden of headache in a patient population from a specialized headache center in Denmark (Vinding et al. 2007) used structured interviews, prospective headache diaries, and standardized self-administered questionnaires. The interview contained a total of 116 questions about the socioeconomic impact of headache disorders and included an extensive description of the influence on working ability, personal impact, utilization of health services, and medicine; it was conducted by a trained medical student blinded to the remaining information about headache diagnosis, frequency, and medication use.

High utilization of the healthcare system and a remarkable absence rate due to headache (about 12 days/year) were reported. Eighty-one percent of patients experienced a marked decrease in work effectiveness. Overall, 91% felt hampered by their headache on a daily basis and 98% had expenses for headache medication.

Further specification could be added to analyses when estimating the burden of headache according to different levels of pain. It has already been said about the classification made by the International Headache Society, which distinguishes three categories for headache.

Results of an extensive survey carried on a sample of 10,585 individuals in the French adult population (data of 1999) showed a prevalence of 17.3% for migraine and nearly 30% for headaches (Auray 2006).

The average expenditure for a headache patient is about €220 (10% for general practitioners consultations, 11% for laboratory evaluations, 17% for specialist consultations, 18% for drugs, and 44% for hospital costs). However, such a costs partition depends largely on the headache category and on individuals' activities and occupational status: although acute headaches lead to the most severe deterioration of quality of life, professional or school activities are not affected in the same way.

Other studies carried out for other European countries show a high prevalence (and high costs) for all types of headache (Radtke and Neuhauser 2009). Finally, a longitudinal survey carried out along 5 years for the USA (14,544 adults were observed) outlined how patients who developed transformed migraine (intending for "transformed migraine" an escalating frequency of migraine of headache attacks) reported more primary care visits, neurologist or headache specialists, etc., costs – $7,750 per year per transformed migraine versus $1,757 per year per episodic migraine – (Munakata et al. 2009).

To sum up, costs of headache, both direct and indirect, are not clearly defined: indirect costs of migraine outweigh the direct costs and, therefore, might represent an obvious target for healthcare intervention, aimed at reducing the burden of migraine (Solomon and Price 1997).

Migraine and Quality of Life

A different approach followed by more recent studies is based on quality of life, rather than analysis of costs.

Despite the prevalence and substantial economic burden of migraine, no standardized measures of quality of life for patients suffering from migraine have been developed so far (Gagne et al. 2007). For example, the Health Plan Employer Data and Information Set, maintained by the National Committee for Quality Assurance is widely used in the US to assess quality of care at the health-plan level, but it does not include any headache- or migraine-related measures. This may be due, in part, to a lack of understanding of migraine or its "underdiagnosis," as it has already been said in the previous section. Migraine, in fact, was not even included in the first Global Burden of Disease in 1990 (Leonardi et al. 2005). The American Migraine Prevalence and Prevention Study found that only 56.2% of those with migraine had ever received a medical diagnosis.

Most existing measures have been developed by the Institute for Clinical Systems Improvement or summarized and reported by the RAND Corporation. Leonardi et al. (2005) summarize classification for disability due to headache according to WHO classification: using disability-adjusted life years (DALYs) as a summary measure of population health (which adds disability to mortality), WHO has shown that mental and neurological disorders collectively account for 30.8% of all years of healthy life lost to disability while migraine alone accounts for 1.4% and is in the top 20 causes of disability worldwide.

This information has to be combined with the increasingly widely accepted belief that disability is a relevant parameter for monitoring the health of nations and that there is an increasing need to measure them.

Classification of Functioning, Disability, and Health applied to headache disorders allows comparability with other health conditions as well as evaluation of the role of the environment as a cause of disability among people with headache.

During the last years an increasing role has been played, moreover, by educational programs on migraine that should lead, as an effect, to lower costs (a study by Page et al. 2009 estimated a diminution of 34.5% for migraine costs and of 14.7% of total medical costs determined by headache after employees of three US companies had followed a migraine screening program).

Migraine in the workplace is an issue related to quality of life (Weiss et al. 2008): management of workplace migraine includes screening, prevention, and effective treatment, in other words, a variety of strategies based on collaborative efforts among workers, occupational health nurses, and other providers.

Treatment of Migraine with New Drugs and Improvements in Terms of Cost Savings and Quality of Life

Appropriate treatment of migraine can decrease the level of costs (Dodick and Lipsy 2004). Prevention and early intervention or effective treatment strategies for headache disorders may be highly cost effective.

Cost-effectiveness models and all aspects of effectiveness (efficacy, tolerability, and cost) have been considered in developing strategies and pharmaceutical treatments to reduce managed care expenditures for migraine treatment.

Economic considerations associated with migraine received little attention prior to the development of triptans, the first effective treatment for acute migraine. Economic research started in 1992, assessing the costs of migraine, both direct and indirect, as well as its economic impact (Stang et al. 2004).

The choice for alternative therapeutic treatments depends on several factors. In evaluating treatment strategies not only the activity of a drug in reaching the main end points (i.e., pain free or headache relief) should be considered, but also the safety and perception of safety by patients, and the cost-effectiveness, including indirect costs compared with personal and social benefits. There are several cost-effectiveness studies aimed at evaluating cost-effectiveness ratios for triptans or other drugs (Wheeler 1998; Blumenfeld 2003; Pini et al. 2005).

Quite recently, the focus has shifted on the cost-effectiveness of preventive treatment. Prophylactic migraine treatment effectiveness has been evaluated by many studies from 1994 on (Adelman and Von Seggern 1995).

Migraine prophylaxis is aimed at preventing frequent attacks and the development of a long-term condition that often incurs heavy costs for abortive treatment, diagnostic services, and medical care (Lainez 2009). Agents approved for migraine prophylaxis include the antiepileptics divalproex and topiramate and the beta blockers propranolol and timolol. Costs vary widely among prophylactic agents.

A new approach to migraine prophylaxis is injection of botulinum toxin (Coloprisco and Martelletti 2003; Mennini et al. 2004). Overall, positive results have been reported concerning the reduction of the duration and the intensity of the attacks.

Since migraine appears to have a direct economic impact on families (medical costs of families with at least one member suffering from migraine were 70% greater than families with no members suffering from headache, Stang et al. 2004), economic analyses should look more in detail at social and familiar environment. An individual approach is, however, required: potential benefits should be weighed against the adverse effects associated with each agent in determining the optimal preventive regimen for individual patients by considering any comorbid condition (Pierangeli et al. 2006).

Moreover, an important role has to be played by the physician as regarding the decision to treat and the choice of prophylactic drug that should be taken with the patient. What is important is to balance expectations and therapeutic realities for each drug (Mennini et al. 2008).

Economics of Headache in Asia and Japan

Migraine is a common disease in Japan and Asians as well as in EU and the US. Prevalence of migraine is 5–10% in Asians (Wang et al. 2008). In Japan, prevalence of migraine among the population aged 15 or over is approximately 8.4% (Sakai and Igarashi 1997).

In 2004, the World Health Organization and the major international headache nongovernmental organizations committed themselves to the Global Campaign against Headache (Lifting The Burden) (Steiner 2004, 2005). In parallel, various effective treatment options have been established, including drug therapy (acute, prophylactic) and nondrug therapy. Despite such organizational efforts and medical innovations, patients suffering serious migraine headache still have few chances to receive adequate medical treatment.

Under the circumstance, further efforts are required in a worldwide scale to raise awareness of the importance of headache treatment.

Several activities have been undertaken: among these, it is possible to mention campaign networks, evidence accumulation, global investigation and research (including education of researchers), that have provided government and relevant bodies with the evidence, developing and executing educational programs.

Likewise, Asians must organizationally accelerate headache treatment to keep pace with the international processes. This was the main reason underlying the 2005 "Kyoto Declaration on Headache," announced at the 12th Congress of the International Headache Society held in Kyoto, Japan. The aim was to assure innovations of headache treatment in cooperation with medical experts and their relevant bodies, to establish and to improve headache care system, and to alleviate burden of headache patients. The declaration was adopted by the chairman of WHA and the chairman of IHS, associated with WHO and The Ministry of Health, Labor and Welfare of Japan.

A large-scale survey for patients visited and/or visiting neurology clinic for the first time took place by eight countries in Asia. The aim was that of enlightening the seriousness of migraineurs' disability in their daily life and to confirm diagnosis and treatment outcomes among neurological outpatients. This survey demonstrated high prevalence of migraine in Asian countries as well, and revealed current status of inadequate diagnosis and treatment despite their high burdens (Wang et al. 2008).

In Korea, quantitative measurement of the burden of migraine was reported using HIT-6 (Headache Impact Test[TM]-6). Among 130 migraineurs, the average of HIT-6 score was 53.4, in which approximately 70% were "moderate" to "severe," which correlated with disabled periods (Shin et al. 2008).

In Japan, SF-36, a generic QoL (Quality of Life) questionnaire, has demonstrated lower QoL in migraineurs compared to epileptic patients. Migraineurs have also found to be more susceptible to anxiety than patients suffering from rheumatism. Hence, these results have demonstrated considerable burden of headache existing in the current Japan society (Sakai et al. 2004; Shimizu et al. 2004). In addition, Japanese migraineur's QoL was investigated using a migraine-specific quality of life questionnaire (MSQ), which indicated that Japanese migraineurs are forced to reschedule their works in a low mood (Sakai et al. 2004). In a comparison with US patients, Japanese migraineurs tend to endure headache compared to US migraineurs in their daily life (Shimizu et al. 2004).

In Taiwan, a large-scale epidemiological study took place with regard to the loss of labor productivity by migraine. The results demonstrated estimated loss of labor of 3.7 million days per year. The loss is predicted to be equivalent to 4.6 billion Taiwanese dollars (equivalent to approximately $145 millions) (Fuh et al. 2008).

In Japan, the economical loss of labor productivity by migraine has been estimated to be 288 billion yen (approximately $3.2 billion) per year (survey in 2005) (Kato et al. 2007; Manaka et al. 2006). Another group investigated the productivity loss among migraineurs under treatment (except migraineurs with no treatment). It has been estimated to be 160 billion yen (approximately $1.8 billion), calculated by multiplying the number of patients (1.067 million) by monthly loss per patient (126,717 yen) and by months per year (Nishimura 2004). Recent investigation of the loss of labor productivity among metropolitan workers has demonstrated that approximately 25% of migraineurs are forced to miss their work, and approximately 60% are taking a stopgap remedy using commercially available drugs instead of an adequate treatment at some medical facility (Suzuki et al. 2009).

About direct costs of headache, there are not, at the present moment, reports investigating the effect of migraine on direct medical costs in Asian countries. Little is known concerning the effect on direct medical costs in Japan as well. Shimizu et al. (2001) investigated direct medical costs by calculating remuneration for medical services in his own clinic: on average of 25 migraineurs, physician visit expenses were 4,225 yen ($47) per visit, emergency room visit costs were 22,680 yen ($252) per visit, and hospitalization costs were 172,298 yen ($1,914) per administration. However, such investigation is based on a small-scale survey in premarketing period, thus interpretation of the results should be taken into consideration.

In addition, since 2003 Diagnosis Procedure Combination (DPC) system, flat payment for acute hospitalization has been introduced in Japan. The system comprehensively evaluates remuneration for medical service based on DPC, one by one for each medical practice including surgery, instead of paying at piece rates. The DPC system has now become widespread in Japan. In 2008, approximately 16% of medical facilities and approximately 50% of beds have been calculated to estimate remuneration for medical practice on acute hospitalization. As of May 2009, hospitalization period of a patient by a DPC category, "migraine, headache syndrome, and others," showed 6 days' increase year by year since 2004 (data from DPC Evaluation Section Committee, Remuneration Survey Group, Social Insurance Council, The Ministry of Health, Labour and Welfare, May 14, 2009). Using 2008 statistics, medical expense claim for one hospitalization can be estimated by DPC points, which amount to 15,425 points (equivalent to 154,250 yen; approximately $1,714).

Moreover, DPC report showed that 129 claims were submitted by the name of DPC diagnostic procedure combination in 2008. In consequence, total medical expense by DPC-specific hospitalization amounts to be 20 million yen (approximately $0.2 million; multiplying 154,250 yen per claim by 129 claims).

About pharmacological treatments for headache, in Asian countries, little is known concerning the effect of triptans on the burden of disease. In Korea, the Health Insurance Review Agency (HIRA) has been established in 2000, in order to review and evaluate reimbursement of medical costs using new drugs by health insurance. A 2009 report (Kim 2009) described that investigation of the effect of drugs for migraine treatment on Korean economy has just started.

In Japan, the effect of sumatriptan tablet 50 mg on RPO for migraine has been investigated by a multi-collaborative clinical study. The results have demonstrated that using MSQ and HIT-6 QoL of migraineurs significantly improved 12 weeks after administration of sumatriptan tablet (Sakai et al. 2005).

A cost-effectiveness analysis regarding sumatriptan therapy for migraine indicated that an incremental cost-effectiveness ratio of sumatriptan versus existing therapy (including commercially available analgesics) was 944,538.9 yen ($10,500) per quality adjusted life years – QALYs gained (Shimizu et al. 2001), conclusively much below the empirical threshold value of 5–6 million yen per QALYs gained (Shiroiwa et al. 2010).

A cost-minimization analysis regarding self-injection of sumatriptan for migraineurs has demonstrated that, on average, it can save 5,918 yen (approximately $66). The number of sumatriptan injection for the treatment of migraine attack has been estimated to be 18,000 per year (data from Japanese Headache Society). In total, it can save 0.17 billion yen per year (saving $1.2 million, obtained multiplying 5,918 yen per treatment by 18,000 treatment) (Mizuho et al. 2009).

Overall, a great commitment against headache started together with the "Global Campaign against Headache": the Japanese Headache Society addresses on a concept of "interhospital cooperation," so that diagnosis and treatment of primary headache should be conducted mainly by primary care doctors, while diagnosis and treatment of secondary and/or intractable headache should be conducted mainly by headache experts.

Compared to US and EU countries, less progress has been made in the evidence accumulation in Asian countries and Japan. Organizational large-scale investigation has still been lagging behind. The effect of migraine on medical expense and the effect of triptans on the burden of diseases are still vague in many respects.

Diligent effort to build up case studies is indispensable, but organizational approach should be taken into account in this respect.

Headache patients should be directed toward primary care doctors, thus at this stage adequate diagnosis and treatment can avoid unfavorable stopgap remedy using commercially available analgesics, and can reduce patients disappointing medical facilities.

The second stage should be to follow up patient suspected to have secondary headache, or utilize headache experts to obtain second opinions.

In this perspective, Japanese Headache Society has been planning to enrich educational program for headache treatment, by establishing educational system leaded by headache experts.

This program aims to establish early-stage headache treatment process by primary care doctors, and also aims their collaboration with headache experts based on the Global Campaign Program.

Conclusion

Headache is well far behind other pathologies, where there is a greater knowledge of the economic aspects of both the pathology-related costs and the likely benefits resulting from different therapeutic approaches.

Notwithstanding the disease costing problems, it is important for the economic analysis to gain ground since there is a growing need to keep account of the available resources and the results attainable in the healthcare policies, from the central to the peripheral levels, where the evaluation tools referred to above prove even more expedient.

Given the social relevance of migraine should be important to increase the knowledge related to the economic consequences of prevention through an increase of availability of health service.

From the analysis of prevalence, incidence, morbidity, and consequence of the state of health caused by headache, and by looking at the Asian experience as well, it seems important to warn the scientific community and policy makers to implement specific "observatories." For this reason, it is useful to increase economic evaluation studies to be able to estimate economic and financial costs of headache and its prevention (as in the Global Campaign against Headache).

References

Adelman JU, Von Seggern R (1995) Cost considerations in headache treatment. Part 1: prophylactic migraine treatment. Headache 35(8):479–487

Auray JP (2006) Socio-economic impact of migraine and headaches in France. CNS Drugs 20(1):37–46

Bigal ME, Rapoport AM, Bordini CA, Tepper SJ, Shftell FD, Speciali JG (2003) Burden of migraine in Brazil: estimate of cost of migraine to the public health system and an analytical study of the cost-effectiveness of a stratified model of care. Headache 43(7):742–754

Blumenfeld A (2003) Botulinum toxin type A treatment of disabling migraine headache: a randomised double-blind, placebo-controlled study. Headache 43:853–860

Cerbo R, Pesare M, Aurilla C, Rondelli V, Barbanti P (2001) Socio-economic costs of migraine. J Headache Pain 2: S15–S19

Clarke CE, MacMillan L, Sondhi S, Wells NE (1996) Economic and social impact of migraine. Quart J Med 89:77–84

Coloprisco G, Martelletti P (2003) Reduction in expenditure on analgesics during one year of treatment of chronic tension headache with BoNT-A. J Headache Pain 4:88–94

Diagnosis Procedure Combination Evaluation Section Committee, Remuneration Survey Group, Social Insurance Council, The Ministry of Health, Labour and Welfare (May 14, 2009). http://www.mhlw.go.jp/shingi/2009/05/s0514-6.html (in Japanese)

Dodick DW, Lipsy RJ (2004) Advances in migraine management: implications for managed care organizations. Manag Care 13(5):45–51

Donia Sofio A, Mazzuca F, Mennini FS (2003) General disease costing principles. J Headache Pain 4(s01): s55–s58

Edmeads J, Findlay H, Tugwell P, Pryse-Phillips W, Nelason RF, Murray TJ (1993) Impact of migraine and tension-type headache on life-style, consulting behaviour, and medication use: a Canadian population survey. Can J Neurol Sci 20:131–137

Fuh JL et al (2008) Impact of migraine on the employed labor force in Taiwan. J Chin Med Assoc 71:74–78, (in Mandarin Chinese), JCMA

Gagne JJ, Leas B, Lofland JH, Goldfarb N, Freitag F, Silberstein S (2007) Quality of care measures for migraine: a comprehensive review. Dis Manage 10(3):138–146

Goetzel RZ, Long SR, Ozminkowski RJ, Hawkins K, Wang S, Lynch W (2004) Health, absence, disability, and presenteeism cost estimates of certain physical and mental health conditions affecting US employers. J Occup Environ Med 46:398–412

Hawkins K, Wang S, Rupnow MF (2007) Indirect cost burden of migraine in the United States. J Occup Environ Med 49(4):368–374

Hazard E, Munakata J, Bigal ME, Rupnow MF, Lipton RB (2009) The burden of migraine in the United States: current and emerging perspectives on disease management and economic analysis. Value Health 12(1):55

Hu XH, Markson LE, Lipton RB, Stewart WF, Berger ML (1999) Burden of migraine in the United States: disability and economic costs. Arch Intern Med 159(8):813–818

Kato Y et al (2007) J Pract Pharmacol 58(7):101–105 (in Japanese)

Kim CY (2009) Health technology assessment in South Korea. Int J Technol Assess Health Care 25(Suppl 1): 219–223

Lafata JE, Moon C, Leotta C, Kolodner K, Poisson L, Lipton RB (2004) The medical care utilization and costs associated with migraine headache. J Gen Intern Med 19(10):1005–1012

Lainez MJ (2009) The effect of migraine prophylaxis on migraine-related resource use and productivity. CNS Drugs 23(9):727–738

Lanteri-Minet M et al (2003) Prevalence and description of chronic daily headache in the general population in France. Pain 102:143–149

Leonardi M, Steiner TJ, Scher AT, Lipton RB (2005) The global burden of migraine: measuring disability in headache disorders with WHO's classification of functioning, disability and health (ICF). J Headache Pain 6(6):429–440

Lipton RB, Stewart WF, Von Korff M (1994) The burden of migraine. A review of cost to society. Pharmacoeconomics 6(3):215–221

Lipton RB, Stewart WF, Von Korff M (1997) Burden of migraine: societal costs and therapeutic opportunities. Neurology 48(3):S4–S9

Lipton RB, Stewart WF, Scher AI (2001) Epidemiology and economic impact of migraine. Curr Med Res Opin 17(1):s4–s12

Manaka S et al (2006) Faculty of Economics. http://homepage2.nifty.com/uoh/gakubu/keizaigakubu.htm (in Japanese)

Mennini FS, Fioravanti L, Piasini L, Palazzo F, Coloprisco G, Martelletti P (2004) A one-year economic evaluation of botulinum toxin type A treatment of chronic tension-type headaches: part I. J Headache Pain 5:188–191

Mennini FS, Gitto L, Martelletti P (2008) Improving care through health economics analyses: cost of illness and headache. J Headache Pain 9:199–206

Mizuho A et al (2009) Pharmacol Stage 8(5):18–23 (in Japanese)

Munakata J, Hazard E, Serrano D, Klingman D, Rupnow MF, Tierce J, Reed M, Lipton RB (2009) Economic burden of transformed migraine: results from the American Migraine Prevalence and Prevention (AMPP) study. Headache 49(4):398–508

Nishimura S (2004) In: Sakai F (ed) Approach to migraine. Sentan Igaku-Sha, Tokyo, pp 56–66 (in Japanese)

Page MJ, Paramore LC, Doshi D, Rupnow MF (2009) Evaluation of resource utilization and cost burden before and after an employer-based migraine education program. J Occup Environ Med 51(2):213–220

Pesa J, Lage MJ (1994) The medical cost of migraine and comorbid anxiety and depression. Headache 34:337–343

Pierangeli G, Cevoli S, Sancisi E, Grimaldi D, Zanigni S, Montagna P, Cortelli P (2006) Which therapy for which patient? Neurol Sci 27(2):S153–S158

Pini LA, Cainazzo MM, Brovia D (2005) Risk benefit and cost-benefit ratio in headache treatment. J Headache Pain 6(4):315–318

Radtke A, Neuhauser H (2009) Prevalence and burden of headache and migraine in Germany. Headache 49(1):79–89

Rasmussen BK (1999) Epidemiology and socio-economic impact of headache. Cephalalgia 19(25):20–23

Sakai F, Igarashi H (1997) Prevalence of migraine in Japan, a nationwide survey. Cephalalgia 17(1):15–22

Sakai T et al (2004) Jpn J Neurol Ther 21:449–458 (in Japanese)

Sakai T et al (2005) Prevalence of migraine in Japan, a nationwide survey. Cephalalgia 25:214–218

Shimizu T et al (2001) Diagn Treat 38(9):3–14 (in Japanese)

Shimizu T et al (2004) Jpn J Headache 31(2):81–83 (in Japanese)

Shin HE, Park JW, Kim YI, Lee KS (2008) Headache Impact Test-6 (HIT-6) scores for migraine patients: their relation to disability as measured from a headache diary. J Clin Neurol 4:158–163

Shiroiwa T et al (2010) International survey on willingness-to-pay (WTP) for one additional QALY gained: what is the threshold of cost effectiveness? Health Econ 19(4):422–437

Solomon GD, Price KL (1997) Burden of migraine. A review of its socioeconomic impact. Pharmacoeconomics 11(1):1–10

Stang PE, Crown WH, Bizier R, Chatterton ML, White R (2004) The family impact and costs of migraine. Am J Manage Care 10(5):313–320

Steiner TJ (2004) Lifting the burden: the global campaign against headache. Lancet Neurol 3(4):204–205

Steiner TJ (2005) Lifting the burden: the global campaign to reduce the burden of headache worldwide. J Headache Pain 6(5):373–377

Stewart WF, Ricci JA, Chee E, Morganstein D, Lipton R (2003) Lost productive time and cost due to common pain conditions in the US workforce. J Am Med Assoc 290:2443–2454

Stovner LJ, Andrée C (2008) Impact of headache in Europe: a review for the Eurolight project. J Headache Pain 9:139–146

Suzuki N et al (2009) Jpn J Headache 36:81 (in Japanese)

Vinding GR, Zeeberg P, Lyngberg A, Nielsen RT, Jensen R (2007) The burden of headache in a patient population from a specialized headache centre. Cephalalgia 27(3):263–270

Volcy-Gomez M (2006) The impact of migraine and other primary headaches on the health system and in social and economic terms. Rev Neurol 43(4): 228–235

Wang SJ, Chung CS, Chankrachang S, Ravishankar K, Merican JS, Salazar G, Siow C, Cheung RT, Phanthumchinda K, Sakai F (2008) Migraine disability awareness campaign in Asia: migraine assessment for prophylaxis. Headache 48(9): 1356–1365

Weiss MD, Bernards P, Price SJ (2008) Working through a migraine: addressing the hidden costs of workplace headaches. AAOHN J 56(12):495–500

Wheeler AH (1998) Botulinum toxin A, adjunctive therapy for refractory headaches associated with pericranial muscle tension. Headache 38(6): 468–471

5 Organization of Headache Services

Timothy J. Steiner[1,5] · *Fabio Antonaci*[2] · *Luiz Paulo Queiroz*[3] · *Sara Van Belle*[4]

[1]Norwegian University of Science and Technology, Trondheim, Norway
[2]University Consortium for Adaptive Disorders and Head Pain (UCADH) and Headache Science Centre, Pavia, Italy
[3]Universidade Federal de Santa Catarina, Florianopólis, SC, Brazil
[4]Prince Leopold Institute of Tropical Medicine, Antwerp, Belgium
[5]Faculty of Medicine, Imperial College London, London, UK

Paolo Martelletti, Timothy J. Steiner (eds.), *Handbook of Headache*, DOI 10.1007/978-88-470-1700-9_5,
© Lifting The Burden 2011

Abstract: Health services rarely meet the health-care needs of most people whose lives are affected by headache disorders. The solution does not lie in throwing additional resources into unstructured services, and in particular it does not lie in the expansion of specialist headache centers in secondary care, to which most people who need care fail to gain access. A regulated three-tier system, with emphasis on primary care, will, it is argued, deliver care more cost-effectively and more responsively to patients' needs.

Introduction: Headache Services – Inefficient and Failing

The World Health Organization (WHO) recognizes headache disorders as a high-priority public health concern (World Health Organization 2000). They are common (Stovner et al. 2007) and in many cases lifelong conditions, associated with recognizable burdens that include personal suffering, disability, and impaired quality of life (Steiner 2000, 2004). Their impact extends beyond those immediately affected (Steiner 2000). Not surprisingly, in countries for which data are available large numbers of people with headache are seen by physicians (Hopkins et al. 1989; Wiles and Lindsay 1996). For example, in a United Kingdom (UK) study, 17% of people aged 16–65 years consulted a primary-care physician because of headache at least once in 5 years; 9% of these were referred to secondary care (Laughey et al. 1999). Neurologists receive by far the most of these referrals: up to a third of all patients consulting neurologists in the UK do so because of headache, more than for any other neurological condition (Hopkins et al. 1989).

Despite this, care is not reaching all who may benefit. In fact, there is a worldwide context of significant need arising from headache disorders set against low priority given to them in the queue for health care (American Association for the Study of Headache and International Headache Society 1998). In wealthy countries such as the United States of America (USA) and UK, only two thirds of adults with migraine are correctly diagnosed (Lipton et al. 2003). While 86% consult at some time, many lapse from care so that only half are currently consulting; yet over 60% of those not consulting nonetheless exhibit high migraine-related disability (Lipton et al. 2003). The same undoubtedly goes for other disabling headache disorders. In poor countries, inevitably, these deficiencies are exacerbated by the general lack of resources. In sub-Saharan Africa, for example, people with the means will find access to specialists in private practice or seek specialist care in the neurology departments of (university) hospitals in capital cities, while organized treatment of headache disorders for the great majority is virtually absent, especially in rural areas. Severe headache, such as might occur in migraine, is commonly assumed to be, and often treated as, a symptom of another disease such as malaria.

Headache-Related Health-Care Needs Assessment

In this context of failing headache services, the large numbers of headache referrals to neurologists in the UK (Hopkins et al. 1989; Wiles and Lindsay 1996; Laughey et al. 1999) and elsewhere should be questioned – and, when this is done, they are impossible to justify. Most headache diagnosis and management requires no more than a basic knowledge of a relatively few very common disorders, and these ought to be wholly familiar to primary-care physicians. Only standard clinical skills, which every physician should have, need to be applied. No special investigations or equipment are usually necessary. In other words, only a small minority of cases of primary headache should not be perfectly well managed in primary care (Steiner 2003).

According to epidemiological evidence, among every one million people living in the world there are 110,000 adults with migraine (Steiner et al. 2003; Stovner et al. 2007), 90,000 of whom are significantly disabled (Lipton et al. 2003). There are up to 600,000 people who have occasional other headaches, the majority being episodic tension-type headache and not significantly disabling. And there are 30,000 with a syndrome of chronic daily headache (Stovner et al. 2007), of whom most are disabled and many have medication-overuse headache. It is reasonable to expect that at least everyone with disabling migraine or chronic daily headache is in need of (i.e., likely to benefit from) good headache care. This means 120,000 adults per million people, or about 15% of the adult population. Empirical data support this: for example, the UK study and general practice consultation and referral rates referred to above (Laughey et al. 1999; Dowson 2003; Dowson et al. 2004). Needs arise in the child population also, but there are fewer data by which to quantify them. Generally, headache disorders are less prevalent in children (Stovner et al. 2007), and the suggestion that headache-care needs arise at about half the rate per head of that in adults (Antonaci et al. 2008) (i.e., 15,000 children per 1,000,000 of the general population) provides a reasonable working basis.

Upon these statistics, with some assumptions about time needed to diagnose correctly and manage optimally, it is possible to make estimates of service requirements, and this has recently been done (Antonaci et al. 2008). While they may be imprecise, the numbers that these calculations generate show beyond any argument that most headache services *must* be provided in primary care (❷ *Table 5.1*) if needs – or even a substantial part of them – are to have any chance of being met.

Primary Care

In WHO's Alma-Ata declaration (World Health Organization International Conference on Primary Health Care 1978; Tarino and Webster 1995; Walley et al. 2008), primary health care is "the first level of contact of individuals, the family and community with the national health system bringing health care as close as possible to where people live and work." In nearly all countries, whatever the overarching system of health care (assuming there is one), primary care has a recognized and important role. In rural areas of sub-Saharan Africa, for example, primary care is the first (and only) point of contact for the majority of patients.

◘ Table 5.1

Estimated service requirements to meet headache-related health-care demand in a population (From Antonaci et al. 2008)

Estimated number of adults/children with headache-care needs per 1,000,000 population (n)	Expected demand in primary care	Expected demand in specialist care
	(hours of medical consultation per week)	
120,000/15,000	780 h (28 full-time equivalents)	140 h (5 full-time equivalents)

The UK has a strong system of primary care (Mainous et al. 2001; Ferris et al. 2001) within its Beveridgian national health service (NHS), which has statutory responsibility for providing comprehensive health care, paid for out of general taxation and essentially free at the point of delivery. Models of health care vary elsewhere in Europe, and throughout the world. Some, still providing free, subsidized or reimbursed care, are supported wholly or in part by insurance-based financial structures operated by the State or in which the State acts as a controlling intermediary. In others, fees for service are levied, which patients may or may not recover, in full or in part, through private or employer-provided insurance. All of these systems are able to accommodate primary care as first port-of-call, and this role of primary care is, usually, emphasized whenever countries undertake health-care reform (Coulter 1995).

There are good reasons for this. Decisions in primary care are best able to take account of patient-related factors such as family medical history and patients' individual expectations and values, of which the continuity and long-term relationships of primary care generate awareness. Continuity of care engenders trust and satisfaction among patients (Mainous et al. 2001). There are other reasons, too, that have to do with efficiency and cost-saving, which are discussed later.

Organizing Headache Services

All of the foregoing lead, inexorably and in a number of separate ways, to resounding awareness of the potential value of primary care – both generally and in optimally delivered headache services in particular. Steiner et al. writing on behalf of the European Headache Federation and *Lifting The Burden*: the Global Campaign against Headache (Steiner et al. 2011), proposed a model for service organization in Europe. Its essential elements are expansion of the contribution from primary care and organization of headache services on three levels, with facilitated but nonetheless controlled pathways between them. The model, slightly adapted, is shown in ❷ *Table 5.2*.

Health-care practitioners in general primary care deliver front-line headache services (level 1), with the benefit to their patients of being locally accessible. They may be primary-care

❐ Table 5.2

Headache services organized on three levels (Adapted from Steiner et al. 2011)

Level 1. General primary care	• Front-line headache services (accessible first contact for most people with headache)
	• Ambulatory care delivered by primary health-care providers (physicians, clinical officers, nurses, and/or pharmacists in some countries)
	• Referring when necessary, and acting as gatekeeper, to:
Level 2. Special-interest headache care	• Ambulatory care delivered by physicians with a special interest in headache
	• Referring when necessary to:
Level 3. Headache specialist centres	• Advanced multidisciplinary care delivered by headache specialists in hospital-based centres

physicians, but this is not essential in a health-care system that relies more on clinical officers, nurses, or pharmacists. Whatever their background, many will need better knowledge of headache for this purpose, but the model does not require *every* primary-care provider to offer level-one headache services if they are able to share case-load between themselves according to their skills and interests. This level should be able to meet the needs of 90% of people consulting for headache, who do not present any particular difficulty (including most of those with migraine and tension-type headache); for the remainder, and reserved for these 10%, the facilitated referral channels to levels 2 and 3 should be utilized.

At an intermediate level are headache clinics staffed by physicians who have developed a special interest. These clinics might be placed in primary or secondary care, according to the structure of health services in a particular country. They should provide care to the 10% of patients who, requiring greater expertise, are referred from level 1 to level 2: more difficult cases of primary headache, and some secondary headache disorders. Ideally they should have access to other services such as neurology, psychology, and physiotherapy. They must have a referral channel to level 3.

Hospital-based specialists are at level 3, providing advanced care for the relatively few patients needing secondary-care management. These should not exceed 1% of all headache patients and, if relieved of the other 99%, specialist headache centers can cover relatively large geographical catchment areas and populations (one full-time specialist per two million people [Steiner et al. 2011]). To perform optimally, and meet all needs at this level, they require full-time inpatient facilities and should support emergency or acute treatment services for patients presenting acutely with serious headache. Furthermore, physicians at this level will ideally work in multidisciplinary teams, with access to equipment and specialists in other disciplines for diagnosis and management of the underlying causes of all secondary headache disorders.

Level 3 is costly, and may be unaffordable, but cost is kept down if access to it is appropriately restricted – a key factor discussed below. On the other hand, if level 3 cannot be fully implemented within this model, or at all, this ought not of itself to detract from the benefits that should be provided to the great majority by levels 1 and 2. Greater problems arise when the focus is on level 3, put in place without due consideration of, or investment in, the essential levels below it.

Equitable distribution is a further challenge. Brazil makes a good example, with 243 "headache specialists" (in 2004/2005 [Department of Health 2003; Masruha et al. 2007]) for a population of about 190 million. While these are more than twice the number needed in a well-functioning three-level model (Steiner et al. 2011), in 5 of Brazil's 27 States there are none at all; the southeast region has 68% of them for 42.6% of the country's population, and the northeast has only 12.4% for 28.1% of the population (Department of Health 2003; Masruha et al. 2007).

The Essential Gate-Keeper Role

The model was developed for Europe (Steiner et al. 2011) and appears suitable for most European countries. With adaptations, perhaps, it may be equally so for most countries worldwide, because its central purpose is to shift demand from secondary-care services and move it to primary care – a move which is not only appropriate from a clinical viewpoint but also, in general, cost-saving (Hossain 1998). The *gate-keeper* role of primary care is the key organizational issue (Dixon et al. 1998; Ferris et al. 2001).

In the UK NHS, GPs have always had this role, controlling access to specialists in secondary care. This is not so in all European countries: in France and Germany, for example, patients may go directly to a specialist, who therefore becomes the first contact. By its nature, specialist care is usually provided in a hospital environment that has the complex technological facilities necessary to perform clinical investigations, surgery, and postoperative care. However, venues such as polyclinics are common also, offering intermediate services, which may be delivered by specialists. Elsewhere in the world there is similar variation. In Brazil, a private health-care system (including 26% of the population who pay for a health-insurance plan [Lucas et al. 2006; Instituto Brasileiro de Geografia e Estatística 2008]) operates alongside the government-funded Unified Health System (UHS). In the private system, people can usually choose their physician: someone with headache may go directly to a "headache specialist." The UHS, on the other hand, offers three levels of health care: level 1 organized and funded by city government, level 2 by State government, and level 3 by Federal government.

Where it is in place, gate-keeping ostensibly guides patients efficiently and in their best interests through the system according to their needs rather than their demands (while needs and demands overlap, they are not the same). However, whatever its supposed purpose, gate-keeping is believed to contribute – and perhaps is essential – to cost containment, in part because of evidence that unrestricted access to specialists induces a demand for costly and sometimes unnecessary services. The effectiveness of this system (Jones et al. 1995), and the equity of it, relies to a great extent on efficiency at the interface between primary and secondary care, a seam in service continuity where breakdowns can occur readily, and detrimentally to patients (Preston et al. 1999).

Clearly there should not be undue system-created delays or other barriers set against those who do need specialist care. The model calls for and its success is dependent upon efficient interfaces between the levels. This is an issue of implementation, best determined according to the context of local health services. At the same time, the model will not be workable if the gate-keeper role is not embedded at level 1, and patients are allowed to go directly to higher levels regardless of need. Patients cannot be blamed for seeking access directly to those they perceive to be experts, and, in many countries, both culture and current health-system organization encourage this behavior. But it is exactly this that breaks down order and, because specialist services are over-loaded, as a direct result denies specialist access to many of those who really need it.

Education

The solution, while not simple, is twofold, and educational in both its parts: changing behavior by improving patients' understanding on the one hand, and – more importantly, and required first – ensuring that the expertise necessary at level 1 is in reality available.

This expertise is no more than standard clinical skills, better knowledge only of the relatively few common headache disorders, and the use of evidence-based guidelines in primary care (Steiner et al. 2007). Duly applied it can keep the great majority of patients at level 1, reducing unnecessary and therefore wasteful demand upon more costly specialist care. This more rational use of health-care resources is the means by which effective care *can* reach many more who need it.

There are, however, major implications for training. These need careful consideration. The start, though it is not easily achieved, is to give more emphasis to headache diagnosis and management in the medical schools undergraduate curriculum. This will ensure at least that newly qualified doctors will have some understanding of a set of burdensome and very common disorders – which is often not the case now. But there will be much more to do beyond that if headache care, when delivered, is to be optimally effective at all levels. Within the three-level care system proposed, a training role for each higher level to the level below can be envisaged. It is likely that the entire structure will depend to some extent upon these roles being developed.

Political Will

Implementing the model may be challenging, but the expectations of successful implementation embrace improved headache services, achieved in a number of complementary ways: extending community-based availability; cutting costs by pulling inappropriate demand in secondary care back into primary care; thereby freeing resources to discover and meet unrecognized headache-related health-care needs in the community. All of these outcomes are politically desirable, and there should, therefore, be political will to achieve them.

Distorted priorities may be at the heart of the current inadequacies. It is likely to be argued, probably correctly, that the creation of a better health-care structure, and the delivery of better care, will stimulate demand with unaffordable results. But it should be recognized that, if this occurs, it is simply unmasking need that is there already. In counter-argument, not only the humanitarian symptom-based burdens (Steiner 2000; Stovner et al. 2007) but, possibly more persuasively, the current huge cost of headache disorders to national economies must be fully acknowledged (Hu et al. 1998). Among headache disorders, migraine alone accounts for an estimated 25 million working days per year lost in the UK (Steiner et al. 2003). Therefore, while major improvement to services requires significant investment, there are opportunities – if even a small part of this lost productivity can be recovered (Lucas et al. 2006) – for substantial savings to offset it.

Looking at the UK again as an example, most patients who cannot be treated effectively in primary care are referred to neurologists, but some may go to other primary-care physicians who have developed a special interest in headache (Department of Health 2003). A few end up in specialized secondary-care or academic headache centers. While these options appear to reflect the three proposed levels, there is no formal organization of UK headache services in this way. Much is ad hoc, and many patients do not progress from level 1 who would benefit from doing so. On the other hand, significant numbers of patients are referred upward who could, and should, be perfectly well managed by a primary-care physician.

In other European countries, intended or unintended controls produce similarly suboptimal outcomes. In Belgium, the role of primary-care physicians in the treatment of headache disorders is unsystematic. Primary-care physicians, if initially consulted, may (over) refer to neurologists as they do in UK, but patients in Belgium also have freedom to seek specialist care directly in polyclinics or hospital-based neurology departments. While this apparently removes control, by greatly undermining any gatekeeper role, specialists' opinions determine the recovery of continuing treatment costs from health-care insurers. A similar result is achieved in the State-funded health-care system in Serbia, where primary care is well-developed but primary-care physicians may not prescribe reimbursable triptans unless a specialist has first formally made the diagnosis of migraine.

These are systems that control demand, presumably to maintain affordability, by, in effect, erecting barriers to access. They place a cap on supply of care because, as the numbers presented earlier demonstrate very clearly, capacity in specialist care is far short of sufficient. Controlling demand of course controls costs, but it is not necessarily efficient in an economic sense, and it elevates the importance of demand over that of need, which is not necessarily clinically efficient. In the Serbian example, costs may be constrained overall, but through a process that ensures triptans reach fewer people than need them, and at higher cost-per-person because of the unnecessary and itself costly requirement for specialist diagnosis.

A problem in Brazil, despite its three health-care levels, is that not all cities or States have the resources or political will to put in place and maintain adequate levels 1 or 2. Varying quality of health care from State to State (even from city to city) is the immediate consequence of this, but it leads also, inevitably, to the wasteful demand upon more costly specialist care referred to earlier.

Conclusions

There are many problems with the current compartmentalized division of headache services between primary and secondary care. The model described seeks vertical integration, while recognizing that headache services not only must, but readily can, be delivered for the most part in primary care. The size of the demand dictates this as the only way forward, but it is a perfectly good way forward in terms of quality of care, and it is capable of adaptation to suit local cultures and health-care systems.

Wherever health-service reform is shifting resources from secondary to primary care (Walley et al. 2008), there is opportunity for change. Beneficial change requires education at a number of levels. These problems, and the priority that should be accorded to headache services, must be acknowledged if political will is to be fostered and harnessed, and change made to happen.

In low- and middle-income countries in particular, treatment of headache disorders may benefit from the current climate, which endows greater priority on care for chronic diseases and shows renewed attention for strengthening primary care (Walley et al. 2008). This, also, is an opportunity, and it calls out to be built on.

References

American Association for the Study of Headache, International Headache Society (1998) Consensus statement on improving migraine management. Headache 38:736

Antonaci F, Valade D, Lanteri-Minet M, Lainez JM, Jensen R, Steiner TJ on behalf of the European Headache Federation and Lifting the Burden: the Global Campaign to Reduce the Burden of Headache Worldwide (2008) Proposals for the organisation of headache services in Europe. Int Emerg Med 3(Suppl 1):S25–S28

Coulter A (1995) Shifting the balance from secondary to primary care. BMJ 311:1447–1448

Department of Health (2003) Guidelines for the appointment of general practitioners with special interests in the delivery of clinical services: headaches. Department of Health, London

Dixon J, Holland P, Mays N (1998) Developing primary care: gatekeeping, commissioning, and managed care. BMJ 317:125–128

Dowson A (2003) Analysis of the patients attending a specialist UK headache clinic over a 3-year period. Headache 43:14–18

Dowson AJ, Bradford S, Lipscombe S et al (2004) Managing chronic headaches in the clinic. Int J Clin Pract 58:1142–1151

Instituto Brasileiro de Geografia e Estatística (2008) Pesquisa Nacional por Amostra de Domicílio 2008. http://www.sidra.ibge.gov.br/bda/tabela/protabl.asp?c=2493&z=pnad&o=9&i=P. Accessed 20 Apr 2010

Ferris TG, Chang Y, Blumenthal D, Pearson SD (2001) Leaving gatekeeping behind – effects of opening access to specialists for adults in a health maintenance organization. NEJM 345:1312–1317

Hopkins A, Menken M, De Friese GA (1989) A record of patient encounters in neurological practice in the United Kingdom. J Neurol Neurosurg Psychiat 52:436–438

Hossain M (1998) The provision of secondary care services in primary care (Diploma dissertation). Imperial College London, London

Hu XH, Markson LE, Lipton RB, Stewart WF, Berger ML (1998) Burden of migraine in the United States: disability and economic costs. Arch Intern Med 159:813–818

Jones R, Lamont T, Haines A (1995) Setting priorities for research and development in the NHS: a case study on the interface between primary and secondary care. BMJ 311:1076–1080

Laughey WF, Holmes WF, MacGregor AE, Sawyer JPC (1999) Headache consultation and referral patterns in one UK general practice. Cephalalgia 19:328–329

Lipton RB, Scher AI, Steiner TJ, Bigal ME, Kolodner K, Liberman JN, Stewart WF (2003) Patterns of health care utilization for migraine in England and in the United States. Neurology 60:441–448

Lucas C, Géraud G, Valade D, Chautard MH, Lantéri-Minet M (2006) Recognition and therapeutic management of migraine in 2004, in France: results of FRAMIG 3, a French nationwide population-based survey. Headache 46:715–725

Mainous AG, Baker R, Love MM, Gray DP, Gill JM (2001) Continuity of care and trust in one's physician: evidence from primary care in the United States and the United Kingdom. Fam Med 33:22–27

Masruha MR, Souza JA, Barreiros H, Piovesan EJ, Kowacs F, Queiroz LP et al (2007) Distribution of "Brazilian headache specialists – analyses of Brazilian headache society members. Einstein 5:48–50

Preston C, Cheater F, Baker R, Hearnshaw H (1999) Left in limbo: patients views on care across the primary/secondary interface. Qual Health Care 8:16–21

Steiner TJ (2000) Headache burdens and bearers. Funct Neurol 15(Suppl 3):219–223

Steiner TJ (2003) Health-care systems for headache: patching the seam between primary and specialist care. J Headache Pain 4(Suppl 1):S70–S74

Steiner TJ (2004) Lifting the burden: the global campaign against headache. Lancet Neurol 3:204–205

Steiner TJ, Scher AI, Stewart WF, Kolodner K, Liberman J, Lipton RB (2003) The prevalence and disability burden of adult migraine in England and their relationships to age, gender and ethnicity. Cephalalgia 23:519–527

Steiner TJ, Paemeleire K, Jensen R, Valade D, Savi L, Lainez MJA, Diener H-C, Martelletti P and Couturier EGM on behalf of the European Headache Federation and Lifting the Burden: The Global Campaign to Reduce the Burden of Headache Worldwide (2007) European principles of management of common headache disorders in primary care. J Headache Pain 8(Suppl 1):S3–S21

Steiner TJ, Antonaci F, Jensen R, Lainez MJA, Lanteri-Minet M, Valade D on behalf of the European Headache Federation and Lifting The Burden: the Global Campaign against Headache (2011) Recommendations for headache service organisation and delivery in Europe. J Headache Pain (DOI: 10.1007/s10194-011-0320-x) (in press)

Stovner LJ, Hagen K, Jensen R et al (2007) Headache prevalence and disability worldwide. Cephalalgia 27:193–210

Tarimo E, Webster EG (1995) Primary health care concepts and challenges in a changing world. Alma-Ata revisited. WHO, Geneva

Walley J, Lawn JE, Tinker A, De Francisco A, Chopra M, Rudan I, Bhutta ZA, Black RE, Lancet Alma Ata Working Group (2008) Primary health care: making Alma Ata reality. Lancet 372:1001–1007

Wiles CM, Lindsay M (1996) General practice referrals to a department of neurology. J Roy Coll Physicians 30:426–431

World Health Organization (2000) Headache disorders and public health. Education and management implications. WHO, Geneva

World Health Organization International Conference on Primary Health Care (1978) Declaration of Alma-Ata. WHO, Geneva

6 "Quality" in Headache Care: What Is It and How Can It Be Measured?

Michele Peters[1] · Crispin Jenkinson[1] · Suraj Perera[2] · Elizabeth W. Loder[3] · Timothy J. Steiner[4,5]
[1]University of Oxford, Oxford, UK
[2]Ministry of Health Care & Nutrition, Colombo, Sri Lanka
[3]Brigham and Women's/Faulkner Hospitals, Boston, MA, USA
[4]Norwegian University of Science and Technology, Trondheim, Norway
[5]Faculty of Medicine, Imperial College London, London, UK

Paolo Martelletti, Timothy J. Steiner (eds.), *Handbook of Headache*, DOI 10.1007/978-88-470-1700-9_6,
© Lifting The Burden 2011

Abstract: Evaluating quality of health care is increasingly recognized as an important contributor to the advancement of health-care delivery, and there is general agreement that achieving and maintaining high quality in health care must be primary aspirations. Yet surprising uncertainty surrounds the meaning of "quality." Undoubtedly, it has multiple dimensions, which is problematic because improvement in one dimension may be at the expense of others. A variety of instruments and a range of methods are available to assess quality of care. These are described here, along with research directed specifically at quality in headache care. Quality indicators for headache developed in the past have been largely limited to diagnosis and treatment in specific health-care settings, or to specific types of headache. They cannot necessarily be transferred between settings; neither is quality of headache care reflected only in accurate diagnosis and appropriate treatment. Adherence to local guidelines, sometimes stipulated as the path to quality, may not achieve quality if these guidelines are not themselves well rooted in quality. For these reasons, a group of health-services researchers and headache specialists have collaborated in formulating a set of quality indicators for headache care, intended to be applicable across countries, cultures, and settings so that deficiencies in headache care worldwide may be recognized and rectified. Equally important is that these indicators will guide the development of headache services in countries that lack them.

Quality in Health Care

It is axiomatic that health-care systems should aspire to high quality of care. All such systems must therefore measure and monitor quality and require methods to do so. Evaluation of health-care quality underpins optimally effective care, efficient use of resources, avoidance of medical errors, service advancement, professional development, and accountability of health professionals and managers (Lawrence et al. 1997). Research into quality improvement, leading to changes in health care in pursuit of it, is a new and important field of health-services research (Grol et al. 2004), which has become central to health care that meets both patients' expectations and patients' needs (Campbell et al. 2003).

Before quality can be assessed, it must first be defined. Quality is not necessarily coupled to financing: There is no direct relationship between better outcomes and the amount spent on health care (McGlynn 2004). Donabedian (1988), in a view now widely endorsed, first suggested that quality of care should be considered in three aspects: "structure," or the attributes of the settings in which care occurs; "process," or the giving and receiving of care; and "outcome," or the effects that care has on health status. Donabedian (1990) also described seven attributes that in his view collectively defined health-care quality: efficacy, effectiveness, efficiency, optimality, acceptability, legitimacy, and equity.

A definition of quality of health care offered by the US Institute of Medicine (IOM) is the following: the degree to which health-care services for individuals and populations increase the likelihood of desired health outcomes and are consistent with current professional knowledge (Institute of Medicine, Committee to Design a Strategy for Quality Review and Assurance in Medicare 1990). This puts the emphasis on outcomes. The IOM specified six attributes of quality, differing somewhat from Donabedian's seven: safety, timeliness, effectiveness, efficiency, equity, and patient/family-centeredness.

Different definitions of quality are both possible and legitimate, as quality clearly includes a variety of elements (Donabedian 1988) and is multidimensional. While this is generally accepted, different stakeholders – patients, health professionals, and managers – may disagree over what the dimensions are, or place different values on them (Marshall and Campbell 2002). Furthermore, there is a tension between dimensions: it is rarely possible to deliver care that is optimal in all of them simultaneously.

How Is Quality Assessed and Improved?

Approaches to improving quality include development and use of quality indicators, standards, or guidelines. Quality indicators are specific, explicitly defined, and employed to assess measurable elements of practice that can be changed to improve health care (Lawrence et al. 1997; Marshall and Campbell 2002; Campbell et al. 2004). Based either on current evidence or on expert consensus, they define standards of care that are realistic and achievable in the specific circumstances (setting, resources, or patient acceptability). Their usefulness has been shown in Denmark, where implementation and use of national indicators are mandatory in all clinical units and departments across a range of conditions (Campbell et al. 2004) and have led to improvements in quality of care between 2000 and 2008 (Mainz et al. 2009). All results from audits are published, with the aim of providing patients with an opportunity to make informed decisions about their care.

Quality indicators are statements about the structure, process, or outcome of care or services provided to patients (McGlynn and Asch 1998). Process indicators (e.g., the proportion of headache patients who receive a timely appointment) are, typically, direct measures of quality of care. Outcome indicators (such as the proportion of patients treated for migraine who report reductions in headache frequency and/or severity after 1 year) are indirect measures of quality of care. Each type has advantages and disadvantages (Mant 2001). Process indicators, being direct, are more sensitive to differences in quality of care, and they are intuitively easy to interpret. However, many care processes are not routinely monitored, and it may not be easy to do so. For example, to know how many patients with migraine are offered triptans requires time-consuming chart review or additional contemporaneous recording during clinical care. Furthermore, there has to be an objective standard based in quality itself. In the example, this knowledge is only useful if it can be stipulated how many *should* be offered triptans. On the other hand, outcome measures commonly are measured routinely. For example, headache clinics may administer and record patient scores on an instrument such as the Migraine Disability Assessment (MIDAS) questionnaire at each clinic visit. Health plans often have administrative information regarding emergency department visits due to headache. This sort of information can be used for evaluation purposes with relatively little effort, particularly when computerized records are kept. An important further advantage of outcome indicators is that they reflect the summary results of all aspects of care, even those that are otherwise difficult to measure such as technical expertise. But a major disadvantage is that outcome measures, being indirect, are influenced by many factors, and changes that may be observed are always much smaller than any changes in the processes that lead to them. This usually means that a larger amount of outcome data is required for analysis. The sample size needed to show a significant improvement in MIDAS scores, to provide a single example, would be much larger than that needed to show an improvement in the number of patients prescribed triptans. Additionally, a clear causal link between processes and outcomes can be difficult to establish.

While strategically chosen indicators provide an understanding of quality achieved by a health-care system (Evans et al. 2009), their use is retrospective. They generate review criteria, by which to assess care provided, on a case-by-case basis to individuals or to populations, and standards, by which to assess outcomes of care or services (Campbell et al. 2004). Thus, quality indicators are essentially different from guidelines, which are statements of good practice used to guide future health care (Marshall and Campbell 2002). Recommendations set out in guidelines are, or should be, based on the best evidence available (Lawrence et al. 1997), but nonetheless guidelines can vary widely between different settings and countries. This is a significant challenge to the argument that quality indicators should be valid across settings and countries (Lawrence et al. 1997).

Few initiatives, described below, have attempted to develop quality indicators in headache care. On the other hand, a wide range of guidelines includes the International Headache Society criteria for diagnosis of headache disorders (Headache Classification Subcommittee of the International Headache Society 2004), country-specific treatment guidelines (e.g., various European national guidelines reviewed by Antonaci et al. (2010), and region-specific guidelines (such as the European Headache Federation guidelines (Steiner and Martelletti 2007)). Guidelines tend to focus on clinical aspects of headache care, with less emphasis on delivery of care or the services responsible for delivering care, despite recent proposals for the organization of European headache services (Antonaci et al. 2008).

As health care is complex, it is unlikely that one method of quality assessment will alone show how quality can be improved. Rather, different methods should be employed together, each tailored appropriately. Some methods are implicit, meaning there are no standards or agreements about what reflects good or poor quality, whereas others use explicit process criteria to determine whether the observed results of care are consistent with the outcome predicted by a model validated on the basis of scientific evidence and clinical judgement (Brook and Appel 1973). With implicit methods, data sources, usually medical records, are reviewed and the following questions answered: (1) was the process of care adequate? (2) could better care have led to improved outcome? (3) was the overall quality of care, in terms of process and outcome, acceptable? (Brook et al. 1996). Analysis of data that are routinely collected, as in many health care settings, is relatively simple, with the advantage that it can be conducted retrospectively (Powell et al. 2004). Caution is needed, however: accuracy and completeness may vary, and changes may occur over time in how data are recorded. Furthermore, there may be chance variation between data sets. Insight into the perspectives of health-care users and attitudes of health-care professionals can be gained by using qualitative methods, such as in-depth interviews or focus-group studies or observational studies (Pope et al. 2004), or by using quantitative measures such as patient-reported outcome measures (Wensing and Elwyn 2004).

A range of methods can evaluate quality of care more explicitly. Systematic reviews critically appraise literature in relation to a clearly specified research question (Grimshaw et al. 2004), or meta-analyses can be conducted on large-scale samples of quality-improvement studies (Grol et al. 2004). Specific studies, usually based on appropriate theoretical, qualitative, and modeling work can be designed to evaluate the effectiveness of change and improvement strategies (Eccles et al. 2004). Ideally these are carried out as randomized designs, but non-randomized designs or quasi-experimental designs can be useful when a randomized study is not possible. Not least important is economic analysis of resources necessary for effective care. Economic evaluations focus on making explicit the relationship between the benefit achieved and the financial resources required (Severens 2004).

Quality in Headache Care

While quality is important in any aspect of health care, for any condition, there are aspects of it that are specific to or of particular importance in headache care. There are strong indications that, generally and worldwide, care for headache is not optimal, so that high levels of disability and work or school absenteeism persist, with huge costs to society (Steiner 2004). Improving the quality of care for headache disorders goes beyond better diagnosis and good treatment, since large numbers of people with headache do not consult doctors and hence will not benefit from improvements in care processes. There is clear evidence of high barriers to care (Sheftell et al. 2005; Ravishankar 2004), and the need to dismantle them is high on the agenda for headache-service quality-improvement.

Research to assess quality in headache care, or to develop methods for assessing it, is so far very limited. The first published use of quality indicators was by an Italian tertiary-care hospital-based headache center, employing the quality-assurance system adopted within all units of the hospital (Ferrari et al. 2000). Aspects that did not conform to the quality objectives were highlighted, and it was possible to rectify these shortcomings. Furthermore, a monitoring system was set up to assess long-term efficacy of the services. Two initiatives only, one in the USA (McGlynn et al. 2003) and one in the UK (O'Flynn and Ridsdale 2002), have sought to develop quality indicators for headache. In both, headache was only one of many conditions for which this was attempted. Of the 21 US headache indicators, only two were outlined in the original article, but the full list is available in a later review (Loder and Sheftell 2005) and online (http://www.rand.org/pubs/monograph_reports/MR1280/mr1280.ch11.pdf). They cover three main domains: symptoms, examinations, and medications (acute and prophylactic). Eleven quality indicators for headache in primary care were developed in the UK, covering diagnosis, referral, and treatment.

There is no published evidence that the UK indicators have ever been used, but the US indicators were applied to health care received by adults (McGlynn et al. 2003). On average, patients consulting physicians because of headache received 45.2% of the recommended care processes, which was below the mean (54.9%) for all of the studied conditions (McGlynn et al. 2003). In a review that specifically focused on the headache data from this study, Loder and Sheftell (2005) concluded that the available evidence was consistent with "widespread systemic deficiencies in headache evaluation and treatment." They recommended that key fundamental processes of headache care needed to be identified and agreed upon with the aim of disseminating this information and fostering their adoption in everyday clinical practice.

To develop a quality measurement specifically for migraine and for use at the health-plan level, Gagne et al. (2007) conducted a review of the literature. Identified measures were grouped as patient-reported or non-patient reported. The US indicators described above were classed as non-patient-reported, whereas patient-reported measures included nine migraine-specific health status measures such as the 24-h Migraine Quality of Life Questionnaire and the MIDAS questionnaire. The review concluded that patient-reported measures, while important, might not provide a feasible method for assessing outcomes at the health-plan level. Subsequently, Leas et al. (2008) developed a "migraine quality measurement set," which included 20 measures focused on diagnosis and utilization (physician visits, emergency department visits, hospitalization, imaging, and use of acute and prophylactic medications).

Although some research has attempted to define or assess quality in headache care, the quality indicators developed have multiple limitations. Those for the US health-plan level, being focused on migraine only, cannot be applied to other recurrent headache disorders. This is an important limitation since, at a population level, tension-type headache accounts for a sizeable proportion of headache-related morbidity and disability. All the indicators or measures are specific to single countries and single settings within each country's health care system – primary care in the UK, or the health-plan level in the USA. All have been developed in relatively wealthy countries with sophisticated medical infrastructures, and are of unclear relevance in resource-poor areas of the world. Furthermore, the indicators have remained focused on diagnosis and treatment, and not taken account of other dimensions of quality such as the provision of patient-centered care, which is a topic of increasing interest in health-services research.

Development of Quality Indicators for Headache Care

In a project within *Lifting The Burden*: the Global Campaign against Headache (Steiner 2004), a group of health-services researchers and headache specialists collaborated first to define "quality" in headache care and then to develop quality indicators. The aim was that these indicators would be applicable across countries, cultures, and health-care settings, so that deficiencies in headache care worldwide might be recognized and rectified. Equally importantly, they would guide the development of headache services in countries that lacked them.

Methods for developing quality indicators include systematic reviews of the evidence from randomized control trials (RCTs) (Campbell and Hacker 2002), but many aspects of health care are not, and probably cannot be, supported by evidence from RCTs. It becomes necessary, therefore, to combine such scientific evidence as is available with the opinions and experiences of relevant experts and stakeholders and, in this work, a panel of international experts was consulted.

Several aspects are of importance when identifying and prioritizing quality indicators: (1) the stakeholder(s) whose perspective(s) the indicators are meant to reflect; (2) the relative importance of structure, process, and outcome; (3) the elements of care that should be assessed; (4) the occurrence and facility of transition points throughout the health system; and (5) the need for and means of testing putative indicators (Campbell et al. 2004; Evans et al. 2009). With these in mind, the domains of quality, and quality indicators addressing them, were identified through three distinct steps: a structured literature review, a qualitative study and a consultation process with stakeholders. These steps are described in turn below. Among many stakeholders, three were considered of key importance: physicians and nurses who deliver headache care, and people with headache who are the recipients of care. In many countries, headache care spans different levels (primary to specialist care), and the intention was that the quality indicators be relevant regardless of who (in terms either of level of care or type of health professional) delivered the care. Since health-care quality indicators are not easily transferred between different countries (Marshall et al. 2003), these indicators were developed by a multinational research group using worldwide consultation. Particular emphasis was placed on making them as independent as possible of health-care settings and systems.

The structured review was conducted to identify research into "health-care quality" of "headache disorders." Only English language articles from 1988 (i.e., publication of the first IHS classification of headache disorders) to January 2008 were included; opinion papers, letters, and drug trials were excluded. The review found four articles that had either developed or used indicators to assess quality. One further review article identified measures that could be used to assess quality. The review also found 28 original research articles that assessed at least one aspect of headache care. Nineteen articles were observational studies (four prospective and 15 retrospective) and nine were interventions, of which six did not have a control group, two were not randomized and one was a randomized control trial. Fourteen studies used existing records as data sources, whereas 19 studies evaluated quality as assessed by the patient and 16 reported quality from the health professional's perspective.

The second step was a qualitative study with representatives of the three stakeholder groups. Three focus groups, one with each stakeholder group, explored how the different stakeholders defined and described "good" quality care for headache. The doctors' group consisted of primary-care physicians and neurologists, all with a special interest in headache. In the nurses' group were specialist nurses working in headache centers. The members of the patients' group experienced headaches at atypically high frequencies so, additionally, two interviews were conducted with people with less frequent headache.

The aim of the review and qualitative study was to extract elements of headache care that were part of quality. The following came out of the review: diagnosis, treatment (acute and prophylactic), headache severity and frequency, referral for care, uptake of care, structure of services, patients' quality of life, disability and satisfaction, and satisfaction of health professionals. The transcribed outputs from the focus groups were analyzed for additional aspects of quality not included in previous lists or used in previous studies. A number of dimensions and themes emerged from the qualitative study and, together with the findings from the review, served as the basis for developing the quality indicators. Education of health-care professionals was viewed as an important part of the delivery of good headache care, both in the literature (Ravishankar 2004) and in the qualitative study. However, it was not included because it was considered beyond the scope of quality indicators to set out criteria for the education of health professionals. Furthermore, guidelines for headache education were already being developed elsewhere (Jensen et al. 2010), and an underlying assumption of these quality indicators was that health-care professionals were trained adequately.

An initial long list of putative quality indicators included 160, in 14 domains. This list was reviewed, refined, and shortened through consultation with 18 stakeholder representatives from 16 countries – neurologists, primary care physicians with special interest in headache, specialist nurses, headache researchers, patient society representatives, and people with headache. This consultation informed a second, wider consultation, to which all members of the International Headache Society were invited by email to participate, along with a large list of people, in all regions of the world, who had professional or personal interests in headache and had initially been recruited by the World Health Organization as contributors to their *Atlas of Headache Disorders*. A total of 157 responded: the majority were headache specialists ($n = 65$, 41.9%) or neurologists ($n = 61$, 40.6%), and the remainder were other medical doctors (including family physicians and pain specialists), nurses, psychologists, physiotherapists, headache patients, and representatives of patient organizations. They came from 45 countries, most frequently the USA ($n = 32$, 20.6%), Italy ($n = 23$, 14.8%), or the UK ($n = 11$, 7.1%). All six WHO regions were represented: 86 (55.5%) from Europe, 501 (32.9%) from the Americas,

◻ **Table 6.1**

The nine domains of quality of headache care, and 30 quality indicators that address them

Domain A. Accurate diagnosis is essential for optimal headache care	
A1	Patients are asked about onset of their headaches
A2	Diagnosis is according to current ICHD criteria
A3	A working diagnosis is made at the first visit
A4	A definitive diagnosis is made at first or subsequent visit
A5	Diagnosis is reviewed during later follow-up
A6	Diaries are used to support or confirm diagnosis
Domain B. Individualized management is essential for optimal headache care	
B1	Waiting-list times for appointments are related to urgency of need
B2	Sufficient time is allocated to each visit for the purpose of good management
B3	Patients are asked about the temporal profile of their headaches
B4	Treatment plans follow evidence-based guidelines, reflecting diagnosis
B5	Treatment plans include psychological approaches to therapy when appropriate
B6	Treatment plans reflect disability assessment
B7	Patients are followed up to ascertain optimal outcome
Domain C. Appropriate referral pathways are essential for optimal headache care	
C1	Referral pathway is available from primary to specialist care
C2	Urgent referral pathway is available when necessary
Domain D. Education of patients about their headaches and their management is essential for optimal headache care	
D1	Patients are given the information they need to understand their headache and its management
D2	Patients are given appropriate reassurance
Domain E. Convenience and comfort are part of optimal headache care	
E1	The service environment is clean and comfortable
E2	The service is welcoming
E3	Waiting times in the clinic are acceptable
Domain F. Achieving patient satisfaction is part of optimal headache care	
F1	Patients are satisfied with their management
Domain G. Optimal headache care is efficient and equitable	
G1	Procedures are followed to ensure resources are not wasted
G2	Patients are not over-investigated
G3	Costs of the service are measured as part of a cost-effectiveness policy
G4	There is equal access to headache services for all who need it
Domain H. Outcome assessment is essential in optimal headache care	
H1	Outcome measures are based on self-reported symptom burden (headache frequency, duration, and intensity)
H2	Outcome measures are based on self-reported disability burden
H3	Outcome measures are based on self-reported quality of life
Domain I. Optimal headache care is safe	
I1	Patients are not overtreated
I2	Systems are in place to be aware of serious adverse events

four (2.6%) from South East Asia, four (2.6%) from Africa, three (1.9%) from Western Pacific and three (1.9%) from Eastern Mediterranean.

What Is Quality in Headache Care?

A multidimensional definition of *quality of headache care* emerged from these three steps, identifying nine domains and 30 quality indicators (**❂** *Table 6.1*), all essential and none claiming especial importance:

▶ Good quality headache care achieves accurate diagnosis and individualized management, has appropriate referral pathways, educates patients about their headaches and their management, is convenient and comfortable, satisfies patients, is efficient and equitable, assesses outcomes and is safe.

The domains reflect several of those proposed by Donabedian (1988), (1990) and the US Institute of Medicine (Institute of Medicine, Committee to Design a Strategy for Quality Review and Assurance in Medicare 1990), both described above, while being specific to headache care.

Summary and Conclusion

It is increasingly important to evaluate quality of health care in order to advance health-care delivery. Maintaining high quality in health care must be a primary aspiration, but a surprising uncertainty surrounds the meaning of "quality." It is generally agreed that quality is multidimensional and dependent on the perspective of the stakeholder (such as health-care professional or health-care recipient).

This chapter reviews definitions of quality in health care and research specifically into quality of headache care. Quality indicators for the latter have been proposed previously, but are largely limited to diagnosis and treatment in specific health-care settings. Guidelines, adherence to which may be stipulated as a quality indicator, are not necessarily themselves well rooted in quality. Here are formulated a set of quality indicators that are specific to headache care but independent of country and setting. They were developed from a review of the "quality in headache care" literature, a qualitative study with stakeholder representatives (health-care professionals and people with headache), and wide consultations. The result of this three-step process is a multidimensional definition of quality in the context of headache care, applicable across countries, cultures, and health-care settings and available to assess headache care worldwide and guide the development of headache services in countries that lack them.

References

Antonaci F, Valade D, Lanteri-Minet M, Lainez JM, Jensen R, Steiner TJ (2008) Proposals for the organisation of headache services in Europe. Intern Emerg Med 3(Suppl 1):S25–S28

Antonaci F, Dumitrache C, De Cillis I, Allena M (2010) A review of current European treatment guidelines for migraine. J Headache Pain 11(1): 13–19

Brook RH, Appel FA (1973) Quality-of-care assessment: choosing a method for peer review. N Engl J Med 288(25):1323–1329

Brook RH, McGlynn EA, Cleary PD (1996) Quality of health care. Part 2: measuring quality of care. N Engl J Med 335(13):966–970

Campbell S, Hacker J (2002) Developing the quality indicator set. In: Marshall M, Campbell S, Hacker J,

Roland M (eds) Quality indicators for general practice. A practical guide to clinical quality for primary care health professionals and managers. Royal Society of Medicine Press Ltd, London, pp 7–13

Campbell SM, Braspenning J, Hutchinson A, Marshall MN (2003) Research methods used in developing and applying quality indicators in primary care. BMJ 326(7393):816–819

Campbell S, Braspenning J, Hutchinson A, Marshall M (2004) Research methods used in developing and applying quality indicators in primary care. In: Grol R, Baker R, Moss F (eds) Quality improvement research. Understanding the science of change in health care. BMJ Books, London, pp 6–28

Donabedian A (1988) The quality of care. How can it be assessed? JAMA 260(12):1743–1748

Donabedian A (1990) The seven pillars of quality. Arch Pathol Lab Med 114(11):1115–1118

Eccles M, Grimshaw J, Campbell M, Ramsay C (2004) Research designs for studies evaluating the effectiveness of change and improvement strategies. In: Grol R, Baker R, Moss F (eds) Quality improvement research. Understanding the science of change in health care. BMJ Books, London, pp 97–114

Evans SM, Lowinger JS, Sprivulis PC, Copnell B, Cameron PA (2009) Prioritizing quality indicator development across the healthcare system: identifying what to measure. Intern Med J 39(10):648–654

Ferrari A, Baraghini GF, Sternieri E, Cavazzuti L, Roli L (2000) Quality assurance system using ISO 9000 series standards to improve the effectiveness and efficacy of the Headache Centre. Funct Neurol 15(Suppl 3):230–236

Gagne JJ, Leas B, Lofland JH, Goldfarb N, Freitag F, Silberstein S (2007) Quality of care measures for migraine: a comprehensive review. Dis Manag 10(3):138–146

Grimshaw J, Mcauley LM, Bero LA, Grilli R, Oxman AD, Ramsay C et al (2004) Systematic reviews of the effectiveness of quality improvement strategies and programmes. In: Grol R, Baker R, Moss F (eds) Quality improvement research. Understanding the science of change in health care. BMJ Books, London, pp 79–96

Grol R, Baker R, Moss F (2004) Quality improvement research: the science of change in health care. In: Grol R, Baker R, Moss F (eds) Quality improvement research. Understanding the science of change in health care. BMJ Books, London, pp 1–5

Headache Classification Subcommittee of the International Headache Society (2004) The international classification of headache disorders: 2nd edition. Cephalalgia 24(Suppl 1):9–160

Institute of Medicine, Committee to Design a Strategy for Quality Review and Assurance in Medicare (1990) Medicare: a strategy for quality assurance, vol 1. National Academies, Washington, DC

Jensen R, Mitsikostas DD, Valade D, Antonaci F (2010) Guidelines for the organization of headache education in Europe: the headache school II. J Headache Pain 11(2):161–165

Lawrence M, Olesen F, for the EQuiP working party on indicators (1997) Indicators of quality in health care. Eur J Gen Pract 3:103–108

Leas BF, Gagne JJ, Goldfarb NI, Rupnow MF, Silberstein S (2008) Assessing quality of care for migraineurs: a model health plan measurement set. Popul Health Manag 11(4):203–208

Loder EW, Sheftell F (2005) The quality of headache treatment in the United States: review and analysis of recent data. Headache 45(7):939–946

Mainz J, Hansen AM, Palshof T, Bartels PD (2009) National quality measurement using clinical indicators: the Danish National Indicator Project. J Surg Oncol 99(8):500–504

Mant J (2001) Process versus outcome indicators in the assessment of quality of health care. Int J Qual Health Care 13(6):475–480

Marshall M, Campbell S (2002) Introduction to quality assessment in general practice. In: Marshall M, Campbell S, Hacker J, Roland M (eds) Quality indicators for general practice. a practical guide to clinical quality indicators for primary care health professionals and managers. Royal Society of Medicine Press Ltd, London, pp 1–6

Marshall MN, Shekelle PG, McGlynn EA, Campbell S, Brook RH, Roland MO (2003) Can health care quality indicators be transferred between countries? Qual Saf Health Care 12(1):8–12

McGlynn EA (2004) There is no perfect health system. Health Aff (Millwood) 23(3):100–102

McGlynn EA, Asch SM (1998) Developing a clinical performance measure. Am J Prev Med 14(3 Suppl):14–21

McGlynn EA, Asch SM, Adams J, Keesey J, Hicks J, DeCristofaro A et al (2003) The quality of health care delivered to adults in the United States. N Engl J Med 348(26):2635–2645

O'Flynn N, Ridsdale L (2002) Headache. In: Marshall M, Campbell S, Hacker J, Roland M (eds) Quality indicators in general practice. a practical guide to clinical quality indicators for primary health care professionals and managers. Royal Society of Medicine Press Ltd, London, pp 112–120

Pope C, van Royen P, Baker R (2004) Qualitative methods in research on healthcare quality. In: Grol R, Baker R, Moss F (eds) Quality improvement research. Understanding the science of change in health care. BMJ Books, London, p 1

Powell A, Davies H, Thomson R (2004) Using routine comparative data to assess the quality of health care:

understanding and avoiding common pitfalls. In: Grol R, Baker R, Moss F (eds) Quality improvement research. Understanding the science of change in health care. BMJ Books, London, p 1

Ravishankar K (2004) Barriers to headache care in India and efforts to improve the situation. Lancet Neurol 3(9):564–567

Severens JL (2004) Value for money of changing healthcare services? Economic evaluation of quality improvement. In: Grol R, Baker R, Moss F (eds) Quality improvement research. Understanding the science of change in health care. BMJ Books, London, pp 203–218

Sheftell FD, Tepper SJ, Bigal ME (2005) Migraine: barriers for care. Neurol Sci 26(Suppl 2):s140–s142

Steiner TJ (2004) Lifting the burden: the global campaign against headache. Lancet Neurol 3(4):204–205

Steiner TJ, Martelletti P (2007) Aids for management of common headache disorders in primary care. J Headache Pain 8(Suppl 1):S2

Wensing M, Elwyn G (2004) Research on patients' views in the evaluation and improvement of quality of care. In: Grol R, Baker R, Moss F (eds) Quality improvement research. Understanding the science of change in health care. BMJ Books, London, pp 64–78

Part 3

The Causes of Headache

7 Genetic Contributors to Headache

Pasquale Montagna[1,†] · Boukje de Vries[2] · Markus Schürks[3,4] · Joost Haan[2,5] · Gisela M. Terwindt[2]
[1]University of Bologna, Bologna, Italy
[2]Leiden University Medical Centre, Leiden, The Netherlands
[3]Brigham and Women's Hospital, Harvard Medical School, Boston, MA, USA
[4]University Hospital, Essen, Germany
[5]Rijnland Hospital, Leiderdorp, The Netherlands

[†]Deceased

Paolo Martelletti, Timothy J. Steiner (eds.), *Handbook of Headache*, DOI 10.1007/978-88-470-1700-9_7,
© Lifting The Burden 2011

Abstract: The primary headaches carry a substantial hereditary liability, as shown by twin and family studies. Hereditary factors account for an important proportion of the phenotypic variance in migraine with aura (MA) and without aura (MO) and tension-type headache (TTH), while the disease risk is also considerably increased for first-degree relatives of cluster headache (CH) patients. The patterns of inheritance are complex, which means that both genetic and environmental factors contribute. Familial hemiplegic migraine (FHM), a monogenic subtype of MA, has an autosomal dominant pattern of inheritance, and so far can be ascribed to mutations in three genes, *CACNA1A*, *ATP1A2*, and *SCN1A*, all coding for ion channels. Available studies have not provided clear evidence that these genes are also involved in the more common forms of migraine (MA and MO). Genome-wide linkage studies and genetic association studies based on candidate genes, but no genome-wide association studies, have been performed in migraine, leading to the discovery of several chromosomal loci. Underlying genes, however, have yet to be discovered. This also applies to studies in TTH and CH. Current research tackles methodological flaws in former studies by using large patient cohorts, multivariate statistical methods, and reducing clinical heterogeneity by the introduction of more refined methods of phenotyping, such as latent class analysis and trait component analysis. Also, gene expression profiles by detecting reliable biomarkers of disease will be helpful in the future. Results of large genome-wide association studies for migraine are expected soon. Future fields of headache research pertain to individual response and adverse effects to therapeutic drugs (pharmacogenetics), and the study of epigenetic factors.

Established Knowledge

Introduction

The International Classification of Headache Disorders (Headache Classification Subcommittee of the International Headache Society 2004) distinguishes between primary and secondary headaches. Primary headaches are nosological entities that display specific characteristics and clinical features apparently original and not derived from, caused by, or dependent on other pathogenic mechanisms (Shorter Oxford English Dictionary 2007) and will be the topic of this review. The Headache Classification Subcommittee (HCS) recognizes three main primary headaches: migraine, tension-type headache (TTH), and cluster headache (CH). *Migraine* affects 15% of the adult general population (Launer et al. 1999), and occurs three times more often in women than men. It is characterized by recurrent attacks of moderate to severe headache, often unilateral and/or pulsating, aggravated by routine physical activity and associated with nausea, vomiting, and/or photo- and phonophobia, which last several hours to days (migraine without aura, MO). In one-third of patients focal neurological symptoms, mostly visual (e.g., fortifications, scotomata, hemianopia), precede the headache (migraine with aura, MA) (Headache Classification Subcommittee of the International Headache Society 2004).

TTH is typically a bilateral headache of mild to moderate intensity, often felt as a pressure or tightness around the head or in the neck. In 2–3% of adults TTH may become chronic, occurring on ≥15 days per month for >3 months. *CH* is characterized by short-lasting attacks (15–180 min) of severe headache around the eye, recurring typically ≥1 daily and, when episodic, in bouts of 6–12 weeks duration (clusters). Attacks display marked autonomic features (red and watering eye, running or blocked nostril, miosis and ptosis) and marked agitation. Clusters may occur up to twice a year with remission in between. In the absence of remissions between clusters we speak of chronic CH. CH affects up to 3 in 1,000 men and up to 1 in 2,000 women.

Genetic Epidemiology of the Primary Headaches: The Migraines

The primary headaches often recur in families and a genetic background has long been hypothesized. First-degree relatives of people with MO have about twice the risk to also get MO and 1.4-times the risk for MA compared to the general population (Russell et al. 1996). First-degree relatives of MA patients carry a four times increased risk for MA. Twin studies further suggest that about half of the phenotypic variance for migraine is attributable to genetic factors. Heritability estimates were about 52% in female twin pairs raised together or apart (Ulrich et al. 1999; Russell et al. 2002). However, segregation studies did not favor a clear pattern of inheritance, and even in families with an apparent autosomal dominant mode of transmission no Mendelian pattern was detected (Devoto et al. 1986; Mochi et al. 1993; Ulrich et al. 1997). The data rather suggested a multifactorial inheritance pattern, where several genes, each with a small effect, interact with environmental factors to cause the migraine phenotype (Ulrich et al. 1997).

The Genetics of Familial Hemiplegic Migraine (FHM) and Sporadic Hemiplegic Migraine (SHM)

FHM is classified by the Headache Classification Subcommittee of the International Headache Society (2004) as a monogenic subtype of MA that includes motor weakness during the attack and, to make the diagnosis, at least one first- or second-degree relative must have migraine with hemiplegic aura attacks. When a patient has migraine attacks with hemiplegia, but a familial history of HM is lacking, sporadic HM (SHM) should be diagnosed. The HCS definition for FHM is restrictive, since FHM patients can have additional clinical features such as cerebellar ataxia, disturbances of vigilance, coma, fever, CSF pleocytosis, epilepsy, and mental retardation.

FHM displays an autosomal dominant transmission pattern. Currently, based on genetic mutational data three types of FHM are distinguished: FHM1, FHM2, and FHM3. Moreover, there are families that are not linked to any of these loci. The gene for FHM1 is located on chromosome 19 (Joutel et al. 1993), with various different missense mutations in conserved functional domains of the *CACNA1A* (formerly *CACNAL1A4*) gene coding for the alpha subunit of a neuronal P/Q-type Ca^{2+} channel (Ophoff et al. 1996). All the 19 known FHM1 mutations are missense mutations (❷ *Fig. 7.1*). The T666M mutation is the most frequent *CACNA1A* mutation in FHM (Kors et al. 2003). Mutations in the same gene were also discovered to account for a variant of episodic ataxia (EA type 2) (Ophoff et al. 1996) while mutations with polyglutamine expansions at the COOH terminal of *CACNA1A* account for spinocerebellar ataxia type 6 (SCA6) (Zhuchenko et al. 1997). Some members of FHM1 families have other phenotypic features, such as delayed cerebral edema and fatal coma after minor head trauma, related to a C>T mutation causing the substitution of serine for lysine at codon 218 (S218L) of *CACNA1A* (Kors et al. 2001), and primary generalized epilepsy, cerebellar ataxia, and mild learning difficulties with a heterozygous C5733T point mutation

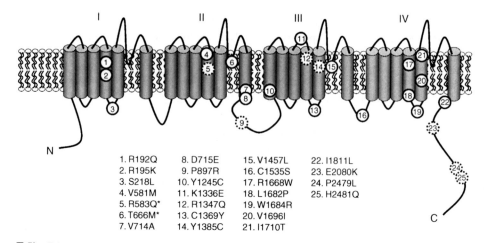

1. R192Q	8. D715E	15. V1457L	22. I1811L
2. R195K	9. P897R	16. C1535S	23. E2080K
3. S218L	10. Y1245C	17. R1668W	24. P2479L
4. V581M	11. K1336E	18. L1682P	25. H2481Q
5. R583Q*	12. R1347Q	19. W1684R	
6. T666M*	13. C1369Y	20. V1696I	
7. V714A	14. Y1385C	21. I1710T	

▫ Fig. 7.1

Schematic representation of HM mutations in the α1A subunit of the voltage-gated Ca$_V$2.1 Ca^{2+} channel encoded by the FHM1 *CACNA1A* gene (Genbank Ac. nr. X99897). The protein is located in the plasma membrane and contains four repeated domains, each encompassing six transmembrane segments. Symbols: Circle with solid line, FHM; circle with dotted line, SHM. Asterisk, mutation for which also SHM was reported (de Vries et al. 2009. With kind permission from Springer Science+Business Media)

introducing a premature stop codon (R1820stop) (Jouvenceau et al. 2001). Kors et al. (2004) reported epilepsy associated with a heterozygous nt 5404 T>C substitution in exon 33, causing FHM1 and cerebellar ataxia, while Chan et al. (2008) and Stam et al. (2009a) found epilepsy in FHM with a *CACNA1A* S218L mutation. Beauvais et al. (2004) described status epilepticus in FHM1, and a region in the *CACNA1A* gene (in exon 8) was found to predispose to idiopathic generalized epilepsy (Chioza et al. 2002). Other clinical features observed in FHM1 families include paroxysmal psychosis, mental retardation (Freilinger et al. 2008), and benign paroxysmal torticollis of infancy (Giffin et al. 2002; Roubertie et al. 2008). These observations led to the concept that migraine, ataxia, and epilepsy represent a spectrum of genetically determined calcium channelopathies, and that monogenic subtypes of this disorder may be successfully used to identify candidate genes for the more common, but genetically more complex, migraine forms (Terwindt et al. 1998).

Functional studies of the effect of *CACNA1A* mutations were performed in a knock-in mouse model carrying the human FHM1 R192Q mutation (van den Maagdenberg et al. 2004). Multiple gain-of-function effects were found, including increased Ca(v)2.1 current density in cerebellar neurons, enhanced neurotransmission at the neuromuscular junction, and a reduced threshold and increased velocity of cortical spreading depression, the mechanism likely responsible for the migraine aura. These observations indicate that the FHM1 mutant mice are useful models to study the pathophysiology of migraine in vivo. Remarkably, blocking the P/Q-type calcium channels in the periaqueductal gray modified nociceptive transmission in the trigeminal nucleus caudalis and facilitated trigeminal nociception. Therefore, P/Q-type calcium channels in the periaqueductal gray appear to play a role in modulating trigeminal nociception and might be involved in migraine pathophysiology (Knight et al. 2002).

Other FHM families were linked to chromosome 1q23 (Gardner et al. 1997; Ducros et al. 1997), and the causative gene for FHM2, coding for the alpha 2 subunit of the Na$^+$/K$^+$-ATPase (*ATP1A2*) was identified. There are now over 30 FHM2 mutations, most found in single families (❷ *Fig. 7.2*). The discovery of several mutations in this gene expanded the spectrum of the phenotypic variety: basilar migraine, benign familial infantile convulsions, permanent mental retardation, recurrent episodes of coma, epileptic seizures, alternating hemiplegia of infancy, and even cerebellar symptoms and mental retardation (De Fusco et al. 2003; Jurkat-Rott et al. 2004; Vanmolkot et al. 2003; Vanmolkot et al. 2006; Echenne et al. 1999; De Fusco et al. 2003; Swoboda et al. 2004; Cevoli et al. 2002; Spadaro et al. 2004).

A third gene, *SCN1A*, coding for a sodium channel, was found to account for FHM3 (Dichgans et al. 2005) (❷ *Fig. 7.3*). FHM3 remains rare (Thomsen et al. 2007); only five FHM3 mutations have been identified that all change amino acid residues (Dichgans et al. 2005; Vanmolkot et al. 2007; Castro et al. 2009; Vahedi et al. 2009). Most known mutations in *SCN1A* are associated with severe childhood epilepsy without migraine. Recently, epilepsy in an FHM family was reported in FHM3 (L263V mutation, Castro et al. 2009). Elicited repetitive daily blindness represents a new phenotype associated with FHM3 (Vahedi et al. 2009). Functional studies remain contradictory: While the *SCN1A* Q1489K mutation exhibited a predominantly

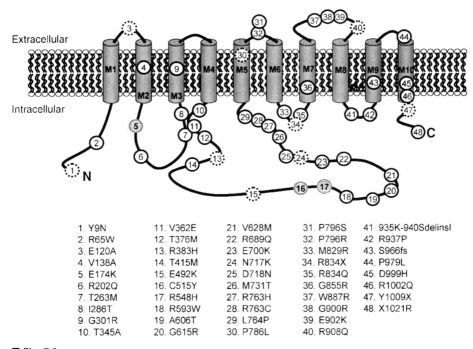

1. Y9N	11. V362E	21. V628M	31. P796S	41. 935K-940SdelinsI
2. R65W	12. T376M	22. R689Q	32. P796R	42. R937P
3. E120A	13. R383H	23. E700K	33. M829R	43. S966fs
4. V138A	14. T415M	24. N717K	34. R834X	44. P979L
5. E174K	15. E492K	25. D718N	35. R834Q	45. D999H
6. R202Q	16. C515Y	26. M731T	36. G855R	46. R1002Q
7. T263M	17. R548H	27. R763H	37. W887R	47. Y1009X
8. I286T	18. R593W	28. R763C	38. G900R	48. X1021R
9. G301R	19. A606T	29. L764P	39. E902K	
10. T345A	20. G615R	30. P786L	40. R908Q	

❑ **Fig. 7.2**

Schematic representation of HM mutations in the α2 subunit of the Na$^+$, K$^+$ ATPase encoded by the FHM2 *ATP1A2* gene (Genbank Ac. nr. NM_000702). The protein is located in the plasma membrane and contains ten transmembrane segments. Symbols: *Circle with solid line,* FHM; *circle with dotted line,* SHM; *circle with horizontal striped pattern,* basilar-type migraine; *circle with vertical striped pattern,* common migraine (de Vries et al. 2009. With kind permission from Springer Science+Business Media)

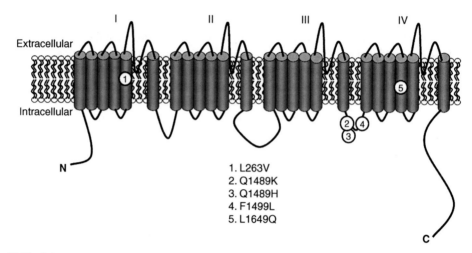

Fig. 7.3

Schematic representation of FHM mutations in the α1 subunit of the voltage-gated $Na_V1.1$ Na^+ channels encoded by the FHM3 *SCN1A* gene (Genbank Ac. nr. NM_006920). The protein is located in the plasma membrane and contains four repeated domains (de Vries et al. 2009. With kind permission from Springer Science+Business Media)

loss-of-function phenotype, the L263V mutation exhibited gain-of-function features. Notably, while the mutations exhibiting loss of function were linked to pure FHM, the gain-of-function mutation occurred in a family having both FHM and a high incidence of generalized epilepsy (Kahlig et al. 2008).

In some FHM families none of these mutations are found, and in others the pattern of transmission is not autosomal dominant (Thomsen et al. 2007). A new locus for FHM has recently been mapped to 14q32 (Cuenca-León et al. 2009). However, genetic information of six FHM patients and seven patients with MO or MA was combined to reach significant LOD scores. Further studies are needed to show whether this locus contains a gene that causes both FHM and common migraine.

FHM accounts for only a minority of all HM cases. Most of the patients occur as sporadic cases (SHM). Only a small percentage of SHM patients carry FHM mutations. Terwindt et al. (2002) found that only 2 out of 27 SHM patients had mutations in the *CACNA1A* gene, while Thomsen et al. (2008) found *CACNA1A* or *ATP1A2* mutations in only 8 out of 100 cases of SHM. De Vries et al. (2007) found any of the known FHM mutations in only 7 out of 39 SHM cases, mostly in *CACNA1A* and *ATP1A2*. For clinical practice, however, it can be important to identify mutations in SHM patients in order to diagnose HM with certainty and prevent unnecessary diagnostics and treatments.

FHM as a Genetic Model for Migraine?

The clinical resemblance of FHM with the common forms of migraine led to the hypothesis that the FHM genes could also be implicated in MA and MO. A number of studies have investigated the role of FHM genes. Some reported an involvement of *CACNA1A* in common

migraine (May et al. 1995; Terwindt et al. 2001; Todt et al. 2005; D'Onofrio et al. 2009); however, most studies reported negative findings (Hovatta et al. 1994; Monari et al. 1997; Kim et al. 1998; Jones et al. 2001; Brugnoni et al. 2002; Noble-Topham et al. 2002; Wieser et al. 2003; Jen et al. 2004; Curtain et al. 2005; von Brevern et al. 2006; Kirchmann et al. 2006; Netzer et al. 2006). Today, no known FHM mutation has been discovered in individuals with MA or MO from families without hemiplegic aura. However, these studies hypothesized that mutations found in FHM may cause common migraine, while it is more likely that "milder," less penetrant, DNA variants are involved. A comprehensive study including almost 3,000 migraine patients tested whether common DNA variants in ion transporter genes are involved in common migraine (Nyholt et al. 2008). Over 5,000 SNPs in 155 ion transporter genes (including the FHM genes) were studied, but no replicated significant SNP was encountered. From this study it seems that common variants in ion transporter genes do not play a major role in the common forms of migraine. Rarer variants or variants with smaller effect size could not be detected with this study design.

This may cast doubt on the hypothesis that FHM represents a good genetic model for MA and MO, thereby questioning the classification of FHM as a subtype of MA (Headache Classification Subcommittee of the International Headache Society 2004; Montagna 2008a). One could argue that several of the clinical signs and symptoms observed in FHM patients are not characteristic for common forms of migraine. This may indicate that FHM might be better classified as a multisystem neurological syndrome, where migraine develops in the context of a wider clinical constellation (Montagna 2008a). However, one could also argue that the main clinical symptoms of headache and aura are similar in FHM and common migraine, and therefore they may share a common pathophysiology (Ferrari et al. 2007).

Monogenetic Syndromes Associated with Migraine

It is remarkable that migraine is a prominent part of the phenotype of several genetic vasculopathies, including cerebral autosomal dominant arteriopathy with subcortical infarcts and leukoencephalopathy (CADASIL), retinal vasculopathy with cerebral leukodystrophy (RVCL) and hereditary infantile hemiparesis, retinal arteriolar tortuosity, and leukoencephalopathy (HIHRATL) (Stam et al. 2009b). The mechanisms by which these genetic vasculopathies give rise to migraine are still unclear. Common genetic susceptibility, increased susceptibility to CSD, and vascular endothelial dysfunction are among the possible explanations. Another nosological entity with co-occurrence of migraine is mitochondrial myopathy, encephalopathy, lactic acidosis, and stroke-like episodes syndrome (MELAS). All these syndromes have a genetic cause and display prominent features of MA or MO in many patients (Montagna 2008b, c).

Linkage and Genetic Association Studies in Common Forms of Migraine

Association Studies in Common Forms of Migraine

In common disorders, such as migraine, many common genetic factors (present in more than 1–5% of the population) are thought to play a role in disease susceptibility. This is known as the *common disease, common variant* hypothesis. A frequently used strategy to identify these common gene variants for common disorders is to perform case–control association studies. These studies test for significant differences in allele frequencies between cases and controls. Many candidate gene association studies have been performed in migraine research, mainly of genes involved in the serotonin and dopamine pathways – but also of other genes with an already suspected function in migraine pathophysiology. Unfortunately, the majority of the associations could not be replicated, suggesting that many of the original findings may in fact represent false positive findings (for review see de Vries et al. 2009). Studies often contained rather low numbers of cases and controls. A positive exception is a recent study that analyzed several SNPs in ten different genes from the dopamine system in over 600 MA cases and controls using a two-step design and showed a positive association with single SNPs in *DBH*, *DRD2*, and the *SLC6A3* genes, also after correction for multiple testing (Todt et al. 2009). Functional consequences of any of these associated SNPs are still unknown.

Another promising association finding seems to be with the 5′,10′-methylenetetrahydrofolate reductase (MTHFR) gene. MTHFR is a key enzyme in folate and homocysteine metabolism. Most studies found an association of the T-allele of the MTHFR 677C>T polymorphism with migraine, although negative findings have been reported as well. The T-allele results in moderately increased levels of homocysteine that may cause migraine through a vascular endothelium dysfunction effect, but evidence for this hypothesis is still lacking. Recently, two meta-analyses summarized studies on the association between the MTHFR 677C>T polymorphism and migraine (Rubino et al. 2009; Schürks et al. 2009). Both studies revealed that the T-allele is associated with MA, but not with MO or migraine overall. However, when the results in one of the meta-analysis were stratified for ethnicity, the results were driven by studies in non-Caucasian populations (Schürks et al. 2009). Other frequently investigated gene variants were the insertion/deletion polymorphism in the angiotensin-converting enzyme (ACE) gene (Schürks et al. 2009), the 5-HTTLPR polymorphism in the serotonin transporter (SLC6A4) gene (Schürks et al. 2010a), and various sex hormone receptor polymorphisms (Schürks et al. 2010b). For a summary of the association studies see ❷ *Table 7.1*.

Linkage Studies in Common Forms of Migraine

A major genetic strategy to identify migraine susceptibility genes has been classical linkage analysis that aims to find linked chromosomal loci using a family-based approach. Over the years, a number of chromosomal loci have been identified using either MO or MA patients diagnosed according to the International Headache Classification Criteria (Headache Classification Subcommittee of the International Headache Society 2004) (❷ *Table 7.2*). However, with a few exceptions, replication of initial findings was often unsuccessful. One of the most promising migraine susceptibility loci resides on chromosome 4: Initial linkage to chromosome 4q24 in Finnish MA families (Wessman et al. 2002) was replicated in an Icelandic sample of MO patients (Björnsson et al. 2003). Although the Finnish and Icelandic migraine loci are not identical, but seem to overlap, it is yet unclear whether they harbor different migraine susceptibility genes. Lack of success with the linkage approach probably is due to the high prevalence of migraine making it difficult to ascertain "clean" pedigrees where migraine genes from spouses do not interfere with the analysis.

In the last few years, linkage studies made use of alternative phenotyping approaches that are based either on individual migraine traits in *trait component analysis* (TCA) or that use

◻ Table 7.1

Summary of association studies performed for migraine that contained at least 275 cases and controls (de Vries et al. 2009. With kind permission from Springer Science+Business Media)

Gene	DNA variant[a]	Cases (n)[b] migraine (MA/MO)	Controls (n)	Associated allele with phenotype (p-value)[c]	Remarks	Reference
5',10'-Methylenetetrahydrofolate reductase (MTHFR)						
MTHFR	c.677C>T (C677T)	652 (465/187)	320	677T: NS (p=0.017/–)	Combined single cases and families; p-values based on initial cohort of 270 migraine cases and 270 controls; replication provided	Lea et al. (2004)
MTHFR	c.677C>T (C677T)	413 (187/226)	1,212	677T: – (p<0.006/NS)		Scher et al. (2006)
MTHFR	c.677C>T (C677T)	898 (898/–)	900	677T: – (NS/–)		Kaunisto et al. (2006)
MTHFR	c.677C>T (C677T)	2,961 (2,170/791)	3,844	677T: NS (p=0.0005/NS)	Meta-analysis	Rubino et al. (2009)
MTHFR	c.667C>T (C677T)	4,577 (1,275/1,951)	20,424	677T: p=0.03 (p=0.02/NS)	Protective effect of 677T	Schurks et al. (2008)
Dopaminergic system; catechol-O-methyltransferase (COMT), dopamine β-hydroxylase (DBH), dopamine transporter (DAT1)						
COMT	c.472A>G (Val158Met)	305	1,468	NS		Hagen et al. (2006)
DBH	–1021C>T	830 (588/242)	500	–1021T: p=0.004 (p=0.011/NS)	p-Values based on initial cohort of 275 migraine cases and 275 controls; replication provided; protective effect of T-allele	Fernandez et al. (2009)
DBH	+1603C>T			NS (NS/NS)		

Table 7.1 (Continued)

Gene	DNA variant[a]	Cases (n)[b] migraine (MA/MO)	Controls (n)	Associated allele with phenotype (p-value)[c]	Remarks	Reference
DBH	rs2097629 (A>G) intron 9	650 (650/—)	650	c.1434+1579G: – (p=0.01/–)	Two-step design (haplotype-tagging); 35 SNPs tested in dopamine pathway; corrected p-values based on total cohort	Todt et al. (2009)
DRD2	rs7131056 (T>G) intron 1			c.−32+16024T – (p=0.006/–)		
SLC6A3	rs40184 (G>A) intron 14			c.1840−204A: – (p=0.03/–)		
DRD1	rs251937 (T>C)	543 (318/225)	587	0.0261 (−/−)	Two-step design (haplotype-tagging); no significant association for these SNPs in the replication cohort	Corominas et al. (2009)
DRD2	rs2283265 (G>T)			0.0030 (p=0.037/p=0.0081)		
DRD3	multiple SNPs tested			0.0033 (−/−)		
DRD5	multiple SNPs tested			NS (−/−)		
DBH	multiple SNPs tested			NS (−/−)		
COMT	multiple SNPs tested			NS (−/−)		
SLC6A3	multiple SNPs tested			NS (−/−)		
TH	rs2070762 (T>C)			0.0035 (NS/p=0.023)		
SLC6A3	VNTR in intron 8	550 (401/149)	550	NS (NS/NS)	SLC6A3 is also known as DAT1	McCallum et al. (2007)
Serotonergic system						
HTR2C	c.69G>C (Cys23Ser)	275	275	NS		Johnson et al. (2003)
	c.2831T>G (T2831G)			NS		

Gene	Variant	N (cases/controls)	N	Result	Notes	Reference
HTR2C	c.69G > C (Cys23Ser)	335 (184/151)	335	NS (NS/NS)		Oterino et al. (2007)
HTR2C	c.69G > C (Cys23Ser)	561 (561/—)	1,235	NS (NS/—)	Meta-analysis	Oterino et al. (2007)
HTR2B	rs16827801T-rs10194776G	528 (220/308)	528	— (—/p=0.0017)	19 Serotonin-related genes covered by 122 SNPs. None of the individual SNPs was significant after multiple testing correction.	Corominas et al. (2010)
DDC	rs2329340A-rs11974297C-rs2044859T-rs11761683G			— (p=0.0019/—)		
MAOA	rs3027400G-rs2072743C			— (—/p=0.006)		
Gamma-aminobutyric acid type A (GABA-A) receptor system; GABA-A receptor α5 (GABRA5), β3(GABRB3), receptor ε (GABRE), γ3 (GABRG3), receptor θ (GABRQ) subunits						
GABRA5	Multiple variants tested	898 (898/—)	900	— (NS/—)	34 SNPs in region 15q11-q13 (haplotype-tagging)	Oswell et al. (2008)
GABRB3	Multiple variants tested			— (NS/—)		
GABRG3	Multiple variants tested			— (NS/—)		
GABRA5	Multiple variants tested	649 (649/—)	652	— (NS/—)	56 SNPs tested in region 15q11-q12 (haplotype-tagging); p-values for two cohorts	Netzer et al. (2008a)
GABRB3	Multiple variants tested			— (NS/—)		
GABRG3	Multiple variants tested			— (NS/—)		

◻ Table 7.1 (Continued)

Gene	DNA variant[a]	Cases (n)[b] migraine (MA/MO)	Controls (n)	Associated allele with phenotype (p-value)[c]	Remarks	Reference
GABRE	Multiple variants tested	384 (254/130)	275	NS (NS/NS)	3 SNPs tested in GABRE	Fernandez et al. (2008)
GABRQ	c.1432T>A (I478F)			NS (NS/NS)		
Hormone receptor system; estrogen receptor 1 and 2 (ESR1 and ESR2), follicle stimulating hormone receptor (FSHR), androgen receptor (AR), CYP19 aromatase polypeptide A1 (CYP19A1), nuclear receptor-interacting protein 1 (NRIP1), progesterone receptor (PGR)						
ESR1	c.594G>A (G594A)	484 (360/124)	484	594A: $p=0.003$ ($p=0.01/p=0.02$)	Two cohorts combined; p-values based on initial cohort of 224 migraine cases and 224 controls	Colson et al. (2004)
ESR1	c.2014G>A (G2014A)	898 (898/−)	900	− (NS/−)		Kaunisto et al. 2006
ESR1	c.325G>C (G325C)	356 (198/158)	374	325C: $p=0.03$ ($p=0.045$/NS)		Oterino et al. (2008)
ESR2	c.2100A>G (A2100G)			2100A: NS ($p=0.03$/NS)		
FSHR	c.2039G>A (Ser680Asn)			2039G: NS ($p=0.01$/NS)		
CYP19A1	c.1672C>T (C1672T)			NS (NS/NS)		
NRIP1	c.225G>A (Gly75Gly)			NS (NS/NS)		
AR	CAG repeat in exon 1	509 (371/138)	454	NS (NS/NS)	p-Values based on initial cohort of 275 migraine cases and 275 controls; PROGINS was replicated	Colson et al. (2005)
PGR	PROGINS ins in intron 7			PROGINS ins: $p=0.02$ (NS/$p=0.008$)		

Inflammation-related genes; tumor necrosis factor-α and -β (TNFA and TNFB) and lymphotoxin α (LTA)

Gene	Variant			Result	Notes	Reference
TNFA	c.308G>A (G308A)	299 (38/261)	306	308G: $p<0.001$ (NS/$p<0.001$)		Rainero et al. (2004)
TNFA	Multiple variants tested	439 (65/327)	382	NS	15 SNPs were tested	Lee et al. (2007)
LTA	−294T>C (rs2844482; promoter)			−294C: $p=0.0002$ ($p=0.006$/$p=0.0008$)		
TNFA	c.308G>A (G308A)	299 (−/299)	278	− (−/NS)		Asuni et al. (2009)
TNFB	c.252G>A (G252A)			252A: − (−/$p=0.018$)		

Insulin receptor gene (INSR)

Gene	Variant			Result	Notes	Reference
INSR	c.2946-713C>A (SNP84; intron 15)	827 (377/450)	765	c.2946-713A: NS ($p=0.002$/NS)	48 SNPs tested in region 19p13; SNP84: rs2860172; SNP90: rs2860174; SNP274: rs1799817/ His1085His; p-values based on 331 migraine cases and 466 controls	McCarthy et al. (2001)
	c.2842+1451T>A (SNP90; intron 14)			c.2842+1451A: NS ($p=0.007$/NS)		
	c.3255C>T (SNP274)			c.3255T: NS ($p=0.008$/NS)		
INSR	c.2842+1451T>A (rs2860174; intron 14)	1,278 (1,278/−)	1,337	c.2842+1451T: − ($p=0.005$/−)	Two-step design (haplotype-tagging); 35 SNPs tested in region 19p13; p-values based on total cohort	Netzer et al. (2008b)

Angiotensin-converting enzyme (ACE), angiotensin receptor 1 (AGTR1) and angiotensin (AGT)

Gene	Variant			Result	Notes	Reference
ACE	Ins/del (rs1799752; intron 15)	342 (187/155)	403	NS (NS/NS)		Tronvik et al. (2008)

◘ Table 7.1 (Continued)

Gene	DNA variant[a]	Cases (n)[b] migraine (MA/MO)	Controls (n)	Associated allele with phenotype (p-value)[c]	Remarks	Reference
ACE	Ins/del (rs1799752; intron 15)	3,226 (1,275/1,951)	20,423	NS (NS/NS)		Schürks et al. (2009)
AGTR1	c.1166A > C (A166C)	3,226 (1,275/1,951)	20,423	NS (NS/NS)		Schürks et al. (2010)
AGT	c.803T > C (Met235Thr)			NS (NS/NS)		
Association studies with other genes						
NOS3	c. −51-898G > A (rs1800779; intron 1)	337 (188/149)	341	NS (NS/NS)	NOS3 encodes for endothelial nitric oxide synthase	Toriello et al. (2008)
	c.894T > G (rs1799983)			NS (NS/NS)		
Ion transporter genes	Multiple variants tested	3,676	3,624	NS (NS/NS)	>5,000 SNPs (haplotype-tagging) in 155 ion transporter genes tested in initial cohort; replication cohorts included	Nyholt et al. (2008)

MA migraine with aura; MO migraine without aura; NS not significant; − not tested/not available; SNP single nucleotide polymorphism; Ins insertion; Del deletion; VNTR variable number of tandem repeats

[a]Nomenclature of DNA variant in the original study; for intronic DNA variants, the respective intron number is indicated

[b]Number of cases

[c]p-Values are given for all migraine cases combined or, when specified between brackets, for MA cases only and/or MO cases only

◻ Table 7.2

Summary of relevant linkage results performed for migraine using the International Headache Classification (IHC) classification guidelines (de Vries et al. 2009. With kind permission from Springer Science+Business Media)

Chromosomal locus	Phenotype	Genotyping method	Reference
1q31	MA, MA/MO[a]	Regional microsatellite markers	Lea et al. (2002)
4q21	MO	Genome-wide scan	Björnsson et al. (2003)
4q24	MA	Genome-wide scan	Wessman et al. (2002)
6p12.2-p21.1	MA/MO	Genome-wide scan	Carlsson et al. (2002)
10q22-q23	MA	Genome-wide scan	Anttila et al. (2008)
11q24	MA	Genome-wide scan	Cader et al. (2003)
14q21.2-q22.3	MO	Genome-wide scan	Soragna et al. (2003)
15q11-q13	MA	Regional microsatellite markers	Russo et al. (2005)
19p13	MA	Regional microsatellite markers	Jones et al. (2001)
Xq25-q28	MA/MO	Regional microsatellite markers	Nyholt et al. (1998a, b, 2000)

MA migraine with aura; MO migraine without aura
[a]Only suggestive linkage for MA/MO combined

a combination of clinical migraine features in *latent class analysis* (LCA). Whereas TCA is rather straightforward, LCA involves a complex statistical empirical clustering approach based on factor analysis that combines the information of several migraine symptoms. The classification reflects disease severity and does not specifically separate MO from MA. In principle, TCA, and to a certain degree LCA, reflects the underlying processes in migraine pathophysiology as they utilize the questionnaire-based information in a more optimal manner, compared to the dichotomous HCS end diagnosis (Anttila et al. 2008). By using TCA, the clinical heterogeneity will be reduced, since traits better reflect the biological pathways that are influenced by specific genetic variations. Several migraine loci were identified using this alternative phenotyping strategy (see ❖ *Table 7.3*).

Genetic Studies of the Other Primary Headaches: Tension-Type Headache (TTH) and Cluster Headache (CH)

Genetic epidemiology studies indicated that first-degree relatives of patients with chronic TTH had a significantly increased risk of chronic TTH while spouses had no increased risk, supporting the importance of genetic factors in chronic TTH (Ostergaard et al. 1997). For episodic TTH, twin studies suggested that phenotypic variation is determined by 81% non-shared environmental effects and 19% additive genetic effects (Ulrich et al. 2004). Additional studies in 2,437 monozygotic, 2,720 same sex dizygotic, and 2,203 opposite sex dizygotic twin pairs (without co-occurrence of migraine) gave heritability estimates of 48% in men and 44% in women; association with migraine significantly increased the risk as well as the frequency of TTH (Russell et al. 2007). Genetic effects thus contribute to nearly half of the variance in the

■ Table 7.3

Summary of linkage results performed for migraine grouped for phenotyping methods latent class analysis (LCA) and trait components analysis (TCA) (de Vries et al. 2009. With kind permission from Springer Science+Business Media)

Chromosomal locus	Phenotypic trait (analysis method)[a]	Reference
4q24	Age at onset, photophobia, phonophobia, photo- and phonophobia, pain intensity, unilaterality, pulsation, nausea, and vomiting (TCA)	Anttila et al. (2006)
5q21	Pulsation (LCA)	Nyholt et al. (2005)
10q22-q23	Migrainous headache (LCA)	Anttila et al. (2008)
10q22-q23	Unilaterality, pulsation, pain intensity, nausea/vomiting, photophobia, phonophobia (TCA)	Anttila et al. (2008)
17p13	Pulsation (TCA)	Anttila et al. (2006)

IHS International Headache Society; *LCA* latent class analysis; *TCA* trait component analysis
[a]Order based on level of significance (most significant trait mentioned first)

liability to TTH. Environmental factors seem to be more important for infrequent episodic TTH (Russell et al. 2006; Russell 2007). Complex segregation analysis indicated that chronic TTH has a multifactorial inheritance (Russell et al. 1998).

CH was considered a sporadic disease without relevant familial recurrence until genetic studies documented that first-degree relatives are 5–39 times and second-degree relatives 1–3 times more likely to have CH than the general population (Leone et al. 2001; Russell 2004). The inheritance pattern was suggested to be autosomal dominant with low penetrance in some families (Russell et al. 1995), although autosomal recessive (De Simone et al. 2003) or multifactorial inheritance could also occur. According to El Amrani et al. (2002), no precise mode of inheritance could be derived from the analysis of cases within multiplex families.

Candidate gene based association studies have been performed in CH investigating variants in *CACNA1A*, the mitochondrial DNA, the HLA antigens, the NO synthase gene, receptor genes for elusive amines on chromosome 6q23, CLOCK genes, and genes in the hypocretin system. The 1246G>A polymorphism in the hypocretin receptor 2 gene (*HCRTR2*) is the only variant that has been associated with CH and was subsequently replicated in an independent population (Rainero et al. 2004, 2008; Schürks et al. 2006). However, a negative association with the *HCRTR2* has also been reported (Baumber et al. 2006).

Current Research

Pharmacogenetics of the Primary Headaches

Patients vary in their response to pharmacologic treatments, which is determined by the physiological variability of receptors and enzymes in the absorption, distribution, metabolism, and excretion of drugs. This is largely under genetic control. Pharmacogenetics applies the knowledge of genetic diversity to the prediction of drug response and adverse effects. For instance, genetic variation accounts for 50% of adverse drug reactions encountered in the clinical setting, especially for drugs that are metabolized by enzymes with variants causing slow metabolism.

Pharmacogenetics is just beginning to be applied to the headaches (Tfelt-Hansen and Brøsen 2008). MaassenVanDenBrink et al. (1998a, b) investigated the role of two polymorphisms (G861C and T-261G) in the *5-HT1B*, and the *5-HT1F* receptor gene in sumatriptan response in a small number of migraine patients. The results did not suggest such an association. Likewise, two other studies did not support that the variants F124C, A-161T, T-261G, and G861C in the *5-HT1B* receptor gene are major determinants to triptan response (Mehrotra et al. 2007; Velati et al. 2008). On the other hand, pain relief by triptans in CH patients was significantly modulated by the common C825T variant in the G protein beta3 subunit gene (*GNB3*) (Schürks et al. 2007).

The response to riboflavin (vitamin B2) treatment appeared to be more effective in migraineurs having non-H mitochondrial DNA haplotypes (Di Lorenzo et al. 2009). In a randomized, double-blind placebo-controlled trial of vitamin supplementation (i.e., 2 mg of folic acid, 25 mg vitamin B6, and 400 mg of vitamin B12) in 52 patients with MA, Lea et al. (2009) found that vitamin supplementation reduced homocysteine levels and the prevalence of migraine disability. In addition, they reported that treatment effect was modulated by the *MTHFR* C677T polymorphism. These are only preliminary data and it may be envisaged that future studies on the pharmacogenetics of headaches will take advantage of the recent advances in the genetics of pain and nociception in general (Montagna 2007).

Epigenetic Mechanisms?

Epigenetic mechanisms have been hypothesized to underlie at least part of the genetic predisposition to headaches (Montagna 2008c). Epigenetics refers to changes in phenotype or gene expression that cannot be ascribed to a modification of the DNA nucleotide sequence, but rather to the expression or silencing of particular genes in particular tissues. The best known epigenetic mechanisms are methylation of cytosine residues at C5 in dinucleotide CpG sites that cause silencing of the gene, RNA interference through microRNAs that silence gene expression, or histone protein changes that activate or inactivate genomic regions. Of note, some epigenetic differences may arise with age while others are found in monozygotic twins, thus are heritable (Fraga et al. 2005), or may be induced by particular life styles and even dietary factors (Oommen et al. 2005; McGowan et al. 2008). Epigenetic mechanisms are increasingly considered relevant in memory formation and more generally in cognitive development and behavior. Evidence for epigenetic modulation of behavior was obtained from animal experiments.

There are no current studies of epigenetic mechanisms in primary headaches. However, epigenetic mechanisms, especially those acting in early life or related to infant–mother attachment patterns (Fish et al. 2004; Champagne 2008; Champagne and Curley 2009), have been proposed as relevant for migraine liability arising later in life and for its comorbidity. They may help to explain why applying current genetic models to primary headaches have been largely unsuccessful (Montagna 2008c) and could also explain drug treatment responses that change over time and with frequency of usage (Schürks 2008).

Conclusion

The identification of headache genes is important for our understanding of the pathophysiology of headache disease mechanisms. Studies in FHM, a rare monogenetic autosomal dominant subtype of migraine with aura, yielded three genes, which play a role in controlling ion and neurotransmitter levels in the brain. Genetic studies investigating the common forms of migraine or other primary headache disorders like TTH or CH were unsuccessful. However, the use of alternative phenotyping methods, the use of biomarkers, and of genome-wide association analysis in large cohorts of headache patients will open new avenues.

References

Anttila V, Kallela M, Oswell G, Kaunisto MA, Nyholt DR, Hamalainen E, Havanka H, Ilmavirta M, Terwilliger J, Sobel E, Peltonen L, Kaprio J, Farkkila M, Wessman M, Palotie A (2006) Trait components provide tools to dissect the genetic susceptibility of migraine. Am J Hum Genet 79(1):85–99, Epub 2006 May 10

Anttila V, Nyholt DR, Kallela M, Artto V, Vepsäläinen S, Jakkula E, Wennerström A, Tikka-Kleemola P, Kaunisto MA, Hämäläinen E, Widén E, Terwilliger J, Merikangas K, Montgomery GW, Martin NG, Daly M, Kaprio J, Peltonen L, Färkkilä M, Wessman M, Palotie A (2008) Consistently replicating locus linked to migraine on 10q22-q23. Am J Hum Genet 82(5):1051–1063

Asuni C, Stochino ME, Cherchi A, Manchia M, Congiu D, Manconi F et al (2009) Migraine and tumour necrosis factor gene polymorphism. An association study in a Sardinian sample. J Neurol 256(2):194–197

Baumber L, Sjöstrand C, Leone M, Harty H, Bussone G, Hillert J, Trembath RC, Russell MB (2006) A genome-wide scan and HCRTR2 candidate gene analysis in a European cluster headache cohort. Neurology 66(12):1888–1893

Beauvais K, Cave-Riant F, De Barace C et al (2004) New CACNA1A gene mutation in a case of familial hemiplegic migraine with status epilepticus. Eur Neurol 52:58–61

Björnsson A, Gudmundsson G, Gudfinnsson E, Hrafnsdóttir M, Benedikz J, Skúladóttir S, Kristjánsson K, Frigge ML, Kong A, Stefánsson K, Gulcher JR (2003) Localization of a gene for migraine without aura to chromosome 4q21. Am J Hum Genet 73(5):986–993, Epub 2003 Sep 25

Brugnoni R, Leone M, Rigamonti A, Moranduzzo E, Cornelio F, Mantegazza R, Bussone G (2002) Is the CACNA1A gene involved in familial migraine with aura? Neurol Sci 23:1–5

Cader ZM, Noble-Topham S, Dyment DA, Cherny SS, Brown JD, Rice GP, Ebers GC (2003) Significant linkage to migraine with aura on chromosome

11q24. Hum Mol Genet 12(19):2511–2517, Epub 2003 Jul 29

Carlsson A, Forsgren L, Nylander PO, Hellman U, Forsman-Semb K, Holmgren G, Holmberg D, Holmberg M (2002) Identification of a susceptibility locus for migraine with and without aura on 6p12.2-p21.1. Neurology 59(11):1804–1807

Castro MJ, Stam AH, Lemos C, de Vries B, Vanmolkot KR, Barros J, Terwindt GM, Frants RR, Sequeiros J, Ferrari MD, Pereira-Monteiro JM, van den Maagdenberg AM (2009) First mutation in the voltage-gated Nav1.1 subunit gene SCN1A with co-occurring familial hemiplegic migraine and epilepsy. Cephalalgia 29(3):308–313

Cevoli S, Pierangeli G, Monari L, Valentino ML, Bernardoni P, Mochi M, Cortelli P, Montagna P (2002) Familial hemiplegic migraine: clinical features and probable linkage to chromosome 1 in an Italian family. Neurol Sci 23:7–10

Champagne FA (2008) Epigenetic mechanisms and the transgenerational effects of maternal care. Front Neuroendocrinol 29(3):386–397, Epub 2008 Mar 28

Champagne FA, Curley JP (2009) Epigenetic mechanisms mediating the long-term effects of maternal care on development. Neurosci Biobehav Rev 33(4): 593–600, Epub 2008 Jan 18

Chan YC, Burgunder JM, Wilder-Smith E, Chew SE, Lam-Mok-Sing KM, Sharma V, Ong BK (2008) Electroencephalographic changes and seizures in familial hemiplegic migraine patients with the CACNA1A gene S218L mutation. J Clin Neurosci 15(8): 891–894, Epub 2008 Mar 7

Chioza B, Osei-Lah A, Nashef L, Suarez-Merino B, Wilkie H, Sham P, Knight J, Asherson P, Makoff AJ (2002) Haplotype and linkage disequilibrium analysis to characterise a region in the calcium channel gene CACNA1A associated with idiopathic generalised epilepsy. Eur J Hum Genet 10(12):857–864

Colson NJ, Lea RA, Quinlan S, Macmillan J, Griffiths LR (2004) The estrogen receptor 1 G594A polymorphism is associated with migraine susceptibility in two independent case/control groups. Neurogenetics 5(2):129–133

Colson NJ, Lea RA, Quinlan S, Macmillan J, Griffiths LR (2005) Investigation of hormone receptor genes in migraine. Neurogenetics 6(1):17–23

Corominas R, Ribases M, Camina M, Cuenca-Leon E, Pardo J, Boronat S et al (2009) Two-stage case-control association study of dopamine-related genes and migraine. BMC Med Genet 10:95

Corominas R, Sobrido MJ, Ribases M, Cuenca-Leon E, Blanco-Arias P, Narberhaus B et al (2010) Association study of the serotoninergic system in migraine in the Spanish population. Am J Med Genet B Neuropsychiatr Genet 153B(1):177–184

Cuenca-León E, Corominas R, Montfort M, Artigas J, Roig M, Bayés M, Cormand B, Macaya A (2009) Familial hemiplegic migraine: linkage to chromosome 14q32 in a Spanish kindred. Neurogenetics 10(3):191–198, Epub 2009 Jan 20

Curtain RP, Lea RA, Tajouri L, Haupt LM, Ovcaric M, MacMillan J, Griffiths LR (2005) Analysis of chromosome 1 microsatellite markers and the FHM2-ATP1A2 gene mutations in migraine pedigrees. Neurol Res 27(6):647–652

D'Onofrio M, Ambrosini A, Di Mambro A, Arisi I, Santorelli FM, Grieco GS, Nicoletti F, Nappi G, Pierelli F, Schoenen J, Buzzi MG (2009) The interplay of two single nucleotide polymorphisms in the CACNA1A gene may contribute to migraine susceptibility. Neurosci Lett 453(1):12–15, Epub 2009 Feb 4

De Fusco M, Marconi R, Silvestri L, Atorino L, Rampolli L, Morgante L, Ballabio A, Aridon P, Casari G (2003) Haploinsufficiency of ATP1A2 encoding the Na+/K+ pump alpha 2 subunit associated with familial hemiplegic migraine type 2. Nat Genet 33:192–196

De Simone R, Fiorillo C, Bonuso S, Castaldo G (2003) A cluster headache family with possible autosomal recessive inheritance. Neurology 61(4):578–579

de Vries B, Freilinger T, Vanmolkot KR, Koenderink JB, Stam AH, Terwindt GM, Babini E, van den Boogerd EH, van den Heuvel JJ, Frants RR, Haan J, Pusch M, van den Maagdenberg AM, Ferrari MD, Dichgans M (2007) Systematic analysis of three FHM genes in 39 sporadic patients with hemiplegic migraine. Neurology 69(23):2170–2176

de Vries B, Frants RR, Ferrari MD, van den Maagdenberg AM (2009) Molecular genetics of migraine. Hum Genet 126(1):115–132, Epub 2009 May 20

Devoto M, Lozito A, Staffa G et al (1986) Segregation analysis of migraine in 128 families. Cephalalgia 6:101–105

Di Lorenzo C, Pierelli F, Coppola G, Grieco GS, Rengo C, Ciccolella M, Magis D, Bolla M, Casali C, Santorelli FM, Schoenen J (2009) Mitochondrial DNA haplogroups influence the therapeutic response to riboflavin in migraineurs. Neurology 72(18):1588–1594

Dichgans M, Freilinger T, Eckstein G et al (2005) Mutation in the neuronal voltage-gated sodium channel SCN1A in familial hemiplegic migraine. Lancet 366:371–377

Ducros A, Joutel A, Vahedi K, Cecillon M, Ferreira A, Bernard E, Verier A, Echenne B, de MA Lopez, Bousser MG, Tournier-Lasserve E (1997) Mapping of a second locus for familial hemiplegic migraine to 1q21-q23 and evidence of further heterogeneity. Ann Neurol 42(6):885–890

Echenne B, Ducros A, Rivier F, Joutel A, Humbertclaude V, Roubertie A, Azais M, Bousser MG, Tournier-Lasserve E (1999) Recurrent episodes of coma: an unusual phenotype of familial hemiplegic migraine with linkage to chromosome 1. Neuropediatrics 30:214–217

El Amrani M, Ducros A, Boulan P, Aidi S, Crassard I, Visy JM, Tournier-Lasserve E, Bousser MG (2002) Familial cluster headache: a series of 186 index patients. Headache 42(10):974–977

Fernandez F, Esposito T, Lea RA, Colson NJ, Ciccodicola A, Gianfrancesco F et al (2008) Investigation of gamma-aminobutyric acid (GABA) A receptors genes and migraine susceptibility. BMC Med Genet 9:109

Fernandez F, Colson N, Quinlan S, Macmillan J, Lea RA, Griffiths LR (2009) Association between migraine and a functional polymorphism at the dopamine beta-hydroxylase locus. Neurogenetics 10(3):199–208

Ferrari MD, van den Maagdenberg AM, Frants RR, Goadsby PJ (2007) Migraine as a cerebral ionopathy with impaired central sensory processing. In: Waxman SG (ed) Molecular neurology. Elsevier, Amsterdam, pp 439–461

Fish EW, Shahrokh D, Bagot R, Caldji C, Bredy T, Szyf M, Meaney MJ (2004) Epigenetic programming of stress responses through variations in maternal care. Ann NY Acad Sci 1036:167–180

Fraga MF, Ballestar E, Paz MF, Ropero S, Setien F, Ballestar ML, Heine-Suner D, Cigudosa JC, Urioste M, Benitez J, Boix-Chornet M, Sanchez-Aguilera A, Ling C, Carlsson E, Poulsen P, Vaag A, Stephan Z, Spector TD, Wu YZ, Plass C, Esteller M (2005) Epigenetic differences arise during the lifetime of monozygotic twins. Proc Natl Acad Sci USA 102:10604–10609

Freilinger T, Bohe M, Wegener B, Müller-Myhsok B, Dichgans M, Knoblauch H (2008) Expansion of the phenotypic spectrum of the CACNA1A T666M mutation: a family with familial hemiplegic migraine type 1, cerebellar atrophy and mental retardation. Cephalalgia 28(4):403–407, Epub 2008 Feb 14

Gardner K, Barmada MM, Ptacek LJ, Hoffman EP (1997) A new locus for hemiplegic migraine maps to chromosome 1q31. Neurology 49(5):1231–1238

Giffin NJ, Benton S, Goadsby PJ (2002) Benign paroxysmal torticollis of infancy: four new cases and linkage to CACNA1A mutation. Dev Med Child Neurol 44:490–493

Hagen K, Pettersen E, Stovner LJ, Skorpen F, Zwart JA (2006) The association between headache and Val158Met polymorphism in the catechol-O-methyltransferase gene: the HUNT study. J Headache Pain 7(2):70–74

Headache Classification Subcommittee of the International Headache Society (2004) International classification of headache disorders, 2nd edn. Blackwell Publishing, Oxford. Cephalalgia 24:1–160

Hovatta I, Kallela M, Farkkila M, Peltonen L (1994) Familial migraine: exclusion of the susceptibility gene from the reported locus of familial hemiplegic migraine on 19p. Genomics 23:707–709

Jen JC, Kim GW, Dudding KA, Baloh RW (2004) No mutations in CACNA1A and ATP1A2 in probands with common types of migraine. Arch Neurol 61(6):926–928

Johnson MP, Lea RA, Curtain RP, MacMillan JC, Griffiths LR (2003) An investigation of the 5-HT2C receptor gene as a migraine candidate gene. Am J Med Genet B Neuropsychiatr Genet 117B(1):86–89

Jones KW, Ehm MG, Pericak-Vance MA, Haines JL, Boyd PR, Peroutka SJ (2001) Migraine with aura susceptibility locus on chromosome 19p13 is distinct from the familial hemiplegic migraine locus. Genomics 78:150–154

Joutel A, Bousser MG, Biousse V, Labauge P, Chabriat H, Nibbio A, Maciazek J, Meyer B, Bach MA, Weissenbach J et al (1993) A gene for familial hemiplegic migraine maps to chromosome 19. Nat Genet 5(1):40–45

Jouvenceau A, Eunson LH, Spauschus A, Ramesh V, Zuberi SM, Kullmann DM, Hanna MG (2001) Human epilepsy associated with dysfunction of the brain P/Q-type calcium channel. Lancet 358: 801–807

Jurkat-Rott K, Freilinger T, Dreier JP et al (2004) Variability of familial hemiplegic migraine with novel A1A2 Na+/K+-ATPase variants. Neurology 62:1857–1861

Kahlig KM, Rhodes TH, Pusch M, Freilinger T, Pereira-Monteiro JM, Ferrari MD, van den Maagdenberg AM, Dichgans M, George AL Jr (2008) Divergent sodium channel defects in familial hemiplegic migraine. Proc Natl Acad Sci USA 105(28):9799–9804, Epub 2008 Jul 9

Kaunisto MA, Kallela M, Hamalainen E, Kilpikari R, Havanka H, Harno H et al (2006) Testing of variants of the MTHFR and ESR1 genes in 1798 Finnish individuals fails to confirm the association with migraine with aura. Cephalalgia 26(12):1462–1472

Kim JS, Yue Q, Jen JC, Nelson SF, Baloh RW (1998) Familial migraine with vertigo: no mutations found in CACNA1A. Am J Med Genet 79:148–151

Kirchmann M, Thomsen LL, Olesen J (2006) The CACNA1A and ATP1A2 genes are not involved in dominantly inherited migraine with aura. Am J Med Genet B Neuropsychiatr Genet 141B(3):250–256

Knight YE, Bartsch T, Kaube H, Goadsby PJ (2002) P/Qtype calcium-channel blockade in the periaqueductal gray facilitates trigeminal nociception: a functional genetic link for migraine? J Neurosci 22:213

Kors EE, Terwindt GM, Vermeulen FL, Fitzsimons RB, Jardine PE, Heywood P, Love S, van den Maagdenberg AM, Haan J, Frants RR, Ferrari MD (2001) Delayed cerebral edema and fatal coma after minor head trauma: role of the CACNA1A calcium channel subunit gene and relationship with familial hemiplegic migraine. Ann Neurol 49:753–760

Kors EE, Haan J, Giffin NJ, Pazdera L, Schnittger C, Lennox GG, Terwindt GM, Vermeulen FL, Van den Maagdenberg AM, Frants RR, Ferrari MD (2003) Expanding the phenotypic spectrum of the CACNA1A gene T666M mutation: a description of 5 families with familial hemiplegic migraine. Arch Neurol 60(5):684–688

Kors EE, Melberg A, Vanmolkot KR, Kumlien E, Haan J, Raininko R, Flink R, Ginjaar HB, Frants RR, Ferrari MD, van den Maagdenberg AM (2004) Childhood epilepsy, familial hemiplegic migraine, cerebellar ataxia, and a new CACNA1A mutation. Neurology 63(6):1136–1137

Launer LJ, Terwindt GM, Ferrari MD (1999) The prevalence and characteristics of migraine in a population-based cohort: the GEM study. Neurology 53(3):537–542

Lea RA, Shepherd AG, Curtain RP, Nyholt DR, Quinlan S, Brimage PJ, Griffiths LR (2002) A typical migraine susceptibility region localizes to chromosome 1q31. Neurogenetics 4(1):17–22

Lea RA, Ovcaric M, Sundholm J, Macmillan J, Griffiths LR (2004) The methylenetetrahydrofolate reductase gene variant C677T influences susceptibility to migraine with aura. BMC Med 2(1):3

Lea R, Colson N, Quinlan S, Macmillan J, Griffiths L (2009) The effects of vitamin supplementation and MTHFR (C677T) genotype on homocysteine-lowering and migraine disability. Pharmacogenet Genomics 19(6):422–428

Lee H, Jen JC, Wang H, Chen Z, Mamsa H, Sabatti C, Baloh RW, Nelson SF (2006) A genome-wide linkage scan of familial benign recurrent vertigo: linkage to 22q12 with evidence of heterogeneity. Hum Mol Genet 15(2):251–258, Epub 2005 Dec 5

Lee KA, Jang SY, Sohn KM, Won HH, Kim MJ, Kim JW et al (2007) Association between a polymorphism in the lymphotoxin-a promoter region and migraine. Headache 47(7):1056–1062

Leone M, Russell MB, Rigamonti A, Attanasio A, Grazzi L, D'Amico D, Usai S, Bussone G (2001) Increased familial risk of cluster headache. Neurology 56(9): 1233–1236

MaassenVanDenBrink A, Vergouwe MN, Ophoff RA, Naylor SL, Dauwerse HG, Saxena PR, Ferrari MD, Frants RR (1998a) Chromosomal localization of the 5-HT1F receptor gene: no evidence for involvement in response to sumatriptan in migraine patients. Am J Med Genet 77:415–420

MaassenVanDenBrink A, Vergouwe MN, Ophoff RA, Saxena PR, Ferrari MD, Frants RR (1998b) 5-HT1B receptor polymorphism and clinical response to sumatriptan. Headache 38:288–291

May A, Ophoff RA, Terwindt GM, Urban C, van Eijk R, Haan J, Diener HC, Lindhout D, Frants RR, Sandkuijl LA et al (1995) Familial hemiplegic migraine locus on 19p13 is involved in the common forms of migraine with and without aura. Hum Genet 96:604–608

McCallum LK, Fernandez F, Quinlan S, Macartney DP, Lea RA, Griffiths LR (2007) Association study of a functional variant in intron 8 of the dopamine transporter gene and migraine susceptibility. Eur J Neurol 14(6):706–707

McCarthy LC, Hosford DA, Riley JH, Bird MI, White NJ, Hewett DR et al (2001) Single-nucleotide polymorphism alleles in the insulin receptor gene are associated with typical migraine. Genomics 78(3):135–149

McGowan PO, Meaney MJ, Szyf M (2008) Diet and the epigenetic (re)programming of phenotypic differences in behavior. Brain Res 1237:12–24, Epub 2008 Jul 29

Mehrotra S, Vanmolkot KR, Frants RR, van den Maagdenberg AM, Ferrari MD, MaassenVan-DenBrink A (2007) The phe-124-Cys and A-161T variants of the human 5-HT1B receptor gene are not major determinants of the clinical response to sumatriptan. Headache 47(5):711–716

Mochi M, Sangiorgi S, Cortelli P et al (1993) Testing models for genetic determination in migraine. Cephalalgia 13:389–394

Monari L, Mochi M, Valentino ML, Arnaldi C, Cortelli P, De Monte A, Pierangeli G, Prologo G, Scapoli C, Soriani S, Montagna P (1997) Searching for migraine genes: exclusion of 290 cM out of the whole human genome. Ital J Neurol Sci 18:277–282

Montagna P (2007) Recent advances in the pharmacogenomics of pain and headache. Neurol Sci 28(Suppl 2):S208–S212

Montagna P (2008a) Migraine: a genetic disease? Neurol Sci 29:S47–S51. doi:10.1007/s10072-008-0886-5

Montagna P (2008b) Migraine genetics. Expert Rev Neurother 8:1321–1330

Montagna P (2008c) The primary headaches: genetics, epigenetics and a behavioural genetic model. J Headache Pain 9(2):57–69

Netzer C, Todt U, Heinze A, Freudenberg J, Zumbroich V, Becker T, Goebel I, Ohlraun S, Goebel H, Kubisch C (2006) Haplotype-based systematic association studies of ATP1A2 in migraine with aura. Am J Med Genet B Neuropsychiatr Genet 141B(3):257–260

Netzer C, Freudenberg J, Toliat MR, Heinze A, Heinze-Kuhn K, Thiele H et al (2008a) Genetic association studies of the chromosome 15 GABA-A receptor cluster in migraine with aura. Am J Med Genet B Neuropsychiatr Genet 147B(1):37–41

Netzer C, Freudenberg J, Heinze A, Heinze-Kuhn K, Goebel I, McCarthy LC et al (2008b) Replication study of the insulin receptor gene in migraine with aura. Genomics 91(6):503–507

Noble-Topham SE, Dyment DA, Cader MZ, Ganapathy R, Brown JD, Rice GP, Ebers GC (2002) Migraine with aura is not linked to the FHM gene CACNA1A or the chromosomal region, 19p13. Neurology 59: 1099–1101

Nyholt DR, Dawkins JL, Brimage PJ, Goadsby PJ, Nicholson GA, Griffiths LR (1998a) Evidence for an X-linked genetic component in familial typical migraine. Hum Mol Genet 7(3):459–463

Nyholt DR, Lea RA, Goadsby PJ, Brimage PJ, Griffiths LR (1998b) Familial typical migraine: linkage to chromosome 19p13 and evidence for genetic heterogeneity. Neurology 50(5):1428–1432

Nyholt DR, Curtain RP, Griffiths LR (2000) Familial typical migraine: significant linkage and localization of a gene to Xq24-28. Hum Genet 107(1):18–23

Nyholt DR, Morley KI, Ferreira MA, Medland SE, Boomsma DI, Heath AC, Merikangas KR, Montgomery GW, Martin NG (2005) Genomewide significant linkage to migrainous headache on chromosome 5q21. Am J Hum Genet 77(3):500–512, Epub 2005 Jul 28

Nyholt DR, LaForge KS, Kallela M, Alakurtti K, Anttila V, Färkkilä M, Hämäläinen E, Kaprio J, Kaunisto MA, Heath AC, Montgomery GW, Göbel H, Todt U, Ferrari MD, Launer LJ, Frants RR, Terwindt GM, de Vries B, Verschuren WM, Brand J, Freilinger T, Pfaffenrath V, Straube A, Ballinger DG, Zhan Y, Daly MJ, Cox DR, Dichgans M, van den Maagdenberg AM, Kubisch C, Martin NG, Wessman M, Peltonen L, Palotie A (2008) A high-density association screen of 155 ion transport genes for involvement with common migraine. Hum Mol Genet 17(21):3318–3331, Epub 2008 Aug 2

Oommen AM, Griffin JB, Sarath G, Zempleni J (2005) Roles for nutrients in epigenetic events. J Nutr Biochem 16:74–77

Ophoff RA, Terwindt GM, Vergouwe MN, van Eijk R, Oefner PJ, Hoffman SM, Lamerdin JE, Mohrenweiser

HW, Bulman DE, Ferrari M, Haan J, Lindhout D, van Ommen GJ, Hofker MH, Ferrari MD, Frants RR (1996) Familial hemiplegic migraine and episodic ataxia type-2 are caused by mutations in the Ca^{2+} channel gene CACNL1A4. Cell 87:543–552

Oterino A, Castillo J, Pascual J, Cayon A, Alonso A, Ruiz-Alegria C et al (2007) Genetic association study and meta-analysis of the HTR2C Cys23Ser polymorphism and migraine. J Headache Pain 8(4):231–235

Oterino A, Toriello M, Cayon A, Castillo J, Colas R, onson-Arranz A et al (2008) Multilocus analyses reveal involvement of the ESR1, ESR2, and FSHR genes in migraine. Headache 48(10):1438–1450

Ostergaard S, Russell MB, Bendtsen L, Olesen J (1997) Comparison of first degree relatives and spouses of people with chronic tension headache. BMJ 314(7087):1092–1093

Oswell G, Kaunisto MA, Kallela M, Hamalainen E, Anttila V, Kaprio J et al (2008) No association of migraine to the GABA-A receptor complex on chromosome 15. Am J Med Genet B Neuropsychiatr Genet 147B(1):33–36

Rainero I, Gallone S, Valfrè W, Ferrero M, Angilella G, Rivoiro C, Rubino E, De Martino P, Savi L, Ferrone M, Pinessi L (2004) A polymorphism of the hypocretin receptor 2 gene is associated with cluster headache. Neurology 63(7):1286–1288

Rainero I, Gallone S, Rubino E, Ponzo P, Valfrè W, Binello E, Fenoglio P, Gentile S, Anoaica M, Gasparini M, Pinessi L (2008) Haplotype analysis confirms the association between the HCRTR2 gene and cluster headache. Headache 48(7):1108–1114, Epub 2008 Apr 8

Roubertie A, Echenne B, Leydet J, Soete S, Krams B, Rivier F, Riant F, Tournier-Lasserve E (2008) Benign paroxysmal tonic upgaze, benign paroxysmal torticollis, episodic ataxia and CACNA1A mutation in a family. J Neurol 255(10):1600–1602, Epub 2008 Sep 3

Rubino E, Ferrero M, Rainero I, Binello E, Vaula G, Pinessi L (2009) Association of the C677T polymorphism in the MTHFR gene with migraine: a meta-analysis. Cephalalgia 29(8):818–825, Epub 2007 Aug 21

Russell MB (2004) Epidemiology and genetics of cluster headache. Lancet Neurol 3(5):279–283

Russell MB (2007) Genetics of tension-type headache. J Headache Pain 8(2):71–76, Epub 2007 May 11

Russell MB, Andersson PG, Thomsen LL, Iselius L (1995) Cluster headache is an autosomal dominantly inherited disorder in some families: a complex segregation analysis. J Med Genet 32(12):954–956

Russell MB, Iselius L, Olesen J (1996) Migraine without aura and migraine with aura are inherited disorders. Cephalalgia 16:305–309

Russell MB, Iselius L, Ostergaard S, Olesen J (1998) Inheritance of chronic tension-type headache investigated by complex segregation analysis. Hum Genet 102(2):138–140

Russell MB, Ulrich V, Gervil M, Olesen J (2002) Migraine without aura and migraine with aura are distinct disorders. A population-based twin survey. Headache 42:332–336

Russell MB, Saltyte-Benth J, Levi N (2006) Are infrequent episodic, frequent episodic and chronic tension-type headache inherited? A population-based study of 11 199 twin pairs. J Headache Pain 7(3):119–126, Epub 2006 Jun 15

Russell MB, Levi N, Kaprio J (2007) Genetics of tension-type headache: a population based twin study. Am J Med Genet B Neuropsychiatr Genet 144B(8):982–986

Russo L, Mariotti P, Sangiorgi E, Giordano T, Ricci I, Lupi F, Chiera R, Guzzetta F, Neri G, Gurrieri F (2005) A new susceptibility locus for migraine with aura in the 15q11-q13 genomic region containing three GABA-A receptor genes. Am J Hum Genet 76(2):327–333, Epub 2004 Dec 7

Scher AI, Terwindt GM, Verschuren WM, Kruit MC, Blom HJ, Kowa H et al (2006) Migraine and MTHFR C677T genotype in a population-based sample. Ann Neurol 59(2):372–375

Schürks M (2008) Epigenetics in primary headaches: a new avenue for research. J Headache Pain 9:191–192

Schürks M, Kurth T, Geissler I, Tessmann G, Diener HC, Rosskopf D (2006) Cluster headache is associated with the G1246A polymorphism in the hypocretin receptor 2 gene. Neurology 66(12):1917–1919, Epub 2006 Mar 22

Schürks M, Kurth T, Stude P, Rimmbach C, de Jesus J, Jonjic M, Diener HC, Rosskopf D (2007) Clin Pharmacol Ther 82(4):396–401, Epub 2007 Mar 14

Schürks M, Kurth T, Buring JE, Zee RY (2009) A candidate gene association study of 77 polymorphisms in migraine. J Pain 10(7):759–766

Schürks M, Rist PM, Kurth T (2010) MTHFR 677C>T and ACE D/I polymorphisms in migraine: a systematic review and meta-analysis. Headache 50(4):588–599

Schürks M, Rist PM, Kurth T (2010a) 5-HTTLPR polymorphism in the serotonin transporter gene and migraine: a systematic review and meta-analysis. Cephalalgia 30(11):1296–1305

Schürks M, Rist PM, Kurth T (2010b) Sex hormone receptor gene polymorphisms and migraine: a systematic review and meta-analysis. Cephalalgia 30(11):1306–1328

Schurks M, Zee RY, Buring JE, Kurth T (2008) Interrelationships among the MTHFR 677C>T polymorphism, migraine, and cardiovascular disease. Neurology 71(7):505–513

Shorter Oxford English Dictionary (2007) Shorter Oxford English Dictionary, 6th edn. Oxford University Press, Oxford

Soragna D, Vettori A, Carraro G, Marchioni E, Vazza G, Bellini S, Tupler R, Savoldi F, Mostacciuolo ML (2003) A locus for migraine without aura maps on chromosome 14q21.2-q22.3. Am J Hum Genet 72(1):161–167, Epub 2002 Dec 9

Spadaro M, Ursu S, Lehmann-Horn F, Liana V, Antonini G, Giunti P, Frontali M, Jurkat-Rott K (2004) A G301R Na+/K + ATPase mutation causes familial hemiplegic migraine type 2 with cerebellar signs. Neurogenetics 5:177–185

Stam AH, Haan J, van den Maagdenberg AM, Ferrari MD, Terwindt GM (2009a) Migraine and genetic and acquired vasculopathies. Cephalalgia 29(9): 1006–1017

Stam AH, Luijckx GJ, Poll-Thé BT, Ginjaar IB, Frants RR, Haan J, Ferrari MD, Terwindt GM, van den Maagdenberg AM (2009b) Early seizures and cerebral oedema after trivial head trauma associated with the CACNA1A S218L mutation. J Neurol Neurosurg Psychiatry 80(10):1125–1129, Epub 2009 Jun 10

Swoboda KJ, Kanavakis E, Xaidara A et al (2004) Alternating hemiplegia of childhood or familial hemiplegic migraine? A novel ATP1A2 mutation. Ann Neurol 55:884–887

Terwindt GM, Ophoff RA, Haan J, Sandkuijl LA, Frants RR, Ferrari MD, Dutch Migraine Genetics Research Group (1998) Migraine, ataxia and epilepsy: a challenging spectrum of genetically determined calcium channelopathies. Eur J Hum Genet 6(4):297–307

Terwindt GM, Ophoff RA, van Eijk R, Vergouwe MN, Haan J, Frants RR, Sandkuijl LA, Ferrari MD, Dutch Migraine Genetics Research Group (2001) Involvement of the CACNA1A gene containing region on 19p13 in migraine with and without aura. Neurology 56:1028–1032

Terwindt G et al (2002) Mutation analysis of the CACNA1A calcium channel subunit gene in 27 patients with sporadic hemiplegic migraine. Arch Neurol 59:1016–1018

Tfelt-Hansen P, Brøsen K (2008) Pharmacogenomics and migraine: possible implications. J Headache Pain 9(1):13–18, Epub 2008 Jan 24

Thomsen LL, Kirchmann M, Bjornsson A, Stefansson H, Jensen RM, Fasquel AC, Petursson H, Stefansson M, Frigge ML, Kong A, Gulcher J, Stefansson K, Olesen J (2007) The genetic spectrum of a population-based sample of familial hemiplegic migraine. Brain 130(Pt 2):346–356, Epub 2006 Dec 2

Thomsen LL, Oestergaard E, Bjornsson A, Stefansson H, Fasquel AC, Gulcher J, Stefansson K, Olesen J (2008) Screen for CACNA1A and ATP1A2 mutations in

sporadic hemiplegic migraine patients. Cephalalgia 28(9):914–921, Epub 2008 May 30

Todt U, Dichgans M, Jurkat-Rott K, Heinze A, Zifarelli G, Koenderink JB, Goebel I, Zumbroich V, Stiller A, Ramirez A, Friedrich T, Göbel H, Kubisch C (2005) Rare missense variants in ATP1A2 in families with clustering of common forms of migraine. Hum Mutat 26(4):315–321

Todt U, Netzer C, Toliat M, Heinze A, Goebel I, Nürnberg P, Göbel H, Freudenberg J, Kubisch C (2009) New genetic evidence for involvement of the dopamine system in migraine with aura. Hum Genet 125(3):265–279, Epub 2009 Jan 17

Toriello M, Oterino A, Pascual J, Castillo J, Colas R, onso-Arranz A et al (2008) Lack of association of endothelial nitric oxide synthase polymorphisms and migraine. Headache 48(7):1115–1119

Tronvik E, Stovner LJ, Bovim G, White LR, Gladwin AJ, Owen K et al (2008) Angiotensin-converting enzyme gene insertion/deletion polymorphism in migraine patients. BMC Neurol 8:4

Ulrich V, Russell MB, Ostergaard S, Olesen J (1997) Analysis of 31 families with an apparently autosomal-dominant transmission of migraine with aura in the nuclear family. Am J Med Genet 74:395–397

Ulrich V, Gervil M, Kyvik KO, Olesen J, Russell MB (1999) The inheritance of migraine with aura estimated by means of structural equation modelling. J Med Genet 36:225–227

Ulrich V, Gervil M, Olesen J (2004) The relative influence of environment and genes in episodic tension-type headache. Neurology 62(11):2065–2069

Vahedi K, Depienne C, Le Fort D, Riant F, Chaine P, Trouillard O, Gaudric A, Morris MA, Leguern E, Tournier-Lasserve E, Bousser MG (2009) Elicited repetitive daily blindness: a new phenotype associated with hemiplegic migraine and SCN1A mutations. Neurology 72(13):1178–1183

van den Maagdenberg AM, Pietrobon D, Pizzorusso T, Kaja S, Broos LA, Cesetti T, van de Ven RC, Tottene A, van der Kaa J, Plomp JJ, Frants RR, Ferrari MD (2004) A Cacna1a knockin migraine mouse model with increased susceptibility to cortical spreading depression. Neuron 41(5):701–710

Vanmolkot KR, Kors EE, Hottenga J, Terwindt GM, Haan J, Hoefnagels WA, Black DF, Sandkuijl LA, Frants RR, Ferrari MD, van den Maagdenberg AM (2003) Novel mutations in the Na+/K + -ATPase pump gene ATP1A2 associated with familial hemiplegic migraine and benign familial infantile convulsions. Ann Neurol 54:360–366

Vanmolkot KR, Stroink H, Koenderink JB et al (2006) Severe episodic neurological deficits and permanent mental retardation in a child with a novel FHM2 ATP1A2 mutation. Ann Neurol 59:310–314

Vanmolkot KR, Babini E, de Vries B, Stam AH, Freilinger T, Terwindt GM, Norris L, Haan J, Frants RR, Ramadan NM, Ferrari MD, Pusch M, van den Maagdenberg AM, Dichgans M (2007) The novel p.L1649Q mutation in the SCN1A epilepsy gene is associated with familial hemiplegic migraine: genetic and functional studies. Mutation in brief #957. Online. Hum Mutat 28(5):522

Velati D, Viana M, Cresta S, Mantegazza P, Testa L, Bettucci D, Rinaldi M, Sances G, Tassorelli C, Nappi G, Canonico PL, Martignoni E, Genazzani AA (2008) 5-hydroxytryptamine1B receptor and triptan response in migraine, lack of association with common polymorphisms. Eur J Pharmacol 580(1-2): 43–47, Epub 2007 Oct 30

von Brevern M, Ta N, Shankar A, Wiste A, Siegel A, Radtke A, Sander T, Escayg A (2006) Migrainous vertigo: mutation analysis of the candidate genes CACNA1A, ATP1A2, SCN1A, and CACNB4. Headache 46(7):1136–1141

Wessman M, Kallela M, Kaunisto MA, Marttila P, Sobel E, Hartiala J, Oswell G, Leal SM, Papp JC, Hämäläinen E, Broas P, Joslyn G, Hovatta I, Hiekkalinna T, Kaprio J, Ott J, Cantor RM, Zwart JA, Ilmavirta M, Havanka H, Färkkilä M, Peltonen L, Palotie A (2002) A susceptibility locus for migraine with aura, on chromosome 4q24. Am J Hum Genet 70(3):652–662, Epub 2002 Feb 8

Wieser T, Mueller C, Evers S, Zierz S, Deufel T (2003) Absence of known familial hemiplegic migraine (FHM) mutations in the CACNA1A gene in patients with common migraine: implications for genetic testing. Clin Chem Lab Med 41:272–275

Zhuchenko O, Bailey J, Bonnen P, Ashizawa T, Stockton DW, Amos C, Dobyns WB, Subramony SH, Zoghbi HY, Lee CC (1997) Autosomal dominant cerebellar ataxia (SCA6) associated with small polyglutamine expansions in the alpha 1A-voltage-dependent calcium channel. Nat Genet 15:62–69

8 Lifestyle Contributors to Headache

Werner John Becker[1] · Allison McLean[2] · K. Ravishankar[3,4]

[1]University of Calgary and Alberta Health Services, Calgary, AB, Canada
[2]Alberta Health Services, Calgary, AB, Canada
[3]Jaslok Hospital and Research Centre, Mumbai, India
[4]Lilavati Hospital and Research Centre, Mumbai, India

Paolo Martelletti, Timothy J. Steiner (eds.), *Handbook of Headache*, DOI 10.1007/978-88-470-1700-9_8,
© Lifting The Burden 2011

Abstract: Lifestyle factors and exposure to specific headache triggers can play a significant role in determining headache frequency in many individuals with migraine and tension-type headache. Attention to these aspects of migraine management as part of the treatment plan has the potential to improve overall patient outcomes. Unfortunately, much of the evidence for the importance of lifestyle factors and triggers in migraine and other headache types is based upon anecdotal evidence and clinical experience, rather than formal scientific evidence. The evidence that is available is reviewed in this chapter, and the following observations are based on this evidence and clinical experience.

Lifestyle factors which may be important in influencing the occurrence of attacks in these primary headaches are irregular or insufficient sleep, irregular or skipped meals, excessive caffeine use, lack of exercise, and obesity. Specific headache triggers which may influence migraine frequency, and perhaps to some extent tension-type headaches as well, include stress, hormonal changes in women, weather changes, too little sleep, sleeping in, perfumes, bright lights, alcohol, certain foods, exertion, and caffeine withdrawal. Patients with migraine, tension-type headache, and perhaps some other headache types may benefit from an organized plan to address lifestyle issues and triggers. A formal lifestyle assessment by a health care professional can be part of such a plan, as can behavioral interventions such as relaxation training, stress-management training, and the acquisition of pacing and self-monitoring skills.

Established Knowledge

Introduction

Lifestyle factors have long been known to contribute to headache. Over half a century ago, John R. Graham published his "Ten commandments of migraine prevention," and many of these concern lifestyle factors (Graham 1955; Spierings 2002). For example, he addressed the modern concept of pacing when he commented that, "The most rewarding long-term therapy will result from an adjustment in [sic] patient's means of living within his or her capacities, rather than an endless round of medication." This chapter will discuss the evidence surrounding lifestyle issues and propose management strategies to address them. The patient case history below illustrates how important lifestyle factors can be for some patients.

Case History

A 40-year-old female with a long history of migraine without aura experienced on average six migraine days a month. Her migraines had been much more frequent in the past, when she would experience 12 or more migraine days a month. She was able to maintain her current migraine frequency if she paid strict attention to her lifestyle and also avoided migraine triggers that she had identified over the years. She was careful to maintain a regular sleep schedule, and slept approximately 8 h every night. She maintained a regular meal schedule, never skipped meals, and was careful not to go too long without food. She had discovered that she had significant dietary triggers, and scrupulously avoided foods which contained monosodium glutamate. She ate primarily foods that she baked or cooked herself, and avoided processed food as much as possible. In particular, she avoided processed meats with nitrites, aspartame, carbonated "soft" drinks, wine, and beer. It was also important to her to maintain careful control over her schedule. If she overloaded her schedule and became too busy, she ran the risk of precipitating a migraine attack. This was particularly true if a major weather change was occurring (like a Chinook wind from the nearby Rocky Mountains), or if she was premenstrual. On those days, she would reduce her activities below their usual level in an effort to maintain herself below her migraine threshold despite the presence of triggers which she could not avoid. From past experience, she knew that if she relaxed her vigilance with regard to these lifestyle issues her migraine frequency would increase.

Overview

There is evidence that lifestyle factors play a role in initiating acute headache attacks (Martin and Behbehani 2001; Kelman 2007). Additionally, emerging evidence suggests that some lifestyle factors can contribute to the transition of headache disorders from the episodic to the chronic form (Bigal and Lipton 2006a; Scher et al. 2008).

Lifestyle contributors to headache frequency and intensity can be divided into two categories: lifestyle habits and specific headache triggers. The division between these two categories is somewhat arbitrary, but they are useful when discussing headache precipitants with patients. In this chapter, they will largely be discussed together. This chapter will deal primarily with migraine headaches, as this is a highly prevalent headache type with generally severe attacks, and one for which headache precipitants are perhaps best understood. However, similar headache aggravating factors have been reported to be important in patients with tension-type headache (Spierings et al. 2001). Lifestyle habits and specific headache triggers associated with migraine are listed in ❷ Table 8.1.

Headache Triggers

Definition

A trigger is a factor which temporarily increases the probability that a migraine headache will occur on exposure to that particular trigger. Every migraine patient can be considered to have a "threshold" for the initiation of a migraine attack. A trigger will result in a migraine attack if this threshold is reached. Trigger detection can be difficult because a trigger factor may not reach migraine threshold with each exposure. It will therefore sometimes cause a headache and sometimes not. An important concept is that two or more triggers occurring simultaneously may summate to reach the patient's threshold for a migraine attack. This may explain why apparently similar occurrences of a potential headache trigger will trigger an attack on some occasions and not on others. Many headache attacks experienced by migraine sufferers appear to the patient to be spontaneous, that is, without a recognizable trigger. Whether this reflects reality or whether potential triggers simply go unrecognized is unknown.

The Proportion of Patients Experiencing Migraine Triggers

In a population-based study, it was reported that 64% of individuals with migraine identified one or more trigger factors (Rasmussen 1993). In a headache referral patient sample, 76% of patients affirmed that at least some of their headaches were triggered by some sort of trigger factor

◻ Table 8.1
Potential migraine triggers and aggravating factors

Specific migraine triggers	Lifestyle factors
Stress and emotional upset, fatigue	Irregular sleep or too little sleep
Decreasing estrogen levels (women)	Irregular meals or skipped meals
Weather changes	Excessively stressful lifestyle
Too little sleep	Excessive caffeine consumption
Sleeping late	Lack of exercise
Perfumes and odors	Obesity
Bright sun, fluorescent lights, glare, computer screens	
Smoke	
Alcohol	
Specific foods	
High altitude, flying	
Heat	
Exercise and exertion, sexual activity	
Loud noises	
Caffeine and caffeine withdrawal	
Infections	
Neck pain	

that they had identified. However, when the same patient sample was provided with a list of potential migraine triggers, 95% confirmed that some of the listed triggers at least occasionally triggered headaches for them (Kelman 2007). The mean number of triggers identified by individual patients was 6.7. The five most common triggers identified by patients were stress, missing meals or fasting, weather change, undersleeping, and in women, hormonal changes.

Migraine Triggers

Stress is the headache trigger identified by most migraine sufferers in a headache referral patient population (Robbins 1994; Scharff et al. 1995; Spierings et al. 2001; Kelman 2007), and also in population-based migraine samples (Rasmussen 1993). A further study identified stress as the most commonly reported trigger second only to a combined fatigue/sleeping difficulty factor in a population-based migraine sample (Chabriat et al. 1999).

In clinic-based studies, 72–84% of migraine patients listed stress as a headache trigger (Robbins 1994; Scharff et al. 1995; Spierings et al. 2001; Kelman 2007). In population-based samples, 42–44% listed stress as a trigger (Rasmussen 1993; Chabriat et al. 1999). In general, patients with chronic migraine report similar triggers as compared to those with episodic migraine attacks, although stress appears to be more prevalent in patients with chronic migraine (Kelman 2007; Radat et al. 2009).

Food triggers are generally not among the trigger factors listed most commonly by migraine sufferers and, for example, were identified by 27% (Kelman 2007) and 30% (Robbins 1994) of respondents. In studies where alcohol was examined separately from "foods," alcohol was cited as a trigger by more patients compared to those who implicated foods. For example, alcohol was mentioned by 38% and foods by 27% of respondents in the study by Kelman (2007).

Several other unusual triggers of headache have been reported. Hot baths have been reported to trigger benign headache attacks (Negoro et al. 2000; Mungen and Bulut 2003), although reversible cerebral vasoconstriction has been found in some patients with headache attacks triggered by bathing (Mak et al. 2005). Headache attacks with symptoms consistent with migraine have also been reported to occur in some patients within 10–60 min of hair washing (Ravishankar 2006).

Other migraine triggers have been reported, including water deprivation (dehydration) (Blau 2005), and smoke (Spierings et al. 2001; Kelman 2007). The proportion of patients reporting individual migraine triggers in one large study is shown in ❷ *Fig. 8.1.*

Specific Food Triggers

Foods considered relevant as migraine triggers include red wine, beer, chocolate, monosodium glutamate (Robbins 1994) and alcohol, aspartame, cheese, chocolate, caffeine, and monosodium glutamate (Scharff et al. 1995). Additional triggers on standard lists include many other items, such as tomatoes, cured meats, and in particular strong or aged cheeses. Borkum (2007) lists a number of foods as suspected migraine triggers:

1. Red wine and other alcohol, caffeine
2. Citrus fruits, nuts, onions
3. MSG, nitrites (cured or processed meats), aspartame
4. Aged cheeses, sour cream, yogurt, yeast extracts
5. Smoked fish, pickled herring
6. Chocolate
7. Eggs, dairy products, beans, fatty foods
   (Modified from Borkum 2007)

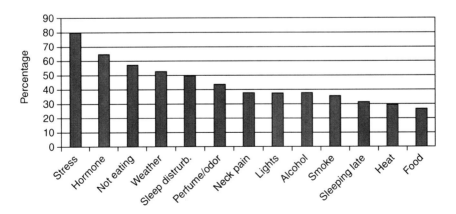

◻ **Fig. 8.1**

Migraine triggers: percentage of patients reporting individual triggers (Clinic-based patient sample) (Kelman 2007)

Although the methodologies used are unique to each study, patients in headache referral populations tend to report alcohol and food related migraine triggers more commonly than individuals with migraine in population-based studies. Alcohol was reported as a migraine trigger by 35%, 42%, and 38% in each of the three clinic-based studies (Scharff et al. 1995; Spierings et al. 2001; Kelman 2007). The corresponding value in a population-based study was 20% (Rasmussen 1993). Similarly, the percentage of patients reporting specific food triggers in clinic-based studies was 27% (Kelman 2007) and 58% (Spierings et al. 2001). In a population-based study, 10% of patients reported specific food triggers (Rasmussen 1993).

Tension-Type Headache Triggers

Many of the headache triggers noted above are often considered characteristic of migraine. However, according to some studies the headache triggers identified by patients with tension-type headaches are quite similar to those in patients with migraine, both in headache referral patient samples (Scharff et al. 1995; Spierings et al. 2001) and in population-based samples (Rasmussen 1993; Chabriat et al. 1999), although some differences have been noted (Rasmussen 1993; Spierings et al. 2001). Triggers common to both include sleep problems, stress, weather, and menstruation (Savi et al. 2002; Wober et al. 2006; Orig et al. 2009). It has also been suggested that approximately 30% of individuals with tension-type headaches are susceptible to foods, most notably alcohol, chocolate, and cheese (Savi et al. 2002).

Lifestyle Factors

Sleep

Headache and sleep problems have been linked in several studies (Spierings and Van Hoof 1997; Boardman et al. 2005). In headache populations, sleep disorders have been "disproportionately observed" in individuals with migraine, tension-type, and cluster headache and include insomnia, hypersomnia, and obstructive sleep apnea (Rains and Poceta 2006). Of 1,283 migraineurs attending a tertiary headache clinic (Kelman and Rains 2005), approximately 50% identified sleep disturbance as a headache trigger, 53% reported difficulties falling asleep, and 51% reported difficulties staying asleep. Further, those with chronic migraine reported greater sleep disturbance than episodic migraineurs, with short sleepers (<6 h per night) experiencing more frequent and more severe headaches. The relationship between headache and sleep is complex. Morning headache, for example, has been reported to occur more frequently in patients with significant obstructive sleep apnea as compared to controls (Goksan et al. 2009). In those with obstructive sleep apnea, however, morning headache was more common in those with a history of a primary headache. The morning headaches varied in phenotype. Many appeared tension-type in nature, but others were suggestive of migraine, with unilateral headache and throbbing pain. Forty percent were reported to be severe.

Sleep hygiene has proven beneficial for children and adolescents with migraine (Bruni et al. 1999). Further, use of sleep hygiene strategies in women with chronic migraine has resulted in statistically significant decreases in headache frequency and intensity, and reversion to intermittent headache patterns (Calhoun and Ford 2007). Rains (2008) has suggested that sleep diary analysis can help determine the best course of treatment. Sleep hygiene is considered appropriate at treatment outset for most patients. Typical recommendations include (1) avoiding daytime naps; (2) eliminating stimulants; (3) maintaining a consistent sleep–wake schedule; (4) having a dark, quiet, comfortable sleep environment; (5) limiting alcohol use; and (6) exercising regularly (at least 5 h before bedtime). Behavioral treatments, including relaxation, sleep restriction, and stimulus control, are recommended for individuals "who spend excessive time in bed not sleeping, those with irregular sleep schedules, or those who exhibit evidence of hyperarousal." Sleep restriction consists of a graduated program of limiting time in bed, and stimulus control involves increasing the conditioned response between the bedroom and sleep. When it is suspected that individuals have "unreal expectations concerning sleep or consequences of not sleeping, anticipatory anxiety, worry, or poor coping skills," referral for cognitive therapy is suggested.

Irregular Meals or Skipped Meals

Postponing a meal or omitting it completely can be a problem for many migraine sufferers (Martin and Behbehani 2001) and some individuals with tension-type headache (Slettbakk et al. 2006). Twenty-one percent of Dutch migraineurs surveyed advised that regular eating and sleeping helped to decrease the impact of their migraines (Vos and Passchier 2003). In a recent focus group, several tension-type headache participants reported the importance of regular eating and drinking as part of their headache management regimen (Slettbakk et al. 2006).

Fasting associated with religious customs such as Ramadan and Yom Kippur has been linked to headache. A recent literature review (Torelli et al. 2009) concluded that in many cases fasting headache is a primary headache, tension-type headache, or migraine without aura that is triggered by fasting. Turkish researchers (Topacoglu et al. 2005) observed that emergency department visits for headache were significantly more frequent during Ramadan months compared with non-Ramadan months. In a study of fasting during Yom Kippur, Mosek and Korczyn (1995) determined that 39% of individuals who fasted reported headache, and that participants with a chronic headache history had a higher incidence of fasting headache than those who did not (66% and 29%, respectively).

Excessively Stressful Lifestyle

In discussing stress, environmental factors or demands which are perceived as demanding or negative are best referred to as stressors, while the term "stress" denotes the individual's reaction to the stressors. The degree to which stressors will elicit a stress response from an individual will vary greatly from person to person, depending on that person's resources and how the environmental demands are perceived (Sauro and Becker 2009). Stress, by acting as a migraine attack trigger, can increase migraine frequency. It can also initiate migraine attacks for the first time in those genetically predisposed to migraine (De Benedittis et al. 1990), and can contribute to the transformation of migraine into a chronic daily headache pattern (chronic migraine) (Scher et al. 2008). When it acts as a migraine trigger, the relationship of stress to migraine is complex, with headaches coming on during a stressful period, but also during the relaxation phase after stress (Spierings et al. 1997). As the stress experienced by the individual is dependant not only upon the stressor, but also upon the individual's reaction to the stressor, stress-management skills and pacing have the potential to be very helpful to the migraine sufferer (Rains et al. 2005; Sauro and Becker 2009).

Excessive Caffeine Consumption

Caffeine may be a problem for migraine sufferers both through the effects of higher doses on the nervous system, and also through the effects of intermittent relative caffeine withdrawal. Higher caffeine consumption has shown some association with the subsequent development of chronic daily headache, particularly for women under age 40 with episodic headache (Scher et al. 2004, 2008; Bigal and Lipton 2006a). As caffeine has analgesic properties (O'Connor et al. 2004), it would perhaps not be surprising if it led to a type of medication overuse headache. Caffeine withdrawal has been shown to be a potent headache precipitant (Silverman et al. 1992), and, along with change in sleep pattern and relaxation after stress, might be a contributor to Saturday morning headache.

Lack of Exercise

Exertion can be a headache trigger in patients with migraine, and this can be a barrier to patients with migraine maintaining a healthy level of fitness. In a population-based study, it was found that there was a strong linear trend toward a higher prevalence of "low" physical activity with increasing headache frequency. It was also found that physically inactive individuals at baseline were more likely to have non-migraine headaches 11 years later (Varkey et al. 2008). However, whether a long-term exercise program can improve headache in patients with migraine is unclear. A program which consisted of a combination of aerobic exercise and progressive muscle relaxation led to a significant reduction of self-rated migraine pain intensity in a randomized clinical trial (Dittrich et al. 2008). Aerobic exercise conditioning programs have been shown to be feasible in patients with migraine and have been reported to lead to improvements in migraine status and quality of life (Varkey et al. 2009). A multidisciplinary program with a heavy emphasis on exercise has been shown to improve migraine status in a randomized trial (Lemstra et al. 2002). However, much more research is needed to clarify what the effects of exercise programs on the course of migraine are (Busch and Gaul 2008).

Obesity

Obesity has been implicated as a factor which can increase migraine headache frequency. Overweight and obese migraine sufferers tend to have a higher headache frequency than those of normal weight (Bigal and Lipton 2006b). Obesity also appears to lead to a greater tendency for those with migraine to develop chronic migraine with a very high headache frequency

(Bigal and Lipton 2006b). Lifestyles which lead to an increased body mass index can therefore have an adverse effect on a patient's migraine.

Approach to Management

Lifestyle Factors

Certain lifestyle factors appear to influence migraine frequency in a high proportion of migraine sufferers, and likely should be seriously addressed by all migraine sufferers with significant disability. If the patient is not convinced that these are important, a headache diary may help to determine if this is indeed true. The following advice, some of which has been summarized by Spierings et al. (2001), should be discussed with all migraine sufferers.

1. Eat regularly during the day, and do not go without food for too long.
2. Go to bed on time (preferably at a similar time each evening). Oversleeping in the morning can trigger headaches. Avoid obtaining too little sleep.
3. Avoid excessive fatigue by pacing activities during the day, as well as in the course of the week.
4. Whenever possible, eat fresh foods to avoid chemicals in processed and preserved foods, and perhaps in foods that have remained too long in the refrigerator.
5. Avoid excessive stress where possible.
6. Maintain regular exercise.

Detection and Avoidance of Specific Triggers

The usual way that individuals with migraine detect specific triggers is to remain vigilant for relationships in time between specific experiences or ingestions and the occurrence of migraine attacks. As a result of such observations, in the experience of one author, few migraine sufferers dare to drink red wine, or if they do so, practice great moderation. Trigger detection can be difficult, however, as exposure to some triggers may result in migraine primarily when this occurs simultaneously with exposure to another trigger. As a result, each of the triggers may not often cause migraine on its own. It may be difficult, therefore, to establish a cause and effect relationship. The relationship between stress and migraine attacks may also be complicated in that the migraine may tend to occur during the relaxation phase once the stressful period is over (Spierings et al. 1997). An understanding of what the usual migraine triggers are, and keeping a careful headache diary which includes potential trigger exposure, can be very useful. In the case of food triggers, a very basic elimination diet can be tried for a time, followed by the introduction of individual foods one by one with careful diary monitoring for headache, but few migraine patients investigate food triggers to this extent.

The complexity of the specific trigger–migraine attack relationship is perhaps best illustrated by patients who regularly experience migraine attacks on Saturday mornings. At least three known headache triggers can be responsible for or contribute to this syndrome. These include caffeine withdrawal if the individual is in the habit of coffee consumption early in the morning on workdays; breaking a regular sleep schedule by sleeping in too long on Saturday morning; and a "let down" headache resulting from relaxation after a stressful work week.

Avoidable Versus Non-Avoidable Migraine Triggers

The degree of exposure to most migraine triggers is potentially modifiable to some extent by most individuals. These clearly include many of the major triggers like alcohol, sleep disturbances, skipping meals, and the like. It may be impossible to completely eliminate stressful life events, but the mastery of pacing and stress-management skills should provide some assistance. Research suggests that greater self-efficacy, defined as the perception that one is able to control one's psychological reactions to stressors, can act as a buffer and make it less likely that a stressful event will trigger a migraine (Marlowe 1998). Hormonal triggers may be difficult to manipulate, but some options are available, for example, continuous use of oral contraceptives without the usual monthly break in some patients with severe menstrual migraine. Even patients with major weather triggers may derive some benefit from ensuring that other more avoidable trigger factors are kept to a minimum when weather triggers are operative so that their presence will not help the weather changes reach the individual's migraine threshold.

The Lifestyle Assessment: A Practical Way to Address Lifestyle and Trigger Issues in Migraine Management

Many migraine sufferers can benefit from a careful review of their lifestyle and trigger management by a health care professional. This need not be a physician, and occupational therapists with special training and experience in headache management are very suited to this role.

Introduction

The lifestyle assessment is conducted utilizing a semi-structured interview. The interview explores typical headache triggers and examines diet, exercise, and sleep habits as well as stress-management strategies. A problem list and treatment plan are established in collaboration with the client. The lifestyle assessment may be completed at the clinic, in the client's home, or over the telephone. Telephone assessments have proven convenient for clients whose schedules prohibit a face-to-face visit and for those who live a considerable distance from the clinic.

The Assessment

The client's headache frequency and intensity are determined. Clients are asked what improves and worsens headaches, and to identify headache triggers. Diaries are reviewed, and potential temporal relationships are explored, such as intensity spikes around exposure to potential triggers or during the menstrual period.

Functional roles are identified, and areas of functional impairment or disability are explored. This discussion extends not only to task performance in general, but to the manner in which functional tasks are potentially overscheduled or avoided altogether. The utilization of adaptive methods to date (such as pacing and energy conservation) is also explored and encouraged.

The individual's exercise routine is examined. Potential barriers to exercise are explored, and strategies to address these issues are determined. Individuals are encouraged to consistently allow for warm up and cool down, to maintain good hydration before and during exercise, and to minimize high-exertion activities. Patients for whom a well-established relationship between head movements and headache is identified are advised to avoid exercise with repetitive and/or static awkward neck movements such as the front crawl swimming stroke or prolonged use of a bicycle requiring a forward flexed posture.

The client is encouraged to eat regularly (ideally every 3–4 h) and to make healthy meal and snack choices. Clients are also encouraged to (1) consult with a registered dietician or (2) analyze diaries for definite or possible triggers, eliminate these items for 3 months, and reintroduce foods if no headache improvement is observed (as per Martin and Behbehani 2001). The client is advised to drink between 1.5 and 2 l of water per day, and suggestions for adherence to this schedule are provided. The client's caffeine intake is reviewed. Clients are strongly encouraged to taper their caffeine intake. One strategy is to decrease by 5 ounces every 3–5 days (Bigal and Lipton 2006a).

A regular sleep–wake schedule is recommended, and instruction in sleep hygiene is provided, including utilization of a pre-sleep routine; relaxation exercises to facilitate falling asleep; eating at least 4 h prior to retiring; restricting fluid intake at least 2 h before retiring; and avoiding naps (Calhoun and Ford 2007). Sleep diaries are provided to establish baselines and to track improvements following implementation of sleep hygiene strategies. Stimulus control and sleep restriction can also be explored (Rains 2008). If there are concerns about snoring or sleep apnea, the client can be referred to an external agency.

Clients occasionally report an association between static and/or dynamic neck, shoulder, or upper back postures and headache. A referral can be made to a community physical therapist, or to an occupational therapist for assistance in adapting home and work environments.

Stress management, relaxation use, and current mood are broached. Instruction in relaxation is provided and an appropriate relaxation CD or tape can be suggested or given to the client to try. The client is challenged to consider all sources of stress, including the headache episode itself and his or her reaction to it. Finally, if the patient reports depressive or anxiety symptoms which are difficult to manage, he or she can be referred to a psychiatrist or psychologist for further assistance. For more information on the lifestyle assessment in the context of an organized headache treatment program, the reader is referred to Sauro and Becker (2008). ❯ *Table 8.2* summarizes the administration of the lifestyle assessment.

◘ Table 8.2
Key elements of the lifestyle assessment

Components	Recommendations
Nutrition/ hydration	• Keep hydrated (i.e., drink ~1.5–2 l of water per day) • Do not skip meals • Eat throughout the day (every 3–4 h) • Limit caffeine intake to 1–2 cups/day. Consider stopping altogether
Sleep	• Keep a regular sleep–wake schedule throughout the week • Track sleep using diaries • Implement sleep hygiene strategies
Exercise	• Include a regular exercise regimen. Allow time for warm up and cool down and maintain hydration throughout
Posture/ function	• Use body mechanics strategies (and assistive devices when necessary) • Adhere to ergonomics principles • Utilize pacing, energy conservation, and rest breaks to maximize productivity
Psychosocial	• Increase awareness of relationship between stress and headache • Incorporate relaxation and stress-management strategies

Current Research

Much remains to be learned about headache triggers, both in migraine and also for other headache types. Most reports which attempt to quantify how often various potential triggers precipitate headache attacks involve patient surveys and patient self-report (Robbins 1994). The epidemiological evidence as to whether many of the commonly reported migraine triggers actually do trigger migraine attacks has been reviewed, and strict scientific evidence is lacking for many putative triggers (Friedman and De Ver Dye 2009). Some migraine triggers, for example, some specific weather changes, have been rigorously studied and confirmed as a trigger factor in a significant proportion of the migraine population (Piorecky et al. 1997; Cooke et al. 2000). More research including randomized trials which assess the ability of specific trigger factors to bring on migraine headaches are needed.

The mechanisms whereby triggers might bring on a migraine attack are not understood, although a number of theories have been proposed (Levy et al. 2009). Recent concepts that cortical spreading depression, or a related phenomenon, may be the initiating factor which triggers the pain phase of the migraine headache (Ayata 2009) suggest that many migraine triggers might affect the balance of inhibition and excitation in the cerebral cortex in a way that makes cortical spreading depression more likely to occur.

Conclusions

Although there is little evidence from scientifically conducted trials as to which factors have the ability to trigger migraine headaches in susceptible individuals, careful surveys carried out in a number of countries over several decades would appear to provide considerable clinical guidance. Patients with significant disability from their migraines, and in particular those whose frequent medication use is placing them at risk for medication overuse headache, should be strongly encouraged to carefully investigate which avoidable triggers and lifestyle factors are influencing their migraine frequency. Patient education, careful use of a headache diary, and behavioral treatment strategies directed at better stress management have the potential to make a significant improvement in migraine frequency. Many of the lifestyle factors which can have an important impact on a patient's migraine were again recognized more than half a century ago by John Graham (Spierings 2002). In his list of errors in living which migraine patients often make, he mentioned overcrowded schedules, lack of breaks, and aiming for impossible goals. A particularly difficult one for migraine sufferers to avoid is one that he called, "making up for lost time," where as soon as the migraine attack is over, the patient rushes to repair the losses and make up for the lost time. Consequently, the next attack comes sooner.

References

Ayata C (2009) Spreading depression: from serendipity to targeted therapy in migraine prophylaxis. Cephalalgia 29:1097–1114

Bigal ME, Lipton RB (2006a) Modifiable risk factors for migraine progression. Headache 46: 1334–1343

Bigal ME, Lipton RB (2006b) Obesity and migraine: a population study. Neurology 66:545–550

Blau JN (2005) Water deprivation: a new migraine precipitant. Headache 45(6):757–759

Boardman HF, Thomas E, Millson DS, Croft PF (2005) Psychological, sleep, and comorbidities associated with headache. Headache 45:657–669

Borkum JM (2007) Chronic headaches: biology, psychology, and behavioral treatment. Lawrence Erlbaum Associates, Mahwah

Bruni O, Galli F, Guidetti V (1999) Sleep hygiene and migraine in children and adolescents. Cephalalgia 19(Suppl 25):57–59

Busch V, Gaul C (2008) Exercise in migraine therapy – is there any evidence for efficacy? A critical review. Headache 48(6):890–899

Calhoun AH, Ford S (2007) Behavioral sleep modifications may revert transformed migraine to episodic migraine. Headache 45:1178–1183

Chabriat H, Danchot J, Michel P, Joire JE, Henry P (1999) Precipitating factors of headache. A prospective study in a national control-matched survey in migraineurs and nonmigraineurs. Headache 39:335–338

Cooke LJ, Rose MS, Becker WJ (2000) Chinook winds and migraine headache. Neurology 54:302–307

De Benedittis G, Lorenzetti A, Piera A (1990) The role of stressful life events in the onset of chronic primary headache. Pain 40:65–75

Dittrich SM, Gunther V, Granz G, Burtscher M, Holzner B, Kopp M (2008) Aerobic exercise with relaxation: influence on pain and psychological well-being in female migraine patients. Clin J Sport Med 18(4):363–365

Friedman DI, De Ver Dye T (2009) Migraine and the environment. Headache 49:941–952

Goksan B, Gunduz A, Karadeniz D, Agan K, Tascilar FN, Tan F, Purisa S, Kaynak H (2009) Morning headache in sleep apnea: clinical and polysomnographic evaluation and response to nasal continuous positive airway pressure. Cephalalgia 29(6):631–641

Graham JR (1955) Treatment of migraine. Little, Brown and Company, Boston

Kelman L (2007) The triggers or precipitants of the acute migraine attack. Cephalalgia 27(5):394–402

Kelman L, Rains JC (2005) Headache and sleep: examination of sleep patterns and complaints in a large clinical sample of migraineurs. Headache 45(7):904–910

Lemstra M, Stewart B, Olszynski WP (2002) Effectiveness of multidisciplinary intervention in the treatment of migraine: a randomized clinical trial. Headache 42(9):845–854

Levy D, Strassman AM, Burstein R (2009) A critical view on the role of migraine triggers in the genesis of migraine pain. Headache 49:953–957

Mak W, Tsang KL, Tsoi TH, Au Yeung KM, Chan KH, Cheng TS, Cheung TF, Ho SL (2005) Bath-related headache. Cephalalgia 25(3):191–198

Marlowe N (1998) Self-efficacy moderates the impact of stressful events on headache. Headache 38(9):662–667

Martin VT, Behbehani MM (2001) Toward a rational understanding of migraine trigger factors. Headache 85(4):911–941

Mosek A, Korczyn AD (1995) Yom Kippur headache. Neurology 45(11):1953–1955

Mungen B, Bulut S (2003) Hot-bath related headache. Cephalalgia 23:846–849

Negoro K, Morimatsu M, Ikuta N, Nogaki H (2000) Benign hot bath-related headache. Headache 40(2):173–175

O'Connor PJ, Motl RW, Broglio SP, Ely RM (2004) Dose-dependent effect of caffeine on reducing leg muscle pain during cycling exercise is unrelated to systolic blood pressure. Pain 109:291–298

Orig JC, Stepanski EJ, Gramling SE (2009) Pain coping strategies for tension-type headache: possible implications for insomnia? J Clin Sleep Med 15(5):52–56

Piorecky J, Becker WJ, Rose MS (1997) Effect of Chinook winds on the probability of migraine headache. Headache 37:153–158

Radat F, Lanteri-Minet M, Nachit-Ouinekh F, Massiou H, Lucas C, Pradalier A, Mercier F, El Hasnaoui A (2009) The GRIM2005 study of migraine consultation in France III: psychological features of subjects with migraine. Cephalalgia 29:338–350

Rains JC (2008) Optimizing circadian cycles and behavioral insomnia treatment in migraine. Curr Pain Headache Rep 12(3):213–219

Rains JC, Poceta JS (2006) Headache and sleep disorders: review and clinical implications for headache management. Headache 36(4):274–275

Rains JC, Penzien DB, McCrory DC, Gray RN (2005) Behavioral headache treatment: history, review of the empirical literature, and methodological critique. Headache 45(Suppl 2):S92–S109

Rasmussen BK (1993) Migraine and tension-type headache in a general population: precipitating factors, female hormones, sleep pattern and relation to lifestyle. Pain 53:65–72

Ravishankar K (2006) "Hair wash" or "head bath" triggering migraine: observation in 94 Indian patients. Cephalalgia 26(11):1330–1334

Robbins L (1994) Precipitating factors in migraine: a retrospective review of 494 patients. Headache 34:214–216

Sauro KM, Becker WJ (2008) Multi-disciplinary treatment for headache in the Canadian healthcare setting. Can J Neurol Sci 35(1):46–56

Sauro KM, Becker WJ (2009) The stress and migraine interaction. Headache 49(9):1378–1386

Savi L, Rainero I, Valfre W, Gentile S, Lo GR, Pinessi L (2002) Food and headache attacks. A comparison of patients with migraine and tension-type headache. Panminerva Med 44(1):27–31

Scharff L, Turk DC, Marcus DA (1995) Triggers of headache episodes and coping responses of headache diagnostic groups. Headache 35(7):397–403

Scher AI, Stewart WF, Lipton RB (2004) Caffeine as a risk factor for chronic daily headache: a population-based study. Neurology 63(11):2022–2027

Scher AI, Midgette LA, Lipton RB (2008) Risk factors for headache chronification. Headache 48:16–25

Silverman K, Evans SM, Strain EC, Griffiths RR (1992) Withdrawal syndrome after the double-blind cessation of caffeine consumption. N Engl J Med 327(16):1109–1114

Slettbakk R, Nilsen CV, Malterud K (2006) Coping with headache. Scand J Prim Health Care 24:22–26

Spierings ELH (2002) Migraine prevention and errors in living: Dr. Graham's lessons for patients and physicians. Headache 42:152–153

Spierings EL, van Hoof MJ (1997) Fatigue and sleep in chronic headache sufferers: an age- and sex-controlled questionnaire study. Headache 37(9):549–552

Spierings EL, Sorbi M, Maassen GH, Honkeep MS (1997) Psychophysical precedents of migraine in relation to the time of onset of the headache: the migraine time line. Headache 37:217–220

Spierings EL, Ranke AH, Honkoop PC (2001) Precipitating and aggravating factors of migraine versus tension-type headache. Headache 41:554–558

Topacoglu H, Karcioglu O, Yuruktumen A, Kivan S, Cimrin AH, Ozucelik DN, Sarileaya S, Soysal S, Torpcu U, Bozkurt S (2005) Impact of Ramadan on demographics and frequencies of disease-related visits in the emergency department. Int J Clin Pract 59(8):900–905

Torelli P, Evangelista A, Bini A, Castellini P, Lambru G, Manzoni GC (2009) Fasting headache: a review of the literature and new hypotheses. Headache 49(5):744–752

Varkey E, Hagen K, Zwart JA, Linde M (2008) Physical activity and headache: Results from the Nord-Trondelag Health Study (HUNT). Cephalalgia 28(12):1292–1297

Varkey E, Cider A, Carlsson J, Linde M (2009) A study to evaluate the feasibility of an aerobic exercise program in patients with migraine. Headache 49(4):563–570

Vos J, Passchier J (2003) Reduced impact of migraine in everyday life: an observational study in the Dutch society of headache patients. Headache 43:645–650

Wober C, Holzhammer J, Zeitlhofer J, Wessel P, Wober-Bingol C (2006) Trigger factors of migraine and tension-type headache: experience and knowledge of the patients. J Headache Pain 7(4):188–195

9 Hormonal Influences on Headache

E. Anne MacGregor[1] · *Astrid Gendolla*[2]
[1]The City of London Migraine Clinic, London, UK
[2]Regionales Schmerzzentrum Essen, Essen, Germany

Paolo Martelletti, Timothy J. Steiner (eds.), *Handbook of Headache*, DOI 10.1007/978-88-470-1700-9_9,
© Lifting The Burden 2011

Abstract: Specific hormonal events during the reproductive years have a profound influence on migraine in women. Onset of migraine is usually postmenarche, during the teens, and early 20s. Migraine prevalence peaks during the early 40s and improves postmenopause. During the reproductive years, migraine is three times more prevalent in women than in men. This is generally considered to be the result of female sex hormones on migraine. Menstruation is a significant migraine trigger with more than 50% of women reporting an association. Attacks are most likely to occur during the 2 days before menstruation and the first 3 days of bleeding. Menstrual attacks are almost invariably *without* aura, even in women who have attacks with aura at other times of the cycle. The majority of attacks can be controlled with symptomatic treatment alone. However, since they are more severe, of longer duration, and more disabling than non-menstrual attacks, targeted prophylaxis may be necessary. Recognition of menstrual migraine as a specific entity has resulted in improved diagnosis and increased research into the condition. However, our understanding of the pathophysiology and the consequent development of effective management strategies remain limited. Clinical and research data support an association between attacks of migraine without aura and "withdrawal" of endogenous or exogenous estrogen, following a period of estrogen priming. Estrogen "withdrawal" migraine can be prevented by maintaining constant levels of estrogen, with or without suppression of the natural menstrual cycle. Further research is necessary to identify if estrogen "withdrawal" is a primary or secondary mechanism. Other mechanisms have also been implicated, particularly prostaglandin release as occurs during migraine associated with dysmenorrhea. Perimenstrual prophylaxis with triptans has shown efficacy. Limited research suggests that high levels of estrogen, such as that occur during pregnancy, with use of combined hormonal contraceptives, and with estrogen replacement therapy, can trigger migraine *with* aura. The pathophysiology of this effect is poorly understood. Genetic susceptibility is a recognized factor in the development of both migraine with and without aura and research for genes involved in hormonal pathways is ongoing.

Established Knowledge

Migraine is a predominantly female disorder; compared with men, 1-year migraine prevalence is nearly threefold higher (17% vs. 6%) in women and lifetime incidence is more than twofold higher (43% vs. 18%) (Lipton et al. 2007; Steiner et al. 2003; Stewart et al. 2008).

The changing hormonal environment during the reproductive years has a significant effect of the frequency, severity, and type of migraine.

During childhood, boys and girls are equally affected by migraine with and without aura (Bille 1962). At puberty, the incidence of migraine without aura rises in females, with 10–20% of women reporting migraine during the same year as menarche (Stewart et al. 1991, 1992). In adolescents, migraine without aura continues to be more prevalent in girls, often accompanying menstruation and with associated dysmenorrhea (Mannix 2008). A retrospective analysis of 896 adolescent girls identified 331 (50.3%) who reported headaches with menstruation of whom 63.6% reported migraine on or between day −2 to +3 of menstruation (Crawford et al. 2009). Of note is that a monthly pattern was apparent in 160 girls even before their first menstrual period (❷ *Table 9.1*).

Throughout the reproductive years, menstruation is one of the most significant risk factors for migraine without aura (Granella et al. 2000; Wober et al. 2007). Compared with all other phases of the menstrual cycle, incidence of migraine without aura is greatest during a 5-day

◘ Table 9.1

Diagnostic criteria for pure menstrual migraine and menstrually related migraine (Adapted from Headache Classification Subcommittee of the International Headache Society (IHS) 2004)

Pure menstrual migraine without aura
Diagnostic criteria
A. Attacks, in a menstruating woman, fulfilling IHS criteria for migraine without aura
B. Attacks occur exclusively on day 1±2 (i.e., days −2 to +3)[a] of menstruation[b] in at least two out of three menstrual cycles and at no other times of the cycle
Menstrually related migraine without aura
Diagnostic criteria
A. Attacks, in a menstruating woman, fulfilling IHS criteria for migraine without aura
B. Attacks occur on day 1±2 (i.e., days −2 to +3)[a] of menstruation[b] in at least two out of three menstrual cycles and additionally at other times of the cycle

[a]The first day of menstruation is day 1 and the preceding day is day −1; there is no day 0
[b]For the purposes of this classification, menstruation is considered to be endometrial bleeding resulting from either the normal menstrual cycle or from the withdrawal of exogenous progestogens, as in the case of combined oral contraceptives and cyclical hormone replacement therapy

window that starts 2 days before the onset of menses and continues through the first 3 days of menstruation (Dzoljic et al. 2002; Johannes et al. 1995; MacGregor and Hackshaw 2004; Stewart et al. 2000). Stewart et al. noted a significantly elevated risk of migraine without aura on the first 2 days of menstruation (OR 2.04; 95% CI 1.49, 2.81) (Stewart et al. 2000). MacGregor et al. reported that women were 25% (RR 1.25) more likely to have migraine in the 5 days leading up to menstruation increasing to 71% (RR 1.71) in the 2 days before menstruation (MacGregor and Hackshaw 2004). The risk of migraine was more than twofold on the first day of menstruation and during the 5 days afterward (RR 2.19). The risk was highest on the first day of menstruation and the following 2 days (RR 2.50).

Compared with migraine at other times of the cycle, menstrual attacks last longer, are more severe, are more likely to relapse, are less responsive to treatment, and are associated with greater disability (Calhoun and Ford 2008; Couturier et al. 2003; Dowson et al. 2005; Granella et al. 2004; MacGregor et al. 2004, 2006b, 2010b; MacGregor and Hackshaw 2004; Pinkerman and Holroyd 2010; Stewart et al. 2000). In a population-based study of over 1,000 women, 84% with menstrual migraine engaged in fewer social activities, 81% had difficulty performing household chores, 58% had to limit family activities, 55% could not engage in sports, and 45% had work-related disability (Couturier et al. 2003). Work-related disability is more often reported for premenstrual migraines than for non-menstrual attacks ($P = 0.006$) (Granella et al. 2004). Similarly, time spent at less than 50% productivity is greater for menstrual than non-menstrual attacks ($P = 0.01$) (Dowson et al. 2005).

Pregnancy provides a brief respite from migraine. Although there is little improvement in the first trimester of pregnancy, during the second and third trimesters up to 80% of women with migraine will experience fewer attacks compared to pre-pregnancy (Aegidius et al. 2009; Granella et al. 2000; Sances et al. 2003). Improvement is more likely with a history of menstrual or menstrually related migraine (Granella et al. 2000; Melhado et al. 2005; Sances et al. 2003). In the week immediately postpartum, headache affects around 30–40% of women (Sances et al. 2003; Scharff et al. 1997; Stein et al. 1984).

Postmenopause is also associated with respite. In a longitudinal study of 404 women enrolled in the Penn Ovarian Aging Study, the percentage of women reporting moderate to severe headache fell from 34% during premenopause to 24% postmenopause ($p = 0.003$) (Freeman et al. 2008). A study of 1,436 women showed a migraine prevalence of 10.5% in spontaneous menopausal women compared with 16.7% in premenopausal and perimenopausal women (OR 0.6, 95% CI 0.4–0.9 $p = 0.03$) (Wang et al. 2003). Time since menopause is associated with improvement (Freeman et al. 2008; Mattsson 2003). This improvement is generally attributed to the absence of variations in sex hormone levels postmenopause.

The type of menopause has a substantial effect on migraine. Natural menopause is associated with a lower prevalence of migraine compared to surgical menopause. In a retrospective questionnaire of 47 postmenopausal women with migraine, eight women (17%) reported new onset of migraine with menopause (Neri et al. 1993). Of those women who had had a physiological menopause, 67% reported improvement or complete remission of migraine postmenopause, 24% reported no change, and 9% reported worsening migraine. Regarding surgical menopause, 33% reported improvement following the procedure, and in 67% migraine was worse. Similarly, a retrospective study of 164 postmenopausal women with migraine without aura attending specialist headache centers in Italy compared surgical and natural menopause (27) Surgical menopause was associated with worsening of migraine ($P < 0.01$); natural menopause was associated with improvement ($P < 0.01$).

Migraine is also affected by whether the ovaries are retained or removed during hysterectomy. In a cross-sectional survey, 15.1% of 986 hysterectomized women with one or both ovaries present reported moderate to severe migraine, compared with 8.8% of 5636 non-hysterectomized women with both ovaries present ($p < 0.001$) (Oldenhave et al. 1993). In a separate study, migraine prevalence was lowest in those with hysterectomy and bilateral oophorectomy, although not to a statistically significant level (hysterectomy only, 28.6%; hysterectomy with unilateral oophorectomy, 36.4%; hysterectomy with bilateral oophorectomy, 15.8%; $p = 0.3$) (Wang et al. 2003). There are no data on the effect of bilateral oophorectomy without hysterectomy.

Pathophysiology

The clinical effect of hormonal events implicates sex hormones in the pathophysiology of migraine. Most of the research to date has studied the effects of the ovarian hormones, progesterone and estrogen.

Insufficient progesterone in the luteal phase was initially considered to be the prime factor responsible for menstrual migraine (Beckham et al. 1992; Gray 1941; Singh and Singh 1947).

During the 1970s, Somerville tested this hypothesis in several studies undertaken on small selected group of women with at least a 6-month history of menstrual migraine. He first used progesterone supplements to maintain mid-luteal phase progesterone levels during the late luteal and menstrual phases. This delayed menstruation in four of six women studied and five experienced migraine at their customary time, irrespective of menstruation (Somerville 1971, 1972b). Somerville also studied the effects of exogenous progesterone in women in whom high serum levels of exogenous estrogen had inhibited ovulation. Neither the administration of progesterone nor its subsequent "withdrawal" resulted in migraine.

Somerville turned his attention to the effect of estrogen "withdrawal" on migraine. He studied two postmenopausal women with a past history of menstrual migraine but who had been free of migraine since the menopause. Migraine was associated with the fall in estrogen following depot estradiol, despite plasma progesterone concentrations never exceeding 1ng/mL (Somerville 1972a).

Somerville undertook several studies in a small group of women who had a history of pure menstrual migraine. He noted that a period of estrogen "priming" with several days of exposure to high estrogen levels is necessary for migraine to result from estrogen "withdrawal" (Somerville 1972a, 1975a, b). Similarly, Lichten et al. primed a group of postmenopausal women with estrogen supplements; falling levels of estrogen were associated with migraine (Lichten et al. 1996).

Epstein et al. noted that the extent of decline from peak to trough estrogen was greater in all 14 women with migraine in their study compared to eight control women who did not have migraine (Epstein et al. 1975). They concluded that variation in hormonal activity might be a potentially relevant factor in all women with migraine; factors additional to the hormonal environment could account for the development of "menstrual" attacks.

MacGregor et al. studied 38 women with pure menstrual or menstrually related migraine aged 29–49 (mean 43) years. Urine was collected daily for assay over three menstrual cycles and analyzed for luteinizing hormone (LH), estrone-3-glucuronide (E_1G), pregnanediol-3-glucuronide (PdG), and follicle-stimulating hormone (FSH) (MacGregor et al. 2006b). Migraine was inversely associated with urinary estrogen levels, across the menstrual cycle. Attacks were significantly more likely to occur in association with falling estrogen in the late luteal/early follicular phase of the menstrual cycle and significantly less likely to occur during the subsequent part of the follicular phase during which estrogen levels rose (❷ *Fig. 9.1*).

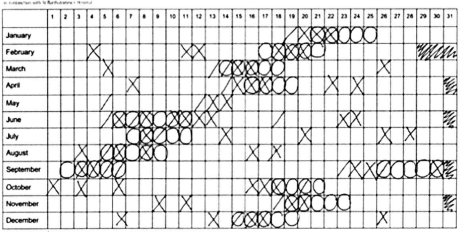

❑ Fig. 9.1

Diary card showing menstrually related migraine (Reproduced with permission from MacGregor 2007)

In summary, the body of research implicates estrogen "withdrawal" triggering migraine. This can occur in the absence of progesterone. If this theory is correct, maintaining stable estrogen levels should prevent migraine. Several studies provide supportive evidence. Somerville showed that migraine could be postponed by maintaining high plasma estradiol levels with an intramuscular injection of long-acting estradiol valerate in oil; migraine subsequently occurred when the plasma estradiol fell (Somerville 1972a). His attempts with oral estrogens and implants failed to provide stable plasma levels of estradiol and were of no benefit to migraine (Somerville 1975a).

De Lignières et al. studied 18 women with menstrual migraine who completed a double-blind placebo-controlled crossover trial using 1.5 mg estradiol gel or placebo daily for 7 days during three consecutive cycles (de Lignieres et al. 1986). Eight menstrual attacks occurred during the 26 estrogen-treated cycles compared with 26 attacks during the 27 placebo cycles. Attacks during estrogen treatment were considerably milder and shorter than those during placebo.

Dennerstein et al. undertook a similar trial with 1.5 mg estradiol gel used by 18 women over four cycles (Dennerstein et al. 1988). Estradiol gel was significantly more effective than placebo, and less medication was used during active treatment.

MacGregor et al. used 1.5 mg estradiol gel in a double-blind placebo-controlled study in 35 women with menstrual migraine (MacGregor et al. 2006a). Each woman treated up to six menstrual cycles (three cycles estradiol; three placebo). Women used the Clearplan® Easy Fertility monitor to identify ovulation. They applied estradiol gel or placebo on the tenth day following ovulation and continued daily until, and including, the second day of menstruation. Estradiol was associated with a 22% reduction in migraine days (RR 0.78 [95% CI 0.62–0.99] $P = 0.04$); these migraines were less severe and less likely to be associated with nausea. As Somerville had found, there was a significant increase in the migraine immediately following cessation of active gel compared to placebo (RR 1.40 [95% CI 1.03–1.92] $P = 0.03$). Possible reasons for this post-gel estrogen "withdrawal" migraine may be that the dose of estradiol was inadequate; the duration of treatment was too short; or perhaps that exogenous estrogen prevents the normal secretion of endogenous estrogen. This study failed to identify a critical "threshold" for estrogen "withdrawal" migraine, in line with the theory that falling levels are more important than absolute levels (Somerville 1972a). However, it seems necessary to maintain estrogen at mid-luteal phase levels, as occurs with 1.5 mg gel or 100 mcg patches. Estrogen doses lower than these are not effective for menstrual migraine prevention (MacGregor and Hackshaw 2002; Pfaffenrath 1993; Pradalier et al. 1994; Smits et al. 1994).

Other Mechanisms

Estrogen and progesterone are neurosteroids, influencing the pain-processing networks and vascular endothelium involved in the pathophysiology of migraine. In particular, estrogen has potent effects on the serotonergic system, increasing serotonergic tone. Serotonin-producing neurons are sensitive to the presence or absence of ovarian hormones (McEwan 2002). This association might account for efficacy of triptans for perimenstrual prophylaxis.

Prostaglandins have also been implicated in menstrual migraine (Horrobin 1977). In particular, entry of prostaglandins into the systemic circulation can trigger throbbing headache, nausea, and vomiting (Carlson et al. 1968). In the uterus, prostaglandins are synthesized primarily by the endometrium. There is a threefold increase in prostaglandin levels in the uterine endometrium from the follicular to the luteal phase, with a further increase during menstruation (Downie et al. 1974). As a result of the "withdrawal" of estrogen and progesterone the endometrium breaks down and prostaglandins are released. This causes vasoconstriction within the endometrium and disruption of endometrial cells, stimulating further prostaglandin synthesis. When an excessive amount of prostaglandins gain entrance to the circulation, other systemic symptoms occur that are characteristically associated with menorrhagia and/or dysmenorrhea such as headache and nausea (Benedetto 1989; Chan 1983). Plasma taken during the premenstrual phase from women with dysmenorrhea and reinfused postmenstruation into the same women resulted in premenstrual symptoms, including headache (Irwin et al. 1981). Thus prostaglandins may have a specific role in migraine associated with dysmenorrhea and/or menorrhagia. In support of this, nonsteroidal anti-inflammatory drugs (NSAIDs), which inhibit prostaglandins, are effective for the prevention of menstrual attacks of migraine (Pradalier et al. 1988).

Implications for Management

Diagnosis

The International Headache Society recognizes two types of menstrual migraine: menstrually related migraine, which is migraine without aura that regularly occurs on or between day −2 to +3 of menstruation, with additional attacks of migraine with or without aura at other times of the cycle; and pure menstrual migraine, which is migraine without aura that occurs only on or between day −2 to +3, i.e., with no attacks at any other time of the cycle (Headache Classification Committee of the International Headache Society 1988; Headache Classification Subcommittee of the International Headache Society (IHS) 2004). For most women with menstrual attacks, migraine also occurs at other times of the month ("menstrually related" migraine) (Headache Classification Subcommittee of the International Headache Society (IHS) 2004; MacGregor et al. 1990). Fewer than 10% of women report migraine exclusively with menstruation and at no other time of the month ("pure" menstrual migraine) (Dzoljic et al. 2002; Granella et al. 1993; Headache Classification Subcommittee of the International Headache Society (IHS) 2004; MacGregor et al. 2004; MacGregor et al. 1990).

To confirm the diagnosis, migraine attacks during the day −2 to +3 window must occur in at least two of three menstrual cycles to establish a relationship that is greater than chance alone. Relying on the history to confirm the diagnosis can be misleading (MacGregor et al. 1997). Use of a 3-month diary to record migraine patterns can reveal the predictable patterns associated with menstrual migraine, aiding diagnosis.

Specific Prophylaxis for Menstrual Migraine

For many women, optimizing symptomatic treatment is all that is necessary to maintain effective control. Only a small percentage of women will have menstrual migraine and wish to consider specific prophylaxis. An understanding of the pathophysiology of menstrual migraine enables prophylaxis to be targeted toward the most likely mechanism. None of the drugs and hormones recommended below is licensed for management of menstrual migraine because, although effective in clinical trials, evidence is limited. Given that there are no investigations to identify the most effective prophylactic, an empirical approach is necessary, prescribing on a "named" patient basis. Because of the fluctuating nature of migraine, it is sensible to try a method for at least three cycles before considering alternative prophylaxis.

Perimenstrual Estrogen Supplements

Several trials have confirmed the efficacy of transcutaneous estradiol for menstrual migraine prophylaxis (de Lignieres et al. 1986; Dennerstein et al. 1988; MacGregor et al. 2006a; Pfaffenrath 1993; Pradalier et al. 1994; Smits et al. 1994). The effective dose is 100 μg patches or 1.5 mg estradiol gel, which produces serum estradiol levels of 75 pg/ml.

Treatment is well tolerated although both MacGregor et al. and Somerville noted a significant increase in the migraine immediately following estradiol treatment (MacGregor et al. 2006a; Somerville 1972a). Although there are no trial data, clinical practice suggests that for these women the duration of supplement use can be extended until day 7 of the cycle, tapering the dose over the last 2 days. Menstrual irregularity can occur, probably due to suppression of endogenous estrogen during treatment (MacGregor et al. 2006a).

Perimenstrual estrogen can be used only when menstruation is regular and predictable. If the woman has an intact uterus, no additional progestogens are necessary, provided that she is ovulating regularly. Ovulation can be confirmed using a home-use fertility monitor, which has the advantage of predicting menstruation (MacGregor et al. 2005).

Safety of estrogens is an important concern. Physiological doses of supplemental estrogens are well tolerated in clinical trials (MacGregor et al. 2006a). There is no evidence that supplements increase the risks of cancer or thrombosis in women who are producing endogenous estrogen (North American Menopause Society 2010). However, supplemental estrogens are not recommended for women who have estrogen-dependent tumors or other estrogen-dependent conditions, including a history of venous thromboembolism.

Perimenstrual Triptans

Trials of frovatriptan, naratriptan, sumatriptan, and zolmitriptan for perimenstrual prophylaxis show efficacy (Brandes et al. 2009; Guidotti et al. 2007; Mannix et al. 2007; Moschiano et al. 2005; Newman et al. 1998, 2001; Silberstein et al. 2004, 2009; Tuchman et al. 2008). Similar to perimenstrual estrogen treatment, "rebound" migraine following treatment with naratriptan, but not frovatriptan, has been noted (Brandes et al. 2009; Mannix et al. 2007). There are no data reported on rebound following treatment with sumatriptan or zolmitriptan.

Patients completing 6–12 months perimenstrual prophylaxis with naratriptan noted that no specific adverse event considered at least possibly to be related to study medication occurred in more than 2% of patients. No serious drug-related adverse events were reported and no patient experienced clinically relevant drug-related changes in 12 lead ECGs, vital signs, or clinical laboratory tests (Brandes et al. 2007).

Long-term safety and tolerability studies with frovatriptan noted that adverse events were generally mild or moderate in severity and were similar to that observed with acute use of triptans (MacGregor et al. 2009). Results of subgroup analyses of women whose medical histories included comorbidities that might suggest increased cardiovascular risk but were not themselves contraindications to frovatriptan, provide preliminary evidence of safety of frovatriptan in this population (MacGregor et al. 2010a).

Nonsteroidal Anti-Inflammatory Drugs

NSAIDs are effective for prophylaxis of menstrual migraine and have the advantage of treating associated dysmenorrhoea (Mannix 2008). Naproxen 550 mg once or twice daily perimenstrually have shown efficacy with good tolerability (Sances et al. 1990). Mefenamic acid 500 mg, three to four times daily, may be started either 2–3 days before the expected onset of menstruation, but is often effective even when started on the first day of bleeding – this is useful if periods are irregular. Treatment is usually only necessary for the first 2–3 days of bleeding (Johnson et al. 1986; Owens 1984).

Other Strategies for Management

Continuous hormonal methods are particularly useful if cycles are irregular, or when the above strategies prove ineffective despite a convincing hormonal link. Contraceptive doses of synthetic estrogens should not be used by women who also have with migraine with aura because of the synergistic increased risk of ischemic stroke (World Health Organization 2009) (❷ Fig. 9.2).

In a small open-label study, 11 women with menstrual migraine were treated with a 28-day cycle of 0.02 mg ethinylestradiol oral contraceptive for 21 days followed by 0.9 mg conjugated equine estrogen daily for 7 days. All women achieved at least a 50% reduction in number of headache days per cycle (mean 77.9% reduction) (Calhoun 2004).

Continuous combined hormonal contraceptives, eliminating the usual monthly hormone-free interval are a safe and effective method of eliminating menstrual symptoms [66] (LaGuardia et al. 2005). They are well tolerated, although unscheduled bleeding is a common reason for withdrawal from clinical trials in the first 6 months of treatment. Continued use induces amenorrhea in 80–100% of women by 10–12 months of treatment (Archer 2006). Women who wish to maintain a monthly "period" may try combined contraceptives with a 2-day hormone-free interval, although data regarding benefit on headache are limited.

The menstrual cycle can also be suppressed using gonadotropin-releasing hormone (GnRH) analogs. Although effective, adverse effects of estrogen deficiency, e.g., hot flushes, restrict their use (Holdaway et al. 1991). The hormones are also associated with a marked reduction in bone density and should not usually be used for longer than 6 months without regular monitoring and bone densitometry. "Add-back" continuous combined estrogen and progestogen can be given to counter these difficulties (Martin et al. 2003; Murray and Muse 1997). Given these limitations, in addition to increased cost, such treatment should be instigated only in specialist departments.

Nice to Know

How Do Estrogens Act in Migraine?

Ovarian steroids cross the blood–brain barrier by passive diffusion, with brain levels mirroring blood levels (Aloisi 2003). They are also produced within the central nervous system (Stoffel-Wagner 1993). As neurosteroids, estrogen and progesterone can influence the

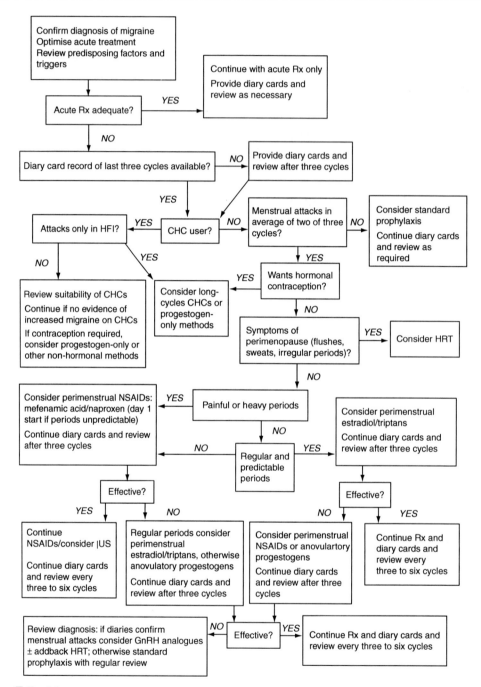

◻ Fig. 9.2

Management strategies for menstrual migraine (Reproduced with permission from MacGregor 2007). *CHC* combined hormonal contraceptives, *GnRH* gonadotrophin-releasing hormone analogue, *HFI* hormone-free interval, *HRT* hormone replacement therapy, *IUS* intrauterine system, *NSAIDs* nonsteroidal anti-inflammatory drugs, *Rx* treatment

pain-processing networks and vascular endothelium involved in the pathophysiology of migraine. Both estrogen and progesterone also have a clinically relevant effect on vascular tone (Sarrel 1999). Further, close interrelationships between estrogens and brain neurotransmitters have been confirmed, including the catecholamines, serotonin, norepinephrine, dopamine, and the endorphins (Facchinetti et al. 1990; Neri et al. 1993).

Estrogen facilitates the glutaminergic system, potentially enhancing neural excitability. This effect is modulated by progesterone, which appears to activate GABAergic systems, suppressing neuronal reactivity (Martin and Behbehani 2006).

Why Are Some Women with Migraine Susceptible to Estrogen "Withdrawal" and Others Are Not?

That estrogens do not affect all women with migraine might be explained by the intrinsic estrogen receptor sensitivity of the hypothalamic neurons. Limited data imply that this may have a genetic basis (Berman et al. 2006). Experimental studies in rats suggest that abnormalities in how estrogen modulates neuronal function in migraine may be due to a mismatch between its gene-regulation and membrane effects. A decline in estrogen levels modulates central sensitization, increasing the pain and disability of the migraine attack (Martin et al. 2007; Welch et al. 2006).

Genes involved in hormonal pathways are also likely to play a role in migraine susceptibility (Colson et al. 2006, 2007) Women who carry a copy of both the progesterone receptor PROGINS and estrogen receptor 1 (ESR1) risk alleles are 3.2 times more likely to suffer from migraine, an effect that is greater than the independent effects of these genetic variants on disease susceptibility.

What Effect Does Estrogen Have on Migraine with Aura?

In contrast to the effect of estrogen "withdrawal" on migraine without aura, migraine with aura is associated with high estrogen states. High levels of estrogen have been reported in women with migraine with aura during the normal menstrual cycle: Mean estradiol levels in women with migraine with aura during the normal menstrual cycle (94.4 ± 28.3 pg/ml) were double those of the control group (50.6 ± 8.9 pg/ml) and women with migraine without aura (41.6 ± 7.1 pg/ml) (Nagel-Leiby et al. 1990). High estrogen states are also associated with the development of migraine with aura in women who have not previously had migraine or who had attacks only of migraine without aura. This occurs in women starting combined oral contraceptives, hormone replacement therapy, and during pregnancy (Bickerstaff 1975; Chancellor et al. 1990; Cupini et al. 1995; Wright and Patel 1986). Resolution of aura typically occurs following a return to lower estrogen states (MacGregor 1999).

Conclusions

The predictable effects of hormonal changes during the reproductive years provide healthcare physicians with specific opportunities to identify and manage migraine in women. Menstrual migraine is a heterogeneous condition. Estrogen "withdrawal," as occurs during the late luteal phase of the menstrual cycle, during the hormone-free interval of combined hormonal contraceptives, and immediately post partum, is associated with increased risk of migraine without aura. In contrast, high estrogen states associated with pregnancy, use of contraceptive ethinylestradiol, and estrogen replacement therapy are associated with increased risk of migraine with aura. Respite follows the natural decline in estrogen postmenopause. Use of estrogen supplements can prevent estrogen "withdrawal" migraine although short-term prevent strategies may be followed by delayed migraine. Where appropriate, continuous hormonal strategies are indicated. Late luteal estrogen "withdrawal" is paralleled by a natural decline in serotonin, which may account for the efficacy of short-term perimenstrual triptan prophylaxis, although the mechanism for response has not been elucidated. Perimenstrual prostaglandin release, associated with dysmenorrheal, is also associated with increased risk of menstrual migraine and responds to treatment with prostaglandin inhibitors. Further research is indicated to identify the differential effect of estrogen on migraine, and to establish genotypes to enable improved diagnosis and management.

References

Aegidius K, Zwart J-A, Hagen K, Stovner L (2009) The effect of pregnancy and parity on headache prevalence: the head-HUNT study. Headache 49:851–859

Aloisi A (2003) Gonadal hormones and sex differences in pain reactivity. Clin J Pain 19:168–174

Archer DF (2006) Menstrual-cycle-related symptoms: a review of the rationale for continuous use of oral contraceptives. Contraception 74:359–366

Beckham JC, Krug LM, Penzien DB, Johnson CA, Mosley TH, Meeks GR, Pbert LA, Prather RC (1992) The relationship of ovarian steroids, headache activity and menstrual distress: a pilot study with female migraineurs. Headache 32:292–297

Benedetto C (1989) Eicosanoids in primary dysmenorrhea, endometriosis and menstrual migraine. Gynecol Endocrinol 3:71–94

Berman NE, Puri V, Chandrala S, Puri S, Macgregor R, Liverman CS, Klein RM (2006) Serotonin in trigeminal Ganglia of female rodents: relevance to menstrual migraine. Headache 46:1230–1245

Bickerstaff ER (1975) Neurological complications of oral contraceptives. Oxford University Press, Oxford

Bille B (1962) Migraine in school children. Acta Paediatr Scand 51:1–151

Brandes JL, Smith T, Diamond M, Ames MH (2007) Open-label, long-term tolerability of naratriptan for short-term prevention of menstrually related migraine. Headache 47:886–894

Brandes JL, Poole A, Kallela M, Schreiber CP, MacGregor EA, Silberstein SD, Tobin J, Shaw R (2009) Short-term frovatriptan for the prevention of difficult-to-treat menstrual migraine attacks. Cephalalgia 29:1133–1148

Calhoun AH (2004) A novel specific prophylaxis for menstrual-associated migraine. South Med J 97:819–822

Calhoun A, Ford S (2008) Elimination of menstrual-related migraine beneficially impacts chronification and medication overuse. Headache J Head Face Pain 48:1186–1193

Carlson LA, Ekelund LG, Oro L (1968) Clinical and metabolic effects of different doses of prostaglandin E1 in man. Prostaglandin and related factors. Acta Med Scand 183:423–430

Chan W (1983) Prostaglandins and nonsteroidal antiinflammatory drugs in dysmenorrhoea. Annu Rev Pharmacol Toxicol 23:131–149

Chancellor AM, Wroe SJ, Cull RE (1990) Migraine occurring for the first time in pregnancy. Headache 30:224–227

Colson NJ, Lea RA, Quinlan S, Griffiths LR (2006) The role of vascular and hormonal genes in migraine susceptibility. Mol Genet Metab 88:107–113

Colson NJ, Fernandez F, Lea RA, Griffiths LR (2007) The search for migraine genes: an overview of current knowledge. Cell Mol Life Sci 64:331–344

Couturier EG, Bomhof MA, Neven AK, van Duijn NP (2003) Menstrual migraine in a representative Dutch population sample: prevalence, disability and treatment. Cephalalgia 23:302–308

Crawford M, Lehman L, Slater S, Kabbouche M, Lecates S, Segers A, Manning P, Powers S, Hershey A (2009) Menstrual migraine in adolescents. Headache J Head Face Pain 49:341–347

Cupini LM, Matteis M, Troisi E, Calabresi P, Bernardi G, Silvestrini M (1995) Sex-hormone-related events in migrainous females. A clinical comparative study between migraine with aura and migraine without aura. Cephalalgia 15:140–144

de Lignieres B, Vincens M, Mauvais-Jarvis P, Mas JL, Touboul PJ, Bousser MG (1986) Prevention of menstrual migraine by percutaneous oestradiol. Br Med J (Clin Res Ed) 293:1540

Dennerstein L, Morse C, Burrows G, Oats J, Brown J, Smith M (1988) Menstrual migraine: a double-blind trial of percutaneous estradiol. Gynecol Endocrinol 2:113–120

Downie J, Poyser N, Wonderlich M (1974) Levels of prostaglandins in human endometrium during normal menstrual cycle. J Physiol 236:465–472

Dowson AJ, Kilminster SG, Salt R, Clark M, Bundy MJ (2005) Disability associated with headaches occurring inside and outside the menstrual period in those with migraine: a general practice study. Headache 45:274–282

Dzoljic E, Sipetic S, Vlajinac H, Marinkovic J, Brzakovic B, Pokrajac M, Kostic V (2002) Prevalence of menstrually related migraine and nonmigraine primary headache in female students of Belgrade University. Headache 42:185–193

Epstein MT, Hockaday JM, Hockaday TD (1975) Migraine and reproductive hormones throughout the menstrual cycle. Lancet 1:543–548

Facchinetti F, Martignoni E, Fioroni L, Sances G, Genazzani AR (1990) Opioid control of the hypothalamus-pituitary-adrenal axis cyclically fails in menstrual migraine. Cephalalgia 10:51–56

Freeman EW, Sammel MD, Lin H, Gracia CR, Kapoor S (2008) Symptoms in the menopausal transition: hormone and behavioral correlates. Obstet Gynecol 111:127–136

Granella F, Sances G, Zanferrari C, Costa A, Martignoni E, Manzoni GC (1993) Migraine without aura and reproductive life events: a clinical epidemiological study in 1300 women. Headache 33:385–389

Granella F, Sances G, Pucci E, Nappi RE, Ghiotto N, Napp G (2000) Migraine with aura and reproductive life events: a case control study. Cephalalgia 20:701–707

Granella F, Sances G, Allais G, Nappi RE, Tirelli A, Benedetto C, Brundu B, Facchinetti F, Nappi G (2004) Characteristics of menstrual and nonmenstrual attacks in women with menstrually related migraine referred to headache centres. Cephalalgia 24:707–716

Gray L (1941) The use of progesterone in nervous tension states. South Med J 34:1004–1005

Guidotti M, Mauri M, Barrila C, Guidotti F, Belloni C (2007) Frovatriptan vs. transdermal oestrogens or naproxen sodium for the prophylaxis of menstrual migraine. J Headache Pain 8:283–288

Headache Classification Committee of the International Headache Society (1988) Classification and diagnostic criteria for headache disorders, cranial neuralgias and facial pain. Cephalalgia 8:1–96

Headache Classification Subcommittee of the International Headache Society (IHS) (2004) The international classification of headache disorders (2nd edition). Cephalalgia 24:1–160

Holdaway IM, Parr CE, France J (1991) Treatment of a patient with severe menstrual migraine using the depot LHRH analogue Zoladex. Aust NZ J Obstet Gynaecol 31:164–165

Horrobin D (1977) Prostaglandins and migraine. Headache 16:113–116

Irwin J, Morse E, Riddick D (1981) Dysmenorrhoea induced by autologous transfusion. Obstet Gynecol 58:286–290

Johannes CB, Linet MS, Stewart WF, Celentano DD, Lipton RB, Szklo M (1995) Relationship of headache to phase of the menstrual cycle among young women: a daily diary study. Neurology 45:1076–1082

Johnson R, Hornabrook R, Lambie D (1986) Comparison of mefenamic acid and propranolol with placebo in migraine prophylaxis. Acta Neurol Scand 73:490–492

LaGuardia KD, Fisher AC, Bainbridge JD, LoCoco JM, Friedman AJ (2005) Suppression of estrogen-withdrawal headache with extended transdermal contraception. Fertil Steril 83:1875–1877

Lichten EM, Lichten JB, Whitty A, Pieper D (1996) The confirmation of a biochemical marker for women's hormonal migraine: the depo-estradiol challenge test. Headache 36:367–371

Lipton RB, Bigal ME, Diamond M, Freitag F, Reed ML, Stewart WF (2007) Migraine prevalence, disease burden, and the need for preventive therapy. Neurology 68:343–349

MacGregor A (1999) Estrogen replacement and migraine aura. Headache 39:674–678

MacGregor EA (2007) Menstrual migraine: a clinical review. J Fam Plann Reprod Health Care 33(1): 36–47

MacGregor EA, Hackshaw A (2002) Prevention of migraine in the pill-free interval of combined oral contraceptives: a double-blind, placebo-controlled pilot study using natural oestrogen supplements. J Fam Plann Reprod Health Care 28:27–31

MacGregor EA, Hackshaw A (2004) Prevalence of migraine on each day of the natural menstrual cycle. Neurology 63:351–353

MacGregor EA, Chia H, Vohrah RC, Wilkinson M (1990) Migraine and menstruation: a pilot study. Cephalalgia 10:305–310

MacGregor EA, Igarashi H, Wilkinson M (1997) Headaches and hormones: subjective versus objective assessment. Headache Q 8:126–136

MacGregor EA, Brandes J, Eikermann A, Giammarco R (2004) Impact of migraine on patients and their families: the Migraine and Zolmitriptan Evaluation

(MAZE) survey – Phase III. Curr Med Res Opin 20:1143–1150

MacGregor EA, Frith A, Ellis J, Aspinall L (2005) Predicting menstrual migraine with a home-use fertility monitor. Neurology 64:561–563

MacGregor EA, Frith A, Ellis J, Aspinall L, Hackshaw A (2006a) Prevention of menstrual attacks of migraine: a double-blind placebo-controlled crossover study. Neurology 67:2159–2163

MacGregor EA, Frith A, Ellis J, Aspinall L, Hackshaw A (2006b) Incidence of migraine relative to menstrual cycle phases of rising and falling estrogen. Neurology 67:2154–2158

MacGregor EA, Brandes JL, Silberstein S, Jeka S, Czapinski P, Shaw B, Pawsey S (2009) Safety and tolerability of short-term preventive frovatriptan: a combined analysis. Headache 49:1298–1314

MacGregor E, Pawsey S, Campbell J, Hu X (2010a) Safety and tolerability of Frovatriptan in the acute treatment of migraine and prevention of menstrual migraine. Gend Med 7(2)88–108

MacGregor E, Victor T, Hu X, Xiang Q, Puenpatom R, Chen W, Campbell J (2010b) Characteristics of menstrual vs nonmenstrual migraine: a post hoc, within-woman analysis of the usual-care phase of a nonrandomized menstrual migraine clinical trial. Headache 50(4):528–538

Mannix LK (2008) Menstrual-related pain conditions: dysmenorrhea and migraine. J Womens Health (Larchmt) 17:879–891

Mannix LK, Savani N, Landy S, Valade D, Shackelford S, Ames MH, Jones MW (2007) Efficacy and tolerability of naratriptan for short-term prevention of menstrually related migraine: data from two randomized, double-blind, placebo-controlled studies. Headache 47:1037–1049

Martin VT, Behbehani M (2006) Ovarian hormones and migraine headache: understanding mechanisms and pathogenesis – part I. Headache 46:3–23

Martin V, Wernke S, Mandell K, Zoma W, Bean J, Pinney S, Liu J, Ramadan N, Rebar R (2003) Medical oophorectomy with and without estrogen add-back therapy in the prevention of migraine headache. Headache 43:309–321

Martin VT, Lee J, Behbehani MM (2007) Sensitization of the trigeminal sensory system during different stages of the rat estrous cycle: implications for menstrual migraine. Headache 47:552–563

Mattsson P (2003) Hormonal factors in migraine: a population-based study of women aged 40 to 74 years. Headache 43:27–35

McEwan B (2002) Estrogen actions throughout the brain. Recent Prog Horm Res 57:357–384

Melhado E, Maciel JA Jr, Guerreiro CA (2005) Headaches during pregnancy in women with a prior history of menstrual headaches. Arq Neuropsiquiatr 63:934–940

Moschiano F, Allais G, Grazzi L, Usai S, Benedetto C, D'Amico D, Roncolato M, Bussone G (2005) Naratriptan in the short-term prophylaxis of pure menstrual migraine. Neurol Sci 26(Suppl 2):s162–s166

Murray SC, Muse KN (1997) Effective treatment of severe menstrual migraine headaches with gonadotropin-releasing hormone agonist and 'add-back' therapy. Fertil Steril 67:390–393

Nagel-Leiby S, Welch KM, Grunfeld S, D'Andrea G (1990) Ovarian steroid levels in migraine with and without aura. Cephalalgia 10:147–152

Neri I, Granella F, Nappi R, Manzoni GC, Facchinetti F, Genazzani AR (1993) Characteristics of headache at menopause: a clinico-epidemiologic study. Maturitas 17:31–37

Newman LC, Lipton RB, Lay CL, Solomon S (1998) A pilot study of oral sumatriptan as intermittent prophylaxis of menstruation-related migraine. Neurology 51:307–309

Newman L, Mannix LK, Landy S, Silberstein S, Lipton RB, Putnam DG, Watson C, Jobsis M, Batenhorst A, O'Quinn S (2001) Naratriptan as short-term prophylaxis of menstrually associated migraine: a randomized, double-blind, placebo-controlled study. Headache 41:248–256

North American Menopause Society (2010) Estrogen and progestogen use in postmenopausal women: 2010 position statement of The North American Menopause Society. Menopause 17:242–255

Oldenhave A, Jaszmann LJ, Everaerd WT, Haspels AA (1993) Hysterectomized women with ovarian conservation report more severe climacteric complaints than do normal climacteric women of similar age. Am J Obstet Gynecol 168:765–771

Owens P (1984) Prostaglandin synthetase inhibitors in the treatment of primary dysmenorrhoea: outcome trials reviewed. Am J Obstet Gynecol 148:96

Pfaffenrath V (1993) Efficacy and safety of percutaneous estradiol vs. placebo in menstrual migraine. Cephalalgia 13:244

Pinkerman B, Holroyd KA (2010) Menstrual and nonmenstrual migraines differ in women with menstrually-related migraine. Cephalalgia 30(10):1187–1194

Pradalier A, Clapin A, Dry J (1988) Treatment review: non-steroidal anti-inflammatory drugs in the treatment and long-term prevention of migraine attacks. Headache 28:550–557

Pradalier A, Vincent D, Beaulieu P, Baudesson G, Launey J-M (1994) Correlation between estradiol plasma level and therapeutic effect on menstrual migraine. In: Rose F (ed) New advances in headache research. Smith-Gordon, London, pp 129–132

Sances G, Martignoni E, Fioroni L, Blandini F, Facchinetti F, Nappi G (1990) Naproxen sodium in menstrual migraine prophylaxis: a double-blind placebo controlled study. Headache 30:705–709

Sances G, Granella F, Nappi RE, Fignon A, Ghiotto N, Polatti F, Nappi G (2003) Course of migraine during pregnancy and postpartum: a prospective study. Cephalalgia 23:197–205

Sarrel PM (1999) The differential effects of oestrogens and progestins on vascular tone. Hum Reprod Update 5:205–209

Scharff L, Marcus DA, Turk DC (1997) Headache during pregnancy and in the postpartum: a prospective study. Headache 37:203–210

Silberstein SD, Elkind AH, Schreiber C, Keywood C (2004) A randomized trial of frovatriptan for the intermittent prevention of menstrual migraine. Neurology 63:261–269

Silberstein SD, Berner T, Tobin J, Xiang Q, Campbell JC (2009) Scheduled short-term prevention with frovatriptan for migraine occurring exclusively in association with menstruation. Headache 49:1283–1297

Singh I, Singh I (1947) Progesterone in the treatment of migraine. Lancet i:745–747

Smits MG, van der Meer YG, Pfeil JP, Rijnierse JJ, Vos AJ (1994) Perimenstrual migraine: effect of Estraderm TTS and the value of contingent negative variation and exteroceptive temporalis muscle suppression test. Headache 34:103–106

Somerville BW (1971) The role of progesterone in menstrual migraine. Neurology 21:853–859

Somerville BW (1972a) The role of estradiol withdrawal in the etiology of menstrual migraine. Neurology 22:355–365

Somerville BW (1972b) The influence of progesterone and estradiol upon migraine. Headache 12:93–102

Somerville BW (1975a) Estrogen-withdrawal migraine II. Attempted prophylaxis by continuous estradiol administration. Neurology 25:245–250

Somerville BW (1975b) Estrogen-withdrawal migraine. I. Duration of exposure required and attempted prophylaxis by premenstrual estrogen administration. Neurology 25:239–244

Stein G, Morton J, Marsh A, Collins W, Branch C, Desaga U, Ebeling J (1984) Headaches after childbirth. Acta Neurol Scand 69:74–79

Steiner TJ, Scher AI, Stewart WF, Kolodner K, Liberman J, Lipton RB (2003) The prevalence and disability burden of adult migraine in England and their relationships to age, gender and ethnicity. Cephalalgia 23:519–527

Stewart WF, Linet MS, Celentano DD, Van Natta M, Ziegler D (1991) Age- and sex-specific incidence rates of migraine with and without visual aura. Am J Epidemiol 134:1111–1120

Stewart WF, Lipton RB, Celentano DD, Reed ML (1992) Prevalence of migraine headache in the United States. Relation to age, income, race, and other sociodemographic factors. JAMA 267:64–69

Stewart WF, Lipton RB, Chee E, Sawyer J, Silberstein SD (2000) Menstrual cycle and headache in a population sample of migraineurs. Neurology 55:1517–1523

Stewart WF, Wood C, Reed ML, Roy J, Lipton RB (2008) Cumulative lifetime migraine incidence in women and men. Cephalalgia 28:1170–1178

Stoffel-Wagner B (1993) Neurosteroid biosynthesis in the human brain and its clinical implications. Ann NY Acad Sci 1007:64–78

Tuchman MM, Hee A, Emeribe U, Silberstein S (2008) Oral zolmitriptan in the short-term prevention of menstrual migraine: a randomized, placebo-controlled study. CNS Drugs 22:877–886

Wang SJ, Fuh JL, Lu SR, Juang KD, Wang PH (2003) Migraine prevalence during menopausal transition. Headache 43:470–478

Welch KM, Brandes JL, Berman NE (2006) Mismatch in how oestrogen modulates molecular and neuronal function may explain menstrual migraine. Neurol Sci 27(Suppl 2):S190–S192

Wober C, Brannath W, Schmidt K, Kapitan M, Rudel E, Wessely P, Wober-Bingol C (2007) Prospective analysis of factors related to migraine attacks: the PAMINA study. Cephalalgia 27:304–314

World Health Organization (2009) Medical eligibility criteria for contraceptive use. WHO, Geneva

Wright G, Patel M (1986) Focal migraine and pregnancy. BMJ 293:1557–1558

10 Comorbidities of Headache Disorders

Markus Schürks[1,2] · *Dawn C. Buse*[3,4] · *Shuu-Jiun Wang*[5,6]
[1]Brigham and Women's Hospital, Harvard Medical School, Boston, MA, USA
[2]University Hospital Essen, Essen, Germany
[3]Albert Einstein College of Medicine of Yeshiva University, Bronx, NY, USA
[4]Montefiore Headache Center, Bronx, NY, USA
[5]Neurological Institute, Taipei Veterans General Hospital, Taipei, Taiwan
[6]National Yang-Ming University School of Medicine, Taipei, Taiwan

Paolo Martelletti, Timothy J. Steiner (eds.), *Handbook of Headache*, DOI 10.1007/978-88-470-1700-9_10,
© Lifting The Burden 2011

Abstract: Headaches are common disorders and migraine is most intensively investigated due to its high prevalence and often highly disabling character. Many conditions that are likewise prevalent have been described comorbid with migraine, and an increase of many comorbid conditions is seen among those with migraine with aura and higher frequency of headache. Well-established comorbidities include cardiovascular, psychiatric, neurological, and other pain disorders. With regard to cardiovascular disorders an association between migraine with aura and ischemic stroke has been most consistently described. Migraine with aura confers a twofold increased risk. Younger age, female gender, smoking, and oral contraceptive use seem to further raise the risk among migraineurs. With regard to psychiatric disorders, those with migraine are at increased risk of major depression, anxiety, panic disorder, bipolar disorder, abuse and neglect, and suicidal ideation or attempts. Common neurologic comorbidities include epilepsy and restless leg syndrome. Potential explanations for increased comorbidities will be explored. The complex network of an association between migraine and many other comorbid conditions is likely due to shared genetic factors that are further modified by environmental factors.

Introduction

Headache disorders are common and affect a large proportion of the population. Among those, tension-type headache (TTH) is most frequent with prevalence up to 80%. Migraine affects "only" 12–16% of the population, but is often more debilitating than TTH. As a consequence migraine has been a more popular research subject than any other form of headache.

Comorbidity may be defined as association between two disorders at a rate higher than expected by coincidence (Feinstein 1970). Studying comorbidity of headache and migraine may provide valuable epidemiological, clinical, and biological insights (Lipton and Silberstein 1994). The clinically heterogeneous picture of migraine with its wide spectrum of signs and symptoms leaves ample room to accommodate various other disorders or conditions into a biological model for migraine. We will put selected comorbidities into perspective and speculate about possible underlying mechanisms. In this chapter we will focus on comorbid conditions that are most frequently investigated and have a high public health impact. We will address and give examples for the following disorders/conditions: cardiovascular disease (CVD), psychiatric disorders, neurological disorders, and chronic pain syndromes.

Established Knowledge

Headache and Cardiovascular Disease

The first case-control study reporting that migraine increases risk for stroke was published in 1975 (Collaborative Group for the Study of Stroke in Young Women 1975). However, it also became apparent that the migraine-stroke association may not be simple, but may differ for ischemic and hemorrhagic events and may be further modified by environmental factors such as oral contraceptives.

The first systematic summary and meta-analysis of studies on the association between migraine and ischemic stroke was published in 2005 (Etminan et al. 2005). The authors reported a twofold increased risk for ischemic stroke among migraineurs, occurring for both migraine with aura (MA) and migraine without aura (MO). Subsequent large studies have added complexity by suggesting, for example, that an increased risk may only occur for MA, but not for MO, and may not be restricted to stroke, but also extend to myocardial infarction, and death due to CVD (Sternfeld et al. 1995; Hall et al. 2004; Velentgas et al. 2004; Ahmed et al. 2006; Kurth et al. 2006, 2007; Liew et al. 2007).

A meta-analysis of studies published until January 2009 reevaluated the evidence on the association between migraine and CVD events, including stroke subtypes, myocardial infarction, and death due to CVD (Schürks et al. 2009b). The authors confirmed an increased risk for ischemic stroke for any migraine (pooled relative risk [RR] = 1.73, 95% confidence interval [CI] 1.31–2.29). But a significantly twofold increased risk appeared only for MA (pooled RR = 2.16, 95% CI 1.53–3.03), and not for MO (pooled RR = 1.23, 95% CI 0.90–1.69). Further subgroup analyses suggested that the association between any migraine and ischemic stroke was more pronounced among women (pooled RR = 2.08, 95% CI 1.13–3.84) than men (pooled RR = 1.37, 95% CI 0.89–2.11). Age <45 years, smoking, and oral contraceptive use were additional factors increasing the risk for ischemic stroke. In contrast, the data did not suggest an increased risk for hemorrhagic stroke (pooled RR = 1.18, 95% CI 0.87–1.60), myocardial infarction (pooled RR = 1.12, 95% CI 0.95–1.32), and death due to CVD (pooled RR = 1.03, 95% CI 0.79–1.34). Result from the most recent population-based case-control study (Bigal et al. 2010) largely agreed with the meta-analysis (Schürks et al. 2009b). The authors reported an increased risk for stroke in MA (adjusted odds ratio [OR] = 2.78, 95% CI 2.02–3.84), but not MO (adjusted OR = 0.97, 95% CI 0.69–1.36). In contrast with the meta-analysis (Schürks et al. 2009b), however, agreeing with previous prospective cohort studies (Kurth et al. 2006, 2007), they found an increased risk for myocardial infarction among migraineurs (adjusted OR = 2.16, 95% CI 1.70–2.76), which was stronger for MA (adjusted OR = 2.86, 95% CI 2.14–3.82) than for MO (adjusted OR = 1.85, 95% CI 1.41–2.42). Of note, in this study CVD events were self-reported and data were only available for overall stroke.

In contrast to data about the relative risk, there is little information about the absolute risk attributable to migraine or MA. Estimates from a case-control study of women aged <45 suggest an incidence rate of 6 ischemic strokes per 100,000 women/year for women without migraine and 19 per 100,000 women/year for women with migraine (Tzourio et al. 1995). This translates into an absolute risk of 13 additional cases of ischemic stroke per 100,000 (or 1.3 per 10,000) women/year due to migraine. Data from the Women's Health Study (women aged ≥45) indicate age-adjusted incidence rates for ischemic stroke of 8.8 per 10,000 women/year among women without migraine and 13.1 per 10,000 women/year among women with MA (Kurth et al. 2006). This translates into 4 additional cases of ischemic stroke per 10,000 women/year due to MA.

In summary, the most firmly established association is between MA and ischemic stroke. Directionality and causality are important aspects to consider (Kurth 2007). In rare cases a migraine attack causes an ischemic stroke (migrainous infarction) or migraine occurs as a result of an ischemic stroke. The majority of cases do not exhibit such tight temporal relationships. Data from prospective cohort studies indicate that MA is associated with incident ischemic stroke (directionality). Causality is less clear, but potential mechanisms include shared susceptibility factors manifesting at different ages and interaction between susceptibility factors for MA and CVD.

Headache and Risk Factors for Cardiovascular Disease

Population-based studies have associated migraine with an unfavorable cardiovascular risk profile including increased lipid levels, diabetes, elevated blood pressure, history of early onset vascular disease, and higher Framingham risk score (FRS) (Scher et al. 2005b; Bigal et al. 2010). This was more pronounced in MA than in MO. These findings prompted speculations that the association between MA and vascular events is confounded by CVD risk factors. However, the association between migraine and ischemic vascular events appears to be independent of many cardiovascular risk factors (Kurth et al. 2006, 2007). Furthermore, the increased risk of ischemic stroke is more apparent among migraineurs without cardiovascular risk factors (Henrich and Horwitz 1989; Kurth et al. 2005; MacClellan et al. 2007) with the exception of smoking and oral contraceptive use (Schürks et al. 2009b).

Several studies have reported on a prothrombotic and inflammatory state in migraine. Among these are elevated levels of prothrombin fragment 1 and 2 (Hering-Hanit et al. 2001), elevated levels of von Willebrand factor (Tietjen et al. 2007a, 2009b), increased platelet activation (D'Andrea et al. 1982; Tietjen et al. 2007a), impaired fibrinolysis (Bianchi et al. 1996), and increased C-reactive protein and markers for oxidative stress (Welch et al. 2006; Vanmolkot and de Hoon 2007; Kurth et al. 2008a; Tietjen et al. 2009b). Most of the findings were more pronounced in MA than MO. These findings agree with results from a population-based study suggesting an increased risk for thromboembolism in migraine (Schwaiger et al. 2008).

Common genetic variants, for example, in the genes coding for the methylenetetrahydrofolate reductase (MTHFR) and the angiotensin-converting enzyme (ACE) have been implicated in both migraine and CVD. Recent meta-analyses, however, found only small effects for migraine (Schürks et al. 2010), ischemic stroke (Casas et al. 2004), and coronary heart disease (Lewis et al. 2005; Zintzaras et al. 2008).

Headache and Vasculopathy

Migraine has been associated with disorders affecting the endothelium/vasculature including Rose angina (Rose et al. 2004), retinal vessel abnormalities (Rose et al. 2007), Raynaud syndrome (O'Keeffe et al. 1993), and – particularly in young female migraineurs – livedo reticularis (Tietjen et al. 2002a, b) and Sneddon's syndrome (Tietjen et al. 2006). Additional studies reported functional impairment of the retinal (Gomi et al. 1989), intracranial (Sakai and Meyer 1979; Totaro et al. 1997; Kastrup et al. 1998; Fiermonte et al. 1999; Silvestrini et al. 2004), and systemic vasculature in migraineurs of recent onset (Vanmolkot et al. 2007). This agrees with reports of dysfunctional vascular smooth muscle cells (Napoli et al. 2009) and a reduced number and impaired function of circulating endothelial progenitor cells in migraine (Lee et al. 2008). The latter findings were more pronounced in MA than MO. Interestingly, coronary and carotid arteries in active migraineurs appear less severely affected by atherosclerosis than in non-migraineurs (Ahmed et al. 2006; Schwaiger et al. 2008), suggesting a systemic vasculopathy rather than atherosclerotic mechanisms underlying the association between migraine and CVD events.

Headache, Silent Brain Infarcts, and White Matter Lesions

A population-based study has reported higher odds of subclinical brain lesions/white matter lesions among patients with migraine (Kruit et al. 2004, 2006). This was restricted to the posterior circulation and predominantly found in MA. Further studies are under way, in particular to evaluate if these brain lesions change over time.

Headache and Patent Foramen Ovale

A potential link between patent foramen ovale (PFO), MA, and risk of ischemic stroke has been discussed (Diener et al. 2007). Paradoxical micro-embolization through a PFO may be a potential mechanism increasing the risk of ischemic stroke in MA (Nozari et al. 2010). The association between migraine and PFO was recently reviewed and the grade of evidence judged as only low to moderate (Schwedt et al. 2008). In addition, recent population-based (Rundek et al. 2008) and clinic-based studies (Garg et al. 2010) did not find an association between migraine and PFO. There is also little evidence whether a PFO modifies the association between MA and ischemic stroke. One study investigated whether the association of MA and ischemic stroke differs by having a PFO or not and the authors did not find a difference (MacClellan et al. 2007). Furthermore, patients with MA and right-to-left shunt did not show an increased white matter lesion load (Adami et al. 2008; Del Sette et al. 2008).

Headache and Psychiatric Disorders

Several psychiatric disorders are established as comorbid with migraine. Such comorbidities have many negative consequences beyond the obvious burden and suffering. They negatively affect quality of life, treatment satisfaction, adherence, success, and clinical course, thus worsening prognosis, increasing headache-related disability, and increasing medical costs (Guidetti et al. 1998; Wang et al. 2001; Pesa and Lage 2004; Lanteri-Minet et al. 2005; Smitherman et al. 2008b; Baskin and Smitherman 2009).

Successfully treating psychiatric comorbidities may positively influence the course of migraine and prevent chronification (Bigal and Lipton 2006a).

Depression

The comorbidity between migraine and depression has been reviewed recently (Hamelsky and Lipton 2006). Several studies report increased ORs for depression ranging from 2.2 to 4.0 among migraineurs (Merikangas et al. 1988; Merikangas et al. 1990; Breslau et al. 1991, 1994a, b, 2000; Breslau and Davis 1993; Merikangas et al. 1994; McWilliams et al. 2004). However, the link is bidirectional, with either disorder increasing the risk of subsequent first onset of the other (Breslau et al. 1994a, 2000). The risk of new onset of migraine in people with depression is increased 2.8–3.5-fold and the risk of new onset of depression in migraineurs 2.4–5.8-fold.

A population-based study reported that 28.5% of subjects with migraine met criteria for depression compared to 12.3% of subjects without migraine (McWilliams et al. 2004). Further, the prevalence appears higher among patients with chronic migraine (CM) than those with episodic migraine (EM). In a clinic-based study, 57% of patients with CM had major depression (Juang et al. 2000). Data from the American Migraine Prevalence and Prevention Study (AMPP) found that CM was associated with increased odds for depression compared to EM (Buse et al. 2010). Respondents with CM were twice as likely to have depression both as measured by the Patient Health Questionnaire-9 (CM 30.2% vs EM 17.2%; OR = 2.0, 95% CI 1.67–2.40) and as reported history of medical diagnosis (CM 42.2% vs EM 25.6%; OR = 2.0, 95% CI 1.68–2.34). Another study confirmed increasing odds of depression with increasing headache frequency (Zwart et al. 2003). Compared to migraine-free controls, the OR (95% CI) of depression in migraineurs with headache on ≤ 7 days/month was 2.0 (1.6–2.5), on 7–14 days/month 4.2 (3.2–5.6), and on ≥ 15 days/month 6.4 (4.4–9.3). Further, a community-based study found that 66% of patients with CM had minor psychiatric disorders as evaluated by Chinese Health Questionnaire compared with 36% of those with chronic TTH (Lu et al. 2001).

The presence of major depression is a predictor of poor treatment outcome in patients with chronic daily headache (Lu et al. 2000) and other forms of headache, and may also play a role in progression of migraine from EM to CM (Ashina et al. 2010a).

Anxiety Disorders

Comorbid anxiety disorders are well documented in migraine (Merikangas et al. 1990; Breslau et al. 1991; Smoller et al. 2003; McWilliams et al. 2004). Patients with migraine more likely have generalized anxiety than those without migraine (9.1% vs 2.5%; OR = 3.9, 95% CI 2.5–6.0) (McWilliams et al. 2004). In addition, young migraineurs have an increased risk for generalized anxiety disorder (OR = 5.3, 95% CI 1.8–15.8) and social phobia (OR = 3.4, 95% CI 1.1–10.9) (Merikangas et al. 1990).

Patients with CM have higher rates of anxiety disorders than those with EM. A recent analysis from the AMPP study reported that those with CM were approximately twice as likely to report history of anxiety compared with those with EM (30.2% vs 18.8%; OR = 1.8, 95% CI 1.51–2.15) (Buse et al. 2010). Other studies reported similar patterns of association (Zwart et al. 2003). Further, anxiety may play a role in migraine chronification (Smitherman et al. 2008a, b; Ashina et al. 2010b).

Panic Disorder

A relationship has been demonstrated between panic and headache disorders (Stewart et al. 1989, 1994; Breslau et al. 1991). In a population-based study, the ORs (95% CI) of panic disorder were 3.7 (2.2–6.2) for migraine and 3.0 (1.5–5.8) for other severe headache disorders compared to non-headache controls (Breslau and Rasmussen 2001). Longitudinal analyses confirmed an association with an increased risk for first onset of panic disorder among persons with migraine (3.5-fold) or severe headache (5.7-fold) compared to controls. Conversely, persons with panic disorder had twofold increased risk for first onset of migraine or severe headache.

Bipolar Disorders

Migraine has been reported comorbid with bipolar disorders (Younes et al. 1986; Merikangas et al. 1990; Breslau et al. 1991; Breslau 1998; Mahmood et al. 1999; Low et al. 2003). ORs for bipolar disorders among migraine patients range from 2.9 to 7.3 (Hamelsky and Lipton 2006). It was reported that 8.8% of migraineurs and 3.3% of controls had a bipolar spectrum disorder as defined by history of a manic or hypomanic episode (OR = 2.9, 95% CI 1.1–8.8) (Merikangas et al. 1990). Among young migraineurs, the OR (95% CI) for Bipolar I was 7.3 (2.2–24.6) and for Bipolar II 5.2 (1.4–19.9) compared with controls (Breslau 1998). In a population sample of 11,904 migraineurs, patient-reported prevalence of bipolar disorder was significantly higher among those with CM compared with EM (4.6% vs 2.8%; OR = 1.56, 95% CI 1.06–2.31) (Buse et al. 2010).

Headache and Suicide

In young adults, history of migraine was associated with increased frequencies of suicidal ideation and suicide attempts (Breslau et al. 1991; Breslau 1992). The association of suicidal ideation and suicide attempts was stronger in MA (2.4-fold and 4.3-fold, respectively) than MO (1.7-fold and 2.7-fold, respectively). A recent community-based study from Taiwan (Wang et al. 2009) in adolescents (aged 13–15) demonstrated that MA (adjusted OR = 1.79) and high headache frequency (>7 days/month) (adjusted OR = 1.69) were associated with suicidal ideation. In addition, 50% of adolescents with chronic daily headache had psychiatric comorbidity and about 20% of them had a high suicide risk (Wang et al. 2007). This association was only demonstrated for MA but not MO and was independent from depression.

Co-Occurring Psychiatric Disorders

Young adults with both major depression and an anxiety disorder are twice as likely to have migraine compared with those with depression only (Merikangas et al. 1990). The researchers proposed that the combination of migraine, anxiety, and depression may constitute a distinct syndrome wherein anxiety is manifested in early childhood, followed by the occurrence of migraine, and then by discrete episodes of depressive disorders in adulthood. Similarly, subjects with anxiety and migraine had very high odds of depression compared with controls without anxiety or migraine (OR = 22.8, 95% CI 12.7–41.2) (Breslau et al. 1991).

In a cohort of adolescents (aged 13–15) with chronic daily headache, 47% had ≥1 assessed psychiatric comorbidity with major depression (21%) and panic disorder (19%) being the most common (Wang et al. 2007). Female gender and older age were found to be associated with depressive disorders. Presence of migraine was associated with psychiatric comorbidities (OR = 3.5, $p = 0.002$) especially in those with MA.

Headache and Neurological Disorders

Restless Legs Syndrome (RLS)

Clinic (Rhode et al. 2007) and population-based (Schürks et al. 2009a) studies have reported that RLS is more prevalent among migraineurs than non-migraineurs. This association appears specific for migraine and is not seen for other primary headache disorders including TTH and cluster headache (Chen et al. 2010). Migraine patients with RLS also had poorer sleep quality than controls. Among patients with migraine, the frequencies of RLS increased with an increasing number of migrainous symptoms (linear-by-linear association, $p < 0.001$), which may be due to shared underlying mechanisms.

Epilepsy

Migraine and epilepsy are both chronic conditions with episodic attacks (Haut et al. 2006). Migrainous headaches frequently occur in temporal relationships with epileptic seizures

(Leniger et al. 2003) and the co-occurrence of migraine and epilepsy has been described, in particular in children (Leniger et al. 2003; Toldo et al. 2010). In addition, MA appears to be a risk factor for seizures (Ludvigsson et al. 2006), suggesting the aura as a common trigger. In certain patients a common genetic disposition has been found (Clarke et al. 2009). However, at the population level the comorbidity of both conditions (Brodtkorb et al. 2008) as well as the shared genetic susceptibility (Ottman and Lipton 1996) are less clear.

Headache and Other Pain Disorders

Migraine often occurs with other pain conditions affecting the head (e.g., TTH, temporomandibular disorder), the musculoskeletal system (e.g., fibromyalgia, chronic fatigue syndrome, arthritis, back pain), and the viscera (e.g., irritable bowel syndrome, endometriosis) (Scher et al. 2005a, 2006; Tietjen et al. 2009a). Further, severity of cutaneous allodynia among migraineurs appears to be associated with various other pain conditions (Tietjen et al. 2009a).

The risk for comorbid pain disorders further increases with headache frequency. The authors of one study reported the following ORs (95% CI) for musculoskeletal symptoms (including pain) among migraineurs (Hagen et al. 2002): women: <7 days/month – 1.5 (1.4–1.6), 7–14 days/month – 3.2 (2.9–3.5), ≥15 days/month – 5.3 (4.4–6.5); men: <7 days/month – 1.7 (1.6–1.8), 7–14 days/month – 3.2 (2.8–3.8), ≥15 days/month – 3.6 (2.9–4.5). Analyses from the AMPP database found similar results with increased odds for chronic pain in CM compared to EM (OR = 2.4; 95% CI 2.0–2.9) (Buse et al. 2010).

Current Research

Headache and Cardiovascular Disease

Much research is devoted to identifying factors that may modify the association between migraine and CVD. In addition to the detrimental effect of younger age, smoking, and oral contraceptive use (Schürks et al. 2009b), migraine attack frequency, vascular risk factors, and certain gene variants appear to further modify this association. This may differ with regard to ischemic stroke and myocardial infarction.

Migraine Attack Frequency

An increasing risk for ischemic stroke has been suggested with rising attack frequency among women with MA (Donaghy et al. 2002; MacClellan et al. 2007). However, the association between migraine attack frequency in MA and CVD may be more complex (Kurth et al. 2009). Risk for ischemic stroke was associated with low attack frequency <monthly (twofold increase) and even stronger with high attack frequency ≥weekly (fourfold increase), but not with monthly attack frequency. In contrast, myocardial infarction was only associated with low attack frequency <monthly (over twofold increase), but not with more frequent attacks.

Vascular Risk Factors

Using the FRS for vascular risk classification of women with MA, those in the lowest FRS group had an almost fourfold increased risk for ischemic stroke, but no elevated risk for myocardial infarction (Kurth et al. 2008b). The association was inverse in the highest risk group. Women with MA had no elevated risk for ischemic stroke, but a more than threefold increased risk for myocardial infarction. In contrast, women with MO did not have increased risk of any vascular event regardless of the FRS risk group they were in.

Obesity is not associated with migraine prevalence (Bigal et al. 2006) or migraine aura (Winter et al. 2009), rather with higher attack frequency, severity, and features like photo- and phonophobia among migraineurs (Bigal et al. 2006; Winter et al. 2009). In addition, obesity is a risk factor for chronic daily headaches (Scher et al. 2003; Bigal and Lipton 2006b).

Gene Variants

The twofold increased risk for CVD among women with MA may be modified by the *MTHFR* 677C > T and *ACE* D/I polymorphisms. Coexistence of MA and the *MTHFR* 677TT genotype selectively raises the risk for CVD. This pattern is driven by a fourfold increased risk for ischemic stroke and not apparent for myocardial infarction (Schürks et al. 2008). Moreover, the twofold increased risk for CVD in MA appears only for carriers of the *ACE* DD/DI genotypes. The risk is not significantly altered among carriers of the II genotype, a pattern similar for myocardial infarction and ischemic stroke (Schürks et al. 2009c).

Headache and Psychiatric Disorders

Abuse, Maltreatment, and Neglect

Recent research has examined the relationship between migraine and childhood abuse, neglect, and maltreatment (Tietjen et al. 2010a, b, c). Migraineurs from headache centers across the USA and Canada reported the following rates of childhood maltreatment: physical abuse 21%, sexual abuse 25%, emotional abuse 38%, physical neglect 22%, and emotional neglect 38%. Migraineurs with history of abuse frequently reported current depression (28%) and anxiety (56%). Those who endorsed three or more categories of childhood mistreatment were more likely to be diagnosed with depression or anxiety (OR = 3.66, 95% CI 2.28–5.88), or both (OR = 6.91, 95% CI 3.97–12.03), when compared with migraineurs without such history. Additionally, emotional abuse in childhood was associated with CM, transformed migraine, continuous daily headache, significantly younger median age of headache onset, severe headache-related disability, and migraine-associated allodynia.

The association of childhood physical maltreatment with migraine could occur early in adolescence (Fuh et al. 2010). Among 3,955 Taiwanese adolescents, those reporting physical maltreatment were more likely to suffer migraine or probable migraine than those reporting no physical maltreatment (30.3% vs 21.3%, OR = 1.6, 95% CI 1.4–1.9). A higher frequency of physical maltreatment was associated with a higher likelihood of migraine (21.3% vs 28.3% vs 38.3%, "never" vs "rarely" vs "sometimes or often maltreated," respectively, $p < 0.001$). In addition, among migraineurs, those reporting physical maltreatment had higher depression scores, a higher frequency of headaches, and a greater proportion of severe headaches.

Physical and Emotional Trauma

Migraine and headache in general have been linked with physical and emotional trauma. Physical trauma such as headache and neck injury (Bekkelund and Salvesen 2003; Sheftell et al. 2007) and post-traumatic stress disorder (PTSD) have been associated with increased rates of headache, higher rates of migraine and chronic daily headache (Couch and Bearss 2001), greater headache-related disability (Tietjen et al. 2007b), and increased risk of migraine chronification (Couch et al. 2007; Tietjen et al. 2010b). The frequency of PTSD in migraineurs is higher than in the general population, and among migraineurs with depression, the prevalence of PTSD is greater in chronic daily headache than in EM (Peterlin 2009).

Discussion

Migraine and other headaches are common and comorbid with many conditions including CVD, psychiatric disorders, neurological disorders, and chronic pain syndromes. Most of these syndromes are likewise frequent. Hence, given the high prevalence we would expect them to often co-occur with migraine and other headaches. However, the picture may not be that simple. For example, the association between migraine, in particular MA, and CVD is not straight and unconditional. Severity of migraine (e.g., attack frequency) appears to play a role and "more" of migraine does not mean "more" of comorbidity as outlined above. It rather depends on which comorbid condition is investigated (e.g., ischemic stroke or myocardial infarction) and likely on additional factors (e.g., smoking, oral contraceptive use).

Comorbidities can be conceptualized in terms of directionality (unidirectional vs bidirectional) and causality (direct causality, indirect causality, or a shared underlying mechanism) (Lipton and Silberstein 1994). For example, to evaluate the comorbid relationship between migraine and depression, a unilateral causal association can be proposed from migraine to depression, in that the experience of pain, disease-related burden and impairment, and feelings of hopeless and helplessness may lead to depression (based on the learned helplessness theory of depression) (Seligman 1975). Conversely, a causal unidirectional hypothesis from depression to migraine may be proposed based upon the psychodynamic theory that pain is an outward somatic manifestation of depression and despair (Dworkin et al. 1990; Von Korff et al. 2005). However, research has demonstrated that the relationship is bidirectional; each disorder predisposes the other, which may be due in part to shared underlying mechanisms such as dysregulation in the serotonergic, noradrenergic, or dopaminergic systems. Other comorbid conditions may share different mechanisms like inflammatory or metabolic syndromes, stressful life events, and/or certain genetic variants with migraine.

The findings of a complex comorbidity network in which migraine and other headaches are single components (i.e., phenotypes) are most compatible with the concept of shared genetic and environmental factors. Let us consider the following: Each of the phenotypes in this network – migraine, ischemic stroke, depression, anxiety, etc. – is likely determined by a large number of gene variants. And each of these variants has a low to moderate impact on the phenotypes. While some genes may only affect one phenotype, others may affect two or more phenotypes. This concept of multiple phenotypes sharing certain genotypes (i.e., pleiotropy) is considered common in many complex disorders. Biological plausibility for this concept in migraine, for example, is supported by rare monogenic syndromes like CADASIL presenting phenotypes of both migraine and ischemic stroke. Furthermore, a recent twin study provided evidence that 20% of the variability in depression and migraine was due to shared genes (Schur et al. 2009). Depending on how many of these exclusive or shared genotypes an individual harbors, the risk for number and severity of phenotypes will be determined. Further complexity is added since environmental factors (e.g., smoking, exogenous hormones, stress) appear to interact with certain gene variants, thus modifying their impact ("epigenetic factors"). This complex network of phenotypes will probably yield many more interesting findings about associations in the future and may offer interesting explanations regarding the mechanisms for each of the disorders including headaches.

Conclusion

Migraine and other headaches are common and comorbid with many other conditions. Some of the best established comorbidity data have focused on CVD, psychiatric disorders, neurologic disorders, and chronic pain syndromes. Rates and specific comorbid conditions vary depending on migraine type and headache frequency as well as environmental and lifestyle factors.

The frequency of comorbid conditions with headaches, in particular migraine, highlights the importance for clinicians to maintain diagnostic vigilance and provide appropriate treatment or referrals when necessary. Beyond the obvious burden and suffering caused by comorbid conditions, comorbidities potentiate the negative consequences of health-related quality of life, negatively impact treatment adherence, patient motivation, and treatment satisfaction, and are related to worse outcomes, which may also include chronification of migraine. Therefore, it is exceptionally important to diagnose and treat comorbidities. They must also be taken into account when formulating safe and effective treatment plans.

Future research involving diligently characterized clinic-based and large population-based cohorts is warranted. Unresolved questions that will fertilize research include the following: (1) Does the huge comorbidity burden specifically affect migraine or are other headache disorders likewise associated with various comorbid conditions? (2) Are migraine patients at a generally increased risk for comorbidities or are there certain subgroups of migraineurs that are more prone to either CVD, depression, or RLS, for example? (3) What is the underlying cause linking migraine with so many other conditions? Specifically which genes and environmental factors increase the risk for comorbidities among migraine/headache patients?

References

Adami A, Rossato G, Cerini R, Thijs VN, Pozzi-Mucelli R, Anzola GP, Del Sette M, Finocchi C, Meneghetti G, Zanferrari C, Group SAMS (2008) Right-to-left shunt does not increase white matter lesion load in migraine with aura patients. Neurology 71:101–107

Ahmed B, Bairey Merz CN, McClure C, Johnson BD, Reis SE, Bittner V, Pepine CJ, Sharaf BL, Sopko G, Kelsey SF, Shaw L (2006) Migraines, angiographic coronary artery disease and cardiovascular outcomes in women. Am J Med 119:670–675

Ashina S, Buse DC, Maizels M, Manack A, Serrano D, Turkel C, Lipton RB (2010a) Depression: a risk factor for migraine chronification: results from the American Migraine Prevalence and Prevention (AMPP) study. 62nd Annual Meeting of the American Academy of Neurology, Toronto

Ashina S, Buse DC, Maizels M, Manack A, Serrano D, Turkel CC, Lipton RB (2010b) Self-reported anxiety as a risk factor for migraine chronification. Results from the American Migraine Prevalence and

Prevention (AMPP) study. 52nd Annual Scientific Meeting of the American Headache Society, Los Angeles

Baskin SM, Smitherman TA (2009) Migraine and psychiatric disorders: comorbidities, mechanisms, and clinical applications. Neurol Sci 30(Suppl 1):S61–S65

Bekkelund SI, Salvesen R (2003) Prevalence of head trauma in patients with difficult headache: the North Norway Headache Study. Headache 43:59–62

Bianchi A, Pitari G, Amenta V, Giuliano F, Gallina M, Costa R, Ferlito S (1996) Endothelial, haemostatic and haemorheological modifications in migraineurs. Artery 22:93–100

Bigal ME, Lipton RB (2006a) Modifiable risk factors for migraine progression. Headache 46:1334–1343

Bigal ME, Lipton RB (2006b) Obesity is a risk factor for transformed migraine but not chronic tension-type headache. Neurology 67:252–257

Bigal ME, Liberman JN, Lipton RB (2006) Obesity and migraine: a population study. Neurology 66:545–550

Bigal ME, Kurth T, Santanello N, Buse D, Golden W, Robbins M, Lipton RB (2010) Migraine and cardiovascular disease: a population-based study. Neurology 74:628–635

Breslau N (1992) Migraine, suicidal ideation, and suicide attempts. Neurology 42:392–395

Breslau N (1998) Psychiatric comorbidity in migraine. Cephalalgia 18(Suppl 22):56–58, discussion 58-61

Breslau N, Davis GC (1993) Migraine, physical health and psychiatric disorder: a prospective epidemiologic study in young adults. J Psychiatr Res 27:211–221

Breslau N, Rasmussen BK (2001) The impact of migraine: Epidemiology, risk factors, and co-morbidities. Neurology 56:S4–S12

Breslau N, Davis GC, Andreski P (1991) Migraine, psychiatric disorders, and suicide attempts: an epidemiologic study of young adults. Psychiatry Res 37:11–23

Breslau N, Davis GC, Schultz LR, Peterson EL (1994a) Joint 1994 Wolff Award Presentation. Migraine and major depression: a longitudinal study. Headache 34:387–393

Breslau N, Merikangas K, Bowden CL (1994b) Comorbidity of migraine and major affective disorders. Neurology 44:S17–S22

Breslau N, Schultz LR, Stewart WF, Lipton RB, Lucia VC, Welch KM (2000) Headache and major depression: is the association specific to migraine? Neurology 54:308–313

Brodtkorb E, Bakken IJ, Sjaastad O (2008) Comorbidity of migraine and epilepsy in a Norwegian community. Eur J Neurol 15:1421–1423

Buse DC, Manack A, Serrano D, Turkel C, Lipton RB (2010) Sociodemographic and comorbidity profiles of chronic migraine and episodic migraine sufferers.

J Neurol Neurosurg Psychiatry. doi:10.1136/jnnp.2009.192492

Casas JP, Hingorani AD, Bautista LE, Sharma P (2004) Meta-analysis of genetic studies in ischemic stroke: thirty-two genes involving approximately 18,000 cases and 58,000 controls. Arch Neurol 61:1652–1661

Chen PK, Fuh JL, Chen SP, Wang SJ (2010) Association between restless legs syndrome and migraine. J Neurol Neurosurg Psychiatry 81(5):524–528

Clarke T, Baskurt Z, Strug LJ, Pal DK (2009) Evidence of shared genetic risk factors for migraine and rolandic epilepsy. Epilepsia 50:2428–2433

Collaborative Group for the Study of Stroke in Young Women (1975) Oral contraceptives and stroke in young women. Associated risk factors. JAMA 231:718–722

Couch JR, Bearss C (2001) Chronic daily headache in the posttrauma syndrome: relation to extent of head injury. Headache 41:559–564

Couch JR, Lipton RB, Stewart WF, Scher AI (2007) Head or neck injury increases the risk of chronic daily headache: a population-based study. Neurology 69:1169–1177

D'Andrea G, Toldo M, Cortelazzo S, Milone FF (1982) Platelet activity in migraine. Headache 22:207–212

Del Sette M, Dinia L, Bonzano L, Roccatagliata L, Finocchi C, Parodi RC, Sivori G, Gandolfo C (2008) White matter lesions in migraine and right-to-left shunt: a conventional and diffusion MRI study. Cephalalgia 28:376–382

Diener HC, Kurth T, Dodick D (2007) Patent foramen ovale, stroke, and cardiovascular disease in migraine. Curr Opin Neurol 20:310–319

Donaghy M, Chang CL, Poulter N (2002) Duration, frequency, recency, and type of migraine and the risk of ischaemic stroke in women of childbearing age. J Neurol Neurosurg Psychiatry 73:747–750

Dworkin SF, Von Korff M, LeResche L (1990) Multiple pains and psychiatric disturbance An epidemiologic investigation. Arch Gen Psychiatry 47:239–244

Etminan M, Takkouche B, Isorna FC, Samii A (2005) Risk of ischaemic stroke in people with migraine: systematic review and meta-analysis of observational studies. BMJ 330:63

Feinstein AR (1970) The pretherapeutic classification of comorbidity in chronic disease. J Chron Dis 23:455–468

Fiermonte G, Annulli A, Pierelli F (1999) Transcranial Doppler evaluation of cerebral hemodynamics in migraineurs during prophylactic treatment with flunarizine. Cephalalgia 19:492–496

Fuh JL, Wang SJ, Juang KD, Lu SR, Liao YC, Chen SP (2010) Relationship between childhood physical maltreatment and migraine in adolescents. Headache 50:761–768

Garg P, Servoss SJ, Wu JC, Bajwa ZH, Selim MH, Dineen A, Kuntz RE, Cook EF, Mauri L (2010) Lack of association between migraine headache and patent foramen ovale: results of a case-control study. Circulation 121:1406–1412

Gomi S, Gotoh F, Komatsumoto S, Ishikawa Y, Araki N, Hamada J (1989) Sweating function and retinal vasomotor reactivity in migraine. Cephalalgia 9:179–185

Guidetti V, Galli F, Fabrizi P, Giannantoni AS, Napoli L, Bruni O, Trillo S (1998) Headache and psychiatric comorbidity: clinical aspects and outcome in an 8-year follow-up study. Cephalalgia 18:455–462

Hagen K, Einarsen C, Zwart JA, Svebak S, Bovim G (2002) The co-occurrence of headache and musculoskeletal symptoms amongst 51 050 adults in Norway. Eur J Neurol 9:527–533

Hall GC, Brown MM, Mo J, MacRae KD (2004) Triptans in migraine: the risks of stroke, cardiovascular disease, and death in practice. Neurology 62:563–568

Hamelsky SW, Lipton RB (2006) Psychiatric comorbidity of migraine. Headache 46:1327–1333

Haut SR, Bigal ME, Lipton RB (2006) Chronic disorders with episodic manifestations: focus on epilepsy and migraine. Lancet Neurol 5:148–157

Henrich JB, Horwitz RI (1989) A controlled study of ischemic stroke risk in migraine patients. J Clin Epidemiol 42:773–780

Hering-Hanit R, Friedman Z, Schlesinger I, Ellis M (2001) Evidence for activation of the coagulation system in migraine with aura. Cephalalgia 21:137–139

Juang KD, Wang SJ, Fuh JL, Lu SR, Su TP (2000) Comorbidity of depressive and anxiety disorders in chronic daily headache and its subtypes. Headache 40:818–823

Kastrup A, Thomas C, Hartmann C, Schabet M (1998) Cerebral blood flow and CO2 reactivity in interictal migraineurs: a transcranial Doppler study. Headache 38:608–613

Kruit MC, van Buchem MA, Hofman PA, Bakkers JT, Terwindt GM, Ferrari MD, Launer LJ (2004) Migraine as a risk factor for subclinical brain lesions. JAMA 291:427–434

Kruit MC, Launer LJ, Ferrari MD, van Buchem MA (2006) Brain stem and cerebellar hyperintense lesions in migraine. Stroke 37:1109–1112

Kurth T (2007) Migraine and ischaemic vascular events. Cephalalgia 27:967–975

Kurth T, Slomke MA, Kase CS, Cook NR, Lee IM, Gaziano JM, Diener HC, Buring JE (2005) Migraine, headache, and the risk of stroke in women: a prospective study. Neurology 64:1020–1026

Kurth T, Gaziano JM, Cook NR, Logroscino G, Diener HC, Buring JE (2006) Migraine and risk of cardiovascular disease in women. JAMA 296:283–291

Kurth T, Gaziano JM, Cook NR, Bubes V, Logroscino G, Diener HC, Buring JE (2007) Migraine and risk of cardiovascular disease in men. Arch Intern Med 167:795–801

Kurth T, Ridker P, Buring J (2008a) Migraine and biomarkers of cardiovascular disease. Cephalalgia 28:49–56

Kurth T, Schürks M, Logroscino G, Gaziano JM, Buring JE (2008b) Migraine, vascular risk, and cardiovascular events in women: prospective cohort study. BMJ 337:a636

Kurth T, Schürks M, Logroscino G, Buring JE (2009) Migraine frequency and risk of cardiovascular disease in women. Neurology 73:581–588

Lanteri-Minet M, Radat F, Chautard MH, Lucas C (2005) Anxiety and depression associated with migraine: influence on migraine subjects' disability and quality of life, and acute migraine management. Pain 118:319–326

Lee ST, Chu K, Jung KH, Kim DH, Kim EH, Choe VN, Kim JH, Im WS, Kang L, Park JE, Park HJ, Park HK, Song EC, Lee SK, Kim M, Roh JK (2008) Decreased number and function of endothelial progenitor cells in patients with migraine. Neurology 70:1510–1517

Leniger T, von den Driesch S, Isbruch K, Diener HC, Hufnagel A (2003) Clinical characteristics of patients with comorbidity of migraine and epilepsy. Headache 43:672–677

Lewis SJ, Ebrahim S, Davey Smith G (2005) Meta-analysis of MTHFR 677C->T polymorphism and coronary heart disease: does totality of evidence support causal role for homocysteine and preventive potential of folate? BMJ 331:1053

Liew G, Wang JJ, Mitchell P (2007) Migraine and coronary heart disease mortality: a prospective cohort study. Cephalalgia 27:368–371

Lipton RB, Silberstein SD (1994) Why study the comorbidity of migraine? Neurology 44:S4–S5

Low NC, Du Fort GG, Cervantes P (2003) Prevalence, clinical correlates, and treatment of migraine in bipolar disorder. Headache 43:940–949

Lu SR, Fuh JL, Juang KD, Wang SJ (2000) Repetitive intravenous prochlorperazine treatment of patients with refractory chronic daily headache. Headache 40:724–729

Lu SR, Fuh JL, Chen WT, Juang KD, Wang SJ (2001) Chronic daily headache in Taipei, Taiwan: prevalence, follow-up and outcome predictors. Cephalalgia 21:980–986

Ludvigsson P, Hesdorffer D, Olafsson E, Kjartansson O, Hauser WA (2006) Migraine with aura is a risk factor for unprovoked seizures in children. Ann Neurol 59:210–213

MacClellan LR, Giles W, Cole J, Wozniak M, Stern B, Mitchell BD, Kittner SJ (2007) Probable migraine with visual aura and risk of ischemic stroke: the stroke prevention in young women study. Stroke 38: 2438–2445

Mahmood T, Romans S, Silverstone T (1999) Prevalence of migraine in bipolar disorder. J Affect Disord 52:239–241

McWilliams LA, Goodwin RD, Cox BJ (2004) Depression and anxiety associated with three pain conditions: results from a nationally representative sample. Pain 111:77–83

Merikangas KR, Risch NJ, Merikangas JR, Weissman MM, Kidd KK (1988) Migraine and depression: association and familial transmission. J Psychiatr Res 22:119–129

Merikangas KR, Angst J, Isler H (1990) Migraine and psychopathology. Results of the Zurich cohort study of young adults. Arch Gen Psychiatry 47:849–853

Merikangas KR, Whitaker AE, Isler H, Angst J (1994) The Zurich Study: XXIII. Epidemiology of headache syndromes in the Zurich cohort study of young adults. Eur Arch Psychiatry Clin Neurosci 244: 145–152

Napoli R, Guardasole V, Zarra E, Matarazzo M, D'Anna C, Sacca F, Affuso F, Cittadini A, Carrieri PB, Sacca L (2009) Vascular smooth muscle cell dysfunction in patients with migraine. Neurology 72:2111–2114

Nozari A, Dilekoz E, Sukhotinsky I, Stein T, Eikermann-Haerter K, Liu C, Wang Y, Frosch MP, Waeber C, Ayata C, Moskowitz MA (2010) Microemboli may link spreading depression, migraine aura, and patent foramen ovale. Ann Neurol 67:221–229

O'Keeffe ST, Tsapatsaris NP, Beetham WP Jr (1993) Association between Raynaud's phenomenon and migraine in a random population of hospital employees. J Rheumatol 20:1187–1188

Ottman R, Lipton RB (1996) Is the comorbidity of epilepsy and migraine due to a shared genetic susceptibility? Neurology 47:918–924

Pesa J, Lage MJ (2004) The medical costs of migraine and comorbid anxiety and depression. Headache 44:562–570

Peterlin BL (2009) Post-traumatic stress disorder in migraine: further comments. Headache 49:787

Rhode AM, Hosing VG, Happe S, Biehl K, Young P, Evers S (2007) Comorbidity of migraine and restless legs syndrome–a case-control study. Cephalalgia 27:1255–1260

Rose KM, Carson AP, Sanford CP, Stang PE, Brown CA, Folsom AR, Szklo M (2004) Migraine and other headaches: associations with Rose angina and coronary heart disease. Neurology 63:2233–2239

Rose KM, Wong TY, Carson AP, Couper DJ, Klein R, Sharrett AR (2007) Migraine and retinal microvascular abnormalities: the atherosclerosis risk in communities study. Neurology 68:1694–1700

Rundek T, Elkind MS, Di Tullio MR, Carrera E, Jin Z, Sacco RL, Homma S (2008) Patent foramen ovale and migraine: a cross-sectional study from the Northern Manhattan Study (NOMAS). Circulation 118:1419–1424

Sakai F, Meyer JS (1979) Abnormal cerebrovascular reactivity in patients with migraine and cluster headache. Headache 19:257–266

Scher AI, Stewart WF, Ricci JA, Lipton RB (2003) Factors associated with the onset and remission of chronic daily headache in a population-based study. Pain 106:81–89

Scher AI, Bigal ME, Lipton RB (2005a) Comorbidity of migraine. Curr Opin Neurol 18:305–310

Scher AI, Terwindt GM, Picavet HS, Verschuren WM, Ferrari MD, Launer LJ (2005b) Cardiovascular risk factors and migraine: the GEM population-based study. Neurology 64:614–620

Scher AI, Stewart WF, Lipton RB (2006) The comorbidity of headache with other pain syndromes. Headache 46:1416–1423

Schur EA, Noonan C, Buchwald D, Goldberg J, Afari N (2009) A twin study of depression and migraine: evidence for a shared genetic vulnerability. Headache 49:1493–1502

Schürks M, Zee RY, Buring JE, Kurth T (2008) Interrelationships among the MTHFR 677C>T polymorphism, migraine, and cardiovascular disease. Neurology 71:505–513

Schürks M, Berger K, Glynn RJ, Buring JE, Kurth T (2009a) Association between migraine and restless legs syndrome in women. Neurology 72:A182

Schürks M, Rist PM, Bigal ME, Buring JE, Lipton RB, Kurth T (2009b) Migraine and cardiovascular disease: a systematic review and meta-analysis. BMJ 339:b3914. doi:10.1136/bmj.b3914

Schürks M, Zee RYL, Buring JE, Kurth T (2009c) ACE D/I Polymorphism, migraine, and cardiovascular disease in women. Neurology 72:650–656

Schürks M, Rist PM, Kurth T (2010) MTHFR 677C>T and ACE D/I polymorphisms in migraine: a systematic review and meta-analysis. Headache 50:588–599

Schwaiger J, Kiechl S, Stockner H, Knoflach M, Werner P, Rungger G, Gasperi A, Willeit J (2008) Burden of atherosclerosis and risk of venous thromboembolism in patients with migraine. Neurology 71: 937–943

Schwedt TJ, Demaerschalk BM, Dodick DW (2008) Patent foramen ovale and migraine: a quantitative systematic review. Cephalalgia 28:531–540

Seligman MEP (1975) Helplessness: on depression, development, and death. W.H. Freeman, San Francisco

Sheftell FD, Tepper SJ, Lay CL, Bigal ME (2007) Post-traumatic headache: emphasis on chronic types following mild closed head injury. Neurol Sci 28(Suppl 2):S203–S207

Silvestrini M, Baruffaldi R, Bartolini M, Vernieri F, Lanciotti C, Matteis M, Troisi E, Provinciali L (2004) Basilar and middle cerebral artery reactivity in patients with migraine. Headache 44:29–34

Smitherman TA, Maizels M, Penzien DB (2008a) Headache chronification: screening and behavioral management of comorbid depressive and anxiety disorders. Headache 48:45–50

Smitherman TA, Penzien DB, Maizels M (2008b) Anxiety disorders and migraine intractability and progression. Curr Pain Headache Rep 12:224–229

Smoller JW, Pollack MH, Wassertheil-Smoller S, Barton B, Hendrix SL, Jackson RD, Dicken T, Oberman A, Sheps DS, Women's Health Initiative I (2003) Prevalence and correlates of panic attacks in postmenopausal women: results from an ancillary study to the women's health initiative. Arch Intern Med 163:2041–2050

Sternfeld B, Stang P, Sidney S (1995) Relationship of migraine headaches to experience of chest pain and subsequent risk for myocardial infarction. Neurology 45:2135–2142

Stewart WF, Linet MS, Celentano DD (1989) Migraine headaches and panic attacks. Psychosom Med 51:559–569

Stewart W, Breslau N, Keck PE Jr (1994) Comorbidity of migraine and panic disorder. Neurology 44:S23–S27

Tietjen GE, Al-Qasmi MM, Shukairy MS (2002a) Livedo reticularis and migraine: a marker for stroke risk? Headache 42:352–355

Tietjen GE, Gottwald L, Al-Qasmi MM, Gunda P, Khuder SA (2002b) Migraine is associated with livedo reticularis: a prospective study. Headache 42:263–267

Tietjen GE, Al-Qasmi MM, Gunda P, Herial NA (2006) Sneddon's syndrome: another migraine-stroke association? Cephalalgia 26:225–232

Tietjen GE, Al-Qasmi MM, Athanas K, Utley C, Herial NA (2007a) Altered hemostasis in migraineurs studied with a dynamic flow system. Thromb Res 119:217–222

Tietjen GE, Brandes JL, Digre KB, Baggaley S, Martin V, Recober A, Geweke LO, Hafeez F, Aurora SK, Herial NA, Utley C, Khuder SA (2007b) High prevalence of somatic symptoms and depression in women with disabling chronic headache. Neurology 68:134–140

Tietjen GE, Brandes JL, Peterlin BL, Eloff A, Dafer RM, Stein MR, Drexler E, Martin VT, Hutchinson S, Aurora SK, Recober A, Herial NA, Utley C, White L, Khuder SA (2009a) Allodynia in migraine: association with comorbid pain conditions. Headache 49:1333–1344

Tietjen GE, Herial NA, White L, Utley C, Kosmyna JM, Khuder SA (2009b) Migraine and biomarkers of endothelial activation in young women. Stroke 40:2977–2982

Tietjen GE, Brandes JL, Peterlin BL, Eloff A, Dafer RM, Stein MR, Drexler E, Martin VT, Hutchinson S, Aurora SK, Recober A, Herial NA, Utley C, White L, Khuder SA (2010a) Childhood maltreatment and migraine (Part I). Prevalence and adult revictimization: a multicenter headache clinic survey. Headache 50:20–31

Tietjen GE, Brandes JL, Peterlin BL, Eloff A, Dafer RM, Stein MR, Drexler E, Martin VT, Hutchinson S, Aurora SK, Recober A, Herial NA, Utley C, White L, Khuder SA (2010b) Childhood maltreatment and migraine (Part II). Emotional abuse as a risk factor for headache chronification. Headache 50:32–41

Tietjen GE, Brandes JL, Peterlin BL, Eloff A, Dafer RM, Stein MR, Drexler E, Martin VT, Hutchinson S, Aurora SK, Recober A, Herial NA, Utley C, White L, Khuder SA (2010c) Childhood maltreatment and migraine (Part III). Association with comorbid pain conditions. Headache 50:42–51

Toldo I, Perissinotto E, Menegazzo F, Boniver C, Sartori S, Salviati L, Clementi M, Montagna P, Battistella PA (2010) Comorbidity between headache and epilepsy in a pediatric headache center. J Headache Pain 11(3):235–240

Totaro R, Marini C, De Matteis G, Di Napoli M, Carolei A (1997) Cerebrovascular reactivity in migraine during headache-free intervals. Cephalalgia 17:191–194

Tzourio C, Tehindrazanarivelo A, Iglesias S, Alperovitch A, Chedru F, d'Anglejan-Chatillon J, Bousser MG (1995) Case-control study of migraine and risk of ischaemic stroke in young women. BMJ 310:830–833

Vanmolkot FH, de Hoon JN (2007) Increased C-reactive protein in young adult patients with migraine. Cephalalgia 27:843–846

Vanmolkot FH, Van Bortel LM, de Hoon JN (2007) Altered arterial function in migraine of recent onset. Neurology 68:1563–1570

Velentgas P, Cole JA, Mo J, Sikes CR, Walker AM (2004) Severe vascular events in migraine patients. Headache 44:642–651

Von Korff M, Crane P, Lane M, Miglioretti DL, Simon G, Saunders K, Stang P, Brandenburg N, Kessler R (2005) Chronic spinal pain and physical-mental comorbidity in the United States: results from the national comorbidity survey replication. Pain 113:331–339

Wang SJ, Fuh JL, Lu SR, Juang KD (2001) Quality of life differs among headache diagnoses: analysis of SF-36 survey in 901 headache patients. Pain 89:285–292

Wang SJ, Juang KD, Fuh JL, Lu SR (2007) Psychiatric comorbidity and suicide risk in adolescents with chronic daily headache. Neurology 68:1468–1473

Wang SJ, Fuh JL, Juang KD, Lu SR (2009) Migraine and suicidal ideation in adolescents aged 13 to 15 years. Neurology 72:1146–1152

Welch KM, Brandes AW, Salerno L, Brandes JL (2006) C-reactive protein may be increased in migraine patients who present with complex clinical features. Headache 46:197–199

Winter AC, Berger K, Buring JE, Kurth T (2009) Body mass index, migraine, migraine frequency and migraine features in women. Cephalalgia 29:269–278

Younes RP, DeLong GR, Neiman G, Rosner B (1986) Manic-depressive illness in children: treatment with lithium carbonate. J Child Neurol 1:364–368

Zintzaras E, Raman G, Kitsios G, Lau J (2008) Angiotensin-converting enzyme insertion/deletion gene polymorphic variant as a marker of coronary artery disease: a meta-analysis. Arch Intern Med 168:1077–1089

Zwart JA, Dyb G, Hagen K, Odegard KJ, Dahl AA, Bovim G, Stovner LJ (2003) Depression and anxiety disorders associated with headache frequency. The Nord-Trondelag Health Study. Eur J Neurol 10:147–152

Part 4

Correct and Timely Headache Diagnosis

11 Classification of Headache

Morris Levin[1] · *Jes Olesen*[2]
[1]Dartmouth Headache Center, Dartmouth Hitchcock Medical Center, Lebanon, NH, USA
[2]Glostrup Hospital, University of Copenhagen, Glostrup, Copenhagen, Denmark

Paolo Martelletti, Timothy J. Steiner (eds.), *Handbook of Headache*, DOI 10.1007/978-88-470-1700-9_11,
© Lifting The Burden 2011

Abstract: In order to effectively study and manage headache disorders, diagnosis is crucial. For most patients with headache, an important first step clinically is to rule out curable causes, including those due to vascular, infectious, neoplastic, and other processes. A classification schema for these many causes of headache is an important tool for making a correct diagnosis. Once secondary headache causes are ruled out, it is crucial to determine which primary headache disorder is present. But the problem clinicians encounter here is that primary headaches do not have laboratory markers, so diagnosis is phenomenological. Hence, classification of these headaches is imperative as well. Historical approaches to classifying primary and secondary headache disorders culminated in the *International Classification of Headache Disorders* (ICHD) completed and published in 1988. This was revised as the *International Classification of Headache Disorders*, 2nd edition (ICHD II) in 2004. Currently, the International Headache Society is engaged on a third edition which is projected to be completed in 2013. These classification systems are based on evidence when available, and, fortunately, research in the field of headache medicine has produced useful data applicable to classification of a number of primary and secondary headache disorders. This chapter provides a practical overview of the rationale behind the ICHD and diagnostic features of the primary and secondary headaches.

Headache Classification in History

Migraine descriptions date from ancient Egypt, but the first clear classification is seen in the writings of Aretaeus of Cappadocia, in the first century AD, who divided headaches into *cephalea* (chronic, frequent, severe, long-lasting headaches) and *cephalalgia* (infrequent milder headaches). In his "De Cephalalgia" (1672), Thomas Willis divided headaches along the following parameters: (1) within or without the skull; (2) universal or particular; (3) short, continuous, or intermittent; (4) wandering or uncertain; (5) before, behind, or the side; and (6) occasional or habitual" (Pearce 1986; Isler 1993; Gladstone and Dodick 2004).

The first significant modern attempt at classifying headache disorders was done by an ad hoc committee formed by the US National Institutes of Health (NIH) in 1962, which consisted of a number of prestigious thinkers in headache: Arnold Friedman, Knox Finley, John Graham, Charles Kunkle, Adrian Ostfeld, and Harold Wolff (Ad Hoc Committee 1962). The schema they devised (❷ *Table 11.1*) consisted of brief definitions of a limited number of headache types. With its relatively vague diagnostic definitions, this classification required a great deal of subjective interpretation and relied primarily on accepted ideas of headache diagnostic classes without much in the way of evidence to support them. The "Ad hoc" classification system, with rather idiosyncratic divisions and categories, became accepted worldwide but began to be seen as more of an impediment to advancing headache understanding than a help by the 1970s.

The International Headache Society (IHS), formed in 1982, soon embarked upon the task of classification by forming the Classification committee in 1985 with Dr. Jes Olesen as the chairman. The IHS Classification of Headache Disorders (ICHD) was published in 1988 (IHS 1988). It was 96 pages long and consisted of 165 diagnoses. The effects of the ICHD were dramatic. It served to drive massive amounts of headache research, it unified headache clinicians and researchers worldwide (it was translated into all major languages), and it made a major first step in providing much needed credibility and scientific rigor for the field of Headache Medicine. In addition, a correspondence to the International Classification of Diseases (ICD) of the World Health Organization (WHO) further promoted uniformity and

❏ **Table 11.1**

Classification of headache (Ad Hoc Committee on Classification of Headache of the National Institute of Health 1962)

1. Vascular headache
A. Classic migraine
B. Common migraine
C. Cluster
D. Hemiplegic, ophthalmoplegic migraine
E. Lower-half headache
2. Muscle contraction headache
3. Combined headache: vascular and MCH
4. Headache of nasal vasomotor reaction
5. Headache of delusional, conversion, or hypochondriacal states
6. Nonmigrainous vascular headaches
7. Traction headache
8. Headache due to overt cranial inflammation
9–13. Headache due to diseases of ear, nose, sinus, teeth
14. Cranial neuritides
15. Cranial neuralgias

accuracy in diagnosis. The revision of the IHS's classification was begun in 1999. Input was solicited from headache and other specialists around the world and a limited number of prepublication presentations were made. The *International Classification of Headache Disorders*, 2nd edition (ICHD II), was published in 2004 (HA Classification Committee 2004). The ICHD II is 160 pages long, and contains approximately 200 diagnoses. At the time of writing, the IHS Classification Committee is engaged in creating a third edition, ICHD III.

Basic Organization and Use of the ICHD

The ICHD II, like its predecessor ICHD I, consists of several parts: Part 1: Primary headaches; Part 2: Secondary headaches; Part 3: Cranial neuralgias, central, and primary facial pain and other headache; and The Appendix (❖ *Table 11.2*). Part 1, Primary Headaches, consists of 45 diagnostic categories in Chapters 1–4 and includes migraine, tension-type headache, cluster headache and its relatives, and a group of "other primary headaches." These first four "primary headache" groups are considered to have "no other causative disorder." Part 2, "secondary headaches," consists of 120 diagnostic categories in Chapters 5–12 and includes headaches "caused by another disorder" such as head trauma, vascular disease, abnormal intracranial pressure, mass lesions, hydrocephalus, and so on. In these chapters, there are headaches due to processes involving a number of structures in and around the head including the eyes, nose, sinuses, teeth, and neck. In addition, there is a chapter on headaches presumably caused by psychiatric disorders. Part 3 consists of 29 causes of facial pain or neuralgic illnesses as well as Chapter 14, "empty for now," to serve as a placeholder for any unclassifiable headache types.

◻ **Table 11.2**
International Classification of Headache Disorders, 2nd edition (ICHD II) (Headache Classification Subcommittee of the International Headache Society 2004)

Part 1: Primary headaches, Chapters 1–4 (no other causative disorder)
1. Migraine
2. Tension-type headache
3. Cluster and its relatives (TACs)
4. Other primary headaches
Part 2: Secondary headaches, Chapters 5–12 (caused by another disorder)
5. Posttraumatic
6. Vascular disease
7. Other intracranial pathology
8. Substances
9. CNS infection
10. Homeostatic disorders
11. Cervicogenic, Eyes, ENT, Sinuses, Mouth, Teeth, TMJ
12. Psychiatric
Part 3: Cranial neuralgias, central and primary facial pain, other headaches
13. Neuralgias and neuropathy
14. Other headaches (Empty for now)
Appendix

◻ **Table 11.3**
ICHD II: The Appendix contents

1. Suggested criteria for possible new entities
Example: A1.1: Menstrual migraine; A3.3 SUNA,
2. Alternative diagnostic criteria for certain categories (pending evidence)
Example: A1.5.1: Alternate Chronic Migraine definition
3. Some previously accepted disorders which have not been supported by evidence
Example: A.1.3.4: Alternating hemiplegia of childhood

The Appendix of the ICHD (❷ *Table 11.3*) is an intriguing collection of (1) suggested criteria for possible new entities, (2) alternative diagnostic criteria for certain existing categories, and (3) previously accepted disorders which have not been supported by evidence. The Appendix is thus a list of fertile research topics and a vehicle for eventual incorporation of new evidence into the next edition of the ICHD proper. Here one finds, for example, an alternate definition for chronic migraine, which is preferred by many to the official definition (see "❷ Migraine," in this chapter).

A troublesome, but unavoidable dichotomy encountered in the ICHD is that the definitions for headache disorders are *symptom-based* for primary headaches, but *etiology-based* for secondary headaches. (This will presumably change when etiologies for primary headaches become known). A conscious decision was made to weight specificity over sensitivity in constructing diagnostic criteria. Precise inclusion and exclusion criteria for each diagnosis are enumerated.

The classification is hierarchical, with a decimal system employed for subdivision. Hence in the case of 5.2.2, chronic posttraumatic headache attributed to mild head injury: "5" denotes posttraumatic headache, "5.2" denotes chronic posttraumatic headache, and "5.2.2" denotes that this chronic posttraumatic headache was caused by mild head injury. The hierarchical format allows one to decide how detailed to make the diagnosis. The Classification Committee felt that in primary care settings, 1–2 digits of specificity would be useful (e.g., 2 – tension-type headache) and that for a researcher or specialist, a 3 digit diagnosis would be more appropriate (e.g., 2.1.1 – infrequent tension-type headache with pericranial tenderness).

For a particular diagnosis all criteria must be fulfilled, thus, for example, to be considered 4.4.2 Orgasmic Headache, ALL of the following must be true:

1. Sudden severe ("explosive") headache
2. Occurs at orgasm
3. Not attributed to another disorder

In patients with more than one distinct type of headache, each is coded separately – i.e., a patient may be coded with: 1.1 Migraine w/o aura, 2.2 Frequent episodic tension-type headache, and 8.2 Medication overuse headache. But, if a single headache type fulfills two different sets of explicit criteria, the use of other data to decide is recommended, for example, history of the headache onset, family history, menstrual relationship, etc. Also, the classification of a patient's headache is based upon his or her current phenomenology, or at least that of the last 1 year. This is a bit controversial, since for example, if there were different headaches in the past, for example, migraine with aura several years ago (but not currently), there is the implication that the patient may still have the "trait" for migraine with aura. These considerations may be important in clinical as well as in research settings.

When a headache disorder is felt to result from another condition, the term "attributed to" is used. According to the ICHD II, these secondary headaches (Part 2) should begin to occur close in time to the causative disorder and should go away when the cause is removed. While very rational, there are two problems with these requirements. First, causation may be difficult to determine and there may have been a delay in headache emergence after the supposed causative event. An even more significant problem is that the cause may not be removable, or that even when the original cause has been removed, permanent changes may lead to persistence of the headaches. When there are difficulties in any of these areas, the ICHD encourages the use of "probable" (e.g., "Probable medication overuse headache"), until more clear evidence of causation is found. In the 3rd edition of the ICHD (ICHD III) the requirements for causation in the secondary headaches will be relaxed, allowing for diagnosis even when causative factors cannot be removed or when headache persists after supposed causes have resolved.

Classification of Primary Headaches

Generally accepted types of migraine, tension-type headache, and cluster headache are delineated in the ICHD II, and a number of less common primary headaches have been categorized in subgroups of these basic diagnoses or have been placed in a fourth category – "Other Primary Headaches." The one unifying feature to primary headaches is their unknown link to any other disease process.

Migraine

Migraine diagnosis depends on a rigorous set of criteria (❷ *Table 11.4*), which include at least moderate severity of pain, nausea, photo- and phonosensitivity, and exercise intolerance. In practice, the diagnosis is not difficult, but a number of migraine patients will probably receive only a "probable migraine" diagnosis if ICHD is applied strictly.

The Migraine with aura category (1.2) is subdivided into: Aura with migraine, aura with non-migraine headache, and aura without headache (❷ *Tables 11.5*, ❷ *11.6*). The rationale behind this was to find a consistent way to handle patients with typical aura but whose headache type otherwise did not meet migraine criteria and the patients with auras without headache at all. Motor auras are placed in the separate Hemiplegic Migraine categories with the implication that motor auras are different from other auras. This has been supported by genetic as well as clinical data (Carrera et al. 2001; De Fusco et al. 2003; Kirchmann et al. 2006; Eriksen et al. 2005).

Basilar-type migraine should have symptoms and/or signs suggestive of the posterior cerebral circulation such as bilateral visual symptoms, dysarthria, vertigo, hearing loss, diplopia, or ataxia (❷ *Table 11.7*) and are considered part of migraine with typical aura (Kirchmann). Retinal migraine requires symptoms referable to one eye, such as unilateral

◻ Table 11.4

ICHD II 1.1 Migraine without aura (Headache Classification Subcommittee of the International Headache Society 2004)

A. At least five attacks fulfilling criteria B–D
B. Headache attacks lasting 4–72 h (untreated or unsuccessfully treated)
C. Headache has at least two of the following characteristics:
1. Unilateral location
2. Pulsating quality
3. Moderate or severe pain intensity
4. Aggravation by or causing avoidance of routine physical activity (e.g., walking or climbing stairs)
D. During headache at least one of the following:
1. Nausea and/or vomiting
2. Photophobia and phonophobia
E. Not attributed to another disorder

◻ Table 11.5

ICHD II 1.2 Migraine with aura: subtypes (Headache Classification Subcommittee of the International Headache Society 2004)

1.2.1 Typical aura with migraine headache
1.2.2 Typical aura with non-migraine headache
1.2.3 Typical aura without headache
1.2.4 Familial hemiplegic migraine (FHM)
1.2.5 Sporadic hemiplegic migraine
1.2.6 Basilar-type migraine

◘ Table 11.6

ICHD II 1.2.1 Typical aura with migraine headache (Headache Classification Subcommittee of the International Headache Society 2004)

A. At least two attacks fulfilling criteria B–D
B. Aura consisting of at least one of the following, but no motor weakness:
1. Fully reversible visual symptoms including positive features (e.g., flickering lights, spots or lines) and/or negative features (i.e., loss of vision)
2. Fully reversible sensory symptoms including positive features (i.e., pins and needles) and/or negative features (i.e., numbness)
3. Fully reversible dysphasic speech disturbance
C. At least two of the following:
1. Homonymous visual symptoms and/or unilateral sensory symptoms
2. At least one aura symptom develops gradually over ≥5 min and/or different aura symptoms occur in succession over ≥5 min
3. Each symptom lasts ≥5 and ≤60 min
D. Headache fulfilling criteria B–D for 1.1 *Migraine without aura* begins during the aura or follows aura within 60 min
E. Not attributed to another disorder

◘ Table 11.7

ICHD II 1.2.6 Basilar-type migraine (Headache Classification Subcommittee of the International Headache Society 2004)

A. At least two attacks fulfilling criteria B–D
B. Aura consisting of at least two of the following fully reversible symptoms, but no motor weakness:
1. Dysarthria
2. Vertigo
3. Tinnitus
4. Hypacusia
5. Diplopia
6. Visual symptoms simultaneously in both temporal and nasal fields of both eyes
7. Ataxia
8. Decreased level of consciousness
9. Simultaneously bilateral paresthesias
C. At least one of the following:
1. At least one aura symptom develops gradually over ≥5 min and/or different aura symptoms occur in succession over ≥5 min
2. Each aura symptom lasts ≥5 and ≤60 min
D. Headache fulfilling criteria B–D for 1.1 *Migraine without aura* begins during the aura or follows aura within 60 min
E. Not attributed to another disorder

ocular vision loss or scotomata. Ophthalmoplegic migraine, once felt to be a primary head-ache, is now relegated to the Neuralgia section (13.17) based on radiologic and other evidence that the entity is more closely related to neuralgic syndromes.

While not a diagnostic entity within the ICHD II, primary chronic daily headache (CDH) is generally defined as headaches (not due to underlying systemic or cranial pathology) on 15 or more days/month. CDH is clearly an important public health problem with a surprisingly high prevalence – probably 4% worldwide. Primary CDH is clearly made up of a mixture of several disorders, found in different ICHD chapters, including Chronic Migraine, Chronic tension-type headache, Hemicraina continua, and New Daily Persistent-Headache (NDPH). Many patients with CDH also have an element of medication overuse headache (discussed later) which further complicates diagnosis.

The definition of Chronic migraine (1.5.1) requires that all headaches meet criteria for migraine (❯ *Table 11.8*). Some have objected to this requirement for chronic migraine since there is thus no diagnostic category which applies to the often-encountered patient with previous intermittent migraine, who evolves to a condition with frequent headaches, many of which have minimal migraine features. A new proposed definition of Chronic Migraine is outlined in a recent Appendix category – A1.5.5 – with less stringent requirements that all headaches fulfill migraine criteria. (Headache Classification Committee et al. 2006; Bigal et al. 2006; Levin et al. 2005) (❯ *Table 11.9*).

Migraines associated with menses are not specifically delineated in the ICHD II. Pure menstrual migraine (PMM – headaches only occurring around menses) and Menstrually related Migraine (MRM – headaches not only limited to menses) are included in the Appendix (A1.1.1, A1.1.2).

Status migrainosis 1.5.2, which refers to the uncommon condition of persistent migraine without abatement for 72 h, also requires that migraine criteria be met.

◻ **Table 11.8**

ICHD II 1.5.1 Chronic migraine (Headache Classification Subcommittee of the International Headache Society 2004)

A. Headache fulfilling criteria C and D for 1.1 *Migraine without aura* on ≥15 days/month for >3 months
B. Not attributed to another disorder

◻ **Table 11.9**

Proposed Appendix criteria for a revised chronic migraine category: IHS 2006 (Headache Classification Committee 2006)

A. Headache on 15 or more days each month
B. Diagnosis of Migraine without aura 1.1
C. Eight or more headaches per month meeting criteria for 1.1 Migraine without aura or 1.2 Migraine with aura, or responsive to migraine specific medication before complete migraine symptomatology develops
D. No medication overuse headache, no chronic tension-type headache, no cluster headache, no NDPH
E. No underlying pathology

Three childhood "migraine" syndromes exist in the ICHD II migraine chapter, ostensibly because they are felt to be precursors of migraine. These include 1.3.1 Cyclical vomiting (spells of nausea and vomiting up to 5 days in duration), 1.3.2 Abdominal migraine (recurrent abdominal pain with varying degrees of nausea in school age children), and 1.3.3 Benign paroxysmal vertigo. 1.5.4 Migrainous infarction is included in the "complications of migraine" portion of the chapter. This diagnosis now requires both persistence of aura symptoms for more than 60 min and MRI changes consistent with stroke in the appropriate brain region.

Tension-Type Headache

Not only is the pathophysiology of tension-type headache not well understood, but even the epidemiology is somewhat unclear. In most studies tension-type headache is much more prevalent than migraine, with an apparent lifetime prevalence approaching 80%. Thus, tension-type headache is an important public health problem. Despite this, a paucity of research on tension-type headache has been done, which probably derives in large part from the under-representation of tension-type headache in specialty and academic settings. The ICHD criteria for tension-type headache are notable for their vagueness and the requirements for nonexistence of certain features (e.g., lack of unilaterality of pain, lack of nausea, lack of exercise intolerance) (❷ Table 11.10). On a practical level, however, tension-type headaches are distinguished from migraine by their relatively milder intensity, and lack of any accompanying "aura-like" symptoms (i.e., visual, sensory, motor, vertigo, cognitive).

ICHD divides tension-type headache into three broad categories based on frequency: 2.1 Infrequent episodic tension-type headache (headache episodes on less than 1 day/month on average), 2.2 Frequent episodic tension-type headache (headache episodes on 1–14 days/ month on average), and 2.3 Chronic tension-type headache (headache episodes on 15 or more days/month on average). These frequency-based categories are arbitrary and somewhat controversial. Chronic tension-type headache, such as Chronic Migraine, requires that tension-type headache occurs on 15 days/month or more (❷ Table 11.11).

◻ Table 11.10

ICHD II 2.1 Infrequent episodic tension-type headache (Headache Classification Subcommittee of the International Headache Society 2004)

A. At least 10 episodes occurring on <1 day/month on average (<12 days/year) and fulfilling criteria B–D
B. Headache lasting from 30 min to 7 days
C. Headache has at least two of the following characteristics:
1. Bilateral location
2. Pressing/tightening (non-pulsating) quality
3. Mild or moderate intensity
4. Not aggravated by routine physical activity such as walking or climbing stairs
D. Both of the following:
1. No nausea or vomiting (anorexia may occur)
2. No more than one of photophobia or phonophobia
E. Not attributed to another disorder

◘ Table 11.11

ICHD II 2.3 Chronic tension-type headache (Headache Classification Subcommittee of the International Headache Society 2004)

A. Headache occurring on ≥15 days/month on average for >3 months (≥180 days/year) and fulfilling criteria B–D
B. Headache lasts hours or may be continuous
C. Headache has at least two of the following characteristics:
1. Bilateral location
2. Pressing/tightening (non-pulsating) quality
3. Mild or moderate intensity
4. Not aggravated by routine physical activity such as walking or climbing stairs
D. Both of the following:
1. No more than one of photophobia, phonophobia or mild nausea
2. Neither moderate or severe nausea nor vomiting
E. Not attributed to another disorder

Cluster Headaches and TAC

The term trigeminal autonomic cephalalgia (TAC) was coined to include three headache types felt to be more or less related: cluster headache, paroxysmal hemicrania, and short-lasting unilateral neuralgiform headache attacks with conjunctival injection and tearing (SUNCT). All have headache of brief duration in common, and all may include autonomic abnormalities in the head, such as conjunctival inflammation, tearing, nasal congestion, rhinorrhea, and ptosis with or without miosis. Cluster headache with its intense, brief (15–180 min) periorbital pain occurring in cycles is generally straightforward in diagnosis and treatment (❷ *Table 11.12*), but the chronic form 3.1.2 can be extremely vexing.

Paroxysmal hemicrania (PH) also has an Episodic form (3.2.1, with flurries of attacks separated in time) and a Chronic form (3.2.2 – no remissions). PH is manifested by even briefer attacks than cluster headache – 2–30 min – which generally occurs more than five times daily. PH is nearly unique in the ICHD II (apart from hemicrania continua, see below) in that response to indomethacin is required for diagnosis. This does create the potential to underdiagnose those patients who are unresponsive to indomethacin but with otherwise typical hemicrania continua.

Short-lasting unilateral neuralgiform headache attacks with conjunctival injection and tearing (SUNCT) 3.3 is the third entity in the TAC chapter of ICHD II. It is a rare condition manifested by yet briefer attacks (5–240 s) occurring up to 200 times daily. The Appendix includes an additional category, short-lasting unilateral neuralgiform headache attacks with autonomic symptoms (SUNA), for the proposed group of patients with similar headaches accompanied by other autonomic symptoms besides lacrimation, such as eyelid edema or nasal congestion.

Other Primary Headaches

The fourth chapter in the ICHD II contains a group of miscellaneous unrelated headaches, including the exercise related headaches and a number of other relatively recently defined

□ Table 11.12

ICHD II 3.1 Cluster headache (Headache Classification Subcommittee of the International Headache Society 2004)

A. At least five attacks fulfilling criteria B–D
B. Severe or very severe unilateral orbital, supraorbital and/or temporal pain lasting 15–180 min if untreated
C. Headache is accompanied by at least one of the following:
1. Ipsilateral conjunctival injection and/or lacrimation
2. Ipsilateral nasal congestion and/or rhinorrhoea
3. Ipsilateral eyelid edema
4. Ipsilateral forehead and facial sweating
5. Ipsilateral miosis and/or ptosis
6. A sense of restlessness or agitation
D. Attacks have a frequency from 1 every other day to 8 per day
E. Not attributed to another disorder

□ Table 11.13

"Other" Headaches: ICHD II (Headache Classification Subcommittee of the International Headache Society 2004)

4.1 Primary stabbing headache
4.2 Primary cough headache
4.3 Primary exertional headache
4.4 Primary headache associated with sexual activity
4.4.1 Preorgasmic headache
4.4.2 Orgasmic headache
4.5 Hypnic headache
4.6 Primary thunderclap headache
4.7 Hemicrania continua
4.8 New daily-persistent headache (NDPH)

headache types (❷ *Table 11.13*). Primary stabbing headache (4.1) is known as "jabs and jolts," and presents with sharp pains in areas innervated by the first two divisions of the trigeminal nerve (cheek, orbit, temporal, and parietal regions). Pain is brief, like the pain of PH, but there are no associated autonomic abnormalities. Interestingly, stabbing pains are not uncommon in migraine and cluster patients, so there may be some overlap here. Primary cough headache (4.2) consists of brief head pain brought on by any valsalva maneuver, and thus may closely mimic the headache secondary to Chiari malformation. Primary exertional headache (4.3) is migraine-like, lasts longer than cough headache, and can be induced by any exercise. When the headache fits migraine criteria it should probably be considered a triggered migraine and treated accordingly.

Primary headaches associated with sexual activity (4.4) take one of two forms: 4.4.1, the so-called Preorgasmic headache (formerly known as "dull" sexual headache), characterized by posterior moderately severe aching pain during intercourse; and 4.4.2, the severe Orgasmic headache ("explosive" coital headache), which mimics subarachnoid or intracerebral hemorrhage as well as arterial dissection. Interestingly, case reports and series have revealed a prominent association between benign exertional headache and sex-induced headaches, so there may be shared pathophysiological factors (Pascual et al. 1996). A third sexually-related headache, the "postural" coital headache, occurs after intercourse, worsens with upright posture and can be very prolonged. After a number of case reports suggested that patients with this type of post-coital headache actually had a low CSF pressure state, it was concluded by most investigators that this headache was indeed due to some disruption of dural integrity caused by the strain of intercourse with subsequent CSF leak. Thus it is now included as a secondary headache due to CSF Fistula (7.2.2).

Hypnic headache (4.5) occurs during sleep in elderly persons. It awakens the patient in the middle of the night, generally at the same time of night (hence the nickname "alarm-clock headache"), last for a short time and then abates. While its pathophysiology is unclear, it shares some features with cluster headache: its nocturnal occurrence, which few other headache types exhibit, and response to lithium.

Primary thunderclap headache is a mysterious, sudden, severe headache that mimics subarachnoid hemorrhage. To be diagnosed it cannot meet criteria for any of the above exertion-related headaches and of course must be shown *not* to be due to more serious disease, such as intracranial hemorrhage, subarachnoid hemorrhage, arterial dissection, cerebral venous thrombosis, cerebral arteritis, reversible cerebral vasoconstriction syndrome (Call-Fleming Syndrome), or pituitary apoplexy. Unruptured intracerebral aneurysms, colloid cysts of the third ventricle, CSF hypotension, and acute sinusitis have also been reported to cause severe sudden headaches and thus diagnostic workup should be exhaustive in cases presenting with the thunderclap headache scenario (Dodick 2002).

Hemicrania continua (HC), 4.7, manifests as unilateral continuous pain, often with autonomic features and, like PH, is completely responsive to indomethacin (❯ *Table 11.14*). The resemblance to the TACs might support placement in Chapter 3 rather than in "Other Headaches." HC shares its indomethacin responsiveness with other Chapter 4 headache

◘ Table 11.14

ICHD II 4.7 Hemicrania continua (Headache Classification Subcommittee of the International Headache Society 2004)

A. Headache for >3 months fulfilling criteria B–D
B. All of the following characteristics:
1. Unilateral pain without side-shift
2. Daily and continuous, without pain-free periods
3. Moderate intensity, but with exacerbations of severe pain
C. At least one of the following autonomic features occurs during exacerbations and ipsilateral to the side of pain:
1. Conjunctival injection and/or lacrimation
2. Nasal congestion and/or rhinorrhea
3. Ptosis and/or miosis
D. Complete response to therapeutic doses of indomethacin
E. Not attributed to another disorder

types – cough headache and stabbing headache, suggesting some shared pathophysiology among these types as well.

New Daily-Persistent Headache (NDPH), 4.8, consists of continuous headache, essentially meeting chronic tension-type headache diagnostic criteria, which began spontaneously. Patients can usually pinpoint a specific date when it started. (Goadsby and Boes 2002; Li and Rozen 2002; Vanast 1986). This pattern suggests a secondary cause, and in many cases, antecedent illness or injury can be identified. Here again, as evidence begins to accumulate, clarification of where these patients fit in the overall classification of headache disorders will contribute to our understanding of pathophysiology and hopefully management of these often intractable cases.

Classification of Secondary Headaches

When a headache arises de novo in close temporal relation to another disorder known to potentially cause headache, and goes away when this disorder resolves or is successfully treated, one may easily conclude that the condition is a secondary one. However, as noted above, these criteria are often met with difficulty. Inferences can be made about causality, but in unclear cases, "probable" secondary headache (e.g., "probable posttraumatic headache," "probable medication overuse headache") is the best diagnosis. When a preexisting headache disorder is clearly worsened by the occurrence of another disorder, it is sensible to conclude that the patient has two problems – the initial primary headache and the secondary headache which represents the secondary "component." (e.g., for an individual with preexisting occasional migraine headaches which had clearly increased in frequency and severity following a head injury, a dual diagnosis of 1.1 migraine headache and 5.2 chronic posttraumatic headache would be reasonable).

Posttraumatic Headaches

Diagnosis in this group of headache disorders is relatively obvious when the injury leads quickly to headaches or a worsening of an existing headache disorder. When there are more than a few days between injury and onset of headaches, or when there are complicating factors relating to litigation and other secondary gain related issues, clear diagnoses are more difficult. The ICHD II requires no more than a lag time of 7 days, despite the many reported cases of longer lag times prior to the onset of headaches, even as long as months. There is still no consensus about the effects of litigation and compensation on the natural history of posttraumatic headache although clearly this is a confounding problem (Cassidy et al. 2000).

The ICHD distinguishes between acute posttraumatic headaches (those which persist less than 3 months after injury) and chronic posttraumatic headaches (persisting longer than 3 months), and further divides this headache type into acute and chronic conditions following mild versus severe head trauma. The definitions of what constitutes mild and moderate head injury are based on a number of parameters including Glasgow Coma Scale scores, presence and duration of loss of consciousness, neuroimaging details, and memory loss (see ❥ Table 11.15). The often-debated whiplash induced headache is also included in the latest version of the ICHD but continues to be examined.

❑ Table 11.15

Posttraumatic headache (Headache Classification Subcommittee of the International Headache Society 2004)

5.1 Acute posttraumatic headache
5.1.1 Acute posttraumatic headache attributed to moderate or severe head injury
5.1.2 Acute posttraumatic headache attributed to mild head injury
5.2 Chronic posttraumatic headache
5.2.1 Chronic posttraumatic headache attributed to moderate or severe head injury
5.2.2 Chronic posttraumatic headache attributed to mild head injury
5.3 Acute headache attributed to whiplash injury
5.4 Chronic headache attributed to whiplash injury

Headache Due to Vascular Disorders

The term "vascular headache" was overused in the past, being applied to any migrainous or even cluster-like headache disorder. While the pain of migraine may in part relate to vascular events (in particular, cortical arterial dilation and inflammation), migraine is as much a neural event as a vascular one, and the truly vascular group of headache disorders, including those due to cerebral ischemia, non-traumatic hemorrhage, vascular malformations, arteritis, other arterial and venous disease are considered separately in Chapter 6 of the ICHD II (❍ *Table 11.16*).

Stroke and TIA can certainly produce headache (Portenoy et al. 1984), although generally not in isolation. The most worrisome causes of vascular headache are generally those due to hemorrhage (subarachnoid hemorrhage and intracerebral hemorrhage), arterial dissection (vertebral and carotid), and those due to inflammatory disease of cerebral arteries (isolated cerebral or systemic arteritis). Cerebral venous thrombosis is an important entity for the practitioner to keep in mind since it may produce a nondescript headache syndrome and routine evaluation of headache may fail to reveal the diagnosis. MR venography or CT angiography is generally sufficient and should be considered in any subacute headache presentation.

Post carotid endarterectomy and angioplasty headaches are included in this category and are important as they might herald impending hemorrhage or other sequelae. A puzzling group of headaches are those due to unruptured vascular malformations including saccular aneurysms, AV fistulas, angiomata, and arteriovenous malformations. It is not clear why these produce headache, although vascular distension is suggested by many as the cause. Finally, the genetic diseases Cerebral Autosomal Dominant Arteriopathy with Subcortical Infarcts and Leukoencephalopathy (CADASIL) and Mitochondrial Encephalopathy, Lactic Acidosis, and Stroke-like episodes (MELAS) syndrome, both of which often present initially with headache, are in this category.

Headache Due to Abnormalities of Intracranial Pressure or Neoplastic Disease

Both high CSF and low CSF pressure have been associated with headache, presumably due to traction on pain sensitive structures, particularly the dura mater. High CSF pressure may result

◘ Table 11.16

Vascular causes of headache (Headache Classification Subcommittee of the International Headache Society 2004)

6.1 Headache attributed to ischaemic stroke or transient ischaemic attack
6.1.1 Headache attributed to ischaemic stroke (cerebral infarction)
6.1.2 Headache attributed to transient ischaemic attack (TIA)
6.2 Headache attributed to non-traumatic intracranial hemorrhage
6.2.1 Headache attributed to intracerebral hemorrhage
6.2.2 Headache attributed to subarachnoid hemorrhage (SAH)
6.3 Headache attributed to unruptured vascular malformation
6.3.1 Headache attributed to saccular aneurysm
6.3.2 Headache attributed to arteriovenous malformation (AVM)
6.3.3 Headache attributed to dural arteriovenous fistula
6.3.4 Headache attributed to cavernous angioma
6.3.5 Headache attributed to encephalotrigeminal or leptomeningeal angiomatosis (Sturge Weber syndrome)
6.4 Headache attributed to arteritis
6.4.1 Headache attributed to giant cell arteritis (GCA)
6.4.2 Headache attributed to primary central nervous system (CNS) angiitis
6.4.3 Headache attributed to secondary central nervous system (CNS) angiitis
6.5 Carotid or vertebral artery pain
6.5.1 Headache or facial or neck pain attributed to arterial dissection
6.5.2 Post-endarterectomy headache
6.5.3 Carotid angioplasty headache
6.5.4 Headache attributed to intracranial endovascular procedures
6.5.5 Angiography headache
6.6 Headache attributed to cerebral venous thrombosis (CVT)
6.7 Headache attributed to other intracranial vascular disorder
6.7.1 CADASIL (Cerebral Autosomal Dominant Arteriopathy with Subcortical Infarcts and Leukoencephalopathy
6.7.2 MELAS (Mitochondrial Encephalopathy, Lactic Acidosis and Stroke-like episodes)
6.7.3 Headache attributed to benign angiopathy of the central nervous system
6.7.4 Headache attributed to pituitary apoplexy

from metabolic or toxic causes or may be idiopathic, in the case of benign intracranial hypertension. Low CSF pressure may occur due to traumatic or other cause of CSF leak, such as the post lumbar puncture syndrome. Low CSF pressure, however, can also be idiopathic. Headaches due to hydrocephalus which produces intracranial hypertension are grouped with these other causes of headache.

The ICHD II requires that the CSF pressure be above 200 mm of H_2O for non-obese and greater than 250 mm H_2O for the obese patients, both in primary and secondary intracranial hypertension induced headaches, and for hydrocephalus induced headaches as well.

Low CSF pressure headaches are diagnosed only if the CSF pressure is less than 60 mm H_2O. Headache attributed to Chiari malformation type I is also included in the same ICHD chapter as CSF pressure-related headaches. This is reasonable since traction of intracranial structures is likewise a probable cause of the head pain, but also because of the potential link between Chiari malformation and low CSF pressure, at least in some reported cases (Kasner et al. 1995).

Intracranial neoplasms can cause headache, again by producing increased intracranial pressure which leads to traction of pain sensitive structures. Carcinomatous meningitis and neoplastic causes of hydrocephalus are other possible neoplastic causes of headache.

Headache Due to Medications, Toxins, and Other Substances

There are a number of ways substances can induce or worsen headaches. First, a number of agents are known to produce headache directly after exposure including alcohol, food additives such as MSG, cocaine, cannabis, histamine, hormonal supplements, nitric oxide donor medication (e.g., nitroglycerine) and many other prescription medications. Carbon monoxide and a number of other chemical agents are also known to produce headache, sometimes as the initial manifestation of toxicity, which thus serves as a useful diagnostic warning. Withdrawal from substances also may produce headache. The most common cause of medication related headache though is Medication Overuse Headache (MOH), coded in ICHD II as 8.2, with a number of subtypes. The mechanism of this group of headaches is still unclear, but seems to occur primarily in migraine sufferers who take frequent pain relieving medications.

A number of controversies have arisen over the classification and diagnosis of MOH. Initially, ICHD II defined this syndrome differently for different substances, for instance requiring migraine headache morphology when MOH was due to triptan medications, and tension-type headache morphology when MOH was due to analgesics. Also, different frequency of usage was expected for different agents: >10 days/month usage of ergotamine, triptan medications, combination analgesics or opioids, and >15 days/month for simple analgesics. Another area of debate was requirement for improvement in headaches when the offending substances were removed, with use of the term "Probable MOH" until this evidence was obtained. In a formal revision of the 8.2 definition of MOH and a later proposal for additional changes in the MOH criteria, based on some careful analysis by Bigal and others (Bigal et al. 2004, 2006) most of these controversies were resolved (Silberstein et al. 2005; Headache Classification Committee et al. 2006). In the revised 8.2 criteria, the headache characteristics were removed and a new category for MOH due to a combination of medications was included. In the MOH Appendix criteria, the requirement for resolution of headaches after cessation of medication was deleted. This serves as an example of the potential ability of the ICHD to undergo evidence-driven change in a timely fashion.

Infectious Causes of Headache

Infections may cause headache in a number of ways. Meningitis of any cause typically produces intense headache. Headache is an early manifestation of most of the encephalitides as well. Brain abscess may be so indolent as to present with focal findings before headache but may also present with headache. Subdural empyema is yet another possible infectious cause. HIV infections may cause headache due to (1) the direct effect of CNS parenchymal infection, (2) opportunistic infections including abscesses or meningitis, and (3) the effects of anti-retrovirus and other antibiotic medications. Neurosarcoidosis, carcinomatous, lymphomatous, and aseptic meningitis can mimic infectious causes of headache. A syndrome of "Chronic post-bacterial meningitis headache" has been reported, listed in ICHD as 9.4.1, and an Appendix diagnosis of "Chronic post-non-bacterial meningitis headache" was written to include this as a possible diagnostic entity, based on case reports. Further evidence may clarify these conditions.

Headache Related to Metabolic Disturbances

The ICHD II terms this category "Headaches due to disorders of homeostasis" and includes headaches due to hypoxia and/or hypercapnia, hypertension-related headaches, headaches related to hypothyroidism, and headaches related to fasting. Other endocrinological disorders such as diabetes and prolactinemia were felt to merit inclusion in the classification of headache, but conclusive evidence has not yet emerged.

Hypoxia-related headaches, according to the ICHD II, require that PaO_2 remains below 70 mmHg, as might be seen in patients with chronic pulmonary disease. 10.1.1, high-altitude headache, is considered a component of acute mountain sickness, and is said to occur only at altitudes above 2,500 m. It remains to be seen whether this demarcation has real significance. Diving headache, 10.1.2, may be primarily due to high concentrations of CO_2 that divers may experience, and is cured by 100% oxygen treatment. Sleep apnea headache (10.1.3), which requires a Respiratory Disturbance Index of 5 or greater, is still controversial, and it is unclear whether it is due to hypoxia, hypercapnia, or the general disturbance in sleep.

Severe hypertension, as seen, for example, in pheochromocytoma or in patients with hypertensive encephalopathy, can clearly lead to headache. More controversial, and unsupported by evidence, is the concept that moderate elevations in blood pressure may lead to headache.

Cervicogenic Headache

Clearly, mechanical and other disorders involving structures in the neck can produce headaches. If successful treatment of cervical disease leads to resolution of the headache, post-hoc diagnosis of cervicogenic headache is logical. However this is often not possible. As a result, many authors have tried to establish useful, consistent criteria for diagnosing cervicogenic headache (Bogduk 2001; Antonaci et al. 2001). ICHD II requires that there be evidence of pathology in the neck which might cause head pain and that there be clinical signs that support this as the cause (❷ *Table 11.17*). But controversy rages about what clinical and radiological features and types of pathology are valid causes of secondary headaches. The ICHD is strict: "Tumours, fractures, infections and rheumatoid arthritis of the upper cervical spine...accepted as valid causes when demonstrated to be so in individual cases. Cervical spondylosis and osteochondritis are NOT accepted as valid causes . . . ." It additionally states that if myofascial causes are prominent, the headache should be diagnosed as tension-type headache.

◘ Table 11.17

Cervicogenic headache 11.2.1 (Headache Classification Subcommittee of the International Headache Society 2004)

Diagnostic criteria
A. Pain, referred from a source in the neck and perceived in one or more regions of the head and/or face, fulfilling criteria C and D
B. Clinical, laboratory and/or imaging evidence of a disorder or lesion within the cervical spine or soft tissues of the neck known to be, or generally accepted as, a valid cause of headache
C. Evidence that the pain can be attributed to the neck disorder or lesion based on at least one of the following
1. Demonstration of clinical signs that implicate a source of pain in the neck
2. Abolition of headache following diagnostic blockade of a cervical structure or its nerve supply using placebo- or other adequate controls
D. Pain resolves within 3 months after successful treatment of the causative disorder or lesion

Headaches Related to Ophthalmological, Otolaryngological, and Dental Disease

Inflammation or other disorders of the eyes, nose, sinuses, ears, face, jaw, or teeth can of course produce headache or facial pain. ❷ *Table 11.18* summarizes the basic causes in these areas which have been supported by evidence. Controversial entities include headaches related to chronic paranasal sinus disease, abnormalities of nasal mucosa and septum and temporomandibular joint disorders (TMD). Again, resolution of the headache after successful treatment of the rhinosinusitis or other inflammatory condition in the face or head confirms the diagnosis. But a number of poorly understood otolaryngological entities deserve further investigation as possible causes for chronic headaches. Of note, an Appendix diagnosis A11.5.1, lists criteria for "Mucosal contact point headache," with the requirement that the pain resolves after the endoscopically identified contact point is anesthetized.

Criteria for diagnosing headache related to the jaw are perennially debated. The ICHD II requires both imaging evidence of TMD as well as at least one positive functional test supportive of causality including (1) precipitation of pain by jaw motion, (2) reduced jaw opening, (3) TMJ noise, or (4) TMJ tenderness.

Psychogenic Headaches

Many clinicians believe that many headache conditions can be caused by or at least worsened by psychiatric illness. However, as noted in ICHD II Section 12, "Overall there is very limited evidence supporting psychiatric causes of headache." The only two diagnoses in this chapter are 12.1, Headache attributed to somatisation disorder and 12.2, Headache attributed to psychotic disorder (i.e., a delusional headache). The problem with drawing conclusions even from compelling case series in this area is the enormous comorbidity of psychiatric and psychological illness in patients with primary headaches, particularly migraine (Sheftell and Atlas 2002). The Appendix of the ICHD II does contain a number of proposed psychiatric secondary headache disorders which bear further study including: headache attributed to major depressive disorder, headache attributed to panic disorder, headache attributed

◘ Table 11.18

Headaches related to ophthalmological, otolaryngological, and dental disease (Headache Classification Subcommittee of the International Headache Society 2004)

11.3 Headache attributed to disorder of eyes
11.3.1 Headache attributed to acute glaucoma
11.3.2 Headache attributed to refractive errors
11.3.3 Headache attributed to heterophoria or heterotropia (latent or manifest squint)
11.3.4 Headache attributed to ocular inflammatory disorder
11.4 Headache attributed to disorder of ears
11.5 Headache attributed to rhinosinusitis
11.6 Headache attributed to disorder of teeth, jaws or related structures
11.7 Headache or facial pain attributed to temporomandibular joint (TMJ) disorder

◘ Table 11.19

Proposed headache types related to psychiatric disorders (Headache Classification Subcommittee of the International Headache Society 2004)

A12.3 Headache attributed to major depressive disorder
A12.4 Headache attributed to panic disorder
A12.5 Headache attributed to generalized anxiety disorder
A12.6 Headache attributed to undifferentiated somatoform disorder
A12.7 Headache attributed to social phobia
A12.8 Headache attributed to separation anxiety disorder
A12.9 Headache attributed to posttraumatic stress disorder

to anxiety disorder, headache attributed to generalized anxiety disorder, headache attributed to undifferentiated somatoform disorder, and headache attributed to posttraumatic stress disorder (see ❯ *Table 11.19*).

Neuralgias

Neuralgias are presented in a final section of the ICHD II classification, "Part 3 – Cranial neuralgias and central causes of facial pain." This is a somewhat unusual part of the ICHD since it contains both *primary* (e.g., idiopathic trigeminal neuralgia) and *secondary* (e.g., postherpetic neuralgia) conditions. ❯ *Table 11.20* lists these various conditions.

The ICHD II: Conclusions

The ideal classification of headaches would be hierarchical, with evidence-based unique diagnostic criteria for each diagnostic entity, easy to use, and practical for both clinical work and research. Because of limited understanding of the nature of primary and many of the secondary headaches, the ICHD as yet does not fulfill all of the above criteria. It is hierarchical,

◘ Table 11.20

Neuralgias and other central causes of facial pain (Headache Classification Subcommittee of the International Headache Society 2004)

13.1 Trigeminal neuralgia
13.1.1 Classical trigeminal neuralgia
13.1.2 Symptomatic trigeminal neuralgia
13.2 Glossopharyngeal neuralgia
13.2.1 Classical glossopharyngeal neuralgia
13.2.2 Symptomatic glossopharyngeal neuralgia
13.3 Nervus intermedius neuralgia
13.4 Superior laryngeal neuralgia
13.5 Nasociliary neuralgia
13.6 Supraorbital neuralgia
13.7 Other terminal branch neuralgias
13.8 Occipital neuralgia
13.9 Neck-tongue syndrome
13.10 External compression headache
13.11 Cold-stimulus headache
13.11.1 Headache attributed to external application of a cold stimulus
13.11.2 Headache attributed to ingestion or inhalation of a cold stimulus
13.12 Constant pain caused by compression, irritation or distortion of cranial nerves or upper cervical roots by structural lesions
13.13 Optic neuritis
13.14 Ocular diabetic neuropathy
13.15 Head or facial pain attributed to herpes zoster
13.15.1 Head or facial pain attributed to acute herpes zoster
13.15.2 Post-herpetic neuralgia
13.16 Tolosa-Hunt syndrome
13.17 Ophthalmoplegic "migraine"
13.18 Central causes of facial pain
13.18.1 Anesthesia dolorosa
13.18.2 Central post-stroke pain
13.18.3 Facial pain attributed to multiple sclerosis
13.18.4 Persistent idiopathic facial pain
13.18.5 Burning mouth syndrome

with nesting of diagnostic groups, and it has generally consistent overriding philosophy, but diagnostic criteria and demarcations between definitions are often just based on the opinion of experts in the absence of scientific evidence. Thus further nosographic studies are much needed. As for research purposes, the ICHD has proven very useful, but ironically, when research provides evidence for changes in diagnostic criteria, studies using "old criteria" become to some extent invalid.

However, the ICHD II must be considered one of the most important publications in clinical neurology of the last several decades. As noted before, it has led to far deeper understanding and authentification of the many entities productive of head and facial pain. Moreover, the ICHD II provides a vehicle for much needed further study of headaches. This is particularly true for the primary headaches, many of which remain more or less mysterious in terms of etiology, pathophysiology, and treatment. The Appendix, with its proposed alternative or new diagnoses, is designed to spur such research. As mentioned, the IHS Classification Committee is working to collect and analyze evidence which might help to strengthen diagnostic criteria for the primary and secondary headaches in preparation for the creation of ICHD III. Describing series of patients with very similar morphological presentations is one approach to promoting diagnostic schema. Discovering reproducible diagnostic historical and physical tests will be helpful. Laboratory and genetic markers will of course be even more compelling.

References

Ad Hoc Committee on Classification of Headache of the National Institute of Health (1962) Classification of headache. JAMA 179:717–718

Antonaci F, Ghirmai S, Bono G et al (2001) Cervicogenic headache: evaluation of the original diagnostic criteria. Cephalalgia 21:573–583

Bigal ME, Tepper SJ, Sheftell FD, Rapoport AM, Lipton RB (2004) Chronic daily headache: correlation between the 2004 and the 1988 International Headache Society diagnostic criteria. Headache 44(7):684–691

Bigal ME, Tepper SJ, Sheftell FD, Rapoport AM, Lipton RB (2006) Field testing alternative criteria for chronic migraine. Cephalalgia 26:477–482

Bogduk N (2001) Cervicogenic headache: anatomic basis and pathophysiologic mechanisms. Curr Pain Headache Rep 5:382–386

Carrera P, Stenirri S, Ferrari M et al (2001) Familial hemiplegic migraine: an ion channel disorder. Brain Res Bull 56:239–241

Cassidy JD, Carrol LJ, Cote P, Lemstra M et al (2000) Effect of eliminating compensation for pain and suffering on the outcome of insurance claims for whiplash injury. N Engl J Med 342:1179–1186

De Fusco M, Marconi R, Silvestri L et al (2003) Haploinsufficiency of ATP1A2 encoding the Na+/K+ pump alpha2 subunit associated with familial hemiplegic migraine type 2. Nat Genet 33:192–196

Dodick DW (2002) Thunderclap headache. J Neurol Neurosurg Psychiatry 72:6–11

Eriksen MK, Thomsen LL, Olesen J (2005) Sensitivity and specificity of the new international diagnostic criteria for migraine with aura. J Neurol Neurosurg Psychiatry 76:212–217

Gladstone JP, Dodick DW (2004) From hemicrania lunaris to hemicrania continua: An overview of the revised *International Classification of Headache Disorders*. Headache 44:692–705

Goadsby PJ, Boes C (2002) New daily persistent headache. J Neurol Neurosurg Psychiatry 72(Suppl 2):ii6–ii9

Headache Classification Committee, Olesen J, Bousser M-G, Diener H-C et al (2006) New appendix criteria open for a broader concept of chronic migraine. Cephalalgia 26:742–746

Headache Classification Subcommittee of the International Headache Society (2004) The international classification of headache disorders, 2nd edn. Cephalalgia 24(Suppl 1):1–160

International Headache Society Classification Committee (1988) Classification and diagnostic criteria for headache disorders, cranial neuralgias and facial pain. Cephalalgia 8(suppl 7):1–96

Isler H (1993) Headache classification prior to the Ad Hoc criteria. Cephalalgia 13(Suppl 2):9–20

Kasner SE, Rosenfeld J, Farber RE (1995) Spontaneous intracranial hypotension: headache with a reversible Arnold-Chiari malformation. Headache 35(9):557–559

Kirchmann M, Thomsen LL, Olesen J (2006) Basilar-type migraine – Clinical, epidemiologic, and genetic features. Neurology 66:880–886

Levin M, Peterlin BL, Ward TN (2005) Review of diagnoses of 50 consecutive patients with chronic daily headache using the ICHD II. Cephalalgia 25:999 (abs)

Li D, Rozen TD (2002) The clinical characterisation of new daily persistent headache. Cephalalgia 22:66–69

Pascual J et al (1996) Cough, exertional, and sexual headaches: an analysis of 72 benign and symptomatic cases. Neurology 46:1520–1524

Pearce JMS (1986) Historical aspects of migraine. J Neurol Neurosurg Psychiatry 49:1097–1103

Portenoy RK, Abissi CJ, Lipton RB et al (1984) Headache in cerebrovascular disease. Stroke 15:1009–1012

Sheftell FD, Atlas SJ (2002) Migraine and psychiatric comorbidity: from theory and hypotheses to clinical application. Headache 42(9):843–844

Silberstein SD, Olesen J, Bousser M-G, Diener H-C, Dodick D et al (2005) The International classification of headache disorders: 2nd edition – Revision of criteria for 8.2 medication overuse headache. Cephalalgia 25:460–465

Vanast WJ (1986) New daily persistent headache: Definition of a benign syndrome. Headache 26:317

12 The Medical History: The Key to Correct Headache Diagnosis

E. Anne MacGregor[1] · *K. Ravishankar*[2] · *David Dodick*[3]

[1]The City of London Migraine Clinic, London, UK
[2]Jaslok Hospital and Research Centre, Lilavati Hospital and Research Centre, Mumbai, India
[3]Mayo Clinic Arizona, Phoenix, AZ, USA

Paolo Martelletti, Timothy J. Steiner (eds.), *Handbook of Headache*, DOI 10.1007/978-88-470-1700-9_12,
© Lifting The Burden 2011

Abstract: Effective management of headache depends on correct diagnosis. The presence of warning symptoms should necessitate further investigation to rule out an underlying cause. Once pathology has been excluded, targeted questions and pattern recognition of typical presentations of headache enable more confident diagnosis. With primary headaches being more common in practice than secondary headaches, correct diagnosis is dependent on a good history. A good history is also important to prevent misdiagnosis when there are coexisting headache types.

Introduction

Headache accounts for around 4.4% of consultations in primary care and is the most common cause of referral to neurologists (Bone and Fuller 2002; Latinovic et al. 2006). And since different headaches have different treatments, it is important to arrive at the right diagnosis. (Lipton et al. 1998). History is crucial to effective diagnosis of primary headaches as the examination is essentially normal. Failure to recognize and manage coexisting headaches is a common cause of treatment failure. In a study of patients with a diagnosis of migraine who were referred to a specialist headache clinic, nearly one-third had at least two headache diagnoses (Blau and MacGregor 1995).

Taking a History

The first task is to exclude a condition requiring more urgent intervention by eliciting any warning features in the history (❷ *Table 12.1*). This can enable identification of those who need further investigation to reach a diagnosis and treat specifically.

Changes in a patient with a long-standing history of primary headache are an alert to question further about the development of new, or unusual, symptoms. Age of the patient is important as the likelihood of pathology is greater with elderly patients. Seizure is a cardinal symptom of intracerebral space–occupying lesions; "thunderclap" headache should raise the suspicion of subarachnoid hemorrhage, carotid dissection, cerebral venous sinus thrombosis, and reversible cerebral vasoconstriction syndrome.

Once serious pathology has been excluded, it is appropriate to take a more detailed history. In an ideal world, patients should be allowed to tell their own story. Time constraints rarely make this feasible, and it is necessary to ask a few pertinent questions to structure the consultation. Unless the patient is particularly verbose or several headaches coexist, the diagnosis can usually be made in a few minutes.

Typical responses to a structured history are useful in diagnosing headaches (❷ *Table 12.2*).

"*How many different headaches do you have?*" This can be a useful opening question, particularly for patients with long-standing primary headaches who develop a more insidious secondary headache (Laughey et al. 1993). Most patients can readily distinguish between different headaches as each type usually follows a typical pattern of onset, timing, and symptoms. If more than one pattern of headache is suspected, it is necessary to take a separate history for each.

"*Why are you consulting now?*" This may be because of the severity or frequency of headache, but it can also reveal patients' fears, or external pressure on them to "do something about their headaches" from family or work.

◻ **Table 12.1**

Identifying secondary causes of headache: SNOOP4 (Dodick 2010)

	Ask about	Possible causes
Systematic symptoms/signs	Fever	Giant cell arteritis
	Chills	Infection
	Night sweats	Malignancy
	Myalgias	
	Weight loss	
Systematic disease	History of malignancy	Metastatic disease
	Immunocompromised state	Opportunistic CNS infection
	HIV	
Neurologic symptoms or signs	Focal or global neurological symptoms or signs, including behavioral or personality changes	Neoplasia
		Infection
	Diplopia, transient visual obscurations, pulsatile tinnitus (especially in obese patients)	Inflammation
		Vascular CNS disease
		Idiopathic intracranial hypertension
Onset sudden (thunderclap headache)	How quickly the pain went from 0/10 to 10/10	Vascular crises (stroke, subarachnoid hemorrhage, cerebral venous sinus thrombosis, reversible cerebral vasoconstriction syndrome, arterial dissection)
Onset after age 50 years		Neoplasia
		Infection
		Inflammation
		Giant cell arteritis
Pattern change (if previous history)	Progressive headache with loss of headache-free periods	
	Precipitated by Valsava	Chiari malformation
		Structural lesions which obstruct CSF flow
		CSF leak
	Postural aggravation	Worse when standing or lying: intracranial hypotension from CSF leak; intracranial hypertension
		Worse with certain neck movements; cervicogenic headache
	Papilledema	Intracranial hypertension

"*When did the headache first start?*" Recent new-onset headaches are of greater concern than long-standing headaches. Headache as an isolated symptom for more than 10 weeks is rarely due to brain tumor (Vazquez-Barquero et al. 1994). Around half of migraineurs experience their first attack before age 25 and three-quarter before age 35 years

◻ **Table 12.2**

An approach to the headache history (MacGregor et al. 2010)

1. How many different headaches types does the patient experience?	
Separate histories are necessary for each. It is reasonable to concentrate on the most bothersome to the patient but others should always attract some enquiry in case they are clinically important.	
2. Time questions	(a) Why consulting now?
	(b) How recent in onset?
	(c) How frequent, and what temporal pattern (especially distinguishing between episodic and daily or unremitting)?
	(d) How long lasting?
3. Character questions	(a) Intensity of pain?
	(b) Nature and quality of pain?
	(c) Site and spread of pain?
	(d) Associated symptoms?
4. Cause questions	(a) Predisposing and/or trigger factors?
	(b) Aggravating and/or relieving factors?
	(c) Family history of similar headache?
5. Response to headache questions	(a) What does the patient do during the headache?
	(b) How much is activity (function) limited or prevented?
	(c) What medication has been and is used, and in what manner?
6. State of health between attacks	(a) Completely well, or residual or persisting symptoms?
	(b) Concerns, anxieties, fears about recurrent attacks, and/or their cause?

(Stewart et al. 2008). Frequency of attacks fluctuates during a lifetime, and it is not uncommon for migraine to return after several years of respite (Bille 1997). Cluster headache is frequently misdiagnosed in primary care, with an average of 2–3 years until correct diagnosis (Bahra and Goadsby 2004; van Vliet et al. 2003).

"How many days in a month do you NOT have a headache of any type for the entire day? How many headache days per month are severe/moderate/mild?" Frequent headaches need detailed analysis of the pattern. Cluster headaches follow a stereotypical pattern of daily attacks over several weeks with periods of remission in-between. Daily, progressive headaches are a cause for concern. Daily headaches are not typically migraine but "chronic migraine" may manifest as near-daily headaches. Patients reporting daily should be asked how the pattern has changed over time. Although an underlying pathology needs exclusion, medication overuse is a more common contributory factor.

"Is there any pattern to attacks?" Patients may notice attacks occur more often at weekends or are linked to menstruation, which then needs to be diagnosed and managed accordingly. Cluster headache often wakes the patient a few hours after sleep. Headache associated with medication overuse and raised intracranial pressure are characteristically worse on waking.

"How long does the headache typically last if you don't take treatment, or if treatment is not effective?" Most migraines in adults will last part of a day, up to 3 days. Attacks are typically shorter in children – sometimes less than a couple of hours (Headache Classification

Subcommittee of the International Headache Society (IHS) 2004). Cluster attacks last between 20 and 180 min (usually 60 min); medication-overuse headache is mostly continuous. Tension-type headaches can vary from a few hours to daily symptoms.

"How severe is the pain?"; *"What does the pain feel like?"* The headache of migraine is usually described as a moderate-to-severe throbbing, pounding headache. The pain of cluster headache is extremely severe and prohibits any activity during the attack period.

"Where do you get the pain?" Patients will usually point to one side of the head, which may alternate between or during attacks. Although typically unilateral, bilateral headache does not discount migraine, occurring in about 30% of attacks. The headache can swap sides between and during attacks. Neck pain is also a common symptom before and during migraine, sometimes radiating to the shoulder. A more generalized and unremitting "pressure" headache is more typically associated with tension-type headache and medication-overuse headache. Cluster headache is strictly unilateral, centered on one eye, and while very uncommon, may shift sides.

"What other symptoms have you experienced?" The presence of associated symptoms can help secure a diagnosis. A positive response to the presence of the following symptoms can "PIN" the diagnosis of migraine (Dodick 2010):

- Photophobia: Does light bother you when you have a headache?
- Impairment: Do you experience headaches that impair your ability to function?
- Nausea: Do you feel nauseated or sick to your stomach when you experience a headache?

A positive answer to two or three of these three questions results in a 93% and 98%, respectively, positive predictive value for a diagnosis of migraine (Lipton et al. 2003).

Migraine may be preceded by premonitory symptoms, which occur hours to days before onset of headache and include symptoms such as unusual tiredness, difficulty concentrating, neck stiffness, yawning, and food cravings (Giffin et al. 2003). These generalized symptoms are often confused with the more specific symptoms of aura. Visual aura symptoms are usually symmetrical, affecting one hemifield of both eyes, although subjectively they may appear to affect only one eye – if there is any doubt, patients should be asked to assess their next attack. A migrainous scotoma is typically positive (bright), starting as a small spot gradually increasing in size to assume the shape of a letter C, developing scintillating edges that appear as zigzags (fortifications – a term coined in the late eighteenth century because the visual disturbances resembled a fortified town surrounded by bastions). The aura usually starts at or near the center of fixation, gradually spreading laterally, increasing in size over a period of 5–30 min. In contrast, ischemic events do not generally have the scintillating and spreading features of the visual aura of migraine and the visual loss is usually a monocular negative scotoma (black). Transient monocular blindness is not typical of migraine and prompts urgent investigation. Sensory aura symptoms are commonly positive, that is, a sensation of pins and needles rather than numbness. In an ischemic episode, a sense of numbness or "deadness" is described. Migraine symptoms have a characteristic unilateral distribution affecting one arm, often spreading over several minutes proximally from the hand to affect the mouth and tongue – "cheiro-oral distribution." This spread to involve the tongue is typical with migraine aura and is rarely seen in cerebrovascular ischemic episodes. Even when sensory symptoms occur, the majority of auras include visual symptoms. Hence, a useful screening question may be: *"Do you have visual disturbances that last up to one hour and resolve before or with the onset of headache?"*

Tension-type headache is often described as a "featureless" headache.

Associated symptoms of cluster headache and other trigeminal autonomic cephalalgias are most prominent on the side ipsilateral to the pain, and include lacrimation, conjunctival injection, nasal congestion, rhinorrhea, Horner's syndrome, facial swelling, erythema, or pallor.

"*Have you found any triggers for attacks?*" Most patients with migraine can list at least a couple of triggers spontaneously and will identify several more if prompted with a list. Within a cluster, alcohol, heat, high altitude, and sleep are common triggers.

"*What makes the headache better?*"; "*What makes the headache worse?*" This can elicit a response such as "lying still helps, while movement makes the headache worse" in the case of migraine. For cluster, patients rarely stay still, often crying and pacing restlessly during the pain (Blau 1993).

"*Who else in your family has similar headaches?*" Although a family history can confirm the diagnosis, absence of a family history does not prohibit migraine. Do not assume that the headache is the same as the patients – many family members of cluster headache patients have migraine.

"*What do you do when you have a headache?*" Patients should be encouraged to describe medication taken, as well as what they physically do – go to bed, lie still, sleep, etc. Those who continue working should be questioned on how well they function.

"*What do the headaches stop you from doing?*" Headaches can cause significant disability with time lost from work, household duties, and leisure, particularly if attacks are severe and/or frequent. This has important implications for treatment as disabling attacks require more aggressive therapy.

"*What medication do you treat the headaches with and what have you tried in the past? How many days in a month do you NOT take a medication of any type (prescription or OTC) for headache?*" Many treatments that appear to fail might succeed if taken in adequate doses, sufficiently early in attacks. Establish what has failed in the past, and why, before recommending alternatives. Patients with frequent headaches should be carefully questioned about frequency with which they take acute medications to exclude medication overuse.

"*How do you feel between attacks?*" The response for episodic headache is usually "*Fine.*" Patients with continued symptoms between attacks may have more than one type of headache.

"*What worries you about your headaches?*" Many patients have fears that they find hard to express. A simple question can prevent the patient leaving the consulting room still harboring fear of a brain tumor that they have been frightened to ask about. Isolated headache is rarely caused by an intracranial lesion, and in primary care, the risk of a brain tumor with headache presentation is only 0.09% (Hamilton and Kernick 2007). Directing this question has the advantage of enabling the doctor to know what the patient's ideas are so that they can be reinforced or refuted, and developed into management plans. This can help forge a better bond between doctor and patient. Patients often do not give an immediate answer to the question, but wait until they are being examined. This may be because they feel less vulnerable during a nonthreatening examination. Eye contact is lost and the break in tension may permit the patient to release information or ask questions that are important.

General Questions

Most of the following will already be known to the physician but confirm that there have been no recent changes to the patients' general health.

Systemic Review

Most patients presenting purely with migraine are otherwise fit and well. Symptoms suggestive of systemic disease require more detailed questioning. In particular, symptoms such as fever, night sweats, chills, and weight loss should be elicited.

Past Medical History

There is rarely a relevant medical history for migraine although some patients may time the onset subsequent to a head injury, illness, or emotional upset. In most cases, it is impossible to know if the event was truly the initiator of migraine. Travel sickness and recurrent abdominal pain in childhood have been linked to the development of migraine in later life, but this association is not diagnostic. Comorbid conditions should be considered, particularly depression, which may require specific management. Work difficulties, marital problems, alcoholism, etc., need consideration. Medical conditions relevant to therapy should be considered, for example, peptic ulcer or uncontrolled hypertension would contraindicate NSAIDs or triptans, respectively.

Medications

Headache is listed as a side effect of almost every available drug. However, some drugs have been particularly associated with increased headache. These include the combined oral contraceptive pill, although menstrual migraine sometimes resolves with continued use. Occasionally, increased frequency and severity of headache or migraine may necessitate adjustments to treatment or even withdrawal. Specific drugs, including dipyridamole, trazadone, nitroglycerin, among others, may worsen migraine. A careful drug history is necessary to ensure that there is no incompatibility between drugs used for migraine and those taken for other indications. Frequent use of acute headache treatments can lead to medication-overuse headache.

Social History

Alcohol sometimes triggers migraine and can worsen cluster headaches in the active phase. Several occupations can increase the likelihood of migraine. Stressful jobs create obvious triggers that can be specifically identified. Working at a computer screen for several hours can result in tension headache. Shift work can disrupt sleep and dietary routines. Unemployment and redundancy carry the risk of depression. Personal or family problems may be relevant.

The impact of headache on the patient's life should be discussed. It is not uncommon for patients to fear making arrangements in case they are disrupted by a migraine. This cycle of fear can be broken with effective management but may require additional psychological treatment.

Family History

A family history may be present but is not necessary to confirm the diagnosis. A family history of arterial disease may be relevant if vasoconstrictor drugs are considered.

Examination

The main purpose of the examination is to reassure patients. Patients and their family are often worried that there is a serious cause for the headaches such as brain tumor or stroke. Patients expect a physical examination and may be less likely to agree with the doctor's perspective and subsequent management recommendations if this is not done. The examination can be brief, but should be thorough. In patients seen in a specialist clinic, fewer than 1% have headaches secondary to intracranial disease, and all have signs of it. The mental state will have been assessed while taking the history. Pulse, blood pressure, and auscultation for cardiac abnormalities and bruits should be checked first and are particularly important if vasoconstrictor drugs such as ergotamine or the triptans are considered. Examining the jaw can identify temporomandibular joint dysfunction that can give rise to headache. Examination of the neck and cervical spine may reveal muscle contraction, cervical spondylosis, or even meningism.

While Taking the History

Speech, mood, and memory can be assessed by the patient's response to questions.

At the end of the history, request permission from the patient before the examination.

A Rapid Neurological Examination

It is unnecessary to check every aspect of neurological function, and a routine screen should take no more than 5 min (❯ *Table 12.3*). Particular attention should be paid to examination of the cranial nerves, tendon reflexes, and optic disks. If the history suggests that there is a more sinister cause for the headache, a full neurological appraisal is necessary. It is of great comfort to patients when doctors explain that the findings are "normal." When time is short, a minimum examination should include blood pressure and examination of the optic fundi.

Investigations

In clinical practice, the initial concern is to differentiate primary headaches from sinister secondary headaches. Investigations do not contribute to the diagnosis of primary headaches and are not warranted in children or adults with a defined headache and normal neurological examination (Detsky et al. 2006; Weingarten et al. 1992). Investigations are indicated if secondary headache is suspected OR because of undefined headache, atypical symptoms, persistent neurological or psychopathological abnormalities, abnormal findings on neurologic examination, or recent trauma. A low threshold is indicated for new-onset headaches and if there is significant parental anxiety about a child with headache. Inappropriate investigations can increase morbidity, particularly in the presence of unrelated incidental findings and, with respect to computed tomography, unnecessary radiation exposure. Symptomatic brain abnormalities are identified in up to 14% of an asymptomatic population (Vernooij et al. 2007). Many patients request investigations for the reassurance that they do not have a brain tumor or other serious underlying pathology. This may be avoided if, on the basis of a sound history and examination, the doctor spends time with the patient directly discussing his or her concerns

◘ Table 12.3

The neurological examination (MacGregor and Frith 2008)

While patient is standing	
Ask the patient to:	Tests:
Close your eyes and stand with your feet together (Romberg)	Midline cerebellar; dorsal column; proprioception
Open your eyes and walk heel to toe	Midline cerebellar; dorsal column; proprioception
Walk on your tip-toes	Power of dorsiflexion
Walk on your heels	Power of plantar flexion
Close your eyes and hold your hands out straight in front of you with your palms flat and facing upward	Hemisphere lesions (e.g., left hemisphere lesion, right hand will bend in and drift up)
	Neglect (e.g., left parietal lesion, right hand will drop down)
Keep your eyes closed. Touch your nose with the fingertip that I touch (person testing uses their own finger to touch a couple of the patient's fingertips in turn)	Light touch and finger-nose test (cerebellar or sensory ataxia and light-touch in fingertip)
Open your eyes and with your arms outstretched, pretend to play the piano	Fine finger movements
	Pyramidal and extrapyramidal function
Tap the back of one hand with your other hand. Change hands and repeat.	Ataxia
Screw your eyes up tight and then relax and open your eyes	Pupil dilation and constriction
	Horner's syndrome
	Lower motor neurone lesion
Bare your teeth/grin	Upper motor neurone facial weakness
Stick your tongue out and wiggle it	Bulbar and pseudobulbar palsy
Stare at my face at point at the fingers which move (person testing has arms out to the side with index finger pointing. Arms stop in an arc and index finger is wiggled on each side in turn or together)	Temporal field defects (important visual field defects always involve one or other temporal field)
	Inattention (parietal lobe lesion)
Keeping your head still, stare at my finger and follow my finger up and down with your eyes (person testing draws a wide "H" in the air)	Eye movements (cranial nerves III, IV, and VI)
	Nystagmus; saccadic (jerky) eye movements
While patient is lying down	
Examine:	Tests:
Limb reflexes	Upper motor neurone lesion (brisk)
	Peripheral nerve or nerve root lesion (absent)
Plantar response	Upper motor neurone lesion (Babinski/extensor response)
Abdominal reflexes	Spinal cord disease

◻ Table 12.3 (Continued)

While patient is lying down	
Funduscopy	Raised intracranial pressure (papilledema)
	Optic atrophy
Pulse and BP	Hypertension
If indicated, examine the chest, palpate breasts, and abdomen	Systemic disease, e.g., neoplasia

(Fitzpatrick 1996). Although it may be necessary for a few who will not be reassured in the absence of a "brain scan," any anxiolytic effects of a normal result may not be sustained beyond a few months (Howard et al. 2005).

Full blood count and erythrocyte sedimentation rate may detect the presence of infection, temporal arteritis, or malignancy.

Plain radiography of the skull is normal in most patients with headache but may be indicated if there is a history of head injury or if symptoms/examination are suggestive of a tumor, particularly of the pituitary gland. This has now been largely replaced by imaging studies.

Lumbar puncture confirms infection (meningitis or encephalitis). It should be used if subarachnoid hemorrhage (SAH) is suspected and CT is either unavailable or the results are inconclusive – CT may be normal in 10–15% of all subarachnoid hemorrhage, and its ability to detect SAH declines with time after the onset of symptoms. Lumbar puncture is also useful for the detection of elevated or low intracranial pressure.

Electroencephalography (*EEG*) is of little diagnostic value in headache but may be considered if a clinical diagnosis suggests features of epilepsy, such as loss of consciousness occurring in association with migraine.

Computerized tomography (*CT*) is of limited value for routine evaluation of headache as a number of secondary causes can easily be missed (❷ *Table 12.4*). CT can demonstrate structural lesions including tumor, vascular malformations, hemorrhage, and hydrocephalus. If intracranial or subarachnoid hemorrhage is suspected, CT scan without contrast can detect recent bleeds – MRI may miss fresh blood. It may be necessary to give an intravenous injection of contrast material to highlight a suspected tumor or vascular lesion. Indications for CT are persistent focal neurological deficits, symptoms or signs suggestive of an arteriovenous malformation and hemorrhagic stroke.

Magnetic resonance imaging (*MRI*) produces better definition of soft tissue abnormalities than CT scanning. MRI with gadolinium is the investigation of choice for meningeal pathology. Although CT detects most tumors, MRI is superior to CT when imaging lesions in the region of the posterior fossa, axial tumors, the orbit and the paranasal sinuses, and demyelinating lesions.

Magnetic resonance or CT-angiography is indicated in patients with thunderclap headache when the lumbar puncture and unenhanced CT scan are unremarkable. Noninvasive angiography is reliable in detecting cervicocephalic arterial dissection, cerebral venous sinus thrombosis, dural arteriovenous fistula, reversible cerebral vasoconstriction syndrome, or intracranial aneurysm.

Cerebral angiography is rarely required as a primary investigation and its use is limited by its invasiveness. If CT or MRI confirms arteriovenous malformation, angiography is used to define the extent of the lesion and demonstrate feeding and draining vessels. Angiography is also still a gold standard for identifying the site, size, and morphology of intracranial aneurysms in the setting of subarachnoid hemorrhage.

◻ **Table 12.4**

Secondary causes of headache that may be missed on computed tomography (Dodick 2010)

Vascular	Saccular aneurysms
	Subarachnoid hemorrhage
	Arteriovenous malformations (especially posterior fossa)
	Carotid or vertebral artery dissections
	Ischemic stroke
	Cerebral venous sinus thrombosis
	Vasculitis
	Reversible cerebral vasoconstriction syndrome
Neoplasia	Parenchymal and extra-axial neoplasms (especially in the posterior fossa)
	Meningeal carcinomatosis
	Pituitary tumor and hemorrhage
	Metastatic brain tumor
Cervicomedullary lesions	Chiari malformation
	Foramen magnum meningioma
	Acoustic schwanomma
Infections	Meningoencephalitis
	Cerebritis and brain abscess
Other	CSF leak (intracranial hypotension)
	Intracranial hypertension
	Idiopathic hypertrophic pachymeningitis

Isotope scanning and *doppler flow studies* are only of value for research in headache. Detection of carotid dissection may be possible with carotid Doppler studies when there is an index of suspicion and MR or CT-angiography is not available.

Conclusions: How to Get It Right

Making a diagnosis of headache based on the suggested approach may appear time consuming. However, primary care physicians often have the advantage of treating a patient for several years and so, for many of the questions, the answers will already be known. A brief but thorough neurological examination need not be time consuming, although blood pressure and fundoscopy are mandatory. The diagnosis should be reviewed at follow-up visits, particularly in cases of treatment failure. Be alert to coexisting headaches, which can confuse the picture.

Need to Know

- A new headache needs a new diagnosis.
- All patients presenting with sudden severe headache warrant further investigation.

- Increased frequency of headache should prompt suspicion of medication overuse.
- Unless directly questioned, patients may not reveal the true extent of medication use.
- Listen to symptoms that patients describe, not the diagnosis that they have been given.
- Pattern recognition from the history enables correct diagnosis.
- Different headaches need to be treated differently.

Case Histories

Case 1

PW is a 52-year-old white male. He presented to the emergency department 5 days after the abrupt onset of his "worse ever headache" associated with nausea and photophobia. At the time of review, his headache was less severe but he still felt unwell. He had a history of infrequent migraine without aura but described this recent headache as more severe and more prolonged than his usual attacks. Prescription drugs that usually helped his migraine had not been effective. He had no other relevant medical history and was not on any regular medication. Glasgow Coma Scale was 15, and neurological examination was unremarkable. A computed tomographic (CT) brain scan identified perimesencephalic subarachnoid hemorrhage (SAH), which resolved on serial CTs. Cerebral angiography showed no evidence of arteriovenous malformation or aneurysm. PW was discharged following full recovery.

Comment: Perimesenchephalic hemorrhage is a non-aneurysmal cause that affects around 10% of patients with SAH. The CT scan shows a characteristic pattern of bleeding confined to the midbrain cisterns. The risk of rebleeding is very low, and the long-term prognosis is good.

Case 2

AS is a 44-year-old Asian female. She visited her primary care physician because of weekly attacks of migraine that were not responding to her usual painkillers. The history revealed that her first attack of migraine when she was 12 but attacks were only once or twice a year. Since her 20s, she had experienced migraine once or twice a month. Over the last 4 years, the attacks had become more frequent and in the last 6 months, the attacks were occurring weekly. AS stated that she had a headache most days but could manage these; it was the weekly attacks that were troubling her. Direct questioning revealed that AS was taking painkillers most days, as this could get her through the day. AS was otherwise healthy and took no medication other than for her headaches. Physical and neurological assessments were unremarkable. The doctor considered that, given the frequency of medication use, the most likely diagnosis was medication-overuse headache. After appropriate management, AS stopped daily medication and reverted to a pattern of migraine once or twice a month. She felt well between attacks, which once again responded to their usual treatment.

Comment: Daily headache is associated with medication-overuse headache (MOH) in around 30% of the population and up to 60% of patients attending specialist clinics. It is most prevalent in those aged 40–50 years and affects three times more women than men. Any patient who has headache more than 10 days a month should be questioned about their use of medication. Specific questions should use of analgesics for reasons other than headache; use of over-the-counter as well as prescription drugs; acute medications becoming less effective;

and escalation to using more drugs. Assessment should also search for possible complications of regular drug intake (e.g., recurrent gastric ulcers, anemia).

Case 3

HM, a 35-year-old white male had been referred to the specialist because his migraine had returned and had failed to respond to treatment. The referral letter from the primary care physician stated that codeine-containing analgesia had controlled HM's pain and several standard migraine prophylactics had been prescribed without success. HM said that he had had migraine for the last 10 years. He usually only had them on-and-off for a couple of months but the present bout had started over 4 months ago and showed no signs of letting up. The history revealed attacks that woke HM a couple of hours after going to sleep, most nights. The pain was excruciating, centered on his right eye, which he felt was being pushed out of his skull. The eye looked red and watery, but the left eye was normal. The pain was so severe that he sat on the bed crying and rocking until the symptoms abated a couple of hours later. Normally a heavy social drinker, HM was avoiding alcohol as it almost instantly triggered an attack. No medication worked, and he felt he could not go on. Physical and neurological assessments were unremarkable. The specialist recognized the typical history of cluster headache and arranged appropriate management.

Comment: Cluster headache affects fewer than 1% of the population. It is frequently misdiagnosed as migraine and treated as such. Unlike migraine, it affects more men than women. The typical "clusters" of attacks, "clockwork" timing, severity of pain, and unilateral autonomic symptoms are distinctive symptoms that lead to the correct diagnosis.

Case 4

PN was a 41-year-old Hispanic male who presented with a 4-h history of a severe unremitting occipital headache that started abruptly while he was straining at stool. The headache was associated with nausea, photophobia, and recurrent vomiting. He preferred to lie still as movement worsened the pain. He had a history of episodic migraine with aura since the age of 14 with, usually, two or three attacks each year that were rarely troublesome. He described this new headache as very different from his migraine. There was no other relevant personal or family history. Examination was unremarkable, although PN was in obvious pain. There was no neck stiffness or focal neurological symptoms.

Complete blood count, serum chemistry, urinalysis, urine drug screen, and electrocardio-gram revealed no abnormalities or remarkable findings. Unenhanced brain CT was normal. There was no evidence of subarachnoid hemorrhage, ischemic or intraparenchymal hemor-rhagic stroke, or intracranial mass lesion. Lumbar puncture revealed an opening pressure of 12 cm water, CSF was clear and without red or white blood cells or xanthachromia, and serum-matched total protein and glucose were normal. Gram stain was negative.

The patient was discharged from the emergency department, only to return 2 days later with another abrupt onset, severe headache that occurred during sexual intercourse. Brain MRI, MR venography, and MR-angiography revealed multiple areas of vasoconstriction involving the anterior and posterior cerebral arteries. A diagnosis of reversible cerebral vasoconstriction syndrome (RCVS) was made. Nimodipine was initiated at a dose of 60 mg every 6 h for the first week, then 30 mg every 6 h for the next 3 weeks. MR-angiogram of the head and neck was repeated 4 weeks after the first imaging study and demonstrated complete resolution of the cerebral vasoconstriction.

Comment: The differential diagnosis of sudden-onset severe headache (thunderclap headache: TCH) is important because of the morbidity and mortality associated with the conditions that can present with TCH. The diagnosis may be challenging when the headache occurs in isolation and in the absence of neurological symptoms or signs, thereby lowering the index of suspicion of a sinister secondary cause. Although subarachnoid hemorrhage and hemorrhagic and ischemic stroke are likely to be identified by brain CT and lumbar puncture, other causes such as cerebral venous sinus thrombosis, carotid or vertebral artery dissection, and RCVS require angiography. Hence, the clinical approach to the patient with TCH should be methodical, tailored to evaluate each of these causes in an appropriate and sequential fashion.

TCH associated with RCVS invariably occurs, and commonly recurs, within the first 7–10 days after the initial onset. However, all patients who present for the first time with TCH should be evaluated for RCVS, which is a much less benign condition than is suggested in the International Classification of Headache Disorders (ICHD-II), where it is listed as 6.7.3 *Headache attributed to benign (or reversible) angiopathy of the central nervous system.* Rapid and accurate diagnosis is important since ischemic or hemorrhagic stroke occurs in up to one-third of patients in the ensuing weeks. It is important to note that up to 20% of patients eventually diagnosed with RCVS have normal initial CT- or MR-angiography. RCVS has been associated not only with serious disorders such as pheochromocytoma, severe hypertension, carcinoid, and porphyria but also with pregnancy, exposure to illicit (marijuana, cocaine) and pharmaceutical drugs (e.g., bromocriptine, SSRIs, intravenous immunoglobulin, and over-the-counter medications containing pseudoephedrine). In the absence of a demonstrable precipitating disease or drug, the headache is often triggered by a Valsalva maneuver. It is probably a commonly overlooked cause of TCH, as recent studies indicate that 40–60% of patients who present with TCH and a negative CT and LP have cerebral vasoconstriction on MR-angiography. Initial management includes control of blood pressure, hydration, analgesia, and avoidance of drugs with vasoconstrictor activity (e.g., triptans, ergots). Nimodipine is usually initiated at a dose of 30–60 mg every 6 h, to reverse the vasoconstriction and minimize the risk of stroke, and should be continued until reversal is complete and the patient has been without headache or other symptoms for at least 7 days. Reversal of vasoconstriction is demonstrated by repeated CT- or MR-angiography, and is usually complete by 2–4 weeks after the onset of headache but may take up to 2 months.

References

Bahra A, Goadsby PJ (2004) Diagnostic delays and mismanagement in cluster headache. Acta Neurol Scand 109:175–179

Bille B (1997) A 40-year follow-up of school children with migraine. Cephalalgia 17:488–491

Blau JN (1993) Behaviour during a cluster headache. Lancet 342:723–725

Blau JN, MacGregor EA (1995) Migraine consultations: a triangle of viewpoints. Headache 35:104–106

Bone I, Fuller G (2002) Headache. J Neurol Neurosurg Psychiatry 72(Suppl 2):ii1

Detsky ME, McDonald DR, Baerlocker MO, Tomlinson GA, McCory DC, Booth CM (2006) Does this patient with headache have a migraine or need neuroimaging? J Am Med Assoc 296:1274–1283

Dodick DW (2010) Pearls: headache. Semin Neurol 30(1):74–81

Fitzpatrick R (1996) Telling patients there is nothing wrong. BMJ 313:311–312

Giffin NJ, Ruggiero L, Lipton RB, Silberstein SD, Tvedskov JF, Olesen J, Altman J, Goadsby PJ, Macrae A (2003) Premonitory symptoms in migraine: an electronic diary study. Neurology 60:935–940

Hamilton W, Kernick D (2007) Clinical features of primary brain tumours: a case-control study using electronic primary care records. Br J Gen Pract 57:695–699

Headache Classification Subcommittee of the International Headache Society (IHS) (2004) The international classification of headache disorders (2nd edn.). Cephalalgia 24:1–160

Howard L, Wessely S, Leese M, Page L, McCrone P, Husain K, Tong J, Dowson A (2005) Are investigations anxiolytic or anxiogenic? A randomised controlled trial of neuroimaging to provide reassurance in chronic daily headache. J Neurol Neurosurg Psychiatry 76:1558–1564

Latinovic R, Gulliford M, Ridsdale L (2006) Headache and migraine in primary care: consultation, prescription, and referral rates in a large population. J Neurol Neurosurg Psychiatry 77:385–387

Laughey WF, MacGregor EA, Wilkinson MI (1993) How many different headaches do you have? Cephalalgia 13:136–137

Lipton RB, Stewart WF, Simon D (1998) Medical consultation for migraine: results from the American migraine study. Headache 38:87–96

Lipton RB, Dodick D, Sadovsky R, Kolodner K, Endicott J, Hettiarachchi J, Harrison W (2003) A self-administered screener for migraine in primary care: the ID migraine validation study. Neurology 61: 375–382

MacGregor A, Frith A (eds) (2008) ABC of headache. BMJ Books, London

MacGregor EA, Steiner TJ, Davies PTG (2010) Guidelines for all healthcare professionals in the diagnosis and management of migraine, tension-type, cluster and medication-overuse headache. Available at: http://www.bash.org.uk/. Accessed 31 Jan 2011

Stewart WF, Wood C, Reed ML, Roy J, Lipton RB (2008) Cumulative lifetime migraine incidence in women and men. Cephalalgia 28:1170–1178

van Vliet JA, Eekers PJ, Haan J, Ferrari MD (2003) Features involved in the diagnostic delay of cluster headache. J Neurol Neurosurg Psychiatry 74: 1123–1125

Vazquez-Barquero A, Ibanez FJ, Herrera S, Izquierdo JM, Berciano J, Pascual J (1994) Isolated headache as the presenting clinical manifestation of intracranial tumors: a prospective study. Cephalalgia 14:270–272

Vernooij MW, Ikram MA, Tanghe HL, Vincent AJ, Hofman A, Krestin GP, Niessen WJ, Breteler MM, van der Lugt A (2007) Incidental findings on brain MRI in the general population. N Engl J Med 357:1821–1828

Weingarten S, Kleinman M, Elperin L, Larson EB (1992) The effectiveness of cerebral imaging in the diagnosis of chronic headache. Arch Intern Med 152:2457–2462

13 The Use of Diaries in the Management of Headache

Vera Osipova[1] · Rigmor Jensen[2] · Cristina Tassorelli[3]
[1]Neurological Clinic, Sechenov Moskow Medical Academy,
Moscow, Russian Federation
[2]Glostrup Hospital, University of Copenhagen, Glostrup, Copenhagen,
Denmark
[3]University Consortium for Adaptive Disorders and Head Pain
(UCADH), University of Pavia, Pavia, Italy

Paolo Martelletti, Timothy J. Steiner (eds.), *Handbook of Headache*, DOI 10.1007/978-88-470-1700-9_13,
© Lifting The Burden 2011

Abstract: The diagnosis of primary headache depends mostly on a detailed history and a normal physical examination. In clinical practice, patients often have difficulty recalling their headache characteristics, especially if they experience several types of headache. Headache diaries and calendars make it possible to record precisely, in a contemporaneous manner, the characteristics of every attack, thus minimizing recall bias and increasing accuracy in the description of attack frequency and characteristics. Several types of diagnostic diaries can be used, depending on the purpose of monitoring and the type of headache. They represent a useful tool, for both the doctor and the patient, in the diagnostic process as well as in the management of the disease.

Introduction

Migraine (M), tension-type headache (TTH), cluster headache (CH), and medication overuse headache (MOH) probably represent the four headache disorders responsible for the vast majority of all headache-related burden (Jensen and Stovner 2008; Stovner et al. 2007). In the case of these four types of headache, the criteria defined by the International Headache Society (IHS) in the International Classification of Headache Disorders (2nd edition) (ICHD-II) (Headache Classification Committee of the International Headache Society 2004) are almost exclusively phenomenological that is based on the anamnestic occurrence of well-defined clinical features of headache during the last year and, in the case of MOH, of specific drug intake behaviors in the last 3 months.

Thus, the diagnosis is reached mainly through a detailed patient history, the finding of a negative physical examination, and the exclusion of local or systemic disease(s) that can cause secondary or symptomatic headache. In clinical practice, it is known that patients may not easily identify and recall certain features of their headaches, especially if they experience several types of headache, as well as drugs taken to abort the pain. Furthermore, the episodic nature of the disease may cause bias toward the most severe or recent headache attacks. Thus, during the interview, patients are more likely to report their most severe, full-blown attacks, forgetting to describe incomplete ones. This could interfere with the quantification of the real amount of headache days per month. Moreover, some difficulties are related to the headache syndromes themselves, because clinical features may change during the course of the attacks and from one attack to another. Some situations (i.e., aura symptoms) imply specific problems and require specially designed tools.

Therefore, the use of monitoring instruments – headache diaries and calendars – becomes crucial in the diagnosis of headache syndromes. Headache diaries and calendars make it possible to record prospectively the characteristics of every attack, and this may reduce the recall bias and increase the accuracy of the headache description. Indications and advantages in the use of diagnostic headache diaries are summarized in ❷ *Table 13.1*.

The use of headache diaries seems a valid tool to help both patients and doctors to learn more about headache features and temporal pattern. The headache diary can be seen a valid companion in different moments of the approach to the headache patients, and in these different moments, it has specific indications and roles.

When Is It Indicated to Use Diaries?

Diaries can be used:

1. Before the first visit
2. In the follow-up after the first visit

◻ Table 13.1

Indications and advantages in the use of diagnostic headache diaries

• To provide the physician with information concerning the real frequency and temporal pattern of attacks/days with headache(s)
• To distinguish between coexisting headache types (in patients with two or more headache types)
• To identify possible trigger factors
• To study the natural history of headaches
• To reveal specific associated symptoms
• To reveal the presence, duration, and type of aura symptoms
• To identify clearly episodic and chronic tension-type headache
• To diagnose (different types of) menstrual migraine
• To evaluate the frequency and amount of symptomatic drugs taken by patients
• To obtain baseline information necessary for the evaluation of preventive treatment
• To monitor the response to treatments
• To evaluate patients' compliance
• To educate patients to better manage their headache
• To empower patients through the understanding of how internal and/or external factors may modify their disease

Use of Diaries Before the First Visit

A simplified version of headache diary has been devised and tested in Danish and in Italian, to aid the diagnosis of migraine (M), tension-type headache (TTH), and medication overuse headache (MOH) (Tassorelli et al. 2008). This basic headache diary (❷ Fig. 13.1) was derived from the different formats of diaries used in the everyday practice in the Danish Headache Center and Pavia Headache Centre (❷ Figs. 13.2 and ❷ 13.3) (Nappi et al. 2006; Russell et al. 1992) and was completed by patients in advance of their first visit to the Headache Center. The basic headache diary has been subsequently optimized with the help of an European panel of experts (UK, Russia, Germany, Portugal, Spain, Bulgaria, the Netherlands, Romania, Croatia, Argentina, Chile) and has been tested in a huge population in multilingual versions (manuscript in preparation). Preliminary data suggest that the diary is suitable for diagnosing coexistence of different types of headache, providing their relative frequency, better identifying trigger and precipitant factors, and allowing realistic evaluation of medications taken by patients in a given lapse of time.

This study supports the approach that the scheme "first visit – follow-up with/without diary monitoring – control visit," is more effectively replaced by the scheme "diary monitoring-first visit-follow-up with diary monitoring – control visits" (❷ Fig. 13.4).

Similarly, in primary care, the diary should be given to patient before patient's first consultation. This may provide additional information that can be integrated with the data collected through the interview and may ultimately shorten the time to definite diagnosis and allow a more complete diagnosis (especially in the event of coexisting forms of headache). Patients should fill in the diary each evening on a day with headache. This information should be sufficient to classify the attack according to ICHD-II (Headache Classification Committee of the International Headache Society 2004). Patients should record the date on which the

Name: _____ Birth Date (d/m/y)_____

1. Day and date of the month		Monday	Tuesday	Wednesday	Thursday	Friday	Saturday	Sunday
		___	___	___	___	___	___	___
2. Did you have a headache today? (if no, go directly to question 15)	No Yes							
3. If yes, when did you first notice it?	(hr:min)							
4. When did it finally go?	(hr:min)							
5. In the hour *before* it started, did you notice eyesight interference such as flashing lights, zigzag lines or blind spots?	No Yes							
6. Was the headache on one side of the head or both?	On one side On both sides							
7. What was the headache like?	Throbbing Pressing							
8. Did physical activity (such as walking upstairs) make the headache worse?	No Yes							
9. How bad was your headache overall? (please see instructions)	Not bad Quite bad Very bad							
10. Were you nauseated? (did you feel you were going to be sick)?	No A little More than a little							
11. Did you throw up?	No Yes							
12. Were you bothered by the light?	No Yes							
13. Were you bothered by noise?	No Yes							
14. Did you do anything, or did anything happen, that may have caused the attack?	If yes, please specify:							
15. Did you take any medication(s) today for headache or for any other pain? For each medication, please enter: a) the name b) the number you took c) the time(s) you took it (hr:min)								

Please check that you have filled in every column

◻ **Fig. 13.1**

Basic headache diary (English version) (Evolved from the diary published in reference Tassorelli et al. 2008)

headache occurred, start and end time of the attack, any aura symptoms, quality, location and intensity of pain, aggravation of pain by physical activity, accompanying symptoms – nausea, photophobia, and phonophobia – graded at none, mild, moderate, and severe, and precipitating factors, if known. All drugs taken (including simple pain killers) and the exact time of intake should also be recorded.

To increase compliance in completing diaries, patients need to be motivated and understand that the diary is a useful resource to ensure the best possible management of their disorder. The diary should come with a set of simple, but detailed instructions on how to complete each item. In the instructions, patients are asked to complete the diary each day and to bring it with them on the day of their appointment.

After each question put one X in the box which is most appropriate.

Name: Birthday:

19	Date:	/	/	/	/	/	/	/
When did the headache begin?	Indicate nearest hour:							
Just before the headache began, was there any disturbance of	vision:							
	other senses:							
Was the headache	rightsided:							
	leftsided:							
	both sides:							
Was the headache	pulsating/throbbing:							
	pressing/tightening:							
Was the headache *) See below	mild:							
	moderate:							
	severe:							
Did the headache change with physical activity such as walking stairs	worse:							
	unchanged:							
	better:							
Did you suffer from nausea?	no:							
	mild:							
	moderate:							
	severe:							
Were you bothered by light?	no:							
	mild:							
	moderate:							
	severe:							
Were you bothered by sounds?	no:							
	mild:							
	moderate:							
	severe:							
When did the headache disappear?	Indicate nearest hour:							
Did anything provoke this attack?	specify:							
Did you take any medicine? Mention each different compound, how much you took, and when you took it (nearest hour).	name:							
	how much:							
	time:							
	name:							
	how much:							
	time:							

*Mild: Does not inhibit work performance or other activities
Moderate: Inhibits, but does not prohibit work performance and other activities
Severe: Prohibits work and other activities

Copyright: Foundation for Migraine Research c/o Jes Olesen, Copenhagen, Denmark.

☐ Fig. 13.2
Paper version of the diary in use at the Danish Headache Center since several years (Nappi et al. 2006; Russell et al. 1992)

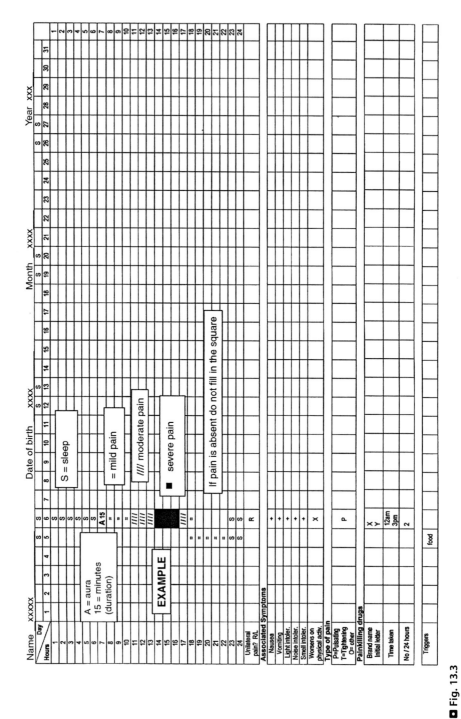

■ Fig. 13.3

Paper version of the diary in use at the Pavia Headache Centre since several years (Nappi et al. 2006)

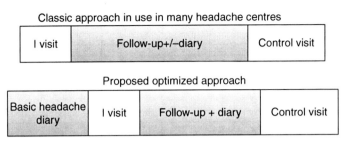

Fig. 13.4

Proposed optimized approach to migraine, tension-type headache, and medication overuse headache with addition of monitoring by means of the basic headache diary before the first visit at the Headache Center

Use of Diaries After the First Visit

The basic headache diary can be continued unless specific needs emerge during the first visit. Otherwise, ad hoc diaries can be used. In general, these diaries seem more helpful when they can show a full month of headache (❯ *Fig. 13.3*).

These diaries can be aimed at better defining a diagnosis (i.e., aura characteristics), identifying trigger or aggravating factors, or to monitor the effect of prescribed treatments, both acute (timing and completeness of effect) and preventive (number of monthly days with headache, monthly number of severe attacks).

Women's headache diary – In women, daily diaries and event logs should be highly detailed comprising menstrual cycle–related symptoms and use of sex hormones, whether for contraception, hormone replacement therapy, or other purposes. A complete record of the characteristics of menstrual bleeding can help define subpopulations of women suffering from pure menstrual migraine or from menstrually related migraine. Diaries are also useful for monitoring migraine during pregnancy and menopause (❯ *Fig. 13.4*, from Nappi et al. 2003, 2006).

Diaries for children – Metsähonkala et al. (1997) evaluated a modified version of the diary designed by Russell et al. (1992) for migraine with separate questions about nausea, vomiting, and loss of appetite. Intensity of pain was described both with words and numbers; other features were not graded. The diary proved more accurate than the interview alone with respect to duration of attacks, detection of other types of headache, presence of aura, etc. In another study, the compliance was quite poor (Richardson et al. 1983), which suggests the need for diaries specifically adapted for children, which are not only simplified but also based on a playful approach such as use of colors or emoticons.

Diary for medication overuse headache – An ongoing multicenter international study will provide insight into the usefulness of an electronic diary that has an alert/alarm system for improving communication between patients and doctors after withdrawal from overused drugs (www.comoestas-project.eu).

Diary for cluster headache – In these patients, some adaptations are necessary to the diary illustrated in ❯ *Fig. 13.3* with respect to listing specific associated autonomic symptoms and the number of attacks per day.

Web diary (electronic format) – A web version of the diary is used at the Pavia Headache Centre (❯ *Fig. 13.3*) and has proven very useful for patients who are familiar with the Internet

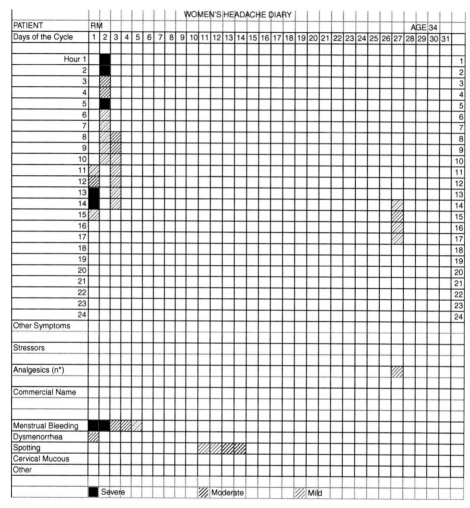

◻ Fig. 13.5
Ad hoc headache diary for women (Nappi et al. 2003, 2006)

(◉ *Fig. 13.5*) (Nappi et al. 2006). It enables clinical monitoring of the patient both prior to the medical examination and during the symptomatic and preventive course of treatment subsequently prescribed. This diary contains the same items as the traditional "paper" version and applies the same criteria for assessing the parameters. Patients fill in the diary on the Net (www.retedeccellenzacefalee.it), download it or submit it to the physician. Descriptive statistics can be performed on the monthly data (i.e., number of days/month with headache, number of headache attacks/month). Furthermore, the system makes it possible to create a bar chart that shows the headache attacks each month, days of menstrual bleeding and, where applicable, days on which the patient took an oral contraceptive. For each month in which the diary is completed, a brief report is developed and sent to the patient, commenting on the course/pattern of the headache.

How Long Is It Necessary to Use Diaries?

Patients should fill in the basic headache diary for at least 1 month before their first appointment to allow a clear picture of the possible headache diagnoses and drug use. One month is realistic and does not unnecessarily prolong the time before the first consultation and treatment recommendations. In tertiary care, the vast majority of patients suffer from chronic or very frequent headaches, so 1 month of diary informating reflects the real headache pattern. However, 1 month may be too short for recording infrequent forms of headache. In this case, the "diary period" could be increased accordingly.

After the first visit, patients should fill in the diary daily until the first follow-up visit. When the physician or the patient agree that the acute treatment is satisfactorily effective, it is possible to switch from the diary to a calendar (❷ Fig. 13.6) (Nappi et al. 2006; Tfelt-Hansen and Welch 2000). Once patients have learned to distinguish between TTH and migraine or other headaches, they are generally able to fill in the calendar correctly. As with epilepsy and other periodic disorders, the use of such calendars is invaluable in the long-term adjustment of the prophylactic strategy.

The calendar is much easier to keep for the patient than the diary and can be carried in a notebook. It contains information from a whole year in one card, and the evolution over time and the response to prophylactic treatment or cessation of daily intake of analgesics can easily be assessed. It is also an important tool in the direct dialogue with patients with respect to annual variations, treatment, and evolution of headaches. Many patients continue to complete calendars after being discharged from clinic (❷ Fig. 13.7).

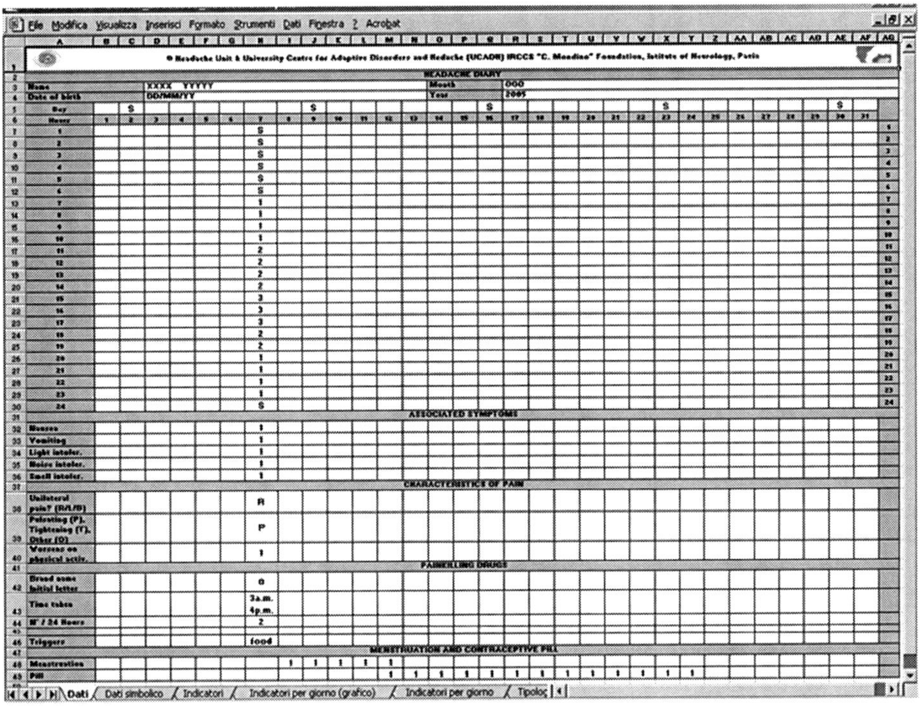

□ Fig. 13.6
Electronic version of paper diary used in Pavia (Nappi et al. 2006)

For your **migraine attacks** indicate the severity as:
1. mild;   2. medium;   3. severe.
1) A mild attack does not inhibit work or other activities.
2) A medium attack inhibits but does not prohibit work or other activities.
3) A severe attack prohibits work and/or other activities.

For your **tension-type headaches** use one or more crosses to indicate severity as defined above:
x. mild;   xx. medium;   xxx. severe.

For attacks of cluster **headache** use letters a, b and c for severity as defined above:
a. mild;   b. medium;   c. severe.

HEADACHE CALENDAR
The year 19_____

The headache calender is used to record all episodes of headache during an entire year. This information will greatly assist your doctor in selecting the best treatment, and it may help yourself to identify factors in your life which worsen or improve your headache condition.
Bring this calender to each consultation with your doctor.

Name:
Social security no.:
Address:
Telephone:

The owner of this card is being treated for headache/migraine by Dr.:

(STAMP)

	Jan.	Feb.	Mar.	Apr.	May	June	July	Aug.	Sept.	Oct.	Nov.	Dec.	
1													1
2													2
3													3
4													4
5													5
6													6
7													7
8													8
9													9
10													10
11													11
12													12
13													13
14													14
15													15
16													16
17													17
18													18
19													19
20													20
21													21
22													22
23													23
24													24
25													25
26													26
27													27
28													28
29													29
30													30
31													31

▢ Fig. 13.7
Calendar for headache in use at the Danish Headache Center (Tfelt-Hansen and Welch 2000)

Otherwise, patients should be instructed to resume filling in diaries whenever the headache starts to worsen in frequency or intensity, or whenever a new type of headache appears.

Other Applications of Headache Diaries and Calendars

In drug trials, diaries and calendars are generally used to evaluate the characteristics and frequency of headache attacks in the run-in period, and the response to symptomatic and preventive treatments. In studies on headache pathogenesis comparing patients and headache-free controls, the use of a headache diary was accidentally helpful also in demonstrating that controls do not always prove so "headache-free" as they are assumed to be (Wittrock et al. 1996). In particular, 34.2% of "headache-free" controls reported multiple headache days in their headache diaries. Many studies have used general diaries or modified diaries tailored to specific objectives to describe the clinical features of migraine including non-headache symptoms and precipitating factors of headache (Giffin et al. 2003; Chabriat et al. 1999).

Diaries have proved indispensable to investigate the relationship between migraine and several physiological parameters. Sleep patterns and the occurrence of migraine attacks were described in a study based on migraine and sleeping diaries (Niederberger et al. 1998). The recurrence of migraine related to female reproductive events (Niederberger et al. 1998; Sances et al. 2003; Johannes et al. 1995; MacGregor and Hackshaw 2004) was investigated using contemporaneous diary cards, which enable recording of headache features, menstruation, medication consumption (symptomatic/prophylactic), and hormonal treatment. A structured migraine diary can also be a valuable aid in improving communication between physicians and patients regarding migraine disability and treatment outcomes (Baos et al. 2005).

Limitations of Headache Diaries

The use of diagnostic headache diaries does have some limitations because the patient's general acceptance is still limited and some subjects are not able to complete them. The episodic nature of the disease causes a bias toward the most severe or recent headache attacks. Moreover, some

▢ Table 13.2
Limitations in the use of diagnostic headache diaries

• The diary cannot replace the clinical interview in the diagnosis of cluster headache and other primary short-lasting headaches
• The diary cannot replace the clinical interview in the diagnosis of secondary headaches
• The diary does not go beyond the first or second diagnostic level
• In case patient has two or more headache types or more than one headache episode per day, there could be some biases in the recording of headache manifestations
• Not all cases and details of migraine aura can be revealed with the diary
• Diaries are difficult to survey
• Time consuming
• The risk of low patient compliance or abilities

difficulties are related to the headache syndromes themselves, because clinical features may change during the course of the attacks and from one attack to another. Some situations (i.e., headaches in children or aura symptoms) imply specific problems and require specially designed tools (❍ *Table 13.2*).

Conclusions

Headache diaries and calendars are important monitoring instruments and are a useful aid in the diagnosis of primary headache syndromes. The combination "*interview + physical examination + headache diary*" should become a "gold standard" in the diagnosis of common headache disorders and replace the former standard "*interview + physical examination*" both in primary and specialized care.

A basic version of headache diary has been validated in an international multicenter study and will be soon available in different languages. This diary could be recommended as a homogeneous, valid support tool in the approach to the process of diagnosing of the most frequent and disabling forms of primary headache disorders in different countries and settings. Integrated with the data collected during the clinical interview, the data collected through the diary can subsequently increase the understanding of headache type(s) in a patient and many other related factors.

Developing new diaries for specific types of primary headache (e.g., migraine with aura, menstrual migraine, trigeminal autonomic cephalalgias) or for particular populations (e.g., children, elderly patients, women) is a necessary and desirable future task. Further studies will need to address these issues.

References

Baos V, Ester F, Castellanos A, Nocea G, Caloto MT, Gerth WC, I-Max Study Group (2005) Use of a structured migraine diary improves patient and physician communication about migraine disability and treatment outcomes. Int J Clin Pract 59:281–286

Chabriat H, Danchot J, Michel P, Joire JE, Henry P (1999) Precipitating factors of headache. A prospective study in a national control-matched survey in migraineurs and nonmigraineurs. Headache 39:335–338

Giffin NJ, Ruggiero L, Lipton RB, Silberstein SD, Tvedskov JF, Olesen J et al (2003) Premonitory symptoms in migraine: an electronic diary study. Neurology 60:935–940

Headache Classification Committee of the International Headache Society (2004) The international classification of headache disorders, 2nd edition. Cephalalgia 24(Suppl 1):1–160

Jensen R, Stovner LJ (2008) Epidemiology and comorbidity of headache. Lancet Neurol 7:354–361

Johannes CB, Linet MS, Stewart WF, Celentano DD, Lipton RB, Szklo M (1995) Relationship of headache to phase of the menstrual cycle among young women: a daily diary study. Neurology 45:1076–1082

MacGregor EA, Hackshaw A (2004) Prevalence of migraine on each day of the natural menstrual cycle. Neurology 63:351–353

Metsähonkala L, Sillanpää M, Tuominen J (1997) Headache diary in the diagnosis of childhood migraine. Headache 37:240–244

Nappi RE, Sances G, Brundu B, Ghiotto N, Detaddei S, Biancardi C et al (2003) Neuroendocrine response to the serotonin agonist M-Chlorphenylpiperazine in women with menstrual status migrainosus. Neuroendocrinology 78:52–60

Nappi G, Jensen R, Nappi RE, Sances G, Torelli P, Olesen J (2006) Diaries and calendars for migraine. A review. Cephalalgia 26:905–916

Niederberger U, Gerber WD, Schiffer N (1998) Sleeping behavior and migraine. An evaluation by daily self-reports. Schmerz 12:389–395

Richardson GM, McGrath PJ, Cunningham SJ, Humphreys P (1983) Validity of the headache diary for children. Headache 23:184–187

Russell MB, Rasmussen BK, Brennum J, Iversen HK, Jensen RA, Olesen J (1992) Presentation of a new instrument: the diagnostic headache diary. Cephalalgia 12:369–374

Sances G, Granella F, Nappi RE, Fignon A, Ghiotto N, Polatti F et al (2003) Course of migraine during pregnancy and postpartum: a prospective study. Cephalalgia 23:197–205

Stovner Lj, Hagen K, Jensen R, Katsarava Z, Lipton R, Scher A, Steiner T, Zwart JA (2007) The global burden of headache: a documentation of headache prevalence and disability worldwide. Cephalalgia 27:193–210

Tassorelli C, Sances G, Allena M, Ghiotto N, Bendtsen L, Olesen J, Nappi G, Jensen R (2008) The usefulness and applicability of a basic headache diary before first consultation: results of a pilot study conducted in two centres. Cephalalgia 28:1023–1030

Tfelt-Hansen P, Welch KMA (2000) General principles of pharmacological treatment of migraine. In: Olesen J, Tfelt-Hansen P, Welch KMA (eds) The headaches. Lippincott Williams & Wilkins, Philadelphia, pp 385–389

Wittrock DA, Ficek SK, Cook TM (1996) Headache-free controls? Evidence of headaches in individuals who deny having headaches during diagnostic screening. Headache 36:416–418

14 "Red Flags" in the Diagnostic Process

Maurice B. Vincent
Universidade Federal do Rio de Janeiro, Rio de Janeiro, RJ, Brazil

Paolo Martelletti, Timothy J. Steiner (eds.), *Handbook of Headache*, DOI 10.1007/978-88-470-1700-9_14,
© Lifting The Burden 2011

Abstract: Most headaches are primary and do not indicate the presence of underlying diseases. There are cases, however, in which head pain is a symptom of a life-threatening disorder. The physician must recognize red flags that indicate the presence of such serious conditions as they require immediate treatment. Potential seriousness indications include recent, particularly intense and very sudden headaches; pain that either are new after the age of 50 or have substantially changed from the previous head pain patterns; headaches that are concomitant with neurological deficits; headache with papilledema, loss of consciousness, seizures or cognitive impairments, meningeal irritation, or other abnormal neurological signs. Neuroimaging is the most important investigation in headache practice, followed by CSF and blood examinations. Imaging must be performed when red flags are present, and further tests such as spinal taps are required when neuroimaging is not elucidative. Venous thrombosis and the reversible cerebral vasoconstriction syndrome are examples of overlooked disorders that frequently present with headache only and require magnetic resonance venography (MRV) and arteriography for a proper diagnosis. Subarachnoid hemorrhage secondary to intracranial aneurysm, cerebral venous thrombosis, idiopathic thunderclap headache, meningitis, reversible cerebral vasoconstriction syndrome, posterior reversible encephalopathy syndrome, acute sinus disease, pituitary apoplexy, primary intracranial hypotension, hydrocephalus, and intracranial occupying lesions are all diseases that may present with headache as the most important or unique symptom.

Established Knowledge

One of the most challenging tasks for the clinician dealing with headache is to safely distinguish benign ailments from life-threatening disorders. Head and facial pain are symptoms frequently related to diseases that cannot be identified by any supplementary neurophysiological, neuroimaging, or laboratory examination. The diagnosis depends on attentiveness, cautiousness, and suspicion – skills physicians develop with practice and time. The majority of the information required for a correct headache diagnosis is available in the case history. The physical examination may sometimes disclose signs that indicate the presence of an underlying disorder. *Therefore, collecting a trustful history is the most important step for a proper headache diagnosis and for identifying relevant red flags.*

Noteworthy is the fact that the diagnostic judgment cannot be satisfactorily accomplished based on isolated red flags. Thus, an intense headache that presents for the first time in a patient during the fifth decade of life without previous history of head pain will necessarily be considered from a totally different perspective than a similar pain at the same age but in someone who claims the headache has been present for the past 20 years. Likewise, a sudden sexual thunderclap headache in its first episode represents a much higher risk than identical headaches occurring during orgasms for many years. A fixed paroxysmal headache fulfilling the diagnostic criteria for migraine in a young woman who suffers from the disease since adolescence must not be interpreted as a dangerous situation, but a fixed headache, especially if recent in time, accompanied by neurological deficits necessarily requires a careful neuroimaging workup. Not only all the variables have to be considered concomitantly, but also must be interpreted individually for every patient.

Two are frequent fears in patients coming to the office because of headache: tumors and aneurysms. The physician must understand the type of apprehensiveness the patient may have. Psychological motivations of this kind may justify the use of neuroimaging not exactly because of a red flag, but to reassure anxious patients that tumors and aneurysms are not present. The doctor will also explain why the supplementary investigation is required when red flags are present, and also why no examination is performed when history and physical examination suffice for a solid diagnostic conclusion. ❷ *Table 14.1* lists important red flags, necessary procedures, and possible associated diagnoses.

The Headache History

Onset and Development

The headache onset is crucial and must be approached first. *In general, the longer is the picture, the less likely is the diagnosis of a secondary disease.* Patients may frequently consider the moment in time when the headache got worse as the disease onset. Thus, right after informing the presumed date of onset, patients must be asked about any previous head pain. Not infrequently the answer will be "I suffered only the normal headaches before," indicating that the history actually started much earlier. *Long-lasting diseases, with clear-cut attacks set apart by asymptomatic intervals point to a benign primary headache, as opposed to recent and progressively aggravating headaches, specially beginning later in life.* Even when the headache is the only initial symptom, tumors, inflammatory and infectious diseases, as well as vascular abnormalities, will sooner or later present with other clinical signs and symptoms indicative of the underlying disorder.

The physician must always be aware of recent changes in the headache pattern. Of course, previous primary benign diseases, such as migraine and tension-type headache, do not preclude the patient from suffering a new life-threatening condition. Particularly tricky is the subject who frequently rings or comes to the office complaining about the same, well-known old primary headache disorder, as the doctor may feel encouraged to minimize the complaints concluding too fast that the diagnosis is still the same. *In fact, any changes in pain location, intensity, suddenness, character, and/or accompanying symptoms and signs must always be carefully considered.* Lack of awareness to such changes may lead to remarkable misconceptions. *Especially after the age of 50, a new headache or a substantial change of the usual headache picture without obvious reasons must be investigated.*

Suddenness

Suddenness is a crucial aspect to consider in headache practice. Most of the benign pictures develop over many hours. *Thus, a headache that reaches its maximum intensity in less than a minute represents one of the most important red flags.* In subarachnoid hemorrhage (SAH), the clinical hallmark is an excruciatingly severe, very sudden in onset headache, present in 50% of the cases. Among SAH patients, two thirds present loss of consciousness and/or focal deficits apart from the head pain. The diagnostic challenge resides in the remainders, as one third will present with nothing more than headache. In 20% of the SAH cases, the headache may develop gradually, over minutes. Valuable is the information that all patients report the present headache as more intense than previous episodes. Transient loss of consciousness, seizure, and double vision may be reported by 26%, 7%, and 5% of the patients, respectively (Linn et al. 1998). Around 20–50% of patients who present with a SAH report a severe headache during the

□ Table 14.1

Red flags requiring investigation of potentially serious headache disorders

Red flag	Additional clinical features	Examination	Possible diagnoses
Unique or multiple thunderclap headaches, irrespectively of trigger factors	Intense headache reaching maximum level within 1–2 min	MR and MRA, MRV CT scans	SAH
			Aneurysm
			RCVS
			Acute hypertensive crisis
			CVT
			Acute sinus disease
			Pituitary apoplexy
			Subdural hematomas
			Primary thunderclap headache
Intense recent unilateral headache	Horner syndrome, possible cervical pain	MRA including cervical arteries	Internal carotid artery dissection
Headache with meningeal irritation, thunderclap headache with normal imaging	Intense, diffuse pulsating headache	Spinal tap	Acute meningitis
			Lyme disease
			Neurosyphylis
			Fungeal meningitis
			Neoplasic leptomeningitis
			Sarcoidosis
			Primary CNS angiitis
			Collagen diseases
Headache after the age of 50	Localized or diffuse headache. Rigid, tender temporal artery	Erythrocyte sedimentation rate, Artery biopsy	Giant cell arteritis
		Duplex-duplex ultrasonography	
Headache onset in the elderly without previous headache tendency	Headache isolated or accompanied by neurological or systemic abnormalities	MR	Secondary headaches including: Cerebral occupying lesion
Recent developing headache, neurological deficits	Headache of relatively mild intensity, poorly localized or diffuse	MR	Cerebral occupying lesion
Headache aggravated by physical exertion, coughing, or Valsalva maneuver	Diffuse headache changing with head position, possible vomiting	MR	Intracranial hypertension – space-occupying lesions
		Spinal tap	
		Ophthalmologic examination (papilledema)	

◻ Table 14.1 (Continued)

Red flag	Additional clinical features	Examination	Possible diagnoses
Orthostastic headache	Possible VI nerve palsy, nuchal rigidity, visual impairment, tinnitus, hypoacusia, photophobia, nausea	MR, include contrasted T1 weighted images Spinal tap	Spontaneous intracranial hypotension
Fixed headache, especially when progressive	Headache that never shifts side, lack of primary headache criteria	MR	Secondary headaches, including tumors
Sexual activity headache	excruciating orgasmic headache	MP	Possible bleeding. Frequent primary headache
Sneezing headache	Short neck on examination	MR	Chiari malformation
Unilateral facial-periauricular-temporal pain	May radiate to neck, head. Limitation in mouth opening. Pain worsening by movement	TMJ MR Odontological examination	TMD
Absolute indomethacin response	Associated autonomic ipsilateral facial abnormalities	MR	Paroxysmal hemicrania
Unilateral frontal headache radiating from the back	Ipsilateal arm pain, triggered by sustained positions or neck movements, local blocks may alleviate the pain	Cervical MR	Cervicogenic headache syndrome
Recent change of headache pattern	Present headache different from the usual pain in location, frequency, duration, intensity, accompanying symptoms or signs	MR	Secondary headaches
		General examination	Chronification of preexisting primary headache
		Spinal tap may be required, as well as blood tests	Mediation overuse headache
Headache and seizure	Seizure during or right after a migrainous aura	MR	Migralepsy
Atypical aura		EEG	Headache as a manifestation of epilepsy
Complex visual phenomena	Headache as a preictal or postictal seizure		Possible parenchymal lesion

◘ Table 14.1 (Continued)

Red flag	Additional clinical features	Examination	Possible diagnoses
Prolonged aura	Headache may occur with motor deficit	MRI, include DWI imaging	TIA, ischemic stroke
Migrainous aura without previous history of migraine			
Headache in a patient with systemic disorder such as HIV, cancer, or infection, or immunodeficiency	Possible concomitant neurological deficit	MRI	Secondary headache
		Blood investigation including immunological and infectious diseases	CNS infection
Delusion, depression, anxiety, or other concomitant psychiatric disorder	Headache not easily comparable to usual clinical patterns	Psychiatric examination	Psychiatric comorbidity
Intense ocular/periorbital pain	Possible conjunctival injection, ptosis, anisocoria, corneal opacity	Ophthalmologic investigation	Acute angle closure glaucoma
	Blurred vision		
Intense ocular/periorbital pain	Proptosis, ocular palsy, conjunctival injection	Orbital MR	Intraorbital myositis
Intense relatively short-lasting headache	Ocular autonomic abnormalities including tearing, conjunctival injection, miosis, semi-ptosis	MR	Trigeminal autonomic cephalalgias

CNS central nervous system, CVT cerebral venous thrombosis, MR magnetic resonance, MRA magnetic resonance angiography, RCVS reverse cerebral vasoconstriction syndrome, SAH subarachnoidal hemorrhage, TIA transient ischemic attack, TMJ temporomandibular joint, TMD temporomandibular dysfunction

days or weeks preceding the very bleeding. This headache, referred as "warning" or "*sentinel headache*," has been considered as the result of "warning leaks" or small SAH. However, it has been found that only 11% of patients present such type of pain during the month preceding the SAH (Linn et al. 2000).

Although SAH has traditionally been considered the natural possibility in a subject suffering from a sudden and intense headache, hemorrhage is present in only 10–43% of such cases (Demaerschalk and Dodick 2003). Other diagnoses must, therefore, be taken into consideration in this context. Thunderclap headaches with extreme severity constitute the most important symptom in *Reversible Cerebral Vasoconstriction Syndrome* (RCVS). Indeed, a severe recent headache may be the only abnormality in 51% of these subjects. Multiple previous thunderclap headaches for some days are present in 94% of the patients, a pattern that may also occur preceding an aneurysm bleeding. The peak duration ranges from 5 min to 36 h; and 79% of the patients reported a trigger factor, including sexual intercourse (29%), defecation (21%), sudden emotion (19%), physical exertion (16%), urination without effort (11%), cough (11%), sneezing (11%), bathing or showering (10%), and sudden head movement (9%). Other neurological signs were noticed in 24% of the patients, mostly focal deficits and, less frequently, seizures (Ducros et al. 2007). *This is in accordance with the statement that headache associated with neurological deficits constitutes a major red flag.* In the so-called *posterior reversible encephalopathy syndrome* (PRES), similarly to RCVS, sudden headache may occur, with confusion, seizures, and cortical blindness. The diagnosis is supported by the typical MR images (Hinchey et al. 1996).

Headache is the most frequent and first symptom in *internal carotid artery dissection,* present in as much as 75% of the subjects (Schievink 2001). The pain, which may be sudden and very intense in 13% of the cases, tends to be unilateral to the anterior part of the head, and may be associated with ipsilateral Horner syndrome (Dodick 2002). This picture always demands an MRA investigation, with special attention to the cervico-cranial vasculature.

Instantaneous headache may also occur in *spontaneous intracranial hypotension.* The pain tends to be bilateral and typically improves with recumbency. Visual impairment, tinnitus, hypoacusia, photophobia, nausea, cranial nerve dysfunctions such as a VI nerve palsy and nuchal rigidity may accompany the pain. The MR scan may show the following typical abnormalities: subdural fluid collections, enhancement of the pachymeninges, engorgement of venous structures, pituitary hyperemia, and sagging of the brain (Schievink 2006).

Idiopathic, benign *thunderclap headaches* are well known. In these patients, neuroimaging and spinal taps are normal despite the typical unexpected excruciating headache, which lasts up to several hours, followed by a mild headache that may persist for weeks. The thunderclap headache may recur repeatedly over 1–2 weeks, or even over subsequent months to years (Dodick 2002). *Before classifying a thunderclap headache as primary, however, the attending physician must rule out by appropriate neuroimaging and spinal tap the diagnoses mentioned above, and notice particularly that some of the so-called idiopathic thunderclap headaches may be associated with diffuse segmental vasospasm (RCVS), a diagnosis that is largely overlooked.*

Location

Isolated location should not be considered a red flag in headache practice. *More relevant in this respect is the tendency for a pain to remain fixed as opposed to headaches that occur in varying positions.* Basically, headaches may be bilateral or holocranial; they may occur unilaterally, but shift sides from one attack to the other; or may be unilateral and never occur at the contralateral side. *Generally, a migratory, non-fixed pain much more likely is not related to underlying anatomical lesions.* When a given structure is anatomically responsible for the genesis of pain in the head, chances are higher for the headache to remain fixed, distributed around the area where the pain arising from that particular structure usually project. *A red flag must therefore be raised in case of an atypical, localized pain, particularly if recent, as opposed to patients suffering from headaches of unfixed locations, especially for a very long time.* When this last pattern is found, neuroimaging has few chances to be of any use, and therefore should not be considered. Concerning specifically tumors, there is no consistent clinical pattern associated with this kind of disease. Moreover, the tumor position does not predict the location of the pain (Kernick et al. 2008). In a series of 206 patients with brain tumor, 98 complained of headache, and in only 13, the headache proved to have a localizing correspondence with the underlying tumor (Valentinis et al. 2010). Headaches at the vertex may indicate parasellar or pituitary lesions, including tumor.

Severity

Headache intensity may represent a red flag, especially in sudden, new, and unexpected cases. However, repeated attacks of short-lasting, excruciating pain hardly indicate the presence of a secondary headache. Many of the extremely intense recurring headache attacks correspond to trigeminal autonomic cephalalgias, notably cluster headache and paroxysmal hemicrania. Life-threatening diseases, such as brain tumors, may induce head pain less frequently than one may suppose. Headache occurs 32.2–71% of patients with *brain tumors*. Besides, tumor-associated headaches do not tend to be particularly excruciating. In a recent prospective study, 47% of the brain tumor patients suffered from headaches, and the presence of increased intracranial pressure showed only a marginally significant association to a greater risk of developing intracranial tumor-attributed headache (Valentinis et al. 2010).

Considering only the "worst headache ever" subjects, SAH may be present in only 12% of the cases (Morgenstern et al. 1998); and 25% if abnormal examinations are also included (Linn et al. 1994). In SAH, the pain is typically described as the worst ever, often followed by transient loss of consciousness and vomiting. The physical examination may disclose retinal hemorrhages, nuchal rigidity, restlessness, consciousness deficits, and focal neurologic signs. An incorrect diagnosis may be given to 23–37% of the SAH patients, especially among those with less marked symptoms and normal physical examination (Edlow and Caplan 2000). In such cases, suspicion must be based only on the headache severity, suddenness, and/or recent change in the headache pattern. Interestingly, up to 20–50% of patients with SAH may complain of a different and often severe warning headache days or weeks before the bleeding (Jakobsson et al. 1996). In cerebral venous thrombosis (CVT), the intensity is usually very high, although it may vary. Diffuse rather than localized pain precedes the neurological deficits in 70–75% of the cases. This diagnosis should be typically considered in a patient presenting with headache, blurred vision secondary to papilledema, intracranial hypertension, and vomiting, as seen in 20–40% of the subjects (Masuhr et al. 2004).

Headaches that get worse in morning hours or cause early morning waking have long been considered as an indication of possible space-occupying lesions. This is supposedly due to increased intracranial pressure during the night because of the lying position and hypoventilation. In fact, only 5% of the patients present all the classic criteria for intracranial tumor headache: severe pain intensity, morning occurrence, and association with nausea or vomiting (Valentinis et al. 2010). Headache is not mandatory in brain tumors, occurring in about half of the cases, and may be relatively mild. Headaches that increase in frequency and severity without a clear-cut reason may indicate the presence of a tumor or a subdural hematoma. Quality, intensity, and location of the head pain are not distinctive in patients with increased intracranial pressure (Valentinis et al. 2010).

Precipitating Factors

A fundamental aspect of headache histories is the information of precipitating, alleviating, and aggravating factors. Pain that typically gets worse in upright positions and disappears during recumbency is indicative of idiopathic intracranial hypotension. Worsening when the head bends forward may be present in primary headaches such as migraine, cervicogenic headache, and paroxysmal hemicrania. Headache induced by Valsalva maneuver, coughing, or sneezing may be related with space-occupying lesions. Sneezing-induced pain may be related to

Chiari malformation in some patients. Space-occupying lesions may induce pain by bending forward or Valsalva maneuver. Sexual activity headache is frequently described as thunderclap headache (Pascual et al. 1996), which may also be induced by hot baths (Negoro et al. 2000). Cough and exertional headaches may be related to intracranial lesions, and therefore should always be investigated with neuroimaging. Secondary causes of cough headache include Chiari I malformation, CSF volume depletion (low CSF pressure headache or spontaneous intracranial hypotension), middle cranial fossa or posterior fossa meningiomas, medulloblastoma, pinealoma, chromophobe adenoma, midbrain cyst, basilar impression, platybasia, and subdural hematoma (Cutrer and Boes 2004).

The most frequent abnormalities in temporomanibular dysfunction (TMD) include unilateral facial pain – sometimes radiating to the ears, temporal and periorbital regions, angle of the mandible, and even the neck – limitation in mouth opening and pain worsening by movement, such as chewing, talking, or yawning. TMD may be suspected specially when such complains are worse in the morning, particularly in patients with clenching or grinding of the teeth (Scrivani et al. 2005). Facial lancinating pain of a neuralgic, shock-like nature evoked by talking, touching, chewing, or swallowing points to trigeminal neuralgia. Movement limitation in trigeminal neuralgia may occur too, specially during paroxysms of pain, when eating of drinking may be particularly painful (Bennetto et al. 2007).

Response to Medication

Although response to medication is considered by some clinicians as an indicator of the headache seriousness, data supporting such practice are lacking (American College of Emergency Physicians 2002). In SAH, for example, the headache may improve either spontaneously or following analgesic administration. The response to specific medication may lead to firm diagnostic conclusions regardless of pain severity. This is the case of indomethacin, a drug expected to completely abolish the pain in *paroxysmal hemicrania* and *hemicrania continua* (Dodick 2004). Corticosteroids are effective and help in the diagnosis of *giant cell arteritis, Tolosa–Hunt syndrome,* and *intraorbital myositis.*

The Physical and Mental Examination: Concomitant Signs and Symptoms

The general and neurological examinations are seldom abnormal in headache practice especially outside the emergency yard. Of course, this does not mean that a careful examination may not be performed routinely. Several abnormalities in the physical examination may point to the possibility of serious underlying conditions if a concomitant headache is present. As for the cranial nerves, the optic fundus may show evidence of glaucoma, hemorrhages, inflammatory disorders as well as intracranial hypertension. Tumors, hydrocephalus, abscess, and other space-occupying lesions will be suspected by examination of the optic fundus. In the so-called *Foster–Kennedy syndrome,* the patient presents unilateral ipsilateral optic nerve atrophy with contralateral papilledema sometimes associated with central scotoma, and anosmia. This syndrome is indicative of a frontal lobe tumor or a meningioma of the optic nerve. Among the possible symptoms, the affected subjects may have headache, dizziness, vertigo, and frontal lobe signs.

The ocular intrinsic and extrinsic muscles must be examined with attention. Third nerve palsies, sometimes with only anisocoria, may be observed in aneurisms, and VI nerve dysfunctions may occur in spontaneous intracranial hypotension, for example. An acute headache occurring together with gaze abnormalities, orbital and periorbital pain, diplopia, swollen eyelids, conjunctival injection, and proptosis points to the diagnosis of *intraorbital myositis* (Costa et al. 2009). The pain is mostly unilateral, affecting preferably females.

The likelihood of *brain tumors* in headache patients increase significantly if the subject also presents with papilledema, alterations in consciousness, memory dysfunction, confusion, incoordination, and seizures. New-onset trigeminal autonomic cephalalgias also require imaging, as secondary cases are well known.

A history of cancer elsewhere in a patient with recent headache episodes increases significantly the chances of a cerebral metastasis. Less important tumor risk factors include headaches with no clear diagnostic pattern after 8 weeks from presentation, headache aggravated by exertion or Valsalva-like maneuver, headaches associated with vomiting, headaches present for some time that change significantly, particularly a rapid increase in frequency, a new headache in a patient over 50 years, headaches that wake the patient from sleep, and confusion (Kernick et al. 2008).

Signs of *meningeal irritation* are indicative of possible underlying diseases when present in a headache patient. Acute meningitis is relatively easier to recognize in a patient presenting with headache. Prompt diagnosis with CSF examination and treatment is mandatory in this case. *Chronic meningitis*, defined as a leptomeningeal disease present for more than 1 month, on the other hand, may present a diagnostic challenge, as the fever, if present, is usually low, the meningeal irritation is mild, and the neurological deficits are much less dramatic than in acute meningitis. The occurrence of chronic headache in such patients may lead to the misdiagnosis of "chronic daily headache," which is a syndromic, nonspecific diagnostic term. Tuberculous meningitis may present with long-lasting, intermittent headache. Cranial nerve deficits are present in 40% of these cases. The differential diagnosis must include Lyme disease, neurosyphylis, fungal meningitis, neoplasic leptomeningitis, sarcoidosis, primary CNS angiitis, and collagen diseases (Hildebrand and Aoun 2003).

Vomiting is common in migraine. Taken as an isolated sign, it should not be considered as a red flag, but may be a warning phenomenon if present in a patient with thunderclap headache, concomitant neurological deficits, or systemic abnormalities such as fever.

The examination of the ocular region may be of pivotal importance in headache diagnosis. A semi-ptosis may indicate the presence of a Claude Bernard-Horner-like syndrome, usually present in trigeminal autonomic cephalalgias. A levator muscle dehiscence will be differentiated from true ptosis by the observation of an elevated lid crease. Examples of disorders leading to *Lagophthalmos* include facial nerve palsy, Graves' disease, and trauma. *Lid Lag* may be observed in Grave's disease, as well as some form of ptosis (Martin and Yeatts 2000). In *acute angle closure glaucoma*, a mostly unilateral condition that may present with headache, signs, and symptoms often occur in the evening, as reduced ambient illumination provokes mydriasis leading to block the narrow angle outflow of aqueous humor. Patients experience then a rapid increase of intraocular pressure, with redness of the eye and moderate-to-severe pain. The closed lids must be palpated as relatively hardness often suggests increased pressure in the involved eye. The redness is most pronounced in the area *adjacent* to the limbus, contrary to the redness present in Horner syndrome. The pupil at the symptomatic side may be moderately dilated and unreactive to light. Corneal edema causes the iris to appear less markedly than those of the normal eye. The vision becomes blurred, and the patient complains of seeing haloes around lights. An ophthalmologist must be contacted immediately in such cases dye to the possibility of vision loss (Leibowitz 2000).

Psychiatric disorders may be related to headaches in many ways. First, bidirectional comorbidity exists between migraine and affective disorders such as depression. Second, headache is one of the possible symptoms of psychiatric disorders, which represents a potential red flag for the clinician. Headache as a *somatization disorder* will often be present for many years sometimes together with multiple physical complaints hard to be explained by a medical condition, substance use, or medication effects. According to the Diagnostic and Statistical Manual of Mental Disorders, Fourth Edition, Text Revision (DSM-IV-TR), unexplained physical complaints must include at least four pain symptoms, two non-pain gastrointestinal symptoms, one non-pain sexual/reproductive symptom, and one non-pain pseudoneurological symptom (e.g., conversion symptoms, dissociative symptoms, or loss of consciousness other than fainting). Headache attributed to psychotic disorder, or "delusional headache," is linked with schizophrenia, delusional disorder, major depressive episode/manic episode with psychotic features. In this case, patients have a very strong belief of a brain tumor, a serious underlying mysterious disease, a foreign body alien or other delusional idea (Smitherman and Baskin 2008). Suspicion during examination of a comorbid psychiatric disorder indicates the necessity of a formal psychiatric examination. As a general rule, nonpsychiatric headaches will much more easily fit known clinical patterns, with coherent onset and evolution over time, contrary to strange, anatomically and physiologically non-justifiable type of pain in case of psychiatric generated headache.

Malingering not infrequently involves headache complains. In such cases, sooner or later during the interview, the subject will tell the physician his/her intentions. Particularly relevant in this context is the whiplash-related headache following a car accident, often used to claim compensation (Obeliene et al. 1998). The subjects also ask for documents stating that they cannot work, as they are too disabled by the daily headache. In such cases, it is important to observe the patient when he or she is not under direct scrutiny. The way he or she talks or interacts with other patients or family before or after the exam may indicate a much less disabling pain than actually claimed. The doctor may face a subject who hardly moves; but an object falling on the floor, if immediately caught by the patient, shows that the pain told to totally prevent bending or moving the head because of its intensity actually is not so awful.

Diagnostic Tests

Lumbar Puncture

Examination of the spinal fluid should be considered in case of intense, thunderclap-like headaches of obscure origin with normal neuroimaging to rule out subarachnoid hemorrhage and in cases, where meningitis is suspected. A lumbar puncture must be performed in patients with recent headache at risk of or known to suffer from AIDS. Adult patients with headache with signs of increased intracranial pressure including papilledema, funduscopic lack of venous pulsations, altered mental status, or focal neurologic deficits should undergo a neuroimaging study before having an LP (2002). In RCVS, the CSF was abnormal in 58% of the subjects, showing slightly elevated white blood cells and/or protein levels (Ducros et al. 2007). Meningitis, encephalitis, Lyme disease, systemic infection, and collagen vascular disease may by suspected when headache occurs together with signs of systemic disorders, such as fever or stress.

Blood Tests

Apart from routine blood examination, specific tests may be relevant for headache investigation. Above the age of 50, *giant cell arteritis* must be considered even in the lack of clear temporal artery abnormities in the case of a new-onset headache, which is the most frequent symptom and occurs in two thirds of the patients. Apart from headache, 50% of the patients suffer from fever, malaise, anorexia and weight loss (Cantini et al. 2008). The diagnosis may be reinforced by a high erythrocyte sedimentation rate, positive C-reative protein, abnormal temporal artery color-duplex ultrasonography, and suggestive temporal artery biopsy. High-resolution magnetic resonance scans may disclose changes in the walls of the superficial temporal arteries.

Electroencephalography

EEG will rarely be of any use in headache practice. This investigation becomes relevant only when epilepsy is suspected. Atypical migraine aura may sometimes represent a diagnostic challenge. However, aura and epilepsy are frequently distinguishable based on symptom duration. Migraine aura manifests during many minutes, usually more than 10, up to 60, whereas a seizure typically lasts for few minutes. Visual symptoms are rarely a manifestation of epilepsy. The nature of the visual abnormalities differ too, as in migraine the positive phenomena tend to be colorless, non-complex, and involve teichopsia-like lines and angles. Less typically, migraine patients may experience complex visual abnormalities such as lilliputian hallucinations (vision of either people or objects as miniatures or small fantastic little animals or creatures) have been described (Podoll and Robinson 2001), as well as splitting or mis-interpretations of the body image (Podoll and Robinson 2000), macro and microsoma-toagnosia (Lippman 1952; Evans and Rolak 2004). In visual epilepsy, the positive images are more frequently colored, present as round shapes more frequently, and may involve complex visual scenes. Epileptic patients may experience headache both as a preictal phenomenon (Yankovsky et al. 2005) as well as a postictal (Ito et al. 2004) phenomenon. In both cases, the headache may present migrainous features. Although headache is often overlooked in epileptic patients, in a series of 341 epilepsy patients, 115 (34%) experienced headache, and seizures were always accompanied by headache in as much as 69 (60%) of them (Leniger et al. 2001).

Migralepsy is defined as migraine fulfilling criteria for migraine with aura together with a seizure fulfilling diagnostic criteria for one type of epileptic attack occurring during or within 1 h after the migraine aura (Sances et al. 2009). If the case history suggests migralepsy, EEG investigation is mandatory. Finally, although evidence exists suggesting that headache may occur as the only symptom in epilepsy (Piccioli et al. 2009), this possibility must be regarded as very exceptional by the attending physician.

Neuroimaging

Neuroimaging is the most important investigation for headache. Among difficult decisions when dealing with headache patients is the indication for neuroimaging. Although only 1% of patients presenting to the emergency yard because of headache have significant underlying diseases requiring emergent diagnosis (Dhopesh et al. 1979) and 10% have secondary headaches (Sobri et al. 2003), it is mandatory to investigate these patients in order to detect treatable serious conditions, such as subarachnoid, brain, or ventricular hemorrhages; cerebral venous thrombosis (CVT); subdural hematoma; infarcts (particularly in the cerebellum); RCVS; aneurysms; hydrocephalus; tumors; acute sinusitis; cervical arteries dissections; acute hypertensive crisis; and pituitary apoplexy. *Three red flags proved to be statistically linked to abnormal neuroimaging in headache patients: papilledema; drowsiness, confusion, memory impairment or loss of consciousness; and paralysis* (Sobri et al. 2003).

Thunderclap headache is certainly the most important phenotype in this context, a clinical picture that may be investigated with CT scans, conventional angiography, digital subtraction angiography (DSA), MR, Magnetic resonance angiography (MRA), CT angiography (CTA), and multidetector CT (MDCT). This condition may be indicative of serious underlying disorders, although primary cases are well known.

Among nontraumatic SAH patients, 80% have a ruptured saccular aneurysm (Edlow and Caplan 2000). This indicates that a search of aneurysm is obligatory in every SAH case. To detect SHA, noncontrast CT scans must be performed using 3-mm cuts instead of 10-mm cuts through the base of the skull to avoid missing small blood collections (Latchaw et al. 1997). Besides, the CT sensitivity decreases with time, from 92% at the first day to 58% five days later (Kassell et al. 1990). DSA is considered the gold standard for diagnosing SAH secondary to aneurysms and vasospasm (Marshall et al. 2010). The vast majority of patients with thunderclap headache and normal CT and CSF examinations will not have a symptomatic cerebral aneurysm (Dodick 2002).

In RCVS, the MRA shows diffuse segmental arterial constriction in 88% of patients, and MRI scans are abnormal in 28% of the cases. On the contrary, computerized tomography (CT) scans is abnormal in only 12% of the patients, indicating that MR and MRI are preferable in this situation (Ducros et al. 2007).

The magnetic resonance venography (MRV) must be performed in such cases as otherwise cerebral venous thrombosis (CVT) may be overlooked. Headache is the most frequent symptom in CVT, occurring in up to 75–95% of the cases. The headache may precede other symptoms for days or even weeks. The pain in mostly insidious, increasing over some days, but typical thunderclap headache may occur in 14% of the subjects.

In children, 10% of *brain tumors* will present with headache only, which is the most frequent presenting symptom (Wilne et al. 2006). Thus, a decision about neuroimaging to rule out brain tumors specifically in children with headache is frequently required. *Red flags for tumors in children with headache have been ranked in a decreasing order of importance as follows: headache history of less than 6 months; recent change of headache characteristics; referral age less than 6 years; headaches occurring always on the same side of the head; headaches on awakening; confusion during headache attacks; ophthalmological signs or symptoms; headaches causing sleep interruption, and unusual headache location (e.g., occipital)* (Ahmed et al. 2010).

Cervicogenic headache syndrome is suspected in patients who present typically fixed, unilateral headache, located to the first trigeminal branch area. It tends to start at the posterior part of the head and/or neck and spread to the front following the scalp, over or around the ear, or through the upper part of the mandible and/or the zygomatic area. An ipsilateral, non-radicular numbness at the ipsilateral shoulder and arm may occur. Digital pressure over trigger points at the occipital-nuchal area, including the greater occipital nerve or the transverse process of the upper vertebrae, may generate attacks similar to the naturally occurring episodes. Triggering factors include positioning or moving the head in particular ways. In such cases, a cervical MR must always be performed (Vincent 2010).

❷ *Table 14.1* shows the indications of neuroimaging as far as headache red flags are concerned. CT scans are not superior to MR in any situation, probably except when detection of acute bleeding is necessary at the emergency yard. When there is no MR contraindication, for example, metal implants, for all the other situations where neuroimaging is necessary, MR must be the preferred choice. The physician can interact with the neuroradiologist before performing the scans, as a better protocol may be suggested depending on the case.

Current Research

Red flags play an important role in headache care as many headache disorders lack diagnostic biomarkers and depend on clinical observations. Research in this field may include three different fronts. First, observational studies are performed to find and confirm the validity of red flags in headache care. Second, data on red flags are used to create recommendations for a better headache care. Third, technology may lead to better diagnostic tests for life-threatening headache disorders. Based on these approaches, recommendations for headache investigation have been proposed (Clinch 2001; Sobri et al. 2003; Kernick et al. 2008; Ahmed et al. 2010). Hopefully, the new neuroimaging advances in migraine research (Schwedt and Dodick 2009) will serve as diagnostic markers in everyday practice. Neuroimaging studies showing structural changes in primary headaches (May 2009) suggest that this technology may be improved and used in the future for practical diagnosis. Faster image acquisitions and sequences are important MR innovations for the diagnosis in the emergency context.

References

Ahmed M, Martinez A, Cahill D, Chong K, Whitehouse WP (2010) When to image neurologically normal children with headaches: development of a decision rule. Acta Paediatr 99(6):940–943

American College of Emergency Physicians (2002) Clinical policy: critical issues in the evaluation and management of patients presenting to the emergency department with acute headache. Ann Emerg Med 39:108–122

Bennetto L, Patel NK, Fuller G (2007) Trigeminal neuralgia and its management. BMJ 334:201–205

Cantini F, Niccoli L, Nannini C, Bertoni M, Salvarani C (2008) Diagnosis and treatment of giant cell arteritis. Drugs Aging 25:281–297

Clinch CR (2001) Evaluation of acute headaches in adults. Am Fam Physician 63:685–692

Costa RM, Dumitrascu OM, Gordon LK (2009) Orbital myositis: diagnosis and management. Curr Allergy Asthma Rep 9:316–323

Cutrer FM, Boes CJ (2004) Cough, exertional, and sex headaches. Neurol Clin 22:133–149

Demaerschalk B, Dodick DW (2003) Recognizing sentinel headache as a premonitory symptom in patients with aneurysmal subarachnoid haemorrhage. Cephalalgia 23:933–934

Dhopesh V, Anwar R, Herring C (1979) A retrospective assessment of emergency department patients with complaint of headache. Headache 19:37–42

Dodick DW (2002) Thunderclap headache. J Neurol Neurosurg Psychiatry 72:6–11

Dodick DW (2004) Indomethacin-responsive headache syndromes. Curr Pain Headache Rep 8:19–26

Ducros A, Boukobza M, Porcher R, Sarov M, Valade D, Bousser MG (2007) The clinical and radiological spectrum of reversible cerebral vasoconstriction syndrome. A prospective series of 67 patients. Brain 130:3091–3101, England

Edlow JA, Caplan LR (2000) Avoiding pitfalls in the diagnosis of subarachnoid hemorrhage. N Engl J Med 342:29–36

Evans RW, Rolak LA (2004) The Alice in Wonderland syndrome. Headache 44:624–625

Hildebrand J, Aoun M (2003) Chronic meningitis: still a diagnostic challenge. J Neurol 250:653–660

Hinchey J, Chaves C, Appignani B, Breen J, Pao L, Wang A, Pessin MS, Lamy C, Mas JL, Caplan LR (1996) A reversible posterior leukoencephalopathy syndrome. N Engl J Med 334:494–500

Ito M, Adachi N, Nakamura F, Koyama T, Okamura T, Kato M, Kanemoto K, Nakano T, Matsuura M, Hara S (2004) Characteristics of postictal headache in patients with partial epilepsy. Cephalalgia 24:23–28

Jakobsson KE, Saveland H, Hillman J, Edner G, Zygmunt S, Brandt L, Pellettieri L (1996) Warning leak and management outcome in aneurysmal subarachnoid hemorrhage. J Neurosurg 85:995–999

Kassell NF, Torner JC, Haley EC Jr, Jane JA, Adams HP, Kongable GL (1990) The international cooperative study on the timing of aneurysm surgery. Part 1: overall management results. J Neurosurg 73:18–36

Kernick DP, Ahmed F, Bahra A, Dowson A, Elrington G, Fontebasso M, Giffin NJ, Lipscombe S, MacGregor A, Peatfield R, Weatherby S, Whitmarsh T, Goadsby PJ (2008) Imaging patients with suspected brain tumour: guidance for primary care. Br J Gen Pract 58:880–885

Latchaw RE, Silva P, Falcone SF (1997) The role of CT following aneurysmal rupture. Neuroimaging Clin N Am 7:693–708

Leibowitz HM (2000) The red eye. N Engl J Med 343: 345–351

Leniger T, Isbruch K, von den Driesch S, Diener HC, Hufnagel A (2001) Seizure-associated headache in epilepsy. Epilepsia 42:1176–1179

Linn FH, Wijdicks EF, van der Graaf Y, Weerdesteyn-van Vliet FA, Bartelds AI, van Gijn J (1994) Prospective study of sentinel headache in aneurysmal subarach-noid haemorrhage. Lancet 344:590–593

Linn FH, Rinkel GJ, Algra A, van Gijn J (1998) Headache characteristics in subarachnoid haemorrhage and benign thunderclap headache. J Neurol Neurosurg Psychiatry 65:791–793

Linn FH, Rinkel GJ, Algra A, van Gijn J (2000) The notion of "warning leaks" in subarachnoid haemorrhage: are such patients in fact admitted with a rebleed? J Neurol Neurosurg Psychiatry 68:332–336

Lippman CW (1952) Certain hallucinations peculiar to migraine. J Nerv Ment Dis 116(4):346–351

Marshall SA, Kathuria S, Nyquist P, Gandhi D (2010) Noninvasive imaging techniques in the diagnosis and management of aneurysmal subarachnoid hem-orrhage. Neurosurg Clin N Am 21:305–323

Martin TJ, Yeatts RP (2000) Abnormalities of eyelid posi-tion and function. Semin Neurol 20:31–42

Masuhr F, Mehraein S, Einhaupl K (2004) Cerebral venous and sinus thrombosis. J Neurol 251:11–23

May A (2009) Morphing voxels: the hype around structural imaging of headache patients. Brain 132: 1419–1425, England

Morgenstern LB, Luna-Gonzales H, Huber JC Jr, Wong SS, Uthman MO, Gurian JH, Castillo PR, Shaw SG, Frankowski RF, Grotta JC (1998) Worst headache and subarachnoid hemorrhage: prospective, modern computed tomography and spinal fluid analysis. Ann Emerg Med 32:297–304

Negoro K, Morimatsu M, Ikuta N, Nogaki H (2000) Benign hot bath-related headache. Headache 40: 173–175

Obeliene D, Bovim G, Schrader H, Surkiene D, Mickeviàiene D, Miseviàiene I, Sand T (1998) Headache after whiplash: a historical cohort study outside the medico-legal context. Cephalalgia 18: 559–564

Pascual J, Iglesias F, Oterino A, Vazquez-Barquero A, Berciano J (1996) Cough, exertional, and sexual headaches: an analysis of 72 benign and symptom-atic cases. Neurology 46:1520–1524, EUA

Piccioli M, Parisi P, Tisei P, Villa MP, Buttinelli C, Kasteleijn-Nolst Trenite DG (2009) Ictal headache and visual sensitivity. Cephalalgia 29:194–203

Podoll K, Robinson D (2000) Illusory splitting as visual aura symptom in migraine. Cephalalgia 20:228–232

Podoll K, Robinson D (2001) Recurrent Lilliputian hal-lucinations as visual aura symptom in migraine. Cephalalgia 21:990–992

Sances G, Guaschino E, Perucca P, Allena M, Ghiotto N, Manni R (2009) Migralepsy: a call for a revision of the definition. Epilepsia 50:2487–2496

Schievink WI (2001) Spontaneous dissection of the carotid and vertebral arteries. N Engl J Med 344: 898–906

Schievink WI (2006) Spontaneous spinal cerebrospinal fluid leaks and intracranial hypotension. J Am Med Assoc 295:2286–2296

Schwedt TJ, Dodick DW (2009) Advanced neuroimaging of migraine. Lancet Neurol 8:560–568

Scrivani SJ, Mathews ES, Maciewicz RJ (2005) Trigeminal neuralgia. Oral Surg Oral Med Oral Pathol Oral Radiol Endod 100:527–538

Smitherman TA, Baskin SM (2008) Headache secondary to psychiatric disorders. Curr Pain Headache Rep 12:305–310

Sobri M, Lamont AC, Alias NA, Win MN (2003) Red flags in patients presenting with headache: clinical indications for neuroimaging. Br J Radiol 76: 532–535

Valentinis L, Tuniz F, Valent F, Mucchiut M, Little D, Skrap M, Bergonzi P, Zanchin G (2010) Headache attributed to intracranial tumours: a prospective cohort study. Cephalalgia 30(4):389–398

Vincent MB (2010) Cervicogenic headache: a review comparison with migraine, tension-type headache, and whiplash. Curr Pain Headache Rep 14:238–243

Wilne SH, Ferris RC, Nathwani A, Kennedy CR (2006) The presenting features of brain tumours: a review of 200 cases. Arch Dis Child 91:502–506

Yankovsky AE, Andermann F, Mercho S, Dubeau F, Bernasconi A (2005) Preictal headache in partial epilepsy. Neurology 65:1979–1981, EUA

Part 5

Migraine

15 How Migraine Presents

Susan W. Broner[1] · *Lisa Yablon*[2]
[1]St. Luke's-Roosevelt Hospital, New York, NY, USA
[2]New York Headache Center, New York, NY, USA

Paolo Martelletti, Timothy J. Steiner (eds.), *Handbook of Headache*, DOI 10.1007/978-88-470-1700-9_15,

Abstract: Migraine is a very common disorder affecting millions of people globally, with significant personal and societal impact. Recognizing this disorder and the different ways in which it can present is crucial to treating patients appropriately and reducing the burden of the disease.

   This chapter reviews migraine, its subtypes, and their presentations. The discussion encompasses diagnosis of migraine with and without aura, basilar-type migraine, hemiplegic migraine (both the inherited and sporadic forms), retinal migraine, and chronic migraine. Various presentations and complications are described, as well as what are believed to be childhood precursors to migraine.

Overview of Migraine

Migraine is a very common neurological disorder. In the USA, its prevalence has remained steady over the years with about 17% of women and 6% of men affected (Lipton et al. 2007). Globally, prevalence estimates indicate that more than 10% of adults have the disorder (Stovner et al. 2007).

   Although incidence studies are relatively few, a recent study shows peak incidence between the ages of 20 and 24 years in women and between 15 and 19 years in men, with four of every ten women and two of every ten men contracting migraine in their lifetimes, most before the age of 35 years (Stewart et al. 2008). In an earlier study, the peak onset was seen in girls aged 12–17 years and in boys aged 5–10, dependent on whether or not they had aura (onset is typically 5 years earlier for migraine with aura than for migraine without aura) (Stewart et al. 1991). When it develops in childhood, migraine presents earlier in boys than in girls, with boys slightly more often affected, but by puberty this ratio shifts and, as adolescence turns to adulthood, women become disproportionately more affected than men in a ratio of about 3:1 (Bille 1962; Waters and O'Connor 1971).

   Migraine can have a devastating impact on the life of a migraine sufferer, personally, financially, and socially, so it is crucial to recognize and treat it appropriately. Given its high prevalence and the very heavy socioeconomic burden that it imposes, the World Health Organization (WHO) ranks migraine as the 19th most disabling disorder worldwide and, in women, the 12th most disabling.

   Migraine is typically an episodic disorder, and its diagnosis depends upon a history of several stereotypical episodes (attacks) with pain characteristics and features meeting criteria laid down in the International Classification of Headache Disorders – Second Edition (ICHD-2) (Headache Classification Committee of the International Headache Society 2004). Importantly, making the diagnosis also requires exclusion of other causes of headache. The patient with migraine will have a normal neurological examination (unless he or she has another disorder); rarely, this alone does not suffice for diagnostic certainty, and brain imaging and laboratory tests are required.

   Attack frequency varies not only from person to person but also within an individual during his or her lifetime. Of women with migraine, at least 60% have menstrually related migraine, and hormonal changes throughout life also lead to varying frequency.

   Migraine without aura is the most common subtype of migraine, but there are several others that are important to recognize because treatment may vary depending on the subtype. Most subtypes include the symptoms of migraine without aura and some, in addition, include neurological symptoms.

Migraine Without Aura

Migraine without aura was previously known as "common migraine" because it is the most prevalent form of migraine. The diagnosis can be made after five attacks have occurred and other causes have been considered and ruled out (Headache Classification Committee of the International Headache Society 2004). The headache must have at least two of four pain characteristics: one-sided, throbbing, moderate to severe intensity, and aggravated by or causing avoidance of routine physical activity. Associated features include at least one of light and sound sensitivity (photo- and phonophobia) or nausea or vomiting. The attack lasts from 4 to 72 h untreated and patients typically prefer to rest in a dark and quiet place during at least part of it.

The pain can be experienced in any part of the head, and it is common for it to shift location. It may be accompanied by autonomic symptoms such as ptosis, nasal congestion or rhinorrhea, conjunctival injection, or lacrimation, sometimes falsely leading to diagnoses of sinus or cluster headache. Indeed, in some countries, migraine is commonly misdiagnosed as "sinus headache" (Cady and Schreiber 2002).

Preceding the onset of headache, some patients experience premonitory symptoms (prodrome). These may consist of yawning, cravings, mood changes, overwhelming fatigue, or difficulty with concentration, lasting minutes to hours or longer. The prodrome differs from aura (see below). After the headache, some patients report a postdrome of fatigue or a "hangover" feeling. Once this final phase is over, the attack is fully resolved and sufferers are entirely well until the next.

Trigger factors may incite particular attacks, such as the menstrual cycle, lack of sleep, certain foods, and so forth, and these may explain a given patient's migraine pattern. Aggravating factors also occur: these include stressors, certain lifestyle habits, and some medications.

Migraine with Aura

About 20% of people with migraine experience an aura as part of some or all attacks. Although aura is sometimes thought to be the sine qua non of migraine diagnosis, this is not the case and most migraine sufferers never have aura. The diagnosis of migraine with aura can be made after at least two similar attacks of headache, usually similar to that of migraine without aura but preceded by or, occasionally, having its onset at the same time as stereotypical focal neurological symptoms (Headache Classification Committee of the International Headache Society 2004). These include visual and/or sensory and/or speech disturbances, and the phenomena may be positive or negative (e.g., tingling or numbness). The most common is visual aura, experienced by 99% of those with aura (Russel and Olesen 1996).

Visual aura is seen homonymously in both eyes and, because of this, is believed to arise from the occipital cortex. It often appears as a scintillating scotoma that gradually enlarges across the visual field. Patients commonly describe this as an expanding white or colored arc to one or other side of their visual field, or as an obscuration of part of their visual field with shimmering zigzag lines around this. Other descriptions include phosphenes (simple flashes of light), heat waves, geometric shapes, and visual distortions including micropsia, macropsia, zoom vision (expanding or contracting in size of an object), mosaic vision (the image appears fractured), and metamorphopsia (the object changes shape or becomes distorted).

Paresthesias are the second most common aura symptom, with unilateral tingling around the lips and mouth, sometimes also involving the hand and forearm and less commonly the leg.

Most people who experience sensory aura also have visual aura. Speech disturbances range from aphasia to dysphasias, but are more difficult to categorize unless witnessed or recorded. Rarely, people can experience olfactory hallucinations and there have been reports of aural hallucinations (Rubin et al. 2002).

Aura develops gradually over 5–20 min and can last up to 60 min. When it lasts for more than an hour, it is considered to be prolonged and this has important treatment implications and medication contraindications (see below). Once the aura has run its course, the sufferer returns to his or her baseline neurological status (Silberstein et al. 2001). In patients for whom aura is a new symptom, a careful history and examination must ensure other causes are not responsible, with brain imaging and laboratory testing as indicated.

Prolonged Aura

New onset of prolonged aura calls for investigation of possible causes, such as anticardiolipin antibody syndrome, lupus anticoagulant, pro-thrombotic states, or other disorders. Patients who experience aura that lasts longer than an hour are believed to be at a higher risk of stroke; therefore, they must not receive triptans or ergots, which increase the risk further. Prolonged aura in the face of recently initiated hormonal treatment requires its immediate discontinuation and urgent evaluation.

Aura with Non-Migraine Headache

Some patients experience stereotypical aura but have headaches that do not meet criteria for migraine. The clinician must be vigilant in excluding ischemic or other causes of aura when it presents without typical migraine headache (Krymchantowski 2005).

Aura Without Headache

This subtype can occur in patients with or without a history of migraine headache, and in all age groups, but is most common in older people with a history of migraine with aura at a younger age (Zeigler and Hassanein 1990). Prevalence estimates of aura without headache vary from around 1–2% to more than 13% of the population (Fleming et al. 2000; Kunkel 2005; Aiba et al. 2010). Patients experience an otherwise typical aura but no headache with or after it. Other disorders, such as transient ischemic attack, seizure, and retinal disease, must be considered and ruled out by appropriate testing, especially in patients with no history of migraine or with vascular risk factors.

Basilar-Type Migraine

Basilar-type migraine is an uncommon subtype of migraine with aura in which aura signs and symptoms are localizable to either the brainstem or both cerebral hemispheres, without associated weakness. It mainly afflicts adolescent girls (Bickerstaff 1961), although there are reports in all age groups, with around 65% of patients experiencing their first attack in the second or third decade (Sturzenegger and Meienberg 1985). Female predominance is similar to that seen in migraine without aura.

Basilar-type migraine fulfills criteria for migraine without aura, with headache that is frequently occipital in location. In addition, aura starts up to 1 h before or during the headache, lasts 5–60 min, and includes at least two of the following fully reversible symptoms: dysarthria, vertigo, tinnitus, hypacusia (reduced hearing), diplopia, simultaneously bilateral visual symptoms, ataxia, decreased level of consciousness, or simultaneously bilateral paresthesias. The diagnosis can be made after at least two attacks, and other causes have been ruled out (Headache Classification Committee of the International Headache Society 2004).

Most patients with basilar-type migraine also experience other episodes of migraine with aura without basilar symptoms (Kirchmann et al. 2006). A quarter also have attacks of basilar-type aura without headache.

Although the aura symptoms associated with basilar-type migraine are referable to the posterior cerebral circulation, no association has ever been proven with basilar artery dysfunction, and there remains some controversy as to whether it is truly a distinct disorder from migraine with aura. A family history of migraine is present in 86% of patients with basilar-type migraine (Lapkin and Golden 1978), and a large Danish study found that, among families with migraine with aura, it is very rare to have more than one family member with basilar-type migraine (Kirchmann et al. 2006).

Hemiplegic Migraine

Hemiplegic migraine is a subtype of migraine with aura in which the aura is characterized by varying degrees of motor weakness lasting from minutes to 1 week. It exists in familial and sporadic forms, both of which typically have their onset in childhood and persist until adulthood, sometimes developing into migraine with and without aura later in life.

Familial hemiplegic migraine (FHM) is a rare autosomal dominantly inherited condition with broad clinical variability, characterized by aura including fully reversible motor weakness and at least one other aura symptom (visual, sensory, or speech disturbance) (Headache Classification Committee of the International Headache Society 2004). These symptoms develop gradually over 5 min or longer and may occur in succession, and overall each aura typically lasts for more than 5 min but less than 24 h, either preceding headache by up to 60 min or beginning during a headache attack that has all the characteristics of migraine without aura. For this diagnosis, a first or second degree relative must also have the disorder.

Patients may also experience attacks of migraine without aura, migraine with typical aura, and migraine with prolonged aura (Silberstein et al. 2001).

Three known genetic mutations, all of which encode for transmembrane ion channels, are known to cause this migraine subtype and each mutation may be associated with other clinical manifestations apart from their shared hemiplegic migraine.

Familial Hemiplegic Migraine 1. Around 50% of patients with FHM have FHM1, carrying one of four mutations in the CACNA1A gene on chromosome 19p13, which encodes for the alpha-1A subunit of the P/Q type calcium channel (Ophof et al. 1998). About one third of these patients have severe attacks with impaired consciousness (Ophoff et al. 1996). Rarely, clinical features include transient cerebral edema and hemispheric cerebral atrophy (Ducros et al. 1997; Ambrosini et al. 2005). Of note, episodic ataxia type 2, characterized by interictal nystagmus and attacks of generalized ataxia, and spinocerebellar ataxia type 6 have the same gene mutation.

Spinocerebellar ataxias are slowly progressive cerebellar ataxias that begin between the ages of 20 and 60. Up to 50% of patients with FHM1 may develop one of the spinocerebellar ataxias, developing permanent cerebellar signs, including gaze-evoked nystagmus or mild ataxia.

Familial Hemiplegic Migraine 2. FHM2 is associated with mutations in the ATP1A2 gene on chromosome 1q23, which encodes for a sodium/potassium ATPase (Ducros et al. 2001). Various mutations in this gene have been linked with different phenotypes, including epilepsy, severe and long-lasting attacks of hemiplegia, recurrent coma, and mental retardation (Jurkat-Rott et al. 2004).

Familial Hemiplegic Migraine 3. A mutation in SCN1A, a sodium channel gene, has been described in several FHM pedigrees without mutations in either A1A or ATP1A2 (Dichgans et al. 2005).

Retinal Migraine

Retinal migraine (RM) is a rare condition in which patients experience monocular visual disturbances for up to 60 min either before or during a migraine headache. The transient disturbances vary from patient to patient and may include scotomas, scintillations, fortification spectra, partial vision loss, or blindness. Many patients confuse a homonymous visual field defect with a monocular visual disturbance, and should alternately cover each eye during an attack to confirm its bilateral or unilateral nature. A complete ophthalmologic evaluation should reveal normality between attacks, and other causes of transient monocular blindness, such as cardioembolic and other vascular diseases, must be ruled out.

The prevalence of this disorder is unknown but it is believed to be very rare, with fewer than 100 reports of it in the literature (Manzoni and Stovner 2010). It appears to affect women more than men, and presents in early adulthood. Although ICHD-2 defines RM as a reversible condition (Headache Classification Committee of the International Headache Society 2004), one survey found that some patients experienced prolonged symptoms of more than 1 h and some went on to developing permanent visual loss, suggesting vulnerability for migrainous infarction (Grosberg et al. 2005).

Chronic Migraine

People who have migraine in any of its subtypes may present in different ways, but episodic migraine is most common. Frequency is highly variable, from headaches every few years to weekly headaches or more, between individuals and within an individual's lifetime. An increase in frequency is commonly seen during times of increased stress or changes in the hormonal milieu, and may be gradual or abrupt.

Chronic migraine is recognized, although there is not yet agreement on its definition, or on its features. According to ICHD-2 criteria (Headache Classification Committee of the International Headache Society 2004), the diagnosis of chronic migraine requires 15 or more days of headache per month for at least 3 months. Not all of these days need, individually, to meet the criteria for migraine. A recently proposed revision to ICHD-2 requires this on only 8 or more days per month (Olesen et al. 2006): headache with at least two of the four pain characteristics (unilateral, throbbing, moderate to severe intensity, aggravated by or causing avoidance of routine physical activity) and at least one of the associated features (light and sound sensitivity or nausea or vomiting).

Chronic migraine is currently described as a complication of migraine (Headache Classification Committee of the International Headache Society 2004), evolving over time from the episodic form. Risk factors for this include body mass index of 30 or greater, female gender, Caucasian race, low educational level, habitual snoring, high caffeine intake, stressful life events including a history of childhood maltreatment (Tietjen et al. 2010), presence of other painful conditions such as arthritis or diabetes, high headache frequency, and medication overuse (Levin 2008). Frequency of medication use tends, for obvious reasons, to increase with frequency of headache. In the presence of medication overuse, diagnosis is complicated by the likelihood of medication-overuse headache (see ❷ Chap. 50).

Other Complications of Migraine

These include status migrainosus (a migraine attack persisting for more than 72 h), persistent aura without infarction (typical aura lasting for more than 1 week), migrainous infarction (aura lasting for longer than an hour, and an ischemic stroke developing in a corresponding area of the brain), and migraine-triggered seizure (an epileptic attack occurring during or in the aftermath of a migraine headache). Of these, status migrainosus is encountered not uncommonly in clinical practice, but the others are rare and require careful evaluation to exclude the possibility of serious underlying causes.

Childhood Migraine Variants

Three syndromes of childhood are believed to be related to migraine: cyclical vomiting, abdominal migraine, and benign paroxysmal vertigo of childhood.

Cyclical vomiting is a disorder that primarily affects infants and children, and is believed to be a variant of migraine. It is a benign, recurrent condition characterized by at least five attacks of intense nausea and vomiting lasting between 1 h and 5 days. The vomiting is profuse, occurring at least four times per hour. Abdominal pain, not part of the diagnostic criteria, may be present and severe, making this diagnosis easily confused with abdominal migraine (below). A prodrome of nausea and pallor is common, occurring within an hour before the attack.

Common migraine triggers including times of stress or excitement, lack of sleep, certain foods, and changes in the hormonal milieu may initiate attacks. Interestingly, positive stressors, such as birthdays and vacations, are more commonly reported as triggers than negative stressors. Between attacks, patients are completely symptom free (Li and Balint 2000).

The majority of people who suffer from cyclical vomiting have a family history of migraine headaches and over a quarter develop migraine later in life (Li and Misiewicz 2003; Boles et al. 2009). Because the condition is so debilitating, it exacts a significant cost in Emergency Department visits, medical investigations to rule out other possible causes of the symptoms, and lost school time (Li and Balint 2000).

Abdominal migraine is characterized by bouts of abdominal pain lasting 1–72 h occurring episodically. The pain is typically periumbilical but may be poorly localized. It has a dull or "sore" quality and is moderate to severe in intensity. Along with the pain come anorexia, nausea, vomiting, and/or pallor, and ICHD-2 criteria require at least two of these symptoms

(Headache Classification Committee of the International Headache Society 2004). During attacks, patients tend to be withdrawn, often have photophobia, and may have mild headache (Cuvellier and Lépine 2010).

Triggers can include stress, motion sickness, and physical exhaustion. As in cyclical vomiting, patients are completely healthy between attacks.

The majority of patients with abdominal migraine develop symptoms between 7 and 12 years of age, and the disorder may affect 1–4% of the population in this age range. Girls are affected more than boys. There is usually a family history of migraine. Abdominal migraine is typically a self-limiting disorder, with most children outgrowing it; it rarely persists into adulthood (Popovich et al. 2010).

Benign paroxysmal vertigo of childhood typically presents in young children, often between 2 and 4 years of age. Symptoms include a sudden onset of vertigo that occurs without warning. The child may look anxious or fearful and may sway, grasp onto nearby support, or sit down abruptly. Nystagmus may be seen and the child may look pale, perspire, and put his or her head in an unusual position. Nausea may also occur. Attacks are usually brief, seconds to 5 min, but rarely can last a few hours. They recur episodically from between once a day to once every few months, often becoming less frequent with time.

Triggers may include typical migraine triggers such as fatigue or stress, but physical activity that involves motion may also initiate an attack. A family history of migraine is often present, and the child may also suffer from motion sickness (Cuvellier and Lépine 2010). Although children are completely normal between attacks, other possible causes should be excluded.

References

Aiba S, Tatsumoto M, Saisu A et al (2010) Prevalence of typical migraine aura without headache in Japanese ophthalmology clinics. Cephalalgia 30(8): 962–967

Ambrosini A, D'Onofrio M, Grieco GS et al (2005) Familial basilar migraine associated with a new mutation in the ATP1A2 gene. Neurology 65:1826–1828

Bickerstaff ER (1961) Basilar artery migraine. Lancet 1:15–17

Bille B (1962) Migraine in school children. Acta Paediatr Scand 51(suppl 136):1–151

Boles RG, Zaki EA, Lavenbarg T et al (2009) Are pediatric and adult-onset cyclic vomiting syndrome (CVS) biologically different conditions? Relationship of adult-onset CVS with the migraine and pediatric CVS-associated common mtDNA polymorphisms 16519T and 3010A. Neurogastroenterol Motil 21(9):936–e72

Cady RK, Schreiber CP (2002) Sinus headache or migraine?: considerations in making a differential diagnosis. Neurology 58:S10–S14

Cuvellier JC, Lépine A (2010) Childhood periodic syndromes. Pediatr Neurol 42(1):1–11

Dichgans M, Freilinger T, Eckstein G et al (2005) Mutation in the neuronal voltage-gated sodium channel SCN1A in familial hemiplegic migraine. Lancet 366:371–377

Ducros A, Joutel A, Vahedi K et al (1997) Familial hemiplegic migraine: mapping of the second gene and evidence for a third locus. Cephalalgia 17:232

Ducros A, Denier C, Joutel A et al (2001) The clinical spectrum of familial hemiplegic migraine associated with mutations in a neuronal calcium channel. N Engl J Med 345:17–24

Fleming JB, Amos AJ, Desmond RA (2000) Migraine aura without headache: prevalence and risk factors in a primary eye care population. Optometry 71(6):381–389

Grosberg BM, Solomon S, Lipton RB (2005) Retinal migraine. Curr Pain Headache Rep 9(4):268–271

Headache Classification Committee of the International Headache Society (2004) The International Classification of Headache Disorders: 2nd edition. Cephalalgia 24(Suppl 1):112

Jurkat-Rott K, Freilinger T, Dreier JP et al (2004) Variability of familial hemiplegic migraine with novel A1A2 Na+/K+-ATPase variants. Neurology 62:1857–1861

Kirchmann M, Thomsen LL, Olesen J (2006) Basilar-type migraine: clinical, epidemiologic and genetic features. Neurology 66:880–886

Krymchantowski AV (2005) Aura with Non-migraine headache. Curr Pain Headache Rep 9:264–267

Kunkel RS (2005) Migraine aura without headache: benign, but a diagnosis of exclusion. Cleve Clin J Med 72(6):529–534

Lapkin ML, Golden GS (1978) Basilar artery migraine: a review of 30 cases. Am J Dis Child 132:278–281

Levin M (ed) (2008) Comprehensive review of headache medicine. Oxford University Press, Oxford

Li BU, Balint JP (2000) Cyclic vomiting syndrome: evolution in our understanding of a brain-gut disorder. Adv Pediatr 47:117–160

Li BU, Misiewicz L (2003) Cyclic vomiting syndrome: a brain-gut disorder. Gastroenterol Clin North Am 32:997–1019

Lipton RB, Bigal ME, Diamond M et al (2007) Migraine prevalence, disease burden and the need for preventative therapy. Neurology 68(5): 343–349

Manzoni GC, Stovner LG (2010) Epidemiology of headache. Handb Clin Neurol 97:3–22

Olesen J, Bousser M-G, Diener H-C et al (2006) New appendix criteria open for a broader concept of chronic migraine. Cephalalgia 26:742–746

Ophof FRA, Haan J et al (1998) Variable clinical expression of mutations in the P/Q-type calcium channel gene in familial hemiplegic migraine. Dutch Migraine Genetics Research Group. Neurology 50:1105–1110

Ophoff RA, Terwindt GM, Vergouwe MN et al (1996) Familial hemiplegic migraine and episodic ataxia type-2 are caused by mutations in the Ca2+ channel gene CACNL1A4. Cell 87:543–552

Popovich DM, Schentrup DM, McAlhany AL (2010) Recognizing and diagnosing abdominal migraines. J Pediatr Health Care 24(6):372–377

Rubin D, McAbee GN, Feldman-Winter LB (2002) Auditory hallucinations associated with migraine. Headache 42(7):646–648

Russel MB, Olesen J (1996) A nosographic analysis of the migraine aura in a general population. Brain 119:335–361

Silberstein SD, Lipton RB, Dalessio DJ (eds) (2001) Wolff's headache and other head pain, 7th edn. Oxford University Press, New York

Stewart W, Linet M, Celentano D et al (1991) Age-and sex-specific incidence rates of migraine with and without visual auras. Am J Epidemiol 134:11110–11120

Stewart W, Wood C, Reed M et al (2008) Cumulative lifetime migraine incidence in women and men. Cephalalgia 28:1170–1178

Stovner LJ, Hagen K, Jensen R et al (2007) The global burden of headache: a documentation of headache prevalence and disability worldwide. Cephalalgia 27:193–210

Sturzenegger MH, Meienberg O (1985) Basilar artery migraine: a follow-up study of 82 cases. Headache 25:408–415

Tietjen GE, Brandes JL, Peterlin BL et al (2010) Childhood maltreatment and migraine (part II). Emotional abuse as a risk factor for headache. Headache 50(1):32–41

Waters WE, O'Connor PJ (1971) Epidemiology of headache and migraine in women. J Neurol Neurosurg Psychiatry 34:148–153

Zeigler DK, Hassanein RS (1990) Specific headache phenomena: their frequency and coincidence. Headache 30:152–156

16 Mechanisms of Migraine and Its Treatment

Lars Edvinsson[1] · *Antoinette Maassen van den Brink*[2] · *Carlos M. Villalón*[3]
[1]Lund University Hospital, Lund, Sweden
[2]Erasmus University Medical Center, Rotterdam, The Netherlands
[3]Cinvestav-Coapa, México, DF, Mexico

Paolo Martelletti, Timothy J. Steiner (eds.), *Handbook of Headache*, DOI 10.1007/978-88-470-1700-9_16,
© Lifting The Burden 2011

Abstract: Migraine is characterized by recurrent unilateral headaches, accompanied by nausea, vomiting, photophobia, and/or phonophobia, and in some cases facial symptoms. Current theories suggest that the initiation of a migraine attack involves a primary CNS event, putatively involving mutations in ion channels that render the individuals more sensitive to environmental factors, resulting in a wave of cortical spreading depression when the attack is initiated. Early positron emission tomography (PET) suggested the involvement of a migraine active region in the brainstem. In migraine attacks, data suggest that the pain is associated with the activation of the trigeminal nerve and the release of calcitonin gene-related peptide (CGRP) from the trigeminovascular system. Administration of triptans (5-HT$_{1B/1D}$ receptor agonists) causes the headache to subside and the levels of CGRP to normalize. Administration of CGRP receptor antagonists aborts the headache by specifically blocking the CGRP receptors located within the trigeminovascular system. Modern acute migraine therapy involves modulation of both CGRP and 5-HT$_{1B/1D}$ receptors.

Introduction

Migraine headaches are ascribed as neurovascular disorders that world-wide afflict up to 15–20% of the general population and with a considerable impact on productivity and quality of life. Migraine is characterized by attacks of moderate to severe headache that last for 4–72 h, often unilateral, pulsating, and associated with photophobia/phonophobia and/or nausea/vomiting (Olesen et al. 2006). In migraine with aura, the headache is preceded by transient focal neurological symptoms, most often contralateral to the pain (Goadsby et al. 2002).

Although the exact causes of the primary headaches remain unknown, some pieces of the pathophysiological puzzle are starting to fall into place, particularly after a series of elegant positron emission tomography (PET) studies (May and Goadsby 1999). During the last 20 years, there has been a heated debate whether the primary headaches are neurogenic or vascular in origin. However, molecular and functional studies suggest a way to incorporate the different aspects into an integrated hypothesis as neurovascular headaches (Goadsby et al. 2002; Pietrobon and Striessnig 2003; Edvinsson and Uddman 2005).

In susceptible individuals, changes in environmental or physiological states trigger the migraine headache attack. Migraine susceptibility is linked to mechanisms regulating central sensitization. The systems that govern neuronal excitability involve homeostatic mechanisms and intracellular signaling pathways. The demonstration of mutations in the calcium channel gene CACNA1A, in approximately 50% of families suffering from familial hemiplegic migraine (FHM), suggests that there is also a molecular genetic cause of the more common types of migraine (Ophoff et al. 1996; Terwindt et al. 1998). However, the central nervous system (CNS) is devoid of sensory pain receptors and intracranially only blood vessels in the dura mater and the circle of Willis are supplied with sensory nerves and receptors that can respond to thermal, mechanical, or distension stimuli (Ray and Wolff 1940; Olesen et al. 2006).

Where Does the Attack Start?

In the Brain?

On the basis of the original cerebral blood flow studies, early researchers suggested that migraine is a disease comprised of two main subtypes, migraine with aura and migraine without aura. In the former, the aura is characterized most often by visual field disturbances, but sometimes also by additional somatosensory disturbances. In three spontaneous attacks of migraine with aura that were captured within 20 min of the onset of visual symptoms, blood oxygenation level dependent (BOLD) data revealed increases in the amplitude of the MR signal (Hadjikhani et al. 2001). A plausible explanation for the blood flow changes seen in association with the aura in a migraine attack is that they are the result of spreading depression – a transient marked reduction in electrical activity in the grey matter, which advances across the cortical surface. The rate of advance is consistent with the spread of symptoms observed and is associated with decreases in blood flow (Lauritzen 1994). One conclusion raised from these studies is that the migraine aura is not evoked by ischemia, but evoked by aberrant firing of neurones and related cellular elements. Probably, the genetic background can make a migraine patient more prone to alterations in the intracranial circulation, since with certain mutations (as seen in FHM) ion channels may be more easily activated (due to altered membrane potential and/or function) and result in excitation of neurons in situations where they are exposed to excessive stress.

An important question is how the event is linked to activation of the trigeminovascular reflex (McCulloch et al. 1986). One tempting way would be to link the cortical spreading depression to neurogenic inflammation in the dura mater and from there activation of sensory and autonomic reflexes (Bolay et al. 2002). However, the dura mater is an extracerebral structure, separated from the brain by, for example, CSF and pial and arachnoid connective tissues; it is nourished by the external carotid artery (Olesen et al. 2006). Alternatively, specific cell bodies projecting from the brainstem to cerebral vessels, such as the extensive adrenergic and serotonergic efferent nerve fibers from neurons in the locus ceruleus and from the raphe nuclei, respectively, could be involved. In fact there are some anatomical data to support this suggestion (Edvinsson et al. 1983; Bradley et al. 2002) showing a close association between intracerebral nerve fibers and cerebral blood vessels.

In patients with migraine without aura, the situation is somewhat more intricate (Weiller et al. 1995). During attacks, small increases in blood flow were observed in the cingulate, auditory and visual association cortices, and in brainstem regions. These changes (except in the brainstem) normalized after injection of sumatriptan and induced complete headache relief. However, the changes were small and could only be significant if the PET data from all nine subjects were normalized, thus being in agreement with previous negative studies with the [133]xenon method that lacks the precision of PET (Olesen et al. 1990). Further support for the importance of a brainstem region was obtained in a patient that developed a migraine attack without aura after glyceryl trinitrate administration. Bahra and colleagues (Bahra et al. 2001) observed activation in the dorsal rostral brainstem region and hence reproduced the data seen previously by Weiller and colleagues (Weiller et al. 1995). In addition, the authors observed a neuronally driven vasodilatation and activation of regions associated with pain processing (Weiller et al. 1995; Bahra et al. 2001). During acute attacks, increased local blood flow was observed in brainstem regions (specifically midbrain and pons). The brainstem activation persisted after injection of sumatriptan. These findings suggest that the pathogenesis of migraine (and the associated emesis) involves an imbalance in the activity of brainstem nuclei regulating nociception and vascular control. On the other hand, it could equally well be an activation of the periaqueductal grey area (PAG) acting as a filter to inhibit the pain (Fields and Basbaum 1994). The study revealed activation of the dorsal raphe nucleus (DRN) and the locus ceruleus (LC). Indeed, these centers have a dense supply of serotonergic and adrenergic fibers, respectively, which may evoke vasoconstriction (via catecholamines or 5-HT) and hence explain the connection with the trigeminovascular reflex. Alternatively, the DRN and LC may send descending fibers to the trigeminal nucleus caudalis (TNC) and dorsal root ganglia where they act in a gate-control function and the PAG acts to inhibit this. Thus, sensory transmission associated with the TNC appears to be regulated by a complex system. It is still unclear whether the brainstem findings reveal the origin of the disease or if it is an accompanying activation designed to limit the symptoms of the migraine headache.

In the Dura Mater?

Application of individual peptides on the dura results in no meaningful activation of cells in the TNC region (Levy et al. 2005), while the application of the "inflammatory soup" causes activation and increased c-fos immunoreactivity (Burstein et al. 1998; Hoffmann et al. 2009). Thus, massive stimulation of the Aδ- and C-fibers in the dura mater may elicit a neuronal response in the brainstem while more normal doses of the agonists do not. Does this ever occur in the clinical situation? The systemic administrations (intravenous) of the above molecules as well as of other vasoactive compounds tested in the "migraine model" by the Danish group have basically revealed that CGRP, PACAP, nitric oxide (nitroglycerine), histamine, sildenafil, and alcohol, inter alia, elicit a weak transient headache in both healthy volunteers and migraine patients, but in a proportion of migraineurs also a more pronounced headache with a maximum at 2–4 h after the drug administration (Olesen 2008). Recent studies of administrations of, e.g., prostacyclin (Wienecke et al. 2010), prostaglandin E_2 (Wienecke et al. 2009), carbachol (Schytz et al. 2010), and VIP/PACAP (Rahmann et al. 2008; Schytz et al. 2009) show the early headache and increases in superficial temporal artery diameter, and some of them a mild late headache resembling "migraine-like." When comparing the headache intensity with that of genuine attacks (Linde et al. 2006), the induced attacks are relatively mild. It is hypothesized that these agents cause their headache effect via the endothelium, mediated by the release of nitric oxide (Olesen 2008). However, it is well known that they use many different other signaling pathways. It is perhaps more reasonable to suggest that the change in vessel tone may excite differently the perivascular sensory nerve fibers to signal dromically to the TG and the TNC.

Nerves in the Walls of Intracranial Blood Vessels

Since intracranial blood vessels are the only source for eliciting intracranial pain (Ray and Wolff 1940), the understanding of the vascular supply by autonomic and sensory nerves is a prerequisite for the understanding of intracranial pain as it occurs in primary headaches. Intracranial blood vessels are supplied with nerve fibers that emanate from cell bodies in ganglia belonging to the sympathetic, parasympathetic, and sensory nervous systems (Gulbenkian et al. 2001). In addition, cerebral resistance vessels may be innervated by fibers that originate within the brain itself, thereby representing an intrinsic nerve supply (Edvinsson and Krause 2002).

Cerebrovascular Autonomic Nerves

The sympathetic nerves (storing noradrenaline and neuropeptide Y) supply the cerebral blood vessels with perivascular adrenergic nerves that arise from the ipsilateral superior cervical ganglion (Nielsen and Owman 1967), while some nerve fibers that supply the vertebral and basilar arteries originate from the inferior cervical ganglion and the stellate ganglion (Arbab et al. 1988). The activation of these fibers results in vasoconstriction, modulation of cerebrovascular autoregulation, reduction of intracranial pressure, and a decrease in cerebral blood volume and cerebrospinal fluid production (Edvinsson and Krause 2002).

The "classical" neurotransmitter in parasympathetic nerves is acetylcholine (ACh) and their cell bodies contain acetylcholinesterase (AChE). Cerebral blood vessels have perivascular nerves that display AChE activity (Edvinsson et al. 1972; Hara et al. 1985; Suzuki et al. 1990). In several species, ACh induces constriction of isolated cerebral arteries without endothelium, while transmural nerve stimulation predominantly induces relaxation in the same preparations (Lee 1980). The neurogenic vasodilatation in these preparations is not blocked by atropine and is thus non-cholinergic (Lee 1980, 1982). Hence, additional substances may be released together with ACh to mediate dilatation (Lee 1980, 1982; Saito et al. 1985), including VIP, pituitary adenylate cyclase activating polypeptide (PACAP), and nitric oxide (NO), which produce cerebral vasodilatation in vitro and in vivo (Uddman et al. 1993; Jansen-Olesen et al. 1994; Goadsby et al. 1996). In fact, NO might be the last link in cholinergic transmission. Another possibility may be that ACh mainly acts prejunctionally to inhibit neurotransmitter release from the adrenergic nerves (Edvinsson et al. 1977; Lee 2000). The vast majority of parasympathetic nerve fibers to cerebral vessels originates in sphenopalatine and otic ganglia (Suzuki et al. 1988; Edvinsson et al. 1989).

Sensory Nervous System

Most sensory fibers to cranial structures derive from the trigeminal ganglion. In the human trigeminal ganglion, CGRP-immunoreactive neurones occur in high numbers (40% of all neuronal cells) whereas SP-immunoreactive neurones are less numerous (18%). In situ hybridization has revealed that 40% of all nerve cell bodies contain CGRP and CGRP mRNA (Edvinsson et al. 1998a; Tajti et al. 1999). CGRP and SP are potent vasodilators in vivo and in vitro, the former being 10–1,000 times more potent (Edvinsson et al. 1981; McCulloch et al. 1986; Edvinsson et al. 1987; Jansen et al. 1991). Several studies have suggested that SP is involved in plasma extravasation from postcapillary venules in the dura mater during primary headaches (Markowitz et al. 1987). While neurokinin receptor antagonists are potent inhibitors of neurogenic inflammation (Shepheard et al. 1993; Shepheard et al. 1995; Phebus et al. 1997), they were ineffective in the acute treatment of migraine (Goldstein et al. 1997). Furthermore, while CGRP is released during the headache phase of a migraine attack, SP is not (Goadsby et al. 1990; Goadsby and Edvinsson 1993). In addition, SP is now considered not to be involved in vascular nociception in humans (Holthusen et al. 1997). This view is supported by intravital microscopy studies demonstrating that vasodilatation during perivascular stimulation of the middle meningeal artery in vivo was blocked by a CGRP antagonist, but unaffected by neurokinin agonists or antagonists (Williamson et al. 1997). Immunocytochemistry has revealed the expression of PACAP not only in parasympathetic but also in sensory ganglia (Moller et al. 1993; Tajti et al. 1999), suggesting that PACAP may act as a neuromodulator in the sensory systems (Moller et al. 1993). There is a moderate supply of PACAP immunoreactive nerve fibers in the cat cerebral circulation (Uddman et al. 1993). In the rat, the majority of the PACAP-containing fibers around cerebral blood vessels originates in the sphenopalatine ganglion (Edvinsson et al. 2001). In the human trigeminal ganglion,

PACAP-containing cell bodies are more numerous than in laboratory animals, amounting to 15–20% (Tajti et al. 1999). Double immunostaining has revealed that PACAP co-localizes with CGRP in some cell bodies in the trigeminal ganglion. PACAP dilates cerebral arteries and can increase cerebral blood flow (Uddman et al. 1993; Jansen-Olesen et al. 1994; Seki et al. 1995). Activation of the trigeminovascular system results in co-release of CGRP and PACAP into the cat jugular vein (Zagami et al. 1990), a model used in studies of migraine (Goadsby et al. 1988). It is also possible that PACAP may participate in antidromic vasodilatation following activation of the trigeminal vascular reflex (McCulloch et al. 1986).

NO has been suggested as an important molecule for initiation of migraine attacks (Olesen et al. 1995). The expression of NOS in trigeminal nerve cell bodies supports this suggestion. NO released from the endothelium (eNOS), from perivascular nerves (nNOS), or inducible NOS (iNOS) may activate the guanylate cyclase system in smooth muscle cells. This results in a decrease in the local intracellular Ca^{++} level, giving rise to vasodilatation, which may activate the pain sensitive structures around the cranial vessels (Olesen et al. 1995). Few trigeminal neurones express NOS in animals (Nozaki et al. 1993; Edvinsson et al. 1998b; Edvinsson et al. 2001), while the human trigeminal ganglia has about 15% of the cell bodies containing NOS (Tajti et al. 1999). Double immunostaining of the cat trigeminal ganglion has revealed that only few CGRP neurones (less than 5%) are NOS positive (Edvinsson et al. 1998b). The relative functional role of CGRP and NO in the trigeminal ganglion has been studied in the cat; CGRP blockade markedly attenuates the cerebral blood flow increase following trigeminal nerve activation while NOS blockade was without effect (Edvinsson et al. 1998b). On the other hand, activation of the parasympathetic nerves results in a NO-dependent flow increase (Goadsby et al. 1996), suggesting a physiological role for NO in the parasympathetic vasodilator system.

Release of Neurotransmitters in Migraine

During migraine attacks, there is a marked increase in the plasma levels of CGRP in the external jugular vein (Goadsby et al. 1990). At the same time, there is no change of CGRP in peripheral blood or in the levels of NPY, VIP, or SP in the jugular vein (❑ *Table 16.1*). Furthermore, there is no difference between migraine with aura or migraine without aura, as both result in substantial increases in venous CGRP levels at the same time as the patients exhibit pain

❑ Table 16.1

Overview of changes in perivascular neuropeptide levels occurring in acute attacks of primary headache disorders

	NPY	VIP	Substance P	CGRP
Migraine without aura	±0	±0	±0	↑
Migraine with aura	±0	±0	±0	↑
Trigeminal neuralgia	±0	±0	±0	↑
Cluster headache	±0	↑	±0	↑
Chronic paroxysmal headache	±0	↑	±0	↑

±0, no change from before headache, ↑ significant increase in neuropeptide level

(Goadsby et al. 1990; Goadsby and Edvinsson 1993; Gallai et al. 1995). Even when blood samples were taken from the cubital fossa vein, increased CGRP levels in migraine patients were observed, both outside attacks (Ashina et al. 2000) and after nitroglycerine-induced attacks (Juhasz et al. 2003). Triptans have been demonstrated to normalize the CGRP levels in spontaneous (Goadsby and Edvinsson 1993; Stepien et al. 2003) as well as triggered (Juhasz et al. 2005) migraine attacks. The mechanisms behind this reduction in elevated plasma CGRP in humans may be due to the presence of $5\text{-}HT_{1B}$ and $5\text{-}HT_{1D}$ receptors expressed on the trigeminal ganglion cells and fibers (Longmore et al. 1997; Hou et al. 2001), which may, during stimulation, cause inhibition of sensory nerve activity (Wang et al. 2010). CGRP analysis is notoriously difficult in biological fluids and negative studies have appeared, however (Friberg et al. 1994; Tvedskov et al. 2005). This may simply reflect that the methodology of analysis, including the use of HPLC fractionation and rapid cool-centrifugation and freezing of the samples, is crucial as evident from several studies (Edvinsson 2004). Recently, it was verified that saliva also can be used to demonstrate the relation between headache attacks and CGRP release; interestingly a CGRP elevation predicted a positive effect of a triptan (Cady et al. 2009). The reason why SP is not released in migraine might be due to a much lower level of SP than of CGRP within the trigeminovascular system to the intracranial vasculature. Direct electrical stimulation of the trigeminal ganglion in humans, however, results in co-release of CGRP and SP (Goadsby et al. 1988), possibly because here the entire sensory system to the head is activated.

Central Mechanisms in Migraine

Once the trigeminovascular reflex is initiated, resulting in an antidromic activation that involves release of CGRP, the central part of this pathway, the TNC, and/or its reciprocal parts at the C1 and C2 levels are also activated. Experiments in laboratory animals as well as in humans have shown that direct stimulation of either the superior sagittal sinus or the trigeminal ganglion results in activation of cells in this region (Goadsby and Zagami 1991; Goadsby and Edvinsson 1994).

How Is the Trigeminovascular Reflex Initiated?

Following the identification of the trigeminal vascular pathway and its dependence on neuro-peptides (Uddman et al. 1985), functional studies showed that denervation does not alter the regional cerebral blood flow or cerebral metabolism, the cerebral vascular responses to carbon dioxide or autoregulation (Edvinsson and Krause 2002). However, vasoconstrictor responses elicited by noradrenaline (McCulloch et al. 1986), alkaline pH, $PGF_{2\alpha}$, $BaCl_2$, subarachnoid blood, or capsaicin are modified (Edvinsson et al. 1990; Edvinsson et al. 1995). The general picture is that following denervation there is no alteration in the maximum contractile response to either of the above agents, but the time to return to the initial basal tone is markedly prolonged. It is hypothesized that vasoconstriction triggers an antidromic release of the sensory neuronal messengers, which results in normalization of the vascular tone. Subsequent studies using antagonists in combination with denervation have shown that CGRP has a significant role in this response (Edvinsson et al. 1995; Edvinsson et al. 1990). Vasodilatation of cortical arterioles induced by acidic pH is not modified by trigeminal denervation (Edvinsson et al. 1995). Thus, if the primary headache attack involves cortical spreading depression with subsequent vasoconstriction of cerebral vessels, the trigeminal vascular system may have a counter-balancing effect designed to normalize cerebrovascular tone. The activation of this system is noted clinically as an increase in cranial venous outflow of CGRP during the attacks (Goadsby et al. 1988; Goadsby et al. 1990; Goadsby and Edvinsson 1993). In an experimental study of spreading depression, it was demonstrated that CGRP is in part involved in the local dilatation (Wahl et al. 1994). In contrast, spreading depression per se in monkeys did not result in enhanced jugular venous CGRP levels (Piper et al. 1993), which agrees well with patient data (Kruuse et al. 2010). If the patient is in a "latent period" (Fanciullacci et al. 1995), then the spreading depression may induce a strong reflex vasoconstriction that may activate the trigeminovascular reflex (McCulloch et al. 1986) as observed in acute primary headaches (Fanciullacci et al. 1997). The connection may be either functional as suggested by Bolay (Bolay et al. 2002) or anatomical (Cohen et al. 1996).

What Is the Role of the Trigeminocervical Complex?

The nociceptive input from cerebral blood vessels and the dura mater to the first synapse in the brainstem is transmitted by small-diameter Aδ- and C-fiber afferents in the ophthalmic division of the trigeminal nerve via the trigeminal ganglion to nociceptive second-order neurons to the superficial and deep layers of the medullar dorsal horn of the trigeminocervical complex (Liu et al. 2004; Liu et al. 2008). This system extends from the trigeminal nucleus caudalis to the C2–C3 segments. To understand the pathophysiology of primary headaches, it is essential to identify the human brain regions that may process the signs of the disorder. Indeed, there is a rich supply of SP-immunoreactive fibers in the marginal layer and in the substantia gelantinosa of the subnucleus caudalis of the TNC and the Rexed's lamina I and II of the C1 and C2 segments of the human spinal cord (Uddman et al. 2002). In addition, there is a moderate supply of CGRP and PACAP fibers in these areas while NOS or VIP fibers were not seen (Christiansen et al. 2003).

Migraine attacks involve changes that are characterized by pain and nausea, symptoms that are mediated by the sensory system and by centers in the brainstem. The vascular components of the disorder are mediated via the trigeminal nerve. Mechanical or electrical stimulation of the dura mater or of cranial blood vessels reproduces signs of migrainous pain (Ray and Wolff 1940). The central structures that process craniovascular pain have been mapped to some degree. Electrical stimulation of the cat superior sagittal sinus leads to increased metabolic activity in the TNC and in the C2 region of the spinal cord (Goadsby and Zagami 1991). A marked increase of the immediate early gene c-fos in lamina I and II of the TNC and in the superficial layers of the C1 and C2 regions can be seen upon stimulation of the middle meningeal artery, the superior sagittal sinus, or the trigeminal ganglion in monkeys and cats (Kaube et al. 1993; Goadsby and Hoskin 1997; Hoskin et al. 1999). However, the expression of neuropeptides in the brainstem is unaltered during 2 h of superior sagittal sinus stimulation (Christiansen et al. 2003). The c-fos response is reduced by antimigraine drugs such as triptans (Knyihar-Csillik et al. 1997, 2000). In humans, evidence for a central site of action of the triptans has come from binding studies that demonstrate their association with the superficial lamina of the caudal part of the TNC and the cervical dorsal horn as well as of the nucleus of the tractus solitarius. In an attempt to characterize the receptors involved, it has been suggested that 5-HT$_{1B}$ receptors are present in very low concentrations in all these nuclei in humans (below 12% of total specific binding), while 5-HT_{1D} receptors account for about 50% of the total specific sumatriptan binding (Longmore et al. 1997). In addition, a significant amount of 5-HT_{1F}-binding sites can be seen (Castro et al. 1997; Pascual et al. 1996). The 5-HT_{1F} site has been examined using the specific agonist LY334370 (Shepheard et al. 1999). This agonist had no contractile effect nor did it inhibit CGRP release. Interestingly, it has recently been suggested that inhibition of another 5-HT receptor, the 5-HT_7 receptor, may partially reduce CGRP release (Wang et al. 2010). These data imply that the antimigraine actions could in part be exerted centrally on these nuclei. In humans, the immunocytochemical distribution of CGRP, SP, and PACAP coincides with the reported localization of the $5\text{-HT}_{1B/1D}$ binding sites in the TNC and in particular with the distribution of $5\text{-HT}_{1B/1D}$ receptor (Uddman et al. 2002). Thus, it is tempting to suggest that if the triptans can reach the TNC and the C1 and C2 spinal segments, they may also inhibit the central activity of the sensory trigeminal fibers.

Treatment Aspects: Where Do the Triptans and CGRP Antagonists Act?

As discussed above, triptans may display a central action via 5-HT_{1D} or 5-HT_{1F} receptors. Second, their therapeutic action could be mediated via the inhibition of neuropeptide release from perivascular nerve endings (5-HT_{1D} receptors). Finally, triptans could, in agreement with the concept of their development, mediate their antimigraine effects via a direct vasoconstrictor action at 5-HT_{1B} receptors (for review see Goadsby et al. 2002). Similarly, for CGRP receptor antagonists several putative modes of action have been described. Interestingly, in comparing the clinical effects, it is remarkable that both telcagepant and olcegepant required substantially higher plasma concentrations relative to their in vitro pA_2 to achieve clinical efficacy for the acute treatment of migraine (Olesen et al. 2004; Ho et al. 2008). For example, plasma concentrations of telcagepant associated with clinical efficacy are in the micromolar range, which is substantially higher than the pA_2 that we have seen for the cranial vascular effect (in the nanomolar range). Several factors may account for these apparent discrepancies. First, a high protein binding of these compounds; indeed, a considerable protein binding is suggested by the fivefold reduction of the potency of telcagepant in the presence of serum (Salvatore et al. 2008). Second, a concentration of drug equal to the pA_2 value may not be sufficient to decrease functional responses since it only shifts the concentration response curves twofold to the right; most likely, a concentration of a least ten times the corresponding pA_2 would functionally inhibit relaxations to CGRP. Thirdly, as nerve terminals releasing CGRP are located in the adventitia close to the media layer of the blood vessels, the concentration of telcagepant at the receptors may be substantially smaller than that at the lumen of the blood vessel, that is, the plasma concentration. This phenomenon is unlikely to occur in vitro, where the antagonist can reach the CGRP receptors from both the luminal and abluminal sides. Lastly, the therapeutic effect of CGRP receptor antagonists could also be mediated via pathways other than only blockade CGRP-induced vasodilatation. Penetration of telcagepant through the blood-brain barrier may be necessary in addition to the peripheral blockade to achieve antimigraine efficacy (Edvinsson 2008). Arguments in favor of a neuronal mechanism are the lack of presynaptic CGRP receptors in the meninges, which suggests that exogenous CGRP is unlikely to directly modify the innervating sensory nerve fibers (Lennerz et al. 2008). This finding is also in agreement with in vivo data obtained in rats, suggesting that an action of CGRP on the dura mater cannot account for the activation of peripheral afferents during migraine

(Levy et al. 2005). In this study, the effects of CGRP in the meninges, including meningeal vasodilatation, were not sufficient to activate or sensitize meningeal nociceptors. Clearly, further studies are needed to resolve the therapeutic mechanisms involved in CGRP receptor antagonism.

Summary

Current data provide a model in which a central "generator" or an "active region" (different in migraine and in cluster headache) is activated. Following changes in cerebral vascular tone, the trigeminovascular reflex is initiated to counter-balance cerebrovascular constriction in part via release of CGRP and VIP. The study of neuropeptide levels in migraine and cluster headache provides a link between the clinical and the basic research, work that is crucial for the understanding of migraine pathophysiology. Indeed, plasma concentrations of CGRP, but not of other neuropeptides, are elevated during migraine headache (with and without aura) and these are normalized by triptans in parallel with alleviation of headache.

The activation of TNC provides the central link to nociception, pain development, and associated symptoms. Hypothetically, intense activation of central pain pathways may involve the superior salivatory nucleus, resulting in parasympathetic VIP release, and manifestation of additional facial symptoms in, for example, cluster headache. A number of possibilities to interact with the sensory system have recently been shown. It was reported that an adenosine A_1 receptor agonist acts prejunctionally to inhibit sensory neurogenic vasodilatation, CGRP release, and firing of second-order neurones in the TNC (Honey et al. 2002). Its clinical usefulness is now evaluated.

By blocking CGRP receptors postjunctionally, the recently developed CGRP blockers (Edvinsson et al. 2002; Salvatore et al. 2008) have been found to be effective in the acute treatment of migraine (Olesen et al. 2004; Ho et al. 2008). Thus, both in spontaneous cases of migraine and in headache attacks induced by administration of CGRP, the CGRP receptor antagonists were effective without any noticeable side effects, establishing a new principle in the acute treatment of migraine (Edvinsson 2009; Villalón and Olesen 2009).

Acknowledgments

The studies of the authors reviewed here have in part been supported by the Swedish Research Council (project no. 5958).

References

Arbab MA, Delgado T, Wiklund L, Svendgaard NA (1988) Brain stem terminations of the trigeminal and upper spinal ganglia innervation of the cerebrovascular system: WGA-HRP transganglionic study. J Cereb Blood Flow Metab 8:54–63

Ashina M, Bendtsen L, Jensen R, Schifter S, Olesen J (2000) Evidence for increased plasma levels of calcitonin gene-related peptide in migraine outside of attacks. Pain 86:133–138

Bahra A, Matharu MS, Buchel C, Frackowiak RS, Goadsby PJ (2001) Brainstem activation specific to migraine headache. Lancet 357:1016–1017

Bolay H, Reuter U, Dunn AK, Huang Z, Boas DA, Moskowitz MA (2002) Intrinsic brain activity triggers trgeminal meningeal afferents in a migraine model. Nat Med 8(2):136–142

Bradley SR, Pieribone VA, Wang W, Severson CA, Jacobs RA, Richerson GB (2002) Chemosensitive serotonergic neruons are closely associated with large medullary arteries. Nat Neurosci 5:401–402

Burstein R, Yamamura H, Malick A, Strassman AM (1998) Chemical stimulation of the intracranial dura induces enhanced responses to facial stimulation in brain stem trigeminal neurons. J Neurophysiol 79:964–982

Cady RK, Vause CV, Ho TW, Bigal ME, Durham PL (2009) Elevated saliva calcitonin gene-related peptide levels during acute migraine predict therapeutic response to rizatriptan. Headache 49:1258–1266

Castro ME, Pascual J, Romon T, del Arco C, del Olmo E, Pazos A (1997) Differential distribution of [³H] sumatriptan binding sites (5-HT$_{1B}$, 5-HT$_{1D}$ and 5-HT$_{1F}$ receptors) in human brain: focus on brainstem and spinal cord. Neuropharmacology 36:535–542

Christiansen T, Bruun A, Knight YE, Goadsby PJ, Edvinsson L (2003) Immunoreactivity of NOS, CGRP, PACAP, SP and VIP in the trigeminal nucleus caudalis and in the cervical spinal cord C1and C2 of the cat. J Headache Pain 4:156–163

Cohen Z, Bonvento G, Lacombe P, Hamel E (1996) Serotonin in the regulation of brain microcirculation. Prog Neurobiol 50:335–362

Edvinsson L (2004) Blockade of CGRP receptors in the intracranial vasculature: a new target in the treatment of headache. Cephalalgia 24:611–622

Edvinsson L (2008) CGRP blockers in migraine therapy: where do they act? Br J Pharmacol 155:967–969

Edvinsson L (2009) Migraine: telcagepant provides new hope for people with migraine. Nat Rev Neurol 5:240–242

Edvinsson L, Krause DN (2002) Cerebral blood flow and metabolism. Lippincott Williams & Wilkins, Philadelphia

Edvinsson L, Uddman R (2005) Neurobiology in primary headaches. Brain Res Brain Res Rev 48:438–456

Edvinsson L, Nielsen KC, Owman C, Sporrong B (1972) Cholinergic mechanisms in pail vessels. Histochmistry, electron microscopy and pharmacology. Z Zellforsch Mikrosk Anat 134:311–325

Edvinsson L, Falck B, Owman C (1977) Possibilities for a cholinergic action on smooth musculature and on sympathetic axons in brain vessels mediated by muscarinic and nicotinic receptors. J Pharmacol Exp Ther 200:117–126

Edvinsson L, McCulloch J, Uddman R (1981) Substance P: immunohistochemical localization and effect upon cat pial arteries in vitro and in situ. J Physiol 318:251–258

Edvinsson L, Degueurce A, Duverger D, MacKenzie ET, Scatton B (1983) Central serotonergic nerves project to the pial vessels of the brain. Nature 306:55–57

Edvinsson L, Ekman R, Jansen I, McCulloch J, Uddman R (1987) Calcitonin gene-related peptide and cerebral blood vessels: distribution and vasomotor effects. J Cereb Blood Flow Metab 7:720–728

Edvinsson L, Hara H, Uddman R (1989) Retrograde tracing of nerve fibers to the rat middle cerebral artery with true blue: colocalization with different peptides. J Cereb Blood Flow Metab 9:212–218

Edvinsson L, Jansen I, Kingman TA, McCulloch J (1990) Cerebrovascular responses to capsaicin in vitro and in situ. Br J Pharmacol 100:312–318

Edvinsson L, Jansen Olesen I, Kingman TA, McCulloch J, Uddman R (1995) Modification of vasoconstrictor responses in cerebral blood vessels by lesioning of the trigeminal nerve: possible involvement of CGRP. Cephalalgia 15:373–383

Edvinsson L, Gulbenkian S, Barroso CP, Cunhae Sa M, Polak JM, Mortensen A et al (1998a) Innervation of the human middle meningeal artery: immunohistochemistry, ultrastructure, and role of endothelium for vasomotility. Peptides 19:1213–1225

Edvinsson L, Mulder H, Goadsby PJ, Uddman R (1998b) Calcitonin gene-related peptide and nitric oxide in the trigeminal ganglion: cerebral vasodilatation from trigeminal nerve stimulation involves mainly calcitonin gene-related peptide. J Auton Nerv Syst 70:15–22

Edvinsson L, Elsås T, Suzuki N, Shimizu T, Lee TJ (2001) Origin and Co-localization of nitric oxide synthase, CGRP, PACAP, and VIP in the cerebral circulation of the rat. Microsc Res Tech 53:221–228

Edvinsson L, Alm R, Shaw D, Rutledge RZ, Koblan KS, Longmore J et al (2002) Effect of the CGRP receptor antagonist BIBN4096BS in human cerebral, coronary and omental arteries and in SK-N-MC cells. Eur J Pharmacol 434:49–53

Fanciullacci M, Alessandri M, Figini M, Geppetti P, Michelacci S (1995) Increase in plasma calcitonin gene-related peptide from the extracerebral circulation during nitroglycerin-induced cluster headache attack. Pain 60:119–123

Fanciullacci M, Alessandri M, Sicuteri R, Marabini S (1997) Responsiveness of the trigeminovascular system to nitroglycerine in cluster headache patients. Brain 120(Pt 2):283–288

Fields HL, Basbaum AI (1994) Central nervous system mechanisms of pain modulation. In: Wall PD, Melzack R (eds) Textbook of pain. Churchill Livingstone, Edinburgh

Friberg L, Olesen J, Olsen TS, Karle A, Ekman R, Fahrenkrug J (1994) Absence of vasoactive peptide release from brain to cerebral circulation during onset of migraine with aura. Cephalalgia 14(1):47–54

Gallai V, Sarchielli P, Floridi A, Franceschini M, Codini M, Glioti G et al (1995) Vasoactive peptide levels in the plasma of young migraine patients with and without aura assessed both interictally and ictally. Cephalalgia 15:384–390

Goadsby PJ, Edvinsson L (1993) The trigeminovascular system and migraine: studies characterizing cerebrovascular and neuropeptide changes seen in humans and cats. Ann Neurol 33:48–56

Goadsby PJ, Edvinsson L (1994) Human in vivo evidence for trigeminovascular activation in cluster headache. Neuropeptide changes and effects of acute attacks therapies. Brain 117(Pt 3):427–434

Goadsby PJ, Hoskin KL (1997) The distribution of trigeminovascular afferents in the nonhuman primate brain Macaca nemestrina: a c-fos immunocytochemical study. J Anat 190:367–375

Goadsby PJ, Zagami AS (1991) Stimulation of the superior sagittal sinus increases metabolic activity and blood flow in certain regions of the brainstem and upper cervical spinal cord of the cat. Brain 114:1001–1011

Goadsby PJ, Edvinsson L, Ekman R (1988) Release of vasoactive peptides in the extracerebral circulation of humans and the cat during activation of the trigeminovascular system. Ann Neurol 23:193–196

Goadsby PJ, Edvinsson L, Ekman R (1990) Vasoactive peptide release in the extracerebral circulation of humans during migraine headache. Ann Neurol 28:183–187

Goadsby PJ, Uddman R, Edvinsson L (1996) Cerebral vasodilatation in the cat involves nitric oxide from parasympathetic nerves. Brain Res 707:110–118

Goadsby PJ, Lipton RB, Ferrari MD (2002) Migraine–current understanding and treatment. N Engl J Med 346:257–270

Goldstein DJ, Wang O, Saper JR, Stoltz R, Silberstein SD, Mathew NT (1997) Ineffectiveness of neurokinin-1 antagonist in acute migraine: a crossover study. Cephalalgia 17:785–790

Gulbenkian S, Uddman R, Edvinsson L (2001) Neuronal messengers in the human cerebral circulation. Peptides 22:995–1007

Hadjikhani N, Sanchez Del Rio M, Wu O, Schwartz D, Bakker D, Fischl B et al (2001) Mechanisms of migraine aura revealed by functional MRI in human visual cortex. Proc Natl Acad Sci USA 98:4687–4692

Hara H, Hamill GS, Jacobowithz DM (1985) Origin of cholinergic nerves to the rat major cerebral arteries: coexistence with vasoactive intestinal polypeptide. Brain Res Bull 25:179–188

Ho TW, Ferrari MD, Dodick DW, Galet V, Kost J, Fan X et al (2008) Efficacy and tolerability of MK-0974 (telcagepant), a new oral antagonist of calcitonin

gene-related peptide receptor, compared with zolmitriptan for acute migraine: a randomised, placebo-controlled, parallel-treatment trial. Lancet 372:2115–2123

Hoffmann J, Neeb L, Israel H, Dannenberg F, Triebe F, Dirnagl U et al (2009) Intracisternal injection of inflammatory soup activates the trigeminal nerve system. Cephalalgia 29:1212–1217

Holthusen H, Kindgen-Milles D, Ding ZP (1997) Substance P is not involved in vascular nociception in humans. Neuropeptides 31:445–448

Honey AC, Bland-Ward PA, Connor HE, Feniuk W, Humphrey PPA (2002) Study of an adenosine A1 receptor agonist on trigeminally evoked dural blood vessel dilation in the anaesthetized rat. Cephalalgia 22:260–264

Hoskin KL, Zagami AS, Goadsby PJ (1999) Stimulation of the middle meningeal artery leads to Fos expression in the trigeminocervical nucleus: a comparative study of monkey and cat. J Anat 194:579–588

Hou M, Kanje M, Longmore J, Tajti J, Uddman R, Edvinsson L (2001) 5-HT(1B) and 5-HT(1D) receptors in the human trigeminal ganglion: co-localization with calcitonin gene-related peptide, substance P and nitric oxide synthase. Brain Res 909:112–120

Jansen I, Alafaci C, McCulloch J, Uddman R, Edvinsson L (1991) Tachykinins (substance P, neurokinin A, neuropeptide K, and neurokinin B) in the cerebral circulation: vasomotor responses in vitro and in situ. J Cereb Blood Flow Metab 11:567–575

Jansen-Olesen I, Goadsby PJ, Uddman R, Edvinsson L (1994) Vasoactive intestinal peptide (VIP) like peptides in the cerebral circulation of the cat. J Auton Nerv Syst 49(Suppl):S97–S103

Juhasz G, Zsombok T, Modos EA, Olajos S, Jakab B, Nemeth J et al (2003) NO-induced migraine attack: strong increase in plasma calcitonin gene-related peptide (CGRP) concentration and negative correlation with platelet serotonin release. Pain 106:461–470

Juhasz G, Zsombok T, Jakab B, Nemeth J, Szolcsanyi J, Bagdy G (2005) Sumatriptan causes parallel decrease in plasma calcitonin gene-related peptide (CGRP) concentration and migraine headache during nitroglycerin induced migraine attack. Cephalalgia 25:179–183

Kaube H, Keay KA, Hoskin KL, Bandler R, Goadsby PJ (1993) Expression of c-Fos-like immunoreactivity in the caudal medulla and upper cervical spinal cord following stimulation of the superior sagittal sinus in the cat. Brain Res 629:95–102

Knyihar-Csillik E, Tajti J, Samsam M, Sary G, Slezak S, Vecsei L (1997) Effect of a serotonin agonist (sumatriptan) on the peptidergic innervation of the rat cerebral dura mater and on the expression of c-fos in the caudal trigeminal nucleus in an experimental migraine model. J Neurosci Res 48:449–464

Knyihar-Csillik E, Tajti J, Csillik AE, Chadaide Z, Mihaly A, Vecsei L (2000) Effects of eletriptan on the peptidergic innervation of the cerebral dura mater and trigeminal ganglion, and on the expression of c-fos and c-jun in the trigeminal complex of the rat in an experimental migraine model. Eur J Neurosci 12:3991–4002

Kruuse C, Iversen HK, Jansen-Olesen I, Edvinsson L, Olesen J (2010) Calcitonin gene-related peptide (cgrp) levels during glyceryl trinitrate (gtn)-induced headache in healthy volunteers. Cephalalgia 30(4): 467–474

Lauritzen M (1994) Pathophysiology of the migraine aura. The spreading depression theory. Brain 117(Pt 1): 199–210

Lee TJ (1980) Direct evidence against acetylcholine as the dilator transmitter in the cat cerebral artery. Eur J Pharmacol 68:393–394

Lee TJ (1982) Cholinergic mechanism in the large cat cerebral artery. Circ Res 50:870–879

Lee TJ (2000) Nitric oxide and the cerebral vascular function. J Biomed Sci 7:16–26

Lennerz JK, Ruhle V, Ceppa EP, Neuhuber WL, Bunnett NW, Grady EF et al (2008) Calcitonin receptor-like receptor (CLR), receptor activity-modifying protein 1 (RAMP1), and calcitonin gene-related peptide (CGRP) immunoreactivity in the rat trigemino-vascular system: differences between peripheral and central CGRP receptor distribution. J Comp Neurol 507:1277–1299

Levy D, Burstein R, Strassman AM (2005) Calcitonin gene-related peptide does not excite or sensitize meningeal nociceptors: implications for the pathophysiology of migraine. Ann Neurol 58: 698–705

Linde M, Mellberg A, Dahlof C (2006) The natural course of migraine attacks. A prospective analysis of untreated attacks compared with attacks treated with a triptan. Cephalalgia 26:712–721

Liu Y, Broman J, Edvinsson L (2004) Central projections of sensory innervation of the rat superior sagittal sinus. Neuroscience 129:431–437

Liu Y, Broman J, Edvinsson L (2008) Central projections of the sensory innervation of the rat middle meningeal artery. Brain Res 1208:103–110

Longmore J, Shaw D, Smith D, Hopkins R, McAllister G, Pickard JD et al (1997) Differential distribution of $5HT_{1D}$- and $5HT_{1B}$-immunoreactivity within the human trigemino-cerebrovascular system: implications for the discovery of new antimigraine drugs. Cephalalgia 17:833–842

Markowitz S, Saito K, Moskowitz MA (1987) Neurogenically mediated leakage of plasma protein occurs from blood vessels in dura mater but not brain. J Neurosci 7:4129–4136

May A, Goadsby PJ (1999) The trigeminovascular system in humans: pathophysiologic implications for primary headache syndromes of the neural influences on the cerebral circulation. J Cereb Blood Flow Metab 19:115–127

McCulloch J, Uddman R, Kingman TA, Edvinsson L (1986) Calcitonin gene-related peptide: functional role in cerebrovascular regulation. Proc Natl Acad Sci USA 83:5731–5735

Moller K, Zhang YZ, Hakanson R, Luts A, Sjolund B, Uddman R et al (1993) Pituitary adenylate cyclase activating peptide is a sensory neuropeptide: immunocytochemical and immunochemical evidence. Neuroscience 57:725–732

Nielsen KC, Owman C (1967) Adrenergic innervation of pail arteries related to the circle of Willis in the cat. Brain Res 6(4):773–776

Nozaki K, Moskowitz MA, Maynard KI, Koketsu N, Dawson TM, Bredt DS et al (1993) Possible origins and distribution of immunoreactive nitric oxide synthase-containing nerve fibers in cerebral arteries. J Cereb Blood Flow Metab 13:70–79

Olesen J (2008) The role of nitric oxide (NO) in migraine, tension-type headache and cluster headache. Pharmacol Ther 120:157–171

Olesen J, Friberg L, Olsen TS, Iversen HK, Lassen NA, Andersen AR et al (1990) Timing and topography of cerebral blood flow, aura, and headache during migraine attacks. Ann Neurol 28:791–798

Olesen J, Thomsen LL, Lassen LH, Jansen-Olesen I (1995) The nitric oxide hypothesis of migraine and other vascular headaches. Cephalalgia 15:94–100

Olesen J, Diener HC, Husstedt IW, Goadsby PJ, Hall D, Meier U et al (2004) Calcitonin gene-related peptide receptor antagonist BIBN 4096 BS for the acute treatment of migraine. N Engl J Med 350:1104–1110

Olesen J, Goadsby PJ, Ramadan NM, Tfelt-Hansen P, Welch KMA (2006) The headaches, 3rd edn. Lipincott, Williams & Wilkins, Philadelphia

Ophoff RA, Terwindt GM, Vergouwe MN, van Eijk R, Oefner PJ, Hoffman SM et al (1996) Familial hemiplegic migraine and episodic ataxia type-2 are caused by mutations in the Ca2+ channel gene CACNL1A4. Cell 87:543–552

Pascual J, Del Arco C, Romon T, Del Olmo E, Pazos A (1996) [³H]Sumatriptan binding sites in human brain: regional-dependent labelling of $5-HT_{1D}$ and $5-HT_{1F}$ receptors. Eur J Pharmacol 295:271–274

Phebus LA, Johnson KW, Stengel PW, Lobb KL, Nixon JA, Hipskind PA (1997) The non-peptide NK-1 receptor antagonist LY303870 inhibits neurognic dural inflammation in guinea pigs. Life Sci 60:1553–1561

Pietrobon D, Striessnig J (2003) Neurobiology of migraine. Nat Rev Neurosci 4:386–398

Piper RD, Edvinsson L, Ekman R, Lambert GA (1993) Cortical spreading depression does not result in the release of calcitonin gene-related peptide into the external jugular vein of the cat: relevance to human migraine. Cephalalgia 13:180–183

Rahmann A, Wienecke T, Hansen JM, Fahrenkrug J, Olesen J, Ashina M (2008) Vasoactive intestinal peptide causes marked cephalic vasodilation, but does not induce migraine. Cephalalgia 28:226–236

Ray B, Wolff H (1940) Experimental studies on headaches, pain sensitive structures of the heada and their significance in headaches. Arch Surg 41:813–856

Saito A, Wu JY, Lee TJ (1985) Evidence for the presence of cholinergic nerves in cerebral arteries: an immunohistochemical demonstration of choline acetyltransferase. J Cereb Blood Flow Metab 10:399–408

Salvatore CA, Hershey JC, Corcoran HA, Fay JF, Johnston VK, Moore EL et al (2008) Pharmacological characterization of MK-0974 [N-[(3R, 6S)-6-(2, 3-difluorophenyl)-2-oxo-1-(2, 2, 2-trifluoroethyl) azepan-3- yl]-4-(2-oxo-2, 3-dihydro-1H-imidazo [4, 5-b]pyridin-1-yl)piperidine-1-carbox amide], a potent and orally active calcitonin gene-related peptide receptor antagonist for the treatment of migraine. J Pharmacol Exp Ther 324:416–421

Schytz HW, Birk S, Wienecke T, Kruuse C, Olesen J, Ashina M (2009) PACAP38 induces migraine-like attacks in patients with migraine without aura. Brain 132:16–25

Schytz HW, Wienecke T, Olesen J, Ashina M (2010) Carbachol induces headache, but not migraine-like attacks, in patients with migraine without aura. Cephalalgia 30:337–345

Seki Y, Suzuki Y, Baskaya MK, Kano T, Saito K, Takayasu M et al (1995) The effects of pituitary adenylate cyclase-activating polypeptide on cerebral arteries and vertebral artery blood flow in anesthetized dogs. Eur J Pharmacol 275:259–266

Shepheard SL, Williamson DJ, Hill RG, Hargreaves RJ (1993) The non-peptide neurokinin1 receptor antagonist, RP 67580, blocks neurogenic plasma extravasation in the dura mater of rats. Br J Pharmacol 108:11–12

Shepheard SL, Williamson DJ, Williams J, Hill RG, Hargreaves RJ (1995) Comparison of the effects of sumatriptan and the NK1 antagonist CP-99, 994 on plasma extravasation in dura mater and c-fos mRNA expression in trigeminal nucleus caudalis of rats. Neuropharmacology 34:255–261

Shepheard S, Edvinsson L, Cumberbatch M, Williamson D, Mason G, Webb J et al (1999) Possible antimigraine mechanisms of action of the 5HT$_{1F}$ receptor agonist LY334370. Cephalalgia 19:851–858

Stepien A, Jagustyn P, Trafny EA, Widerkiewicz K (2003) Suppressing effect of the serotonin 5HT1B/D receptor agonist rizatriptan on calcitonin gene-related peptide (CGRP) concentration in migraine attacks. Neurol Neurochir Pol 37:1013–1023

Suzuki N, Hardebo JE, Owman C (1988) Origins and pathways of cerebrovascular vasoactive intestinal polypeptide-positive nerves in rat. J Cereb Blood Flow Metab 8:697–712

Suzuki N, Hardebo JE, Owman C (1990) Origins and pathways of choline acetyltransferase=positive parasympathetic nerve fibers to crebral vessels in rat. J Cereb Blood Flow Metab 10:399–408

Tajti J, Uddman R, Moller S, Sundler F, Edvinsson L (1999) Messenger molecules and receptor mRNA in the human trigeminal ganglion. J Auton Nerv Syst 76:176–183

Terwindt GM, Ophoff RA, Haan J, Vergouwe MN, van Eijk R, Frants RR et al (1998) Variable clinical expression of mutations in the P/Q-type calcium channel gene in familial hemiplegic migraine. Neurology 50:1105–1110

Tvedskov JF, Lipka K, Ashina M, Iversen HK, Schifter S, Olesen J (2005) No increase of calcitonin gene-related peptide in jugular blood during migraine. Ann Neurol 58:561–568

Uddman R, Edvinsson L, Ekman R, Kingman T, McCulloch J (1985) Innervation of the feline cerebral vasculature by nerve fibers containing calcitonin gene-related peptide: trigeminal origin and co-existence with substance P. Neurosci Lett 62:131–136

Uddman R, Goadsby PJ, Jansen I, Edvinsson L (1993) PACAP, a VIP-like peptide: immunohistochemical localization and effect upon cat pial arteries and cerebral blood flow. J Cereb Blood Flow Metab 13:291–297

Uddman R, Tajti J, Hou M, Sundler F, Edvinsson L (2002) Neuropeptide expression in the human trigeminal nucleus caudalis and in the cervical spinal cord C1 and C2. Cephalalgia 22:112–116

Villalón CM, Olesen J (2009) The role of CGRP in the pathophysiology of migraine and efficacy of CGRP receptor antagonists as acute antimigraine drugs. Pharmacol Ther 124:309–323

Wahl M, Schilling L, Parsons AA, Kaumann A (1994) Involvement of calcitonin gene-related peptide (CGRP) and nitric oxide (NO) in the pial artery dilatation elicited by cortical spreading depression. Brain Res 637:204–210

Wang X, Fang Y, Liang J, Yin Z, Miao J, Luo N (2010) Selective inhibition of 5-ht$_7$ receptor reduces cgrp release in an experimental model for migraine. Headache 50:579–587

Weiller C, May A, Limmroth V, Juptner M, Kaube H, Schayck RV et al (1995) Brain stem activation in spontaneous human migraine attacks. Nat Med 1:658–660

Wienecke T, Olesen J, Oturai PS, Ashina M (2009) Prostaglandin e_2(pge_2) induces headache in healthy subjects. Cephalalgia 29:509–519

Wienecke T, Olesen J, Ashina M (2010) Prostaglandin i(2) (epoprostenol) triggers migraine-like attacks in migraineurs. Cephalalgia 30:179–190

Williamson DJ, Hargreaves RJ, Hill RG, Shepheard SL (1997) Intravital microscope studies on the effects of neurokinin agonists and calcitonin gene-related peptide on dural vessel diameter in the anaesthetized rat. Cephalalgia 17:518–524

Zagami AS, Goadsby PJ, Edvinsson L (1990) Stimulation of the superior sagittal sinus in the cat causes release of vasoactive peptides. Neuropeptides 16:69–75

17 Treatment and Prevention of Migraine

Paolo Martelletti · Ivano Farinelli
School of Health Sciences, Sapienza University of Rome, Rome, Italy

Paolo Martelletti, Timothy J. Steiner (eds.), *Handbook of Headache*, DOI 10.1007/978-88-470-1700-9_17,
© Lifting The Burden 2011

Abstract: Migraine exerts a significant impact on quality of life. Several drugs are available for acute therapy of migraine attacks, namely, specific such as triptans or generic such as analgesics/anti-inflammatory. In some cases, prophylaxis therapy is taken into account according to both attack frequency and severity. In the past, the most common criterion applied for prophylaxis therapy was represented by the number of attacks per month. Considering such a pattern essential, the suggested number of attacks per month was of five or more episodes. At a later date, demand for prophylaxis also considered consumption of symptomatic drugs as well as increase of migraine frequency in a short period of time. Today, prophylaxis therapy is evaluated according to its impact on patients. Therefore, a general evaluation of the patient in terms of functional disability and quality of life is required to assess the appropriateness of prophylaxis therapy, as well as evaluating the risk of medication overuse or the presence of concomitant pathologies (e.g., hypertension, depression, epilepsy). Furthermore, in cases where the condition reaches a level of chronicity (chronic migraine), new options are available today in prophylaxis therapy.

Established Knowledge

Several treatments are available for both the control of migraine's acute attacks and preventive therapy. Treatment choices should be tailored on single patients, according to existing comorbidities as well as concurrent pathologies.

Acute Treatment

Several drugs are available for acute therapy of migraine attacks, such as triptans or analgesic/anti-inflammatory. Therapeutic guidelines have been published recently (Steiner et al. 2007). Such principles have been extended to Emergency Department settings (Martelletti et al. 2008).

Triptans

Triptans represent the first treatment choice for migraine attacks (❷ *Table 17.1*). Seven different molecules exist to be employed. Contraindications to their use consist in the presence of cardiovascular issues in view of their vasoconstrictive capacity. Frequent adverse events are represented by dizziness, somnolence, asthenia, and chest tightness. Sumatriptan has been the first drug introduced in such treatment; 50 and 100 mg tablets proved to be superior to placebo in headache relief at 4 h (77% vs 39%) (Pfaffenrath et al. 1998).

Eletriptan has been shown to be superior to placebo at dosages of 20 mg (54% vs 24%) and 40 mg (65% vs 24%) in achieving 2-h pain-free response (Goadsby et al. 2000).

Rizatriptan 10 mg proved to be superior to placebo in pain-free response at 2 h (70% vs 22%) (Mathew et al. 2004).

Almotriptan 12.5 mg was considerably more effective than placebo in pain relief (14.9% vs 8.2%) and pain-free response (2.5% vs 0.7%), as early as 30 min after dosing. At 2 h, pain relief for almotriptan 12.5 mg was of 63.7%, compared to placebo 35%; 2-h pain-free response rates were of 36.4% for almotriptan and 13.9% for placebo (Dahlöf et al. 2006).

Zolmitriptan 2.5-mg and 5-mg tablets resulted significantly more effective than placebo in achieving headache relief as well as pain-free response at 2 h, compared to placebo. However,

□ Table 17.1

Specific anti-migraine drugs (availability varies from country to country) (Adapted from Steiner et al. 2007)

Almotriptan	Tablets 12.5 mg
Eletriptan	Tablets 20 mg and 40 mg (80 mg may be effective when 40 mg is not)
Frovatriptan	Tablets 2.5 mg
Naratriptan	Tablets 2.5 mg
Rizatriptan	Tablets 10 mg (and 5 mg, to be used when propranolol is being taken concomitantly); mouth-dispersible wafers 10 mg
Sumatriptan	Tablets and rapidly dissolving tablets 50 mg and 100 mg; suppositories 25 mg; nasal spray 10 mg (licensed for adolescents) and 20 mg; subcutaneous injection 6 mg
Zolmitriptan	Tablets 2.5 mg and 5 mg; mouth-dispersible tablets 2.5 mg and 5 mg; nasal spray 5 mg
Ergotamine tartrate	Tablets 1 mg and 2 mg; suppositories 2 mg

zolmitriptan proved to be inferior to eletriptan 80 mg and rizatriptan 10 mg for sustained pain-free rate (Chen and Ashcroft 2008).

Naratriptan 2.5 mg represents a further therapeutic choice. However, rizatriptan 10 mg and sumatriptan 100 mg resulted more effective than naratriptan in terms of headache relief, while zolmitriptan 2.5 mg showed similar efficacy (Ashcroft and Millson 2004).

Frovatriptan 2.5 mg showed headache response rates ranging from 38% to 40%, compared to placebo 22–35%, at 2 h after administration. At 24 h, headache recurrence for frovatriptan 2.5 mg ranged between 9% and 14%, compared to placebo 18% (Balbisi 2004).

A meta-analysis of 53 trials compared headache responses at 2 h, where sumatriptan 100 mg, rizatriptan 10 mg, and eletriptan 80 mg proved to be higher than naratriptan 2.5 mg, eletriptan 20 mg, and frovatriptan 2.5 mg. Comparing both efficacy and tolerability of triptans with sumatriptan, three drugs show positive results: rizatriptan 10 mg, eletriptan 80 mg, and almotriptan 12.5 mg (Ferrari et al. 2001).

Ergotamine Tartrate

Ergotamine (oral/rectal, and caffeine combination) may be considered in the treatment of selected patients affected by moderate-to-severe migraine. Several small clinical trials provide evidence about the effectiveness of ergotamine as well as its combinations. Nausea and vomiting represent the most commonly observed short-term adverse effects. However, such a drug is not present worldwide (Silberstein and Mc Crory 2003).

NSAIDs

Acetylsalicylic acid effervescent 1,000 mg has been shown to be as effective as sumatriptan 50 mg or ibuprofen 400 mg in the treatment of migraine attacks. The mentioned treatments were all superior to placebo. However, sumatriptan proved to be more effective than acetylsalicylic acid in pain-free response at 2 h after administration. Incidence of upper gastrointestinal tract complications (i.e., bleeding or perforation) in general population is calculated to be 1–2 cases per 1,000 persons per year, with a case fatality rate ranging around 5–10%. Ibuprofen 200 and 400 mg resulted more effective than placebo in reducing pain intensity as well as in removing pain (pain-free) within 2 h in adults affected by moderate or severe migraine attacks (Codispoti et al. 2001) ❷ *Table 17.2* summarizes nonspecific therapy for the management of acute attacks (❷ *Table 17.2*).

Diclofenac at dosages of 50 and 100 mg resulted effective in the relief of migraine headache pain at 2 h in respect to placebo, showing no significant differences between the dosages (The Diclofenac-K/Sumatriptan Migraine Study Group 1999).

Ketoprofen at both dosages of 75 mg (62%) and 150 mg (61%) resulted superior to placebo (28%) in headache relief at 2 h (Dib et al. 2002).

Naproxen sodium showed to be more effective than placebo in the reducing pain intensity as well as pain relief at 2 h, although it proved itself less powerful in respect to other NSAIDs. An incisive combination of naproxen sodium and sumatriptan has been recently ascertained for acute treatment of migraine attacks. Incidence of headache relief at 2 h after administration of this combination (65%) was superior to sumatriptan monotherapy (55%), naproxen sodium monotherapy (44%), and placebo (28%) (Suthisisang et al. 2010; Brandes et al. 2007).

Paracetamol

Paracetamol 1,000 mg produces significant pain reduction at 2 h in respect to placebo (52% vs 32%) (Prior et al. 2010).

Combination Drugs

Several combination drugs are available in different countries. Indoprocaf represents a widespread choice for such treatment. In a recent study, Indoprocaf resulted to be similarly effective as sumatriptan (Sandrini et al. 2007).

▢ Table 17.2

Drugs used in acute migraine treatment (Adapted from Martelletti et al. 2008)

Analgesics	Antiemetics
Acetylsalicylic acid 900–1,000 mg (adults only)	Domperidone 20 mg or
Ibuprofen 400–800 mg or	Metoclopramide 10 mg
Diclofenac 50–100 mg or	
Ketoprofen 100 mg or	
Naproxen 500–1,000 mg	
Indomethacin 50–100 mg	
or (where these are contraindicated)	
Paracetamol 1,000 mg	
Combination drugs	
Indoprocaf (indomethacin 25/50 mg, prochlorperazine 2–8 mg, caffeine 75–150 mg)	

Opiates

In some countries, the use of opiates represents a second-line treatment for migraine attacks. A particular role is played by drugs with codeine association. Their main limitation consists in the possibility of abuse (Taylor 2010).

Preventive Therapy

Preventive therapy should be employed in patients reaching at least 3 migraine days per month. The choice of such therapy depends on the presence of possible comorbidities such as obesity, cardio-cerebrovascular diseases, depression, and psychiatric disorders (❷ Table 17.3).

Beta-Adrenergic Blockers

This drug category represents an established first treatment choice for reducing migraine attacks. In a systematic review in which 26 placebo-controlled trials have been examined, in 17 cases propranolol showed to be more effective compared to placebo. In two trials only, no difference has been detected in favor of propranolol. Therapeutic range varies from 40 mg to 120 mg twice daily (Linde and Rossnagel 2004). Metoprolol at a dosage of 25–100 mg twice daily results as effective as propranolol (Kangasniemi and Hedman 1984). Common side effects are reduced energy and tiredness. The use of both propranolol and metoprolol is contraindicated in patients affected by asthma.

Flunarizine

Flunarizine is a nonselective calcium antagonist that proved to be effective for frequency reduction of migraine attacks in a range dose of 5–15 mg daily (Leone et al. 1991). Common

◻ Table 17.3
Prophylactic drugs with good evidence of efficacy (availability and regulatory approval vary from country to country; use of drugs off-license rests on individual clinical responsibility) (Adapted from Steiner et al. 2007)

Beta-adrenergic blockers without partial agonism	Atenolol 25–100 mg bd or
	Bisoprolol 5–10 mg od or
	Metoprolol 50–100 mg bd or
	Propranolol LA 80 mg od-160 mg bd
Topiramate	25 mg od-50 mg bd
Flunarizine	5–10 mg od
Sodium valproate	600–1,500 mg daily
Amitriptyline	10–100 mg nocte

adverse events are represented by drowsiness, weight gain, depression, and parkinsonism. In a double-blind comparison with propranolol, however, flunarizine resulted slightly less effective (Diener et al. 2002).

Sodium Valproate

Sodium valproate is an anticonvulsant agent superior to placebo in migraine prophylaxis, administered at a dosage of 400–600 mg twice daily (Hering and Kuritzky 1992). Drowsiness, weight gain, tremor, gastrointestinal distress (nausea or vomiting), and hair loss represent the most common adverse events, which, however, are transient. A rare adverse event is hepatotoxicity (Silberstein and Wilmore 1996).

Amitriptyline

Amitriptyline is the only antidepressant agent with fairly consistent findings for efficacy in migraine prevention (Couch and Hassanein 1979). Recommended dosage varies between 25 mg and 50 mg each night. Dosages higher than 50 mg did not prove to be superior in terms of efficacy. Common adverse events are drowsiness, urinary retention, and arrhythmias (Lampl et al. 2009).

Current Research

At present, migraine appears to receive new benefits from basic research for its acute treatment, as well as from promising innovative applications of biological agents for the treatment of chronic migraine. New molecules will be soon introduced in this therapeutic arena for the benefit of a class of sufferers, who have been "orphaned" for decades in the development of new therapies, both safe and effective (Farinelli et al. 2009; Stovner et al. 2009).

Acute Treatment

CGRP Antagonists

MK-0974 at dosages ranging from 25 mg to 600 mg has been evaluated in a randomized, double-blind, placebo-, and active-controlled study (rizatriptan 10 mg or placebo). At 2 h, dosage spectrum from 300 mg to 600 mg showed significance versus placebo (MK-0974 68.1%, rizatriptan 69.5%, and placebo 46.3%). The protocol, a phase-2 trial for migraine prevention, has been interrupted since 13 patients out of 660 reported high ALT or AST >3 beyond the upper limit of normal. Such potential hepatotoxicity risk must be considered prospectively (Ho et al. 2008).

Nitric Oxide Synthase Inhibitors

Nitric oxide synthase (NOS) inhibitor NG-methyl4-arginine hydrochloride (546C88) proved to be effective in the treatment of spontaneous migraine attacks. At present, only the molecules GW 274150 and GW 273629 have been evaluated (Lassen et al. 1997).

Preventive Therapy

Candesartan

Angiotensin type 1 blocker candesartan is a long-acting angiotensin II type receptor antagonist that has been recently examined for migraine prophylaxis. In a randomized, double-blind, placebo-controlled study carried out on 60 patients experiencing two up to six attacks per month, candesartan 16 mg resulted effective and well-tolerated. In 12 weeks, the mean number of headache days has been of 18.5 in the placebo group versus 13.6 in the candesartan group ($P = 0.001$) (Tronvik et al. 2003).

Glutamate NMDA Receptor Antagonists

A randomized, double-blind study on Glutamate NMDA receptor antagonists showed note-worthy clinical correlates for action on the kainite receptor. Such study revealed the antagonist LY466195 to be effective for relief in acute migraine. Adverse events reported were visual problems (Weiss et al. 2006).

Tonabersat

The gap-junction blocker tonabersat at dosages of 20–40 mg, administered daily for 1 week, has been evaluated in a randomized, placebo-controlled, multicenter, parallel group study. Responses indicated a 50% reduction of migraine attacks, specifically 62% for tonabersat and 45% for placebo ($P < 0.05$). Nausea was the most frequent adverse symptom reported (11% of patients) (Goadsby et al. 2009).

Chronic Migraine - Preventive Therapy

Established Knowledge

Topiramate

Topiramate has been initially introduced as anticonvulsant and later on recognized as effective for reducing frequency in migraine attacks, compared to placebo (Diener et al. 2004). After a titration period, dosage has been increased every 8 weeks, starting from 25 mg daily up to 50–200 mg daily. A significant limitation of such prophylaxis therapy relies in adverse events, which can also appear in therapy discontinuation, such as paresthesia, cognitive dysfunction, and weight loss (Brandes et al. 2004).

OnabotulinumtoxinA

OnabotulinumtoxinA is employed for headache prophylaxis in adults affected by chronic migraine. At the primary endpoint, OnabotulinumtoxinA proved to be statistically superior to placebo for what concerns the frequency of headache days relative to baseline (-9.0 OnabotulinumtoxinA/-6.7 placebo, $P < 001$). Frequency of adverse events resulted higher in the OnabotulinumtoxinA group (65.1%) in respect to the placebo group (56.4%). Adverse events reported were mild or moderate severity, resolved without sequelae. Frequent adverse events are represented by neck pain (7.5%) and muscular weakness (5.2%). Eyelid ptosis, myalgia, and musculoskeletal stiffness were also higher (Diener et al. 2010; Aurora et al. 2010). The pooled analysis of both trials showed OnabotulinumtoxinA to be an effective in the prophylaxis of chronic migraine. OnabotulinumtoxinA treatment produced noteworthy improvements compared with placebo in several multiple headache symptom measures, with a significant reduction of headache-related disability and improved functioning, vitality, and overall health-related quality of life. Repeat treatments with OnabotulinumtoxinA proved to be safe and well-tolerated (Dodick et al. 2010).

References

Ashcroft DM, Millson D (2004) Naratriptan for the treatment of acute migraine: meta-analysis of randomised controlled trials. Pharmacoepidemiol Drug Saf 13:73–82

Aurora SK, Dodick DW, Turkel CC et al (2010) OnabotulinumtoxinA for treatment of chronic migraine: results from the double-blind, random-ized, placebo-controlled phase of the PREEMPT I trial. Cephalalgia 30:793–803. doi:10.1177/0333102410364676

Balbisi EA (2004) Frovatriptan succinate, a 5-HT1B/1D receptor agonist for migraine. Int J Clin Pract 58:695–705

Brandes JL, Saper JR, Diamond M et al (2004) Topiramate for migraine prevention: a randomized controlled trial. JAMA 291:965–973

Brandes JL, Kudrow D, Stark SR et al (2007) Sumatriptan-naproxen for acute treatment of migraine: a randomized trial. JAMA 297:1443–1454

Chen LC, Ashcroft DM (2008) Meta-analysis of the effi-cacy and safety of zolmitriptan in the acute treat-ment of migraine. Headache 48:236–247

Codispoti JR, Prior MJ, Fu M et al (2001) Efficacy of nonprescription doses of ibuprofen for treating migraine headache. A randomized controlled trial. Headache 41:665–679

Couch JR, Hassanein RS (1979) Amitriptyline in migraine prophylaxis. Arch Neurol 36:695–699

Dahlöf CG, Pascual J, Dodick DW et al (2006) Efficacy, speed of action and tolerability of almotriptan in the acute treatment of migraine: pooled individual patient data from four randomized, double-blind, placebo-controlled clinical trials. Cephalalgia 26:400–408

Dib M, Massiou H, Weber M et al (2002) Efficacy of oral ketoprofen in acute migraine: a double-blind randomized clinical trial. Neurology 58:1660–1665

Diener HC, Matias-Guiu J, Hartung E et al (2002) Efficacy and tolerability in migraine prophylaxis of flunarizine in reduced doses: a comparison with propranolol 160 mg daily. Cephalalgia 22:209–221

Diener HC, Tfelt-Hansen P, Dahlöf C et al (2004) Topiramate in migraine prophylaxis – results from a placebo-controlled trial with propranolol as an active control. J Neurol 25:943–950

Diener HC, Dodick DW, Aurora SK et al (2010) OnabotulinumtoxinA for treatment of chronic migraine: results from the double-blind, random-ized, placebo-controlled phase of the PREEMPT 2 trial. Cephalalgia 30:804–814

Dodick DW, Turkel CC, DeGryse RE et al (2010) OnabotulinumtoxinA for treatment of chronic migraine: pooled results from the double-blind, randomized, placebo-controlled phases of the PREEMPT clinical program. Headache 50:921–936. doi:10.1111/j.1526-4610.2010.01678.x

Farinelli I, De Filippis S, Coloprisco G et al (2009) Future drugs for migraine. Intern Emerg Med 4:367–373

Ferrari MD, Roon KI, Lipton RB et al (2001) Oral triptans (serotonin 5-HT(1B/1D) agonists) in acute migraine treatment: a meta-analysis of 53 trials. Lancet 358:1668–1675

Goadsby PJ, Ferrari MD, Olesen J et al (2000) Eletriptan in acute migraine: a double-blind, placebo-controlled comparison to sumatriptan. Eletriptan Steering Committee. Neurology 54:156–163

Goadsby PJ, Ferrari MD, Csanyi A et al (2009) Randomized, double-blind, placebo-controlled, proof-of-concept study of the cortical spreading depression inhibiting agent tonabersat in migraine prophylaxis. Cephalalgia 29:742–750

Hering R, Kuritzky A (1992) Sodium valproate in the prophylactic treatment of migraine: a double-blind study versus placebo. Cephalalgia 12:81–84

Ho TW, Mannix LK, Fan X et al (2008) Randomized controlled trial of an oral CGRP receptor antagonist, MK-0974, in acute treatment of migraine. Neurology 70(16):1304–1312

Kangasniemi P, Hedman C (1984) Metoprolol and propranolol in the prophylactic treatment of classical and common migraine. A double-blind study. Cephalalgia 4:91–96

Lampl C, Huber G, Adl J et al (2009) Two different doses of amitriptyline ER in the prophylaxis of migraine: long-term results and predictive factors. Eur J Neurol 16:943–948

Lassen LH, Ashina M, Christiansen I et al (1997) Nitric oxide synthase inhibition in migraine. Lancet 349:401–402

Leone M, Grazzi L, La Mantia L et al (1991) Flunarizine in migraine: a minireview. Headache 31:388–391

Linde E, Rossnagel K (2004) Propranolol for migraine prophylaxis. Cochrane Database Syst Rev 2:D003225

Martelletti P, Farinelli I, Steiner TJ (2008) Acute migraine in the emergency department: extending European principles of management. Intern Emerg Med 3: S17–S24

Mathew NT, Kailasam J, Meadors L (2004) Early treatment of migraine with rizatriptan: a placebo-controlled study. Headache 44:669–673

Pfaffenrath V, Cunin G, Sjonell G et al (1998) Efficacy and safety of sumatriptan tablets (25 mg, 50 mg, and 100 mg) in the acute treatment of migraine: defining the optimum doses of oral sumatriptan. Headache 38:184–190

Prior MJ, Codispoti JR, Fu M (2010) A randomized, placebo-controlled trial of acetaminophen for treatment of migraine Headache. Headache 50(5): 819–933. doi:10.1111/j.1526-4610.2010.01638.x

Sandrini G, Cerbo R, Del Bene E et al (2007) Efficacy of dosing and re-dosing of two oral fixed combinations of indomethacin, prochlorperazine and caffeine compared with oral sumatriptan in the acute treatment of multiple migraine attacks: a double-blind, double-dummy, randomised, parallel group, multicentre study. Int J Clin Pract 61:1256–1269

Silberstein SD, McCrory DC (2003) Ergotamine and dihydroergotamine: history, pharmacology, and efficacy. Headache 43(2):144–166

Silberstein SD, Wilmore LJ (1996) Divalproex sodium: migraine treatment and monitoring. Headache 36:239–242

Steiner TJ, Paemeleire K, Jensen R (2007) European principles of management of common headache disorders in primary care. J Headache Pain 8:S1–S47

Stovner LJ, Tronvik E, Hagen K (2009) New drugs for migraine. J Headache Pain 10:395–406

Suthisisang CC, Poolsup N, Suksomboon N et al (2010) Meta-analysis of the efficacy and safety of naproxen sodium in the acute treatment of migraine. Headache 50:808–818

Taylor FR (2010) Acute treatment of migraine headaches. Semin Neurol 30(2):145–153

The Diclofenac-K/Sumatriptan Migraine Study Group, Bussone G, Grazzi L, D'Amico D (1999) Acute treatment of migraine attacks: efficacy and safety of a nonsteroidal anti-inflammatory drug, diclofenac-potassium, in comparison to oral sumatriptan and placebo. The Diclofenac-K/Sumatriptan Migraine Study Group. Cephalalgia 19:232–240

Tronvik E, Stovner LJ, Helde G et al (2003) Prophylactic treatment of migraine with an angiotensin II receptor blocker: a randomized controlled trial. JAMA 289:65–69

Weiss B, Alt A, Ogden AM, Gates M et al (2006) Pharmacological characterization of the competitive GLUK5 receptor antagonist decahydroisoquinoline LY466195 in vitro and in vivo. J Pharmacol Exp Ther 318:772–781

18 What to Tell Patients About Migraine

Timothy J. Steiner[1,2] · *Paolo Martelletti*[3]
[1]Norwegian University of Science and Technology, Trondheim, Norway
[2]Faculty of Medicine, Imperial College London, London, UK
[3]School of Health Sciences, Sapienza University of Rome, Rome, Italy

Parts of this contribution have also been published as part of a Springer Open Choice article which is freely available at springerlink.com – DOI 10.1007/s10194-007-0428-1

Paolo Martelletti, Timothy J. Steiner (eds.), *Handbook of Headache*, DOI 10.1007/978-88-470-1700-9_18,
© Lifting The Burden 2011

Abstract: Headache disorders are real – they are not just in the mind.

This chapter summarizes information suitable for communication to migraine patients on causes, types, symptoms, triggers, and treatment strategies. The information is aimed at helping them to understand their headache, their diagnosis and their treatment, and to work with their health-care provider in a way that will get best results for them.

Introduction

Migraine is a medical disorder. It takes place in attacks, once or twice a year in some people but up to several times a month in others. The main feature of these attacks is headache, which may be severe. Other common features are feeling sick (nauseated) or being sick (vomiting) and finding light and noise uncomfortable.

If you feel nauseated when you have a headache, or light and noise bother you, or if your headache makes it difficult to carry out your usual daily activities, it is quite likely that it is migraine.

What Causes Migraine?

Migraine comes from the brain. It is a disorder of the parts of the brain that process pain and other sensations. You probably inherited it from one or other parent or from a grandparent.

Who Gets Migraine?

About one in seven adults have migraine, so it is very common. Women are three times more likely to be affected than men. It often starts in childhood or adolescence. In girls in particular, it may start at puberty. Because of inheritance, migraine runs in families.

What Are the Different Types of Migraine?

The commonest is *migraine without aura* (aura is described later). About three-quarters of people with migraine have only this type; one in ten have *migraine with aura*, and twice this many have both types from time to time. Much less common are attacks of aura alone, with no headache. This type of migraine tends to develop in older people. There are other types of migraine, but these are rare.

What Are the Symptoms of Migraine?

Symptoms are present during the attack, which has four stages, although not all of these always happen. Between attacks, most people with migraine are completely well.

The *premonitory phase* comes before any other symptoms of the attack. Only half of people with migraine are aware of this phase. If you are one of these, you may feel irritable, depressed or tired for hours or even 1 or 2 days before the headache begins. However, some people find they are unusually energetic during this time. Some have food cravings. Others "just know" that a migraine attack is about to start.

The *aura*, when it happens, is almost always the next phase. Only a third of people with migraine ever have aura, and it may not be part of every attack even for them. Aura is a signal from the brain, which is being temporarily (but not seriously) affected by the migraine process. It lasts, usually, for 10–30 min, but can be longer. It mostly affects vision. You may notice blank patches, bright or flashing lights or coloured zigzag lines spreading in front of your eyes, usually to one side. Less common are *sensory* symptoms – pins-and-needles or numbness – which generally start in the fingers of one hand, and spread up the arm to affect that side of the face or tongue. When these happen, there are nearly always visual symptoms as well. Difficulty speaking or finding the right words can also be part of the aura.

The *headache phase* is the most troublesome for most people, lasting for a few hours or up to 2 or 3 days. Migraine headache is often severe. It tends to be one-sided, but can be on both sides, and although most commonly at the front or in the temple it can be anywhere in the head. It is usually a throbbing or pounding headache, very often made worse by movement. You probably feel nauseated, and may vomit (which seems to relieve the headache). You may also find light and noise unpleasant and prefer to be alone in the dark and quiet.

The *resolution phase* follows as the headache fades. During this time, you may again feel tired, irritable and depressed, and have difficulty concentrating. It can take a further day before you feel fully recovered.

What Is My "Migraine Threshold"?

Migraine is unpredictable. An attack can start at any time. However, some people are more prone to attacks than others. The higher your *migraine threshold*, the less likely you are to develop an attack, and the lower your threshold the more at risk you are.

So-called *triggers* play a part in this. A trigger will set off an attack (although we do not understand how this happens). It does this more easily if your migraine threshold is low. If your threshold is high, two or three triggers may need to come together for this to happen.

Separate from triggers are *predisposing factors*. These have the effect of lowering your threshold, so that triggers work more easily. Tiredness, anxiety and general stress have this effect, as can menstruation, pregnancy and the menopause in women.

What Are the Triggers?

Everyone wants to know what might trigger his or her migraine. This is often difficult and sometimes impossible to pin down because triggers are not the same for everybody, or even always the same for different attacks in the same person. Many people with migraine cannot identify any triggers. Possible triggers are many and varied.

Diet: some foods (and alcohol), but only in some people; more commonly, delayed or missed or inadequate meals, caffeine withdrawal and becoming dehydrated.

Sleep: changes in sleep patterns, both lack of sleep and sleeping in.

Other life-style: intense exercise, or long-distance travel, especially across time zones.

Environmental: bright or flickering lights, strong smells and marked weather changes.

Psychological: emotional upset or, surprisingly, relaxation after a stressful period.

Hormonal factors in women: menstruation; breaks in hormonal contraception or hormone-replacement therapy (HRT).

The commonest trigger is hunger, or not enough food in relation to needs. This is particularly the case in young people – children prone to migraine should never miss breakfast. In women, hormonal changes associated with the menstrual cycle are important potential triggers.

These, and most other triggers, represent some form of *stress*, and suggest that people with migraine do not respond well to change.

What Treatment Can I Take?

Medications that treat the migraine attack are called *acute* treatments. The right ones can be very effective, but need to be taken correctly and not overused. They include non-prescription painkillers, most of which contain aspirin, ibuprofen or paracetamol. Of these, paracetamol is least effective for most people. In all cases, soluble or effervescent preparations work faster and better.

You can also take medicine called an anti-emetic if you feel nauseated or likely to vomit. Some anti-emetics actually help the painkillers by causing your body to absorb them more quickly. You can have these as suppositories if you feel very nauseated during migraine attacks.

Your pharmacist can give you advice on the best non-prescription treatments to take. If none of these works for you, or you need more than the recommended dose, the pharmacist may suggest you should ask for medical advice.

Your doctor may prescribe one of the specific anti-migraine treatments. You should try these when painkillers and anti-emetics do not relieve your symptoms and get you back into action reasonably quickly. They work quite differently. They do not tackle pain but undo what is happening in your brain to cause an attack. They include ergotamine, widely used in some countries but not others, and a group of newer drugs called triptans. If your doctor advises it, you can use these drugs together with painkillers, anti-emetics or both.

There are some simple measures that can make medication more effective.

Take Medication Early . . .

Always carry at least one dose of the medication that has been recommended by your doctor, nurse or pharmacist. Take it as soon as you know an attack is coming on. Medication taken early is more likely to work well. During a migraine attack, the stomach is less active, so tablets taken by mouth are not absorbed as well into the bloodstream as they would be normally. Eat something if you can, or drink something sweet.

. . . But Not Too Often

Always carefully follow the instructions that come with your medication. In particular, do not take acute treatment too often because you can give yourself a headache from the treatment.

This is called *medication-overuse headache*. To avoid this happening, never take medication to treat headache symptoms *regularly* on more than 2 or 3 days a week.

What if These Don't Work?

If frequent or severe attacks are not well controlled with acute treatment, so-called *prophylactic* medication is an option. Unlike acute treatment, you *should* take this daily because it works in a totally different way – by preventing the migraine process starting. In other words, it raises your migraine threshold.

Your doctor or nurse can give you advice on the choice of medicines available and their likely side-effects. Most were first developed for quite different conditions, so do not be surprised if you are offered a medication described as treatment for high blood pressure, epilepsy or even depression. This is *not* why you are taking it. These medications work against migraine too.

If you are taking one of these, do follow the instructions carefully. Research has shown that a very common reason for this type of medication not working is that patients forget to take it.

What Else Can I Do to Help Myself?

Exercising regularly and keeping fit will benefit you. Avoiding predisposing and trigger factors is sensible, so you should be aware of the full range of possible triggers. You may be able to avoid some triggers even if there are others that you find difficult or impossible to control.

Keep a Diary

Diary cards can record a lot of relevant information about your headaches – how often you get them, when they happen, how long they last and what your symptoms are. They are valuable in helping with diagnosis, identifying trigger factors and assessing how well treatments work.

What if I Think I May Be Pregnant?

You will need advice from your doctor or nurse. Some of the medications used for migraine are unsuitable if you are pregnant.

Do I Need Any Tests?

Most cases of migraine are easy to recognize. There are no tests to confirm the diagnosis, which is based on your description of your headaches and the lack of any abnormal findings when your doctor examines you. A brain scan is unlikely to help. If your doctor is at all unsure about the diagnosis, he or she may ask for tests to rule out other causes of headaches, but these are not often needed.

Will My Migraine Get Better?

There is no known cure for migraine. However, for most people with migraine, attacks become less frequent in later life.

Meanwhile, doing all you can to follow the advice in this leaflet can make the change from a condition that is out of control to one that you can control.

Acknowledgment

The text of this chapter is taken from a leaflet prepared by *Lifting The Burden*: the Global Campaign against Headache. It was drafted by a small writing group, revised following review by an international panel whose principal responsibility was to ensure worldwide cross-cultural relevance and, finally, checked for ease of comprehension by the Campaign for Plain English. The leaflet is endorsed by the World Health Organization and has been published in *Journal of Headache and Pain* (2007).

References

Lifting The Burden. The Global Campaign to Reduce the Burden of Headache Worldwide (2007) Information for people affected by migraine. J Headache Pain 8(Suppl 1):S26–S29

Part 6

Tension-Type Headache

19 How Tension-Type Headache Presents

Lars Bendtsen[1] · *Rigmor Jensen*[1] · *Elizabeth W. Loder*[2]
[1]Glostrup Hospital, University of Copenhagen, Glostrup, Copenhagen, Denmark
[2]Brigham and Women's/Faulkner Hospitals, Boston, MA, USA

Paolo Martelletti, Timothy J. Steiner (eds.), *Handbook of Headache*, DOI 10.1007/978-88-470-1700-9_19,
© Lifting The Burden 2011

Abstract: The substantial societal and individual burdens associated with tension-type headache (TTH) constitute a major public health issue that has previously been overlooked. Tension-type headache is extremely prevalent, affecting up to 78% of the general population; roughly 3% suffer from chronic tension-type headache. Tension-type headache is the most featureless of headaches. An accurate diagnosis, in which the individual headache episode is distinguished from migraine and from a secondary headache, especially medication overuse headache, is essential. The use of a diagnostic headache diary is helpful for treatment planning. Possible triggers and comorbidity with other disorders, in particular depression, should also be assessed before treatment is initiated.

Introduction

Tension-type headache (TTH) is the most common form of headache and is what many people consider as their "normal" headache, in contrast to migraine. Overall direct costs due to medical services and medications are higher for TTH than for migraine due to its higher prevalence (Jensen and Symon 2005), and decreased work effectiveness and abolished social activities is reported by up to 60% of persons with TTH (Schwartz et al. 1997). A recent study found overall increased absence rates for subjects with frequent TTH but not for migraineurs (Lyngberg et al. 2005d). For these reasons, even though this disease is not the most visible type of headache, it is one of the most costly to society. At the same time it is the least studied type of common headache (Bendtsen and Jensen 2006).

Definition

The second version of the International Classification of Headache Disorders (Headache Classification Subcommittee of the International Headache Society 2004) distinguishes among three forms of TTH, mainly on basis of headache frequency. These are (a) infrequent episodic TTH (less than 12 headache days/year), (b) frequent episodic TTH (between 12 and 180 days/year), and (c) chronic TTH (at least 180 days/year) (❷ *Table 19.1*).

Chronic TTH differs not only from the episodic forms in frequency but also with respect to pathophysiology, lack of response to most treatment strategies, more medication overuse, more disability, and higher personal and socioeconomic costs (Bendtsen and Jensen 2006). The infrequent episodic form has very little impact on the individual and can be regarded as trivial, with no need for medical attention. Patients with frequent episodic or chronic TTH, in contrast, encounter considerable disability and often warrant specific intervention.

Diagnosis

TTH is characterized by a bilateral, pressing, tightening pain of mild to moderate intensity, occurring either in short episodes of variable duration (episodic forms) or continuously (chronic form). The headache is not associated with typical migraine features such as vomiting, severe photophobia, or phonophobia. In the chronic form, one symptom of mild nausea, photophobia, or phonophobia may be present (Headache Classification Subcommittee of the International Headache Society 2004) (❷ *Table 19.1*). Due to lack of accompanying symptoms

◘ Table 19.1

Diagnostic criteria for the three subtypes of tension-type headache (ICHD-II) (Headache Classification Subcommittee of the International Headache Society 2004)

2.1 [G44.2] Infrequent episodic tension-type headache
A. At least ten episodes occurring on <1 day/month on average (<12 days/year) and fulfilling criteria B–D
B. Headache lasting from 30 min to 7 days
C. Headache has at least two of the following characteristics:
1. Bilateral location
2. Pressing/tightening (non-pulsating) quality
3. Mild or moderate intensity
4. Not aggravated by routine physical activity such as walking or climbing stairs
D. Both of the following:
1. No nausea or vomiting (anorexia may occur)
2. No more than one of photophobia or phonophobia
E. Not attributed to another disorder
2.2 [G44.2] Frequent episodic tension-type headache
As 2.1 except for:
A. At least ten episodes occurring on ≥1 but <15 days/month for at least 3 months (≥12 and <180 days/year) and fulfilling criteria B–D
2.3 [G44.2] Chronic tension-type headache
A. Headache occurring on ≥15 days/month on average for>3 months (≥180 days/year)[a] and fulfilling criteria B–D
B. Headache lasts hours or may be continuous
C. Headache has at least two of the following characteristics:
1. Bilateral location
2. Pressing/tightening (non-pulsating) quality
3. Mild or moderate intensity
4. Not aggravated by routine physical activity such as walking or climbing stairs
D. Both of the following:
1. No more than one of photophobia, phonophobia, or mild nausea
2. Neither moderate or severe nausea nor vomiting
E. Not attributed to another disorder

[a]*2.3 Chronic tension-type headache* evolves over time from episodic tension-type headache; when these criteria A–E are fulfilled by headache that, unambiguously, is daily and unremitting within 3 days of its first onset, code as 4.8 *New daily persistent headache*

and the relatively milder pain intensity, patients are rarely severely incapacitated by their pain. TTH is the most featureless of the primary headaches and because many secondary headaches may mimic TTH, a diagnosis of TTH should be made only after exclusion of other organic disorders.

A general and neurological examination as well as prospective follow-up using diagnostic headache diaries (Russell et al. 1992) in which all drugs taken are recorded are therefore of utmost importance to reach the diagnosis. There are no imaging or laboratory tests that are reliably useful in the differential diagnosis. Manual palpation of the pericranial muscles and their insertions should be done (Jensen 1999; Bendtsen 2000) to demonstrate a possible muscular factor for the patient and to plan the treatment strategy, where physical training and relaxation therapy are important components.

In the general population, 94% of migraineurs also experience TTH and 56% experience frequent episodic TTH (Lyngberg et al. 2005a). In contrast, TTH occurs with similar prevalence in those with and without migraine, leading to the assumption that migraine may trigger TTH, whereas TTH may not trigger migraine. This comorbidity may explain why there has been so much controversy about TTH as a clinical entity and why the existence of TTH has been questioned.

Epidemiology

TTH varies considerably both in frequency and duration from rare short-lasting episodes of discomfort to frequent, long-lasting, or even continuous disabling headaches. In its infrequent mild form, TTH may be a nuisance, but is not regarded as a disease by the affected persons or their doctors. In its frequent and severe forms, it becomes distressing and socially disturbing due to the constant pain, surpassing on a population level the effects of migraine and cluster headache. Pooling these extremes of mild and severe forms of the disorder together in overall prevalence statistics may therefore be misleading.

The lifetime prevalence of TTH was as high as 78% in a population-based study in Denmark, but the majority (59%) of those affected had infrequent episodic TTH (less than 1 headache day/month) without specific need of medical attention (Lyngberg et al. 2005a). Nevertheless, 24–37% had TTH several times a month, 10% had it weekly and 3–6% of the population had chronic TTH (Rasmussen 1995; Lyngberg et al. 2005a).

The female to male ratio of TTH is 5:4 indicating that, unlike migraine, women are only slightly more affected than men (Andlin-Sobocki et al. 2005; Stovner et al. 2007). The average age of onset of TTH is higher than in migraine, namely 25–30 years in cross-sectional epidemiological studies (Rasmussen 1995). The prevalence peaks between the age of 30–39 years and decreases slightly with age (Rasmussen et al. 1991b).

A recent review of the global prevalence and burden of headaches (Stovner et al. 2007) showed that the disability of TTH was greater than that of migraine, which indicates that the overall cost of TTH is greater than that of migraine. Two Danish studies have shown that the number of workdays missed in the population was three times higher for TTH than for migraine (Rasmussen 1995; Lyngberg et al. 2005d) and a US study has also found that absenteeism due to TTH is considerable (Schwartz et al. 1997). Also, it has been stated that the indirect costs of all headaches are several times higher than those of migraine alone, indicating that the cost of non-migraine headaches (mainly TTH) are higher than that of migraine (Berg and Stovner 2005). The burden is particularly high for the minority who have substantial and complicating comorbidities (Jensen and Stovner 2008).

TTH patients seek less medical help than migraineurs. In a population study only 16% of patients with tension-type headache had been in contact with their general practitioner because of the headache, in contrast to 56% of migraineurs (Rasmussen et al. 1992). When data are corrected for the much higher prevalence of TTH, the total use of medical contacts is 54% higher for tension-type headache than for migraine. Severely affected TTH patients usually see numerous doctors and spend large sums of money on so-called alternative treatments, but the effect is never documented and many patients are left without effective pain relief. One study found that patients with chronic tension-type headache had experienced frequent headaches for an average of 7 years before seeking treatment. While they continued to attend work or school, their performance was severely affected and almost half had severe depression or anxiety. Those with affective problems were more functionally impaired (Holroyd et al. 2000).

The above-mentioned studies were cross-sectional and do not provide information on the important question of what happens to prevalence over time. This was studied by Lyngberg and colleagues, who replicated a cross-sectional study among the young adult population from 1989 (Lyngberg et al. 2005a). The 1-year prevalence of TTH increased significantly from 79% to 87% over a 12-year period, while the increase for the frequent episodic subform was even more pronounced from 29% to 37% (Lyngberg et al. 2005a). These findings suggest that the socioeconomic impact of TTH has markedly increased in the last decade.

How can we explain this increase? To answer this question it is necessary to clarify risk factors in a longitudinal study. Lyngberg et al. interviewed and examined 740 persons from the general population in 1989 and again 12 years later in a follow-up study (Lyngberg et al. 2005b). The annual incidence of frequent TTH was 14.2 per 1,000 persons with a female to male ratio of 2.6:1. The incidence decreased markedly with age, which is clinically important, e.g., when considering the need for diagnostic investigation in an elderly patient presenting with newly developed frequent headaches. Risk factors for the development of TTH were poor self-related health, inability to relax after work, and sleeping few hours per night (Lyngberg et al. 2005c). These findings are interesting because they may lead to new ways of preventing or treating tension-type headaches.

The clinician is often asked by TTH patients how long headaches might continue to be a problem. The natural history of TTH was examined by Lyngberg et al. in a longitudinal study (Lyngberg et al. 2005c). The headache status for the participants from a cross-sectional study performed in 1989 was reevaluated in a follow-up study in 2001. Among subjects with frequent episodic TTH or chronic TTH in 1989, 45% had remission, i.e., experienced infrequent or no headache in 2001, 39% had unchanged frequent episodic TTH, and 16% had a poor outcome, i.e., experienced chronic TTH in 2001. Poor outcome was associated with baseline chronic TTH, coexisting migraine, not being married, and sleeping problems. Thus, patients with frequent episodic TTH can be reassured that the prognosis is fairly favorable, with an almost 50% chance that they will not suffer from frequent headaches over a prolonged period. Intervention studies with specific focus on the identified risk factors in headache disorders have not yet been published.

History

Patients with TTH usually describe their pain as a "dull," "non-pulsating" headache. The pain is typically bilateral (90%) and a strict unilateral location calls for increased attention and secondary causative factors for headache should be considered. The pain quality is pressing and tightening and terms such as a sensation of "tightness," "pressure," or "soreness" are used. The pain is often described as an external pain coming from the outside and some patients refer to a "band" or a "cap" compressing their head, while others mention a heavy "weight" over their head and/or their shoulders.

BASIC HEADACHE DIARY

Name: __Hanne Jensen_____ Birthday: _____

Start of registration period: ___3/2-2010____　　Stop of registration period:____9/2-2010_____

Please complete and tick the most appropriate boxes **every** evening on the days with headache

1.	Date (day/month)		3/2	4/2	5/2	6/2	7/2	8/2	9/2
2.	When did your headache start? (h:m)		7.30	15.00	-	-	6.00	6.30	10.00
3.	When did your headache disappear? (h:m)		14.00	22.30	-	-	22.30	12.00	14.00
4.	Was your headache preceded by any of these symptoms:	Visual:	□	□	□	□	□	□	□
		Sensory:	□	□	□	□	□	□	□
		Speech problems:	□	□	□	□	□	□	□
5.	Was the headache	Bilateral:	x	x	□	□	□	□	x
		Right-sided:	□	□	□	□	x	x	□
		Left-sided:	□	□	□	□	□	□	□
6.	Was the headache	Non-pulsating:	x	x	□	□	□	□	x
		Pulsating:	□	□	□	□	x	x	□
7.	What was the intensity of your headache – (mean value for the whole day see instructions below*)	Mild:	x	□	□	□	□	□	□
		Moderate:	□	x	□	□	□	x	x
		Severe:	□	□	□	□	x	□	□
8.	Did the headache worsen with physical activity – e.g.walking stairs	No:	x	x	□	□	□	□	x
		Yes:	□	□	□	□	x	x	□
9.	Nausea	No:	x	□	□	□	□	□	□
		Mild:	□	x	□	□	□	□	x
		Moderate:	□	□	□	□	□	x	□
		Severe:	□	□	□	□	x	□	□
10.	Light intolerance	No:	x	x	□	□	□	□	x
		Yes:	□	□	□	□	x	x	□
11.	Noise intolerance	No:	x	x	□	□	□	□	x
		Yes:	□	□	□	□	x	x	□
12.	Any possible trigger factor	Specify :					Men-strua-tion		
13.	Did you take any drug for the headache or associated symptoms (for each name: dosage and number of tablets, injections or suppositories and time of intake	Name:	Ibu				Suma	Suma	Ibu
		Dose:	400 mg				50 mg	50 mg	400 mg
		Time:	8.00				6.10	6.45	10.15
		Name:					Ibu	Ibu	
		Dose:					400 mg	600 mg	
		Time:					12.30	10.30	
		Name:					Suma		
		Dose:					50 mg		
		Time:					22.00		

*) mild=does not inhibit work or other activities
moderate=inhibits but does not prohibit work or other activities;
severe=prohibits work and other activities

❏ Fig. 19.1

A diagnostic diary from a TTH patient with coexisting migraine

In one study, TTH was of a pressing quality in 78% of patients, mild or moderate in 99%, bilateral in 90%, and 72% had no aggravation by physical activity (Rasmussen et al. 1991a). The accompanying symptoms of nausea, photophobia, and phonophobia occur only rarely and if present, they are usually mild. The presence of nausea may raise suspicion of migraine or medication overuse. In addition, nausea and aggravation by physical activity are important predictors of a migraine attack. Patients suffering from both conditions can learn to discriminate between TTH and migraine by paying attention to these accompanying symptoms.

For diagnosis the use of headache diaries (Russell et al. 1992) for at least 4 weeks is highly recommended. A detailed diagnostic diary is useful initially with a change to a simplified calendar for the follow-up once a diagnosis is established. An example of a diagnostic diary for a patient suffering from frequent episodic TTH and coexisting migraine without aura is illustrated in ❷ *Fig. 19.1*. Detailed studies of the diagnostic and educational values of such diaries are in progress in Europe (Tassorelli et al. 2008) and could pave the way for further systematic studies between different clinics and countries.

A detailed history of any possible triggers is also of importance, especially in the episodic subforms. As in migraine, elimination of any possible triggers, such as dental pathology, cyclic hormonal relationship, sinus disease, unphysiological working conditions, posture, unbalanced meals, and inadequate sleep, can reduce the frequency of attacks although in practice triggers are sometimes difficult to identify.

◻ Table 19.2

Worrisome features, differential diagnosis, and suggested investigations

Warning feature	Differential diagnosis	Suggested investigation
Thunderclap – abrupt onset of a new headache	Subarachnoid hemorrhage	CT-C and MRA, and if negative a lumbar puncture
Atypical aura (>1 h or motor symptoms)	Migraine, TIA, or stroke	Detailed history, CT-C or MRI
New headache in a patient older than 40 years	Intracranial tumor or temporal arteritis	Detailed history, CT-C or MRI as well as blood tests
New headache in a prepubertal child	Intracranial tumor	Detailed history and eventually MRI
Nausea and progressive headache frequency	Medication overuse headache	Detailed medication registration and a new neurological examination
Intense headache aggravated by physical activity and accompanying symptoms	Migraine	Detailed history and diagnostic diary
Progressive headache accompanied by focal neurological or cognitive symptoms or signs	Intracranial space-occupying lesion	Detailed examination and CT-C or MRI
Progressive pulsating headache, tinnitus, and transient visual disturbances	Idiopathic intracranial hypertension	MRA and MRV and if normal lumbar puncture and opening pressure

In summary, a secondary headache should always be considered in patients consulting for headache. Medication overuse headache is the most frequent secondary headache disorder but serious life-threatening causes of headache also may mimic TTH. The major differential diagnoses are listed in ❯ *Table 19.2.*

Examination

Although diagnostic tests are widely used in patients with TTH, they are seldom indicated unless atypical features are present. In addition to the primary diagnosis, a careful history is important to assess for coexisting diseases such as depression or anxiety. In TTH the general examination should also include manual palpation of the pericranial muscles, particularly the temporal, masseter, sternocleidomastoid, and trapezius muscles plus neck muscle insertions. One or two fingers should be used, with moderate to firm pressure and small rotating movements (Bendtsen et al. 1995). Pain can be scored on a 0–3 scale based on verbal response and observation of the patient (❯ *Fig. 19.2*). This may demonstrate the possible source of pain for the patient and indicate the potential benefit of physical training or relaxation therapy.

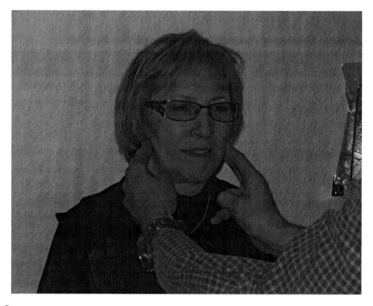

◻ **Fig. 19.2**
Illustration of the muscle palpation technique used in examining headache patients. Use second and third finger and use and exert mild pressure with small rotating movements. Palpate both sides of the head and neck. For palpation of neck insertions support the head with one hand and palpate under the cranium with the other. The muscles that are usually examined are the temporal, masseter, sternocleidomastoid, and trapezius muscles plus neck muscle insertions. The whole examination takes only about 2 min and is very effective in demonstrating the possible source of pain in tension-type headache

Investigations

In case of headache onset after the age of 40 years, recent changes in headache pattern, abnormal neurological findings, weight loss or marked weight increase, or personality or cognitive changes, secondary causes should be sought and blood samples and neuroimaging with CT or MRI should be undertaken. Neuroimaging of cervical and/or lumbar spine is not usually recommended as the specificity in relation to headache is poor and very often misleading.

A complete general and neurological examination including blood pressure, cardiac auscultation, body weight, inspection of the lumbar and cervical spine and fundi is essential in all newly referred headache patients. Abnormalities leading to discovery of a secondary cause of headache are rarely identified, but it is still important to look for symptoms and signs of sinister headaches; this also reassures patients that they have been carefully evaluated by their doctor.

References

Andlin-Sobocki P, Jonsson B, Wittchen HU, Olesen J (2005) Cost of disorders of the brain in Europe. Eur J Neurol 12(Suppl 1):1–27

Bendtsen L (2000) Central sensitization in tension-type headache – possible pathophysiological mechanisms. Cephalalgia 20:486–508

Bendtsen L, Jensen R (2006) Tension-type headache: the most common, but also the most neglected, headache disorder. Curr Opin Neurol 19:305–309

Bendtsen L, Jensen R, Jensen NK, Olesen J (1995) Pressure-controlled palpation: a new technique which increases the reliability of manual palpation. Cephalalgia 15:205–210

Berg J, Stovner LJ (2005) Cost of migraine and other headaches in Europe. Eur J Neurol 12(Suppl 1):59–62

Headache Classification Subcommittee of the International Headache Society (2004) The international classification of headache disorders: 2nd edition. Cephalalgia 24(suppl 1):1–160

Holroyd KA, Stensland M, Lipchik GL, Hill KR, O'Donnell FS, Cordingley G (2000) Psychosocial correlates and impact of chronic tension-type headaches. Headache 40:3–16

Jensen R (1999) Pathophysiological mechanisms of tension-type headache: a review of epidemiological and experimental studies. Cephalalgia 19:602–621

Jensen R, Stovner LJ (2008) Epidemiology and comorbidity of headache. Lancet Neurol 7:354–361

Jensen R, Symon D (2005) Epidemiology of tension-type headaches. In: Olesen J, Goadsby PJ, Ramadan N, Tfelt-Hansen P, Welch KM (eds) The headaches. Lippincott, Williams & Wilkins, Philadelphia, pp 621–624

Lyngberg AC, Rasmussen BK, Jorgensen T, Jensen R (2005a) Has the prevalence of migraine and tension-type headache changed over a 12-year period? A Danish population survey. Eur J Epidemiol 20:243–249

Lyngberg AC, Rasmussen BK, Jorgensen T, Jensen R (2005b) Incidence of primary headache: a Danish epidemiologic follow-up study. Am J Epidemiol 161:1066–1073

Lyngberg AC, Rasmussen BK, Jorgensen T, Jensen R (2005c) Prognosis of migraine and tension-type headache: a population-based follow-up study. Neurology 65:580–585

Lyngberg AC, Rasmussen BK, Jorgensen T, Jensen R (2005d) Secular changes in health care utilization and work absence for migraine and tension-type headache: a population based study. Eur J Epidemiol 20:1007–1014

Rasmussen BK (1995) Epidemiology of headache. Cephalalgia 15:45–68

Rasmussen BK, Jensen R, Olesen J (1991a) A population-based analysis of the diagnostic criteria of the International Headache Society. Cephalalgia 11:129–134

Rasmussen BK, Jensen R, Schroll M, Olesen J (1991b) Epidemiology of headache in a general population – a prevalence study. J Clin Epidemiol 44:1147–1157

Rasmussen BK, Jensen R, Olesen J (1992) Impact of headache on sickness absence and utilisation of medical services: a Danish population study. J Epidemiol Commun Health 46:443–446

Russell MB, Rasmussen BK, Brennum J, Iversen HK, Jensen R, Olesen J (1992) Presentation of a new instrument: the diagnostic headache diary. Cephalalgia 12:369–374

Schwartz BS, Stewart WF, Lipton RB (1997) Lost workdays and decreased work effectiveness associated with headache in the workplace. J Occup Environ Med 39:320–327

Stovner L, Hagen K, Jensen R, Katsarava Z, Lipton R, Scher A, Steiner T, Zwart JA (2007) The global burden of headache: a documentation of headache prevalence and disability worldwide. Cephalalgia 27:193–210

Tassorelli C, Sances G, Allena M, Ghiotto N, Bendtsen L, Olesen J, Nappi G, Jensen R (2008) The usefulness and applicability of a basic headache diary before first consultation: results of a pilot study conducted in two centres. Cephalalgia 28:1023–1030

20 Mechanisms of Tension-Type Headache and Their Relevance to Management

Lars Bendtsen[1] · David Bezov[2] · Sait Ashina[2]

[1]Glostrup Hospital, University of Copenhagen, Glostrup, Copenhagen, Denmark

[2]Albert Einstein College of Medicine, Montefiore Medical Center, Bronx, NY, USA

Paolo Martelletti, Timothy J. Steiner (eds.), *Handbook of Headache*, DOI 10.1007/978-88-470-1700-9_20,
© Lifting The Burden 2011

Abstract: The tenderness of pericranial myofascial tissues is considerably increased in patients with tension-type headache (TTH). The mechanisms responsible for the increased myofascial pain sensitivity have been extensively studied. Peripheral activation or sensitization of myofascial nociceptors could play a role in causing increased pain sensitivity, but firm evidence for a peripheral abnormality is still lacking. Most likely, peripheral mechanisms are of major importance in subjects with episodic TTH. Numerous studies have demonstrated that the central nervous system is sensitized in patients with chronic TTH. Sensitization of pain pathways in the central nervous system due to prolonged nociceptive stimuli from pericranial myofascial tissues seem to be responsible for the conversion of episodic to chronic TTH. The central sensitization explains why patients with chronic TTH are difficult to treat. This delineates two major targets for future treatment strategies: (a) to identify the source of peripheral nociception in order to prevent the development of central sensitization and thereby the conversion of episodic into chronic TTH and (b) to reduce established central sensitization and facilitate descending inhibition of pain.

Introduction

Tension-type headaches (TTH) are very prevalent and are responsible for substantial costs both for the individual and the society (Schwartz et al. 1997). In contrast to migraine, no significant improvement in treatment possibilities has been seen in TTH within the last decades. This may partly be attributed to the fact that the understanding of TTH pathophysiology is less complete than that of migraine. Fortunately, we have gained a significant amount of new knowledge on pathophysiological aspects of TTH within the last decade, and we are now beginning to understand some of the complex mechanisms leading to this prevalent disease (Jensen 1999; Bendtsen 2000; Vandenheede and Schoenen 2002; Ashina 2004; Ashina et al. 2005; Bendtsen and Jensen 2006; Mathew 2006; Fernandez-de-Las-Penas et al. 2007b; Fumal and Schoenen 2008; Bendtsen and Jensen 2009). This is the first step toward the development of more effective treatments. Previously, the research into the mechanisms leading to TTH mainly focused on peripheral factors. More recently, it has become clear that central factors, that is, factors in the central nervous system, play a crucial role in particular in the more chronic forms of the disorder.

Established Knowledge

Genetic Predisposition

Because of the enormous prevalence and variability in frequency and severity of TTH, any inheritance is almost certain to be polygenic. The population-relative risk in relatives compared with normal controls has been calculated in a single study. In chronic TTH, the risk was increased threefold, indicating a genetic predisposition (Østergaard et al. 1997). The transmission observed in this study was suggestive of a complex mode of inheritance of TTH predisposition genes or TTH susceptibility genes (Russell et al. 1998). At present, we adopt the view that the great majority of the population, perhaps all, have the potential to develop TTH if exposed to sufficiently strong environmental factors.

Environmental and Psychological Factors

Headaches are generally reported to occur in relation to emotional conflict and psychosocial stress, but as in migraine the cause–effect relationship is not clear. Stress and mental tension are the most frequently reported precipitating factors (Jensen and Becker 2005). However, they occur with similar frequency in TTH and migraine (Jensen and Becker 2005) and may therefore not be of specific importance for the pathophysiology of TTH. It has recently been demonstrated that stress induces more headache in patients with chronic TTH than in healthy controls probably through hyperalgesic effects on already sensitized pain pathways (Cathcart et al. 2010a). However, stress did not aggravate abnormal temporal summation or diffuse noxious inhibitory control mechanisms (Cathcart et al. 2010b).

In general, there is no increase in anxiety or depression in patients with infrequent TTH, while frequent TTH is associated with higher rates of anxiety and depression (Heckman and Holroyd 2006). As in other chronic pain disorders, psychological abnormalities in TTH may be viewed as secondary rather than primary. It has been demonstrated that depression increases vulnerability to TTH in patients with frequent headaches during and following a laboratory stress test and that the induced headache is associated with elevated pericranial muscle tenderness (Janke et al. 2004). The investigators suggested that depression may aggravate existing central sensitization (discussed later) in patients with frequent headaches (Janke et al. 2004). Thus, there may be a bidirectional relationship between depression and frequent TTH.

Maladaptive coping strategies, e.g., catastrophizing and avoidance, seem to be common in TTH (Heckman and Holroyd 2006). It has been demonstrated that the 1-year prevalence of TTH increased significantly over a 12-year period from 1989 to 2001 (Lyngberg et al. 2005a). Risk factors for the development of TTH were poor self-rated health, an inability to relax after work and sleep disturbances (Lyngberg et al. 2005b).

Peripheral Factors

Myofascial tenderness and hardness. A large number of studies have consistently shown that the pericranial myofascial tissues are considerably more tender in patients with TTH than in healthy subjects, and that the tenderness is positively associated with both the intensity and the frequency of TTH (Jensen 1999; Lipchik et al. 2000; Buchgreitz et al. 2006; Fernandez-de-Las-Penas et al. 2007a). The tenderness is uniformly increased throughout the pericranial region in both patients with episodic and chronic TTH (Langemark and Olesen 1987; Jensen et al. 1998; Buchgreitz et al. 2006). It has also been demonstrated that the consistency of pericranial muscles is increased (Ashina et al. 1999b). Tenderness and hardness have been found to be increased both on days with and without headache (Jensen 1999; Ashina et al. 1999b; Lipchik et al. 2000) indicating that these factors are of primary importance for the development of headache and not only a consequence of the headache.

What could be the pathophysiological basis for the possible pain originating in the myofascial tissues? Under normal conditions, myofascial pain is mediated by thin myelinated (Aδ) fibers and unmyelinated (C) fibers, while the thick myelinated (Aα and Aβ) fibers normally mediate innocuous sensations (Newham et al. 1994). Various noxious and innocuous events such as mechanical stimuli, ischemia and chemical mediators could excite and sensitize Aδ-fibers and C-fibers (Mense 1993) and thereby play a role in producing increased tenderness in TTH.

Muscle contraction. The origin of pain in TTH has traditionally been attributed to increased contraction and ischemia of head and neck muscles. Sustained experimental tooth clenching has been reported to induce more headache in TTH patients than healthy controls (Jensen and Olesen 1996), and TTH patients are more liable to develop shoulder and neck pain in response to static exercise than healthy controls (Christensen et al. 2005). Numerous laboratory-based electromyographic studies have reported normal or only slightly increased muscle activity in TTH (Jensen 1999). However, EMG activity has been reported to be increased in myofascial trigger points (tenderness in a hypersensible spot within a palpable taut band, local twitch response elicited by snapping palpation, and elicited referred pain with palpation) (Hubbard and Berkoff 1993), and it is possible that continuous activity in a few motor units over long time could be sufficient for excitation or sensitization of peripheral nociceptors (Bendtsen 2000).

The existence and importance of trigger points in myofascial pain disorders has long been debated (Fernandez-de-Las-Penas et al. 2007b). A recent series of pilot studies performed in a blinded fashion reported an increased number of active trigger points both in patients with frequent episodic TTH and in patients with chronic TTH (Fernandez-de-Las-Penas et al. 2006a, b, 2007c). In chronic, but not in episodic, TTH the trigger points were positively correlated to headache severity.

Muscle tenderness and hardness at tender muscle sites could also result from a local contracture (i.e., shortening of the contractile apparatus without action potentials in the muscle fibers) rather than normal contraction of motor units (Simons and Mense 1998). This mechanism would explain the lack of EMG abnormalities in TTH, but the mechanisms of peripheral nociceptor activation by a contracture have not yet been studied in enough detail (Mense et al. 2003).

By use of microdialysis technique, Ashina et al. (2002) demonstrated that lactate levels in a tender site in the trapezius muscle did not differ between patients and healthy subjects during rest and static exercise, ruling out muscle ischemia in these patients. However, the increase in muscle blood flow during exercise was lower in patients than in controls. The investigators suggested the altered blood flow was caused by altered sympathetic outflow to blood vessels in striated muscle secondary to plastic changes in the central nervous system (central sensitization) (Ashina et al. 2002).

It can be concluded that the muscle pain in TTH is not caused by generalized excessive muscle contraction and muscle ischemia. However, it cannot be excluded that a locally increased muscle tone without EMG activity (contracture) may result in microtrauma of muscle fibers and tendon insertions or that excessive activity in a few motor units may excite or sensitize peripheral nociceptors.

Peripheral excitation and sensitization. The increased myofascial pain sensitivity in TTH could be due to release of inflammatory mediators resulting in excitation and sensitization of peripheral sensory afferents (Bendtsen 2000). However, Ashina et al. (2003) demonstrated that the in vivo interstitial concentrations of adenosine 5-triphosphate, glutamate, glucose, pyruvate, urea, and prostaglandin E_2 in tender muscles during rest and static exercise did not differ between patients with chronic TTH and healthy controls. The investigators concluded that tender muscle sites in these patients are not sites of ongoing inflammation.

Schmidt-Hansen et al. demonstrated that infusion of hypertonic saline into various pericranial muscles elicits referred pain that is perceived as head pain in healthy subjects (Schmidt-Hansen et al. 2006d). Mork et al. infused a combination of endogenous substances into the trapezius muscle and reported that patients with frequent episodic TTH developed more pain than healthy controls (Mork et al. 2004). Concomitant psychophysical measures indicated that peripheral sensitization of myofascial sensory afferents was responsible for the muscular hypersensitivity in these patients.

Summary on peripheral factors. Pericranial myofascial pain sensitivity is increased in patients with TTH and peripheral mechanisms most likely play a role in the pathophysiology of TTH. Peripheral activation or sensitization of myofascial nociceptors could play a role in the increased pain sensitivity, but firm evidence for peripheral abnormality is still lacking.

Central Factors

Central pain sensitivity. The increased myofascial pain sensitivity in TTH could also be caused by central factors such as sensitization of second-order neurons at the level of the spinal dorsal horn/trigeminal nucleus, sensitization of supraspinal neurons, and decreased antinociceptive activity from supraspinal structures (Bendtsen 2000). The measurement of pain sensitivity to various types of stimuli applied to various parts of the body have provided important information about the nociceptive system in TTH. Pain detection thresholds have been reported normal in patients with episodic TTH in studies performed before the separation between the infrequent and frequent form of TTH was made (Göbel et al. 1992; Bovim 1992; Jensen et al. 1993; Jensen 1996). In contrast, pain detection thresholds have been reported decreased in patients with frequent episodic TTH (Mork et al. 2003; Schmidt-Hansen et al. 2007), and both pain detection and tolerance thresholds were found to be decreased in patients with chronic TTH in studies performed with sufficient sample size (Langemark et al. 1989, 1993; Schoenen et al. 1991; Bendtsen et al. 1996a; Ashina et al. 2006; Sandrini et al. 2006; Schmidt-Hansen et al. 2007; Fernandez-de-Las-Penas et al. 2007a; Lindelof et al. 2009). Ashina et al. (2006) demonstrated that the difference in pain sensitivity is even more pronounced in cephalic and extracephalic regions when recording pain sensitivity to clinically relevant stimuli, namely, suprathreshold stimuli (❷ *Fig. 20.1*). Increased temporal summation to pressure pain (Cathcart et al. 2010b) and trend toward increased temporal summation to electrical pain (Ashina et al. 2006) in patients with chronic TTH compared to controls have also been demonstrated.

Patients with chronic TTH have been found to be hypersensitive to each of the different stimulus modalities examined, namely, pressure (Langemark et al. 1989; Schoenen et al. 1991; Bendtsen et al. 1996a), thermal (Langemark et al. 1989) and electrical (Langemark et al. 1993; Bendtsen et al. 1996a; Ashina et al. 2006; Sandrini et al. 2006; Lindelof et al. 2009) stimuli as well as intramuscular infusions of painful substances (Schmidt-Hansen et al. 2007; Lindelof et al. 2009). Sensitivity to various stimulus modalities is increased both at cephalic and extra-cephalic sites (Langemark et al. 1989, 1993; Schoenen et al. 1991; Bendtsen et al. 1996a; Ashina et al. 2006), to stimulation of various tissues, i.e., muscle, skin, tendons and peripheral nerves (Langemark et al. 1989; Schoenen et al. 1991; Langemark et al. 1993; Bendtsen et al. 1996a; Ashina et al. 2006; Schmidt-Hansen et al. 2007 Lindelof et al. 2009), and both during and outside of headache (Schmidt-Hansen et al. 2007). Together, these studies were suggestive of a generalized increase in pain sensitivity in patients with frequent TTH. The data from these clinical studies were recently confirmed in a population-based study demonstrating a close relation between altered pain perception and chronification of headache (Buchgreitz et al. 2006). In addition, it was demonstrated that a previously reported increase in TTH prevalence over a 12-year period was related to increased pain sensitivity (Buchgreitz et al. 2007a).

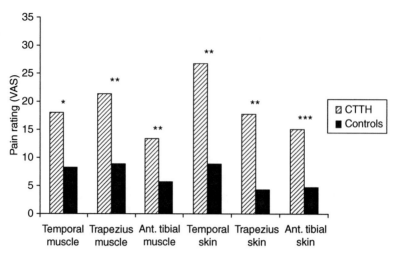

◘ Fig. 20.1

Pain perception study demonstrating pronounced generalized hyperalgesia in patients with chronic tension-type headache (CTTH). Pain ratings to suprathreshold single electrical stimulation (VAS) of skin and muscle in patients with CTTH and healthy controls. *$p < 0.05$, **$p < 0.01$, ***$p < 0.001$ (Data from Ashina et al. 2006)

The fact that chronic TTH patients are hypersensitive to stimuli applied at both cephalic and at extra-cephalic, non-symptomatic locations strongly indicates that synaptic transmission of nociceptive input within the central nervous system is increased in this group of patients. Peripheral sensitization would have more localized effects and cannot alone explain the generalized hyperalgesia seen in patients with chronic TTH (Treede et al. 1992; Milanov and Bogdanova 2004). The expansion of hypersensitivity to other tissues such as skin is consistent with referred hyperalgesia, which may be explained by convergence of multiple peripheral sensory afferents onto sensitized spinal cord neurons. The widespread and non-specific nature of the hypersensitivity, however, suggests that the central sensitization involves supraspinal neurons as well (Bendtsen 2000). Thus, it can be concluded that nociceptive processing in the central nervous system is increased in patients with chronic TTH, while central nociceptive processing seems to be normal in patients with infrequent episodic TTH.

A significant but incomplete correlation between general pain hypersensitivity and pericranial tenderness has been demonstrated (Bendtsen et al. 1996a; Jensen et al. 1998). Indeed, the increase in myofascial tenderness is more pronounced than the increase in generalized pain sensitivity (Bendtsen 2000); therefore, generalized hypersensitivity can only partially account for the increased pericranial tenderness in patients with chronic TTH. It has been demonstrated that the stimulus-response function for pressure versus pain in pericranial muscles is not only quantitatively, but also qualitatively altered in patients with chronic TTH (Bendtsen et al. 1996b). On the basis of results from animal studies this is most likely explained by central sensitization at the level of the spinal dorsal horn/trigeminal nucleus. Thus, the increased tenderness in patients with chronic TTH is probably partly caused by segmental central sensitization.

Decreased antinociceptive activity. Decreased antinociceptive activity from supraspinal structures, i.e., deficient descending inhibition, may also contribute to the increased pain

sensitivity in chronic TTH (Langemark et al. 1993; Pielsticker et al. 2005; Sandrini et al. 2006; Buchgreitz et al. 2008a; Cathcart et al. 2010b). Sandrini et al. (2006) demonstrated deficient diffuse noxious inhibitory control in chronic TTH, and a recent high-density brain EEG mapping study found impaired inhibition of nociceptive input in CTTH patients (Buchgreitz et al. 2008a). Cathcart et al. (2010b) recently reported deficient inhibition of repeated noxious mechanical stimulation in patients with chronic TTH. Impaired descending inhibition could be the primary abnormality or it could contribute to or be a consequence of central sensitization (Bendtsen 2000). Longitudinal studies are needed to clarify this.

Thus, present knowledge strongly suggests that the central nervous system is sensitized both at the level of the spinal dorsal horn/trigeminal nucleus and supraspinally in patients with frequent TTH, while the central pain processing seems to be normal in patients with infrequent episodic TTH.

How Headache May Become Chronic

In healthy subjects, the processing of pain from myofascial tissues is finely regulated, such that the degree of perceived pain is appropriate for the actual situation. The nociceptive system allows the detection of potential harmful events and enables the individual to react appropriately to these, e.g., to avoid unphysiological working positions that cause strain on the pericranial muscles and headache. The painful stimulus from the periphery is usually eliminated by actions from the individual and, if necessary, by local reparative mechanisms in the myofascial tissues. The properties of the nociceptive system will normally not be altered after a short lasting painful episode. This may be representative of the nociceptive system in subjects with rare episodes of TTH (Bendtsen 2000).

Under some conditions, the painful stimulus from the pericranial myofascial tissues may be more prolonged or more intense than normally. The mechanisms behind this are not known, but may include increased muscle activity or the release of various chemical mediators secondary to local pathological conditions. Increased muscle activity secondary to psychogenic stress is likely to be of relevance in this respect. The reason may be because the psychogenic stress condition may cause a prolonged increase of muscle tone via the limbic system and at the same time potentiate pain facilitation from the brain stem to the spinal dorsal horn (Merskey 1994). It is also possible that stress may decrease muscle blood flow via sympathetically mediated vasoconstriction and in this way contribute to aggravation of TTH (Ashina et al. 2002). In most subjects these conditions will be self-limiting due to central pain modulatory mechanisms and local reparative processes and will be experienced as frequent headache episodes for a limited period of time.

In predisposed individuals, the prolonged nociceptive input from the pericranial myofascial tissues may lead to sensitization of nociceptive second order neurons at the level of the spinal dorsal/trigeminal nucleus (Bendtsen 2000). Possible mechanisms include an impaired supraspinal inhibition of nociceptive transmission in the spinal dorsal horn. In the sensitized state, the afferent Aβ-fibers that normally inhibit Aδ- and C-fibers by presynaptic mechanisms in the dorsal horn, will on the contrary stimulate the nociceptive second order neurons. In addition, the effect of Aδ- and C-fiber stimulation of the nociceptive dorsal horn neurons will be potentiated, and the receptive fields of the dorsal horn neurons will be expanded (Coderre et al. 1993). The nociceptive input to supraspinal structures will therefore be considerably increased, which may result in increased excitability of supraspinal neurons as well as decreased inhibition or increased facilitation of nociceptive transmission in the spinal dorsal horn, i.e., in generalized pain hypersensitivity. The central neuroplastic changes may also increase the activity of the motor neurons both at the supraspinal and at the segmental level, resulting in slightly increased muscle activity and in increased muscle hardness. It is possible that low-grade tension that normally does not result in pain does so in the presence of central sensitization. By these mechanisms the central sensitization may be maintained even after the initial eliciting factors have been normalized, and the individual will experience daily headaches. This hypothesis (Bendtsen 2000) may account for the majority, but not all, cases of chronic TTH. In some patients the central dysfunction, e.g., deficient supraspinal descending inhibition, may be the primary abnormality making the individual more susceptible to a normal level of nociceptive input, and in other patients the disorder may be purely central with no interaction with the periphery.

To summarize, it is likely that prolonged nociceptive input from tender pericranial myofascial tissues may result in segmental central sensitization at the level of the upper cervical spinal dorsal horn/trigeminal nucleus with secondary sensitization of supraspinal neurons. This may be responsible for the conversion of episodic to chronic TTH (❯ *Fig. 20.2*) (Bendtsen 2000).

Imaging studies. The above hypothesis was further supported by a recent study demonstrating decrease in volume of gray matter brain structures involved in pain processing in patients with chronic TTH (Schmidt-Wilcke et al. 2005). This decrease was positively correlated with duration of headache and is most likely a consequence of central sensitization generated by prolonged input from pericranial myofascial structures (Schmidt-Wilcke et al. 2005).

Pharmacological studies. The hypothesis of central sensitization in TTH is further supported by clinical pharmacological studies (Bendtsen 2002). Thus, amitriptyline reduces both headache and pericranial myofascial tenderness in patients with chronic TTH (Bendtsen and Jensen 2000). The reduction of myofascial tenderness during treatment with amitriptyline

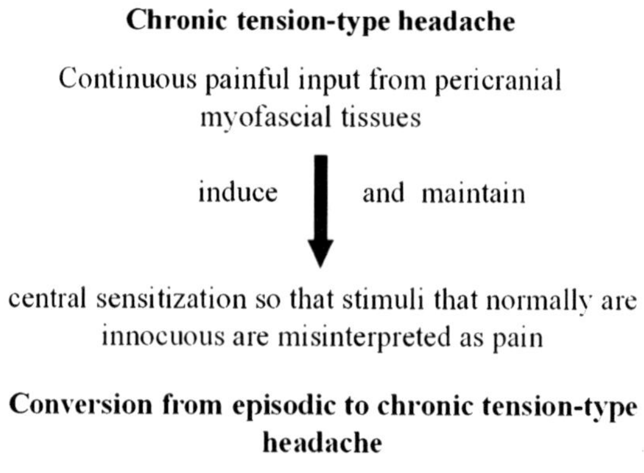

Chronic tension-type headache

Continuous painful input from pericranial
myofascial tissues

induce   and maintain

central sensitization so that stimuli that normally are
innocuous are misinterpreted as pain

**Conversion from episodic to chronic tension-type
headache**

◘ Fig. 20.2
The proposed pathophysiological model of chronic tension-type headache delineates two major aims for future research: (a) to identify the source of peripheral nociception in order to prevent the development of central sensitization in patients with episodic tension-type headache, and (b) to reduce established central sensitization in patients with chronic tension-type headache (Modified from Bendtsen 2000)

may be caused by a segmental reduction of central sensitization in combination with an enhanced efficacy of noradrenergic or serotonergic descending inhibition (Bendtsen and Jensen 2000).

Animal studies have shown that sensitization of pain pathways may be caused by or associated with activation of nitric oxide synthase (NOS) and the generation of nitric oxide (NO) and that the NOS inhibitors reduce central sensitization in animal models of persistent pain (Meller and Gebhart 1993). On the basis of these findings and the hypothesis of central sensitization in chronic TTH, Ashina et al. demonstrated that infusion of the NO donor, glyceryl trinitrate, induces TTH-like headache in patients with chronic TTH (Ashina et al. 2000). In addition, the same group investigated the analgesic effect of the NOS inhibitor N^G-monomethyl-L-arginine hydrochloride (L-NMMA). This drug significantly reduced headache (Ashina et al. 1999c) as well as pericranial myofascial tenderness and hardness (Ashina et al. 1999a) in patients with chronic TTH. Sarchielli et al. reported increased platelet NOS activity in patients with chronic TTH possibly reflecting central up-regulation of NOS (Sarchielli et al. 2002). This pharmacologic data supports the notion that central sensitization is involved in the pathophysiology of chronic TTH. Moreover, these findings suggest that inhibition of NO and thereby central sensitization may become a novel means of future treatment of chronic TTH.

An animal model of TTH has been developed (Makowska et al. 2005a). This model allows investigation of the important interactions between peripheral myofascial factors and central sensitization and may prove to be of major importance for the investigations of pathophysiology (Makowska et al. 2005b) and drug development (Makowska et al. 2006; Panfil et al. 2006) in TTH.

Longitudinal pain sensitivity studies. Final evidence for the cause effect relationship between frequent headache and central sensitization has to come from longitudinal studies. This was recently provided from a 12-year follow-up study demonstrating that patients who developed episodic TTH had increased pericranial myofascial tenderness, but normal general pain sensitivity at follow up, while subjects that developed chronic TTH had normal pain sensitivity at baseline, but developed increased central pain sensitivity at follow up (Buchgreitz et al. 2008b). The investigators concluded that increased pain sensitivity is a consequence of frequent TTH, not a risk factor, and that the results support that central sensitization plays an important role for the chronification of TTH (Buchgreitz et al. 2008b).

Relevance for Management

Our improved knowledge about the mechanisms leading to TTH should be taken advantage of in the management of this disorder, since information about the nature of the disease is important for the majority of patients. It can be explained to the patient that muscle pain may lead to a disturbance of the brain's pain modulating mechanisms, so that normal innocuous stimuli are perceived as painful, with secondary perpetuation of muscle pain and risk of anxiety and depression. Environmental and psychological factors such as non-physiological working positions and psychological stress should be minimized if possible, and co-morbid disorders such as anxiety and depression should be treated, since these factors may contribute to possible chronification of TTH (Bendtsen et al. 2009).

The degree and location of pericranial myofascial tenderness should be examined by manual palpation to demonstrate the possible sources of pain. This may help the health care professional to choose the most relevant of the non-pharmacological managements such as instruction in optimal working positions, relaxation training, EMG biofeedback and physical therapy (Bendtsen et al. 2009). Effective intervention against peripheral factors may possibly prevent the development of central sensitization and thereby the chronification of headache.

When managing patients with frequent or chronic TTH, the ways of reducing the established central sensitization should be considered in addition to the above-mentioned treatments. This may be possible by means of prophylactic medications, such as the tricyclic antidepressants, usually in combination with non-pharmacological treatments such as relaxation training or cognitive-behavioral therapy (Bendtsen et al. 2009).

Current Research

Even in the hands of the best experts, management of chronic TTH is difficult, which may be partly explained by our insufficient knowledge of the mechanisms leading to this disorder (Bendtsen et al. 2009). The recent advances in our understanding of the pathophysiology of TTH have fortunately stimulated much needed further research. Current research concentrates on exploring the basis for the peripheral sensitization and the mechanisms leading to central sensitization. This will hopefully lead to improved treatment possibilities for this widespread disorder.

References

Ashina M (2004) Neurobiology of chronic tension-type headache. Cephalalgia 24:161–172

Ashina M, Bendtsen L, Jensen R, Lassen LH, Sakai F, Olesen J (1999a) Possible mechanisms of action of nitric oxide synthase inhibitors in chronic tension-type headache. Brain 122:1629–1635

Ashina M, Bendtsen L, Jensen R, Sakai F, Olesen J (1999b) Muscle hardness in patients with chronic tension-type headache: relation to actual headache state. Pain 79:201–205

Ashina M, Lassen LH, Bendtsen L, Jensen R, Olesen J (1999c) Effect of inhibition of nitric oxide synthase on chronic tension-type headache: a randomised crossover trial. Lancet 353:287–289

Ashina M, Bendtsen L, Jensen R, Olesen J (2000) Nitric oxide-induced headache in patients with chronic tension-type headache. Brain 123:1830–1837

Ashina M, Stallknecht B, Bendtsen L, Pedersen JF, Galbo H, Dalgaard P, Olesen J (2002) In vivo evidence of altered skeletal muscle blood flow in chronic tension-type headache. Brain 125:320–326

Ashina M, Stallknecht B, Bendtsen L, Pedersen J, Schifter S, Galbo H, Olesen J (2003) Tender points are not sites of ongoing inflammation - in vivo evidence in patients with chronic tension-type headache. Cephalalgia 23:109–116

Ashina S, Bendtsen L, Ashina M (2005) Pathophysiology of tension-type headache. Curr Pain Headache Rep 9:415–422

Ashina S, Bendtsen L, Ashina M, Magerl W, Jensen R (2006) Generalized hyperalgesia in patients with chronic tension-type headache. Cephalalgia 26:940–948

Bendtsen L (2000) Central sensitization in tension-type headache – possible pathophysiological mechanisms. Cephalalgia 20:486–508

Bendtsen L (2002) Sensitization: its role in primary headache. Curr Opin Investig Drugs 3:449–453

Bendtsen L, Jensen R (2000) Amitriptyline reduces myofascial tenderness in patients with chronic tension-type headache. Cephalalgia 20:603–610

Bendtsen L, Jensen R (2006) Tension-type headache: the most common, but also the most neglected, headache disorder. Curr Opin Neurol 19:305–309

Bendtsen L, Jensen R (2009) Tension-type headache. Neurol Clin 27:525–535

Bendtsen L, Jensen R, Olesen J (1996a) Decreased pain detection and tolerance thresholds in chronic tension-type headache. Arch Neurol 53:373–376

Bendtsen L, Jensen R, Olesen J (1996b) Qualitatively altered nociception in chronic myofascial pain. Pain 65:259–264

Bendtsen L, Evers S, Linde M, Mitsikostas DD, Sandrini G, Schoenen J (2009) EFNS guideline on the treatment of tension-type headache – Report of an EFNS task force. Eur J Neurol 17:1318–1325

Bovim G (1992) Cervicogenic headache, migraine, and tension-type headache. Pressure-pain threshold measurements. Pain 51:169–173

Buchgreitz L, Lyngberg AC, Bendtsen L, Jensen R (2006) Frequency of headache is related to sensitization: a population study. Pain 123:19–27

Buchgreitz L, Lyngberg A, Bendtsen L, Jensen R (2007) Increased prevalence of tension-type headache over a 12-year period is related to increased pain sensitivity. A population study. Cephalalgia 27:145–152

Buchgreitz L, Egsgaard LL, Jensen R, Arendt-Nielsen L, Bendtsen L (2008a) Abnormal pain processing in chronic tension-type headache: a high-density EEG brain mapping study. Brain 131:3232–3238

Buchgreitz L, Lyngberg AC, Bendtsen L, Jensen R (2008b) Increased pain sensitivity is not a risk factor but a consequence of frequent headache: a population-based follow-up study. Pain 137:623–630

Cathcart S, Winefield AH, Lushington K, Rolan P (2010a) Noxious inhibition of temporal summation is impaired in chronic tension-type headache. Headache 50(3):403–412

Cathcart S, Petkov J, Winefield AH, Lushington K, Rolan P (2010b) Central mechanisms of stress-induced headache. Cephalalgia 30(3):285–295

Christensen M, Bendtsen L, Ashina M, Jensen R (2005) Experimental induction of muscle tenderness and headache in tension-type headache patients. Cephalalgia 25:1061–1067

Coderre TJ, Katz J, Vaccarino AL, Melzack R (1993) Contribution of central neuroplasticity to pathological pain: review of clinical and experimental evidence. Pain 52:259–285

Fernandez-de-Las-Penas C, Alonso-Blanco C, Cuadrado ML, Gerwin RD, Pareja JA (2006a) Myofascial trigger points and their relationship to headache clinical parameters in chronic tension-type headache. Headache 46:1264–1272

Fernandez-de-Las-Penas C, Alonso-Blanco C, Cuadrado ML, Gerwin RD, Pareja JA (2006b) Trigger points in the suboccipital muscles and forward head posture in tension-type headache. Headache 46:454–460

Fernandez-de-Las-Penas C, Cuadrado ML, Arendt-Nielsen L, Ge HY, Pareja JA (2007a) Increased pericranial tenderness, decreased pressure pain threshold, and headache clinical parameters in chronic tension-type headache patients. Clin J Pain 23:346–352

Fernandez-de-Las-Penas C, Cuadrado ML, Arendt-Nielsen L, Simons DG, Pareja JA (2007b) Myofascial trigger points and sensitization: an updated pain model for tension-type headache. Cephalalgia 27:383–393

Fernandez-de-Las-Penas C, Cuadrado ML, Pareja JA (2007c) Myofascial trigger points, neck mobility, and forward head posture in episodic tension-type headache. Headache 47(5):662–672

Fumal A, Schoenen J (2008) Tension-type headache: current research and clinical management. Lancet Neurol 7:70–83

Göbel H, Weigle L, Kropp P, Soyka D (1992) Pain sensitivity and pain reactivity of pericranial muscles in migraine and tension-type headache. Cephalalgia 12:142–151

Heckman BD, Holroyd KA (2006) Tension-type headache and psychiatric comorbidity. Curr Pain Headache Rep 10:439–447

Hubbard DR, Berkoff GM (1993) Myofascial trigger points show spontaneous needle EMG activity. Spine 18:1803–1807

Janke EA, Holroyd KA, Romanek K (2004) Depression increases onset of tension-type headache following laboratory stress. Pain 111:230–238

Jensen R (1996) Mechanisms of spontaneous tension-type headaches: an analysis of tenderness, pain thresholds and EMG. Pain 64:251–256

Jensen R (1999) Pathophysiological mechanisms of tension-type headache: a review of epidemiological and experimental studies. Cephalalgia 19:602–621

Jensen R, Becker WJ (2005) Symptomatology of episodic tension-type headaches. In: Olesen J, Goadsby PJ, Ramadan N, Tfelt-Hansen P, Welch KM (eds) The headaches. Lippincott Williams & Wilkins, Philadelphia, pp 685–692

Jensen R, Olesen J (1996) Initiating mechanisms of experimentally induced tension-type headache. Cephalalgia 16:175–182

Jensen R, Rasmussen BK, Pedersen B, Olesen J (1993) Muscle tenderness and pressure pain thresholds in headache. A population study. Pain 52:193–199

Jensen R, Bendtsen L, Olesen J (1998) Muscular factors are of importance in tension-type headache. Headache 38:10–17

Langemark M, Olesen J (1987) Pericranial tenderness in tension headache. A blind, controlled study. Cephalalgia 7:249–255

Langemark M, Jensen K, Jensen TS, Olesen J (1989) Pressure pain thresholds and thermal nociceptive thresholds in chronic tension-type headache. Pain 38:203–210

Langemark M, Bach FW, Jensen TS, Olesen J (1993) Decreased nociceptive flexion reflex threshold in chronic tension-type headache. Arch Neurol 50:1061–1064

Lindelof K, Ellrich J, Jensen R, Bendtsen L (2009) Central pain processing in chronic tension-type headache. Clin Neurophysiol 120:1364–1370

Lipchik GL, Holroyd KA, O'Donnell FJ, Cordingley GE, Waller S, Labus J, Davis MK, French DJ (2000) Exteroceptive suppression periods and pericranial muscle tenderness in chronic tension-type headache: effects of psychopathology, chronicity and disability. Cephalalgia 20:638–646

Lyngberg AC, Rasmussen BK, Jorgensen T, Jensen R (2005a) Has the prevalence of migraine and tension-type headache changed over a 12-year period?

A Danish population survey. Eur J Epidemiol 20:243–249

Lyngberg AC, Rasmussen BK, Jorgensen T, Jensen R (2005b) Incidence of primary headache: a Danish epidemiologic follow-up study. Am J Epidemiol 161:1066–1073

Makowska A, Panfil C, Ellrich J (2005a) Long-term potentiation of orofacial sensorimotor processing by noxious input from the semispinal neck muscle in mice. Cephalalgia 25:109–116

Makowska A, Panfil C, Ellrich J (2005b) Nerve growth factor injection into semispinal neck muscle evokes sustained facilitation of the jaw-opening reflex in anesthetized mice – possible implications for tension-type headache. Exp Neurol 191:301–309

Makowska A, Panfil C, Ellrich J (2006) ATP induces sustained facilitation of craniofacial nociception through P2X receptors on neck muscle nociceptors in mice. Cephalalgia 26:697–706

Mathew NT (2006) Tension-type headache. Curr Neurol Neurosci Rep 6:100–105

Meller ST, Gebhart GF (1993) Nitric oxide (NO) and nociceptive processing in the spinal cord. Pain 52:127–136

Mense S (1993) Nociception from skeletal muscle in relation to clinical muscle pain. Pain 54:241–289

Mense S, Simons DG, Hoheisel U, Quenzer B (2003) Lesions of rat skeletal muscle after local block of acetylcholinesterase and neuromuscular stimulation. J Appl Physiol 94:2494–2501

Merskey H (1994) Pain and psychological medicine. In: Wall PD, Melzack R (eds) Textbook of pain. Churchill Livingstone, Edinburgh, pp 903–920

Milanov I, Bogdanova D (2004) Pain and tension-type headache: a review of the possible pathophysiological mechanisms. J Headache Pain 5:4–11

Mork H, Ashina M, Bendtsen L, Olesen J, Jensen R (2003) Induction of prolonged tenderness in patients with tension-type headache by means of a new experimental model of myofascial pain. Eur J Neurol 10:249–256

Mork H, Ashina M, Bendtsen L, Olesen J, Jensen R (2004) Possible mechanisms of pain perception in patients with episodic tension-type headache. A new experimental model of myofascial pain. Cephalalgia 24:466–475

Newham DJ, Edwards RHT, Mills KR (1994) Skeletal muscle pain. In: Wall PD, Melzack R (eds) Textbook of pain. Churchill Livingstone, Edinburgh, pp 423–440

Østergaard S, Russell MB, Bendtsen L, Olesen J (1997) Comparison of first degree relatives and spouses of

people with chronic tension headache. BMJ 12:1092–1093

Panfil C, Makowska A, Ellrich J (2006) Brainstem and cervical spinal cord Fos immunoreactivity evoked by nerve growth factor injection into neck muscles in mice. Cephalalgia 26:128–135

Pielsticker A, Haag G, Zaudig M, Lautenbacher S (2005) Impairment of pain inhibition in chronic tension-type headache. Pain 118:215–223

Russell MB, Iselius L, Olesen J (1998) Inheritance of chronic tension-type headache investigated by complex segregation analysis. Hum Genet 102:138–140

Sandrini G, Rossi P, Milanov I, Serrao M, Cecchini AP, Nappi G (2006) Abnormal modulatory influence of diffuse noxious inhibitory controls in migraine and chronic tension-type headache patients. Cephalalgia 26:782–789

Sarchielli P, Alberti A, Floridi A, Gallai V (2002) L-Arginine/nitric oxide pathway in chronic tension-type headache: relation with serotonin content and secretion and glutamate content. J Neurol Sci 198:9–15

Schmidt-Hansen PT, Svensson P, Jensen TS, Graven-Nielsen T, Bach FW (2006) Patterns of experimentally induced pain in pericranial muscles. Cephalalgia 26:568–577

Schmidt-Hansen PT, Svensson P, Bendtsen L, Graven-Nielsen T, Bach FW (2007) Increased muscle pain sensitivity in patients with tension-type headache. Pain 129:113–121

Schmidt-Wilcke T, Leinisch E, Straube A, Kampfe N, Draganski B, Diener HC, Bogdahn U, May A (2005) Gray matter decrease in patients with chronic tension type headache. Neurology 65:1483–1486

Schoenen J, Bottin D, Hardy F, Gerard P (1991) Cephalic and extracephalic pressure pain thresholds in chronic tension-type headache. Pain 47:145–149

Schwartz BS, Stewart WF, Lipton RB (1997) Lost workdays and decreased work effectiveness associated with headache in the workplace. J Occup Environ Med 39:320–327

Simons DG, Mense S (1998) Understanding and measurement of muscle tone as related to clinical muscle pain. Pain 75:1–17

Treede RD, Meyer RA, Raja SN, Campbell JN (1992) Peripheral and central mechanisms of cutaneous hyperalgesia. Prog Neurobiol 38:397–421

Vandenheede M, Schoenen J (2002) Central mechanisms in tension-type headaches. Curr Pain Headache Rep 6:392–400

21 Management of Tension-Type Headache

Lars Bendtsen[1] · *Christian Lampl*[2] · *Mohammed Al Jumah*[3] · *Rigmor Jensen*[1]
[1]Glostrup Hospital, University of Copenhagen, Glostrup, Copenhagen, Denmark
[2]Headache Center, Konventhospital Barmherzige Brüder Linz, Linz, Austria
[3]KAIMRC/King Saud Bin Abdulaziz University for Health Sciences, Riyadh, Saudi Arabia

Paolo Martelletti, Timothy J. Steiner (eds.), *Handbook of Headache*, DOI 10.1007/978-88-470-1700-9_21,
© Lifting The Burden 2011

Abstract: Management of the acute episode in patients with infrequent tension-type headache (TTH) is often straightforward, but in patients with frequent TTH management is often difficult. Establishment of an accurate diagnosis is important before initiation of any treatment. Nondrug management should always be considered although the scientific basis is limited. Information, reassurance, and identification of trigger factors may be rewarding. EMG biofeedback has a documented effect in TTH, while cognitive-behavioral therapy and relaxation training most likely are effective. Physical therapy and acupuncture may be valuable options for patients with frequent TTH, but there is no robust scientific evidence for efficacy.

Simple analgesics and nonsteroidal anti-inflammatory drugs are recommended for treatment of episodic TTH. Combination analgesics containing caffeine are drugs of second choice. Triptans, muscle relaxants, and opioids should not be used. It is crucial to avoid frequent and excessive use of analgesics to prevent the development of medication-overuse headache. The tricyclic antidepressant amitriptyline is drug of first choice for the prophylactic treatment of chronic TTH. Mirtazapine and venlafaxine are drugs of second choice. The efficacy of the prophylactic drugs is often limited and treatment may be hampered by side effects.

Introduction

Tension-type headache (TTH) is the most prevalent and costly headache with a major impact on quality of life for the individual and society (Stovner et al. 2007). It is a complex disorder where a range of heterogeneous mechanisms are likely to play a role (Bendtsen and Jensen 2006). Management of the acute episode in patients with infrequent TTH is often straightforward, but in patients with frequent headaches, biological mechanisms, in particular increased sensitivity of the central nervous system (Bendtsen 2000), as well as psychological mechanisms often complicate management. It is important to consider which mechanisms may be important for the individual patient and to tailor the treatment accordingly (Bendtsen et al. 2010).

A correct diagnosis should be assured by a clinical neurological examination, description of symptoms and pain quality, as well as by means of a headache diary (Russell et al. 1992) recorded over at least 4 weeks. The diary may also reveal triggers and medication overuse, and it will establish the baseline against which to measure the efficacy of treatments. Identification of a high intake of analgesics is essential as other treatments are largely ineffective in the presence of medication overuse (Katsarava and Jensen 2007). Significant comorbidity, e.g., anxiety or depression, should be identified and treated concomitantly.

In general, non-pharmacological management should always be considered in TTH (Bendtsen et al. 2010). When it comes to pharmacological management, the general rule is that patients with episodic TTH (Headache Classification Subcommittee of the International Headache Society 2004) are treated with symptomatic (acute) drugs, while prophylactic drugs should be considered in patients with very frequent episodic TTH and in patients with chronic TTH (Headache Classification Subcommittee of the International Headache Society 2004). Analgesics are often ineffective in patients with chronic TTH. Furthermore, their frequent use produces risk of medication-overuse headache (Katsarava and Jensen 2007) as well as systemic side effects and toxicity.

It should be explained to the patient that frequent TTH only seldom can be cured, but that a meaningful improvement can be obtained with the combination of nondrug and drug treatments. These treatments are described separately in the following but should go hand in hand.

Established Knowledge

Non-Pharmacological Management

Information, Reassurance, and Identification of Trigger Factors

Nondrug management should be considered for all patients with TTH and is widely used. However, the scientific evidence for efficacy of most treatment modalities is sparse (Bendtsen et al. 2010). The very fact that the physician takes the problem seriously may have a therapeutic effect, particularly if the patient is concerned about serious disease, e.g., brain tumor, and can be reassured by thorough examination. Identification of trigger factors should be performed, since coping with triggers may be of value (Martin and MacLeod 2009). The most frequently reported triggers for TTH are stress (mental or physical), irregular or inappropriate meals, high intake or withdrawal of coffee and other caffeine-containing drinks, dehydration, sleep disorders, too much or too little sleep, reduced or inappropriate physical exercise, psycho-behavioral problems as well as variations during the female menstrual cycle and hormonal substitution (Rasmussen et al. 1992; Ulrich et al. 1996; Nash and Thebarge 2006). It has been demonstrated that stress induces more headache in patients with chronic TTH than in healthy controls probably through hyperalgesic effects on already sensitized pain pathways (Cathcart et al. 2010).

Information about the nature of the disease is important. It can be explained that muscle pain can lead to a disturbance of the brain's pain-modulating mechanisms (Bendtsen 2000; Fumal and Schoenen 2008; Bendtsen and Jensen 2009), so that normally innocuous stimuli are perceived as painful, with secondary perpetuation of muscle pain. The prognosis in the longer run was found to be favorable in a population-based 12-year epidemiological follow-up study, since approximately half of all individuals with frequent or chronic TTH had remission of their headaches (Lyngberg et al. 2005). It is not known whether the same is true for individuals who seek medical consultation.

Psycho-Behavioral Treatments

A large number of psycho-behavioral treatment strategies have been used to treat chronic TTH. EMG biofeedback, cognitive-behavioral therapy, and relaxation training have been investigated the most. However, only few trials have been performed controlled with sufficient power and clear outcome measures (Verhagen et al. 2009).

EMG biofeedback. The aim of EMG biofeedback is to help the patient to recognize and control muscle tension by providing continuous feedback about muscle activity (Holroyd et al. 2005). A recent meta-analysis including 53 studies concluded that bio-feedback has a medium-to-large effect. The effect was found to be long-lasting and enhanced by combination with relaxation therapy (Nestoriuc et al. 2008). The majority of the studies included employed EMG-biofeedback. It was not possible to draw reliable conclusions as to whether the effect differed between patients with episodic and chronic TTH.

Cognitive-behavioral therapy. The aim of cognitive-behavioral therapy is to teach the patient to identify thoughts and beliefs that generate stress and aggravate headaches. These thoughts are then challenged, and alternative adaptive coping self-instructions are considered (Holroyd et al. 2005). One study found cognitive-behavioral therapy, treatment with tricyclic antidepressants, and a combination of the two treatments better than placebo with no significant difference between treatments (Holroyd et al. 2001), while another study reported no difference between cognitive-behavioral therapy and amitriptyline (Holroyd et al. 1991). Cognitive-behavioral therapy may be effective but there is no convincing evidence (Silver 2008; Verhagen et al. 2009).

Relaxation training. The goal of relaxation training is to help the patient to recognize and control tension as it arises in the course of daily activities. A recent review concluded that there is conflicting evidence that relaxation is better than no treatment, waiting list, or placebo (Verhagen et al. 2009).

Noninvasive Physical Therapy

Physical therapy is widely used for the treatment of TTH and includes the improvement of posture, massage, spinal manipulation, oromandibular treatment, exercise programs, hot and cold packs, ultrasound and electrical stimulation, but the majority of these modalities have not been properly evaluated (Jensen and Roth 2005). Active treatment strategies are generally recommended (Jensen and Roth 2005). A recent review concluded that exercise may have a value for TTH (Fricton et al. 2009). A controlled study (Torelli et al. 2004) combined various techniques such as massage, relaxation, and home-based exercises and found a modest effect. It was reported that adding craniocervical training to classical physiotherapy was better than physiotherapy alone (van Ettekoven and Lucas 2006). Spinal manipulation has no effect in episodic TTH (Bove and Nilsson 1998) and no convincing effect in chronic TTH (Hoyt et al. 1979; Boline et al. 1995). Oromandibular treatment with occlusal splints is often recommended but has not yet been tested in trials of reasonable quality and cannot be recommended in general (Graff-Radford and Canavan 2005). There is no firm evidence for efficacy of therapeutic touch, cranial electrotherapy, hypnotherapy, or transcutaneous electrical nerve stimulation (Bronfort et al. 2004; Verhagen et al. 2009).

It can be concluded that there is a huge contrast between the widespread use of physical therapies and the lack of robust scientific evidence for efficacy of these therapies, and that further studies of improved quality are necessary to either support or refute the effectiveness of physical modalities in TTH (Bendtsen et al. 2010).

Acupuncture and Nerve Block

The prophylactic effect of acupuncture has been investigated in several trials in patients with frequent episodic or chronic TTH. A review (Silver 2008) and a meta-analysis (Davis et al. 2008) concluded that there is no evidence for efficacy of acupuncture in TTH, while a recent Cochrane analysis (Linde et al. 2009) concluded that there was overall a slightly better effect from acupuncture than from sham acupuncture. Together, the available evidence suggests that acupuncture could be a valuable option for patients suffering from frequent TTH, but more research is needed before final conclusions can be made (Bendtsen et al. 2010). A recent study reported no effect of greater occipital nerve block in patients with chronic TTH (Leinisch-Dahlke et al. 2005).

Conclusions

Nondrug management should always be considered although the scientific basis is limited. Information, reassurance, and identification of trigger factors may be rewarding. EMG biofeedback has a documented effect in TTH, while cognitive-behavioral therapy and relaxation training most likely are effective, but there is no convincing evidence (Bendtsen et al. 2010). Physical therapy and acupuncture may be valuable options for patients with frequent TTH, but there is no robust scientific evidence for efficacy (Bendtsen et al. 2010).

Pharmacological Management

Acute drug therapy refers to the treatment of individual attacks of headache in patients with episodic and chronic TTH. Most headaches in patients with episodic TTH are mild to moderate and the patients often can self-manage by using simple analgesics (paracetamol or aspirin) or nonsteroidal anti-inflammatory drugs (NSAIDs). The efficacy of the simple analgesics tends to decrease with increasing frequency of the headaches. In patients with chronic TTH, the headaches are often associated with stress, anxiety, and depression, and simple analgesics are usually ineffective and should be used with caution because of the risk of medication-overuse headache at a regular intake of simple analgesics above 14 days a month or triptans or combination analgesics above 9 days a month (Olesen et al. 2006). Other interventions such as nondrug treatments and prophylactic pharmacotherapy should be considered. The following discussion on acute drug therapy mainly addresses treatment of patients with episodic TTH, while the discussion on prophylactic drug therapy addresses treatment of chronic TTH.

Acute Pharmacotherapy

Simple analgesics and NSAIDs. Most randomized placebo-controlled trials have demonstrated that aspirin in doses of 500 mg and 1,000 mg (Steiner et al. 2003b) and acetaminophen 1,000 mg (Prior et al. 2002; Steiner et al. 2003a) are effective in the acute therapy of TTH. One study found no difference in efficacy between solid and effervescent aspirin (Langemark and Olesen 1987). There is no consistent difference in efficacy between aspirin and acetaminophen. The NSAIDs, ibuprofen in doses of 200–800 mg, naproxen sodium 375–550 mg, ketoprofen 25–50 mg and diclofenac potassium 12.5–25 mg have all been demonstrated more effective than placebo in acute TTH (Bendtsen et al. 2010). Most, but not all, comparative studies report that the above-mentioned NSAIDs are more effective than acetaminophen and aspirin (Bendtsen et al. 2010). Among the NSAIDs, it has not been possible to clearly demonstrate superiority of any particular drug (Bendtsen et al. 2010).

There are only few studies investigating the ideal dose for drugs used for the acute treatment of TTH. One study demonstrated a significant dose–response relationship of aspirin with 1,000 mg being superior to 500 mg and 500 mg being superior to 250 mg (Von Graffenried and Nuesch 1980). Ketoprofen 25 mg tended to be more effective than 12.5 mg (Mehlisch et al. 1998), while another study found very similar effects of ketoprofen 25 mg and 50 mg (van Gerven et al. 1996). Paracetamol 1,000 mg seems to be superior to 500 mg, since only the former dose has been demonstrated effective. In lack of evidence, the most effective dose of a drug well tolerated by a patient should be chosen. Suggested doses are presented in ● *Table 21.1*.

Combination analgesics. The efficacy of simple analgesics is increased by combination with caffeine 64–200 mg (Bendtsen et al. 2010). It is possible, but not proven, that combinations of simple analgesics or NSAIDs with caffeine are more likely to induce MOH than simple analgesics or NSAIDs alone. It has therefore been recommended that simple analgesics or NSAIDs are drugs of first choice, and that combinations of one of these drugs with caffeine are drugs of second choice for the acute treatment of TTH (Bendtsen et al. 2010). There are no comparative studies examining the efficacy of combination with codeine. Combinations of simple analgesics with codeine or barbiturates should not be used, because use of the latter drugs increases the risk of developing medication-overuse headache (Scher et al. 2010).

Triptans and muscle relaxants. Triptans have been reported effective for the treatment of interval headaches (Cady et al. 1997), which were most likely mild migraines (Lipton et al. 2002), in patients with migraine, but triptans do not have a clinically relevant effect in patients with episodic TTH (Brennum et al. 1996). Muscle relaxants have not been demonstrated effective in episodic TTH.

Conclusions. Simple analgesics and NSAIDs are the mainstays in the acute therapy of TTH (● *Table 21.1*). Paracetamol 1,000 mg is probably less effective than the NSAIDs, but has a better gastric side-effect profile (Langman et al. 1994). Ibuprofen 400 mg may be recommended as drug of choice among the NSAIDs because of a favorable gastrointestinal side-effect profile compared with other NSAIDs (Langman et al. 1994; Verhagen et al. 2006). Combination analgesics containing caffeine are more effective than simple analgesics or NSAIDs alone but are regarded by some experts (Bigal and Lipton 2009) to more likely induce medication-overuse headache. Physicians should be aware of the risk of developing medication-overuse headache as a result of frequent and excessive use of all types of analgesics in acute therapy (Katsarava and Jensen 2007). Triptans, muscle relaxants, and opioids do not play a role in the treatment of TTH.

■ **Table 21.1**

Recommended drugs for acute therapy of tension-type headache (Bendtsen et al. 2010). There is sparse evidence for optimal doses. The most effective dose of a drug well tolerated by a patient should be chosen

Substance	Dose (mg)	Comment
Ibuprofen	200–800	Gastrointestinal side effects, risk of bleeding
Ketoprofen	25	Side effects as for ibuprofen
Aspirin	500–1,000	Side effects as for ibuprofen
Naproxen	375–550	Side effects as for ibuprofen
Diclofenac	12.5–100	Side effects as for ibuprofen, only doses of 12.5–25 mg tested in TTH
Paracetamol	1,000 (oral)	Less risk of gastrointestinal side effects compared with NSAIDs
Caffeine comb.	65–200	See below[a]

[a]Combination with caffeine 65–200 mg increases the efficacy of ibuprofen and paracetamol, but possibly also the risk for developing medication-overuse headache (Bendtsen et al. 2010)

Although simple analgesics and NSAIDs are effective in episodic TTH, the degree of efficacy has to be put in perspective. For example, the proportion of patients that were pain-free 2 h after treatment with paracetamol 1,000 mg, naproxen 375 mg, and placebo were 37%, 32%, and 26%, respectively (Prior et al. 2002). The corresponding rates for paracetamol 1,000 mg, ketoprofen 25 mg, and placebo were 22%, 28%, and 16% in another study with 61%, 70%, and 36% of subjects reporting worthwhile effect (Steiner and Lange 1998). Thus, efficacy is modest and there is clearly room for better acute treatment of episodic TTH.

Prophylactic Pharmacotherapy

Prophylactic pharmacotherapy should be considered in patients with chronic TTH, and it can be considered in patients with very frequent episodic TTH. Comorbid disorders, e.g., overweight or depression, should be taken into account. For many years, the tricyclic antidepressant amitriptyline has been used. More lately other antidepressants, NSAIDs, muscle relaxants, anticonvulsants, and botulinum toxin have been tested in chronic TTH (Bendtsen et al. 2010).

Amitriptyline. The tricyclic antidepressant amitriptyline is the only drug that has proven to be effective in several controlled trials in chronic TTH. Thus, five out of six placebo-controlled studies found a significant effect of amitriptyline (Bendtsen et al. 2010). The two most recent studies reported that amitriptyline 75 mg/day reduced headache index (duration x intensity) with 30% compared with placebo (Bendtsen et al. 1996; Holroyd et al. 2001). The effect was long-lasting (at least 6 months) (Holroyd et al. 2001) and not related to the presence of depression (Bendtsen et al. 1996).

Other antidepressants. The tricyclic antidepressant clomipramine 75–150 mg daily (Langemark et al. 1990) and the tetracyclic antidepressants maprotiline 75 mg daily (Fogelholm and Murros 1992) and mianserin 30–60 mg daily (Langemark et al. 1990) have been reported more effective than placebo. Interestingly, some of the newer more selective antidepressants with action on serotonin and noradrenaline seem to be as effective as amitriptyline with the advantage that they are tolerated in doses needed for the treatment of a concomitant depression. Thus, the noradrenergic and specific serotonergic antidepressant mirtazapine 30 mg/day reduced headache index by 34% more than placebo in difficult-to-treat patients without depression including patients who had not responded to amitriptyline (Bendtsen and Jensen 2004). The efficacy of mirtazapine was comparable to that of amitriptyline reported by the same group (Bendtsen et al. 1996). A systematic review concluded that the two treatments may be equally effective for the treatment of chronic TTH (Silver 2008). The serotonin and noradrenaline reuptake inhibitor venlafaxine 150 mg/day (Zissis et al. 2007) reduced headache days from 15 to 12 per month in a mixed group of patients with either frequent episodic or chronic TTH. The selective serotonin reuptake inhibitors (SSRIs) citalopram (Bendtsen et al. 1996) and sertraline (Singh and Misra 2002) have not been found more effective than placebo.

Miscellaneous agents. There have been conflicting results for treatment with the muscle relaxant tizanidine (Fogelholm and Murros 1992; Murros et al. 2000), while the NMDA-antagonist memantine was not effective (Lindelof and Bendtsen 2009). Botulinum toxin has been extensively studied. It was concluded in a systematic review that botulinum toxin is likely to be ineffective or harmful for the treatment of chronic TTH (Silver 2008).

▣ Table 21.2

Recommended drugs for prophylactic therapy of tension-type headache (Bendtsen et al. 2010)

Substance	Daily dose (mg)
Drug of first choice	
Amitriptyline	30–75
Drugs of second choice	
Mirtazapine	30
Venlafaxine	150
Drugs of third choice	
Clomipramine	75–150
Maprotiline	75
Mianserin	30–60

The prophylactic effect of daily intake of simple analgesics has not been studied in trials that had this as the primary efficacy parameter, but explanatory analyses indicated that ibuprofen 400 mg/day was not effective in one study (Bendtsen et al. 2007). On the contrary, ibuprofen increased headache compared with placebo indicating a possible early onset of medication-overuse headache (Bendtsen et al. 2007). Topiramate (Lampl et al. 2006) and buspirone (Mitsikostas et al. 1997) have been reported effective in open-label studies.

Conclusions. Amitriptyline has a clinically relevant prophylactic effect in patients with chronic TTH and should be the drug of first choice (Bendtsen et al. 2010) (❱ *Table 21.2*). Mirtazapine or venlafaxine are probably effective, while the older tricyclic and tetracyclic antidepressants clomipramine, maprotiline, and mianserin may be effective. A recent systematic review (Silver 2008) concluded that amitriptyline and mirtazapine are the only forms of treatment that can be considered proven beneficial for the treatment of chronic TTH. However, the last search was performed in 2007 before publication of the study on venlafaxine (Zissis et al. 2007).

Amitriptyline should be started at low dosages (10–25 mg/day) and titrated by 10–25 mg weekly until the patient has either good therapeutic effect or side effects are encountered. It is important that patients are informed that this is an antidepressant agent but has an independent action on pain. The maintenance dose is usually 30–75 mg daily administered 1–2 h before bedtime to help to circumvent any sedative adverse effects. A significant effect of amitriptyline may be observed already in the first week on the therapeutic dose (Bendtsen et al. 1996). It is therefore advisable to change to other prophylactic therapy, if the patient does not respond after 4 weeks on maintenance dose. The side effects of amitriptyline include dry mouth, drowsiness, dizziness, obstipation, and weight gain. Mirtazapine, of which the major side effects are drowsiness and weight gain, or venlafaxine, of which the major side effects are vomiting, nausea, dizziness, and loss of libido, should be considered if amitriptyline is not effective or not tolerated. Discontinuation should be attempted every 6–12 months. The physician should keep in mind that the efficacy of preventive drug therapy in TTH is often modest, and that the efficacy should outweigh the side effects.

Current Research

Previous and current research on management of TTH is very limited compared with other major headache disorders, e.g., migraine. There is an urgent need for more research in non-pharmacological as well as pharmacological treatment possibilities to improve the management of this common disorder.

References

Bendtsen L (2000) Central sensitization in tension-type headache – possible pathophysiological mechanisms. Cephalalgia 20:486–508

Bendtsen L, Jensen R (2004) Mirtazapine is effective in the prophylactic treatment of chronic tension-type headache. Neurology 62:1706–1711

Bendtsen L, Jensen R (2006) Tension-type headache: the most common, but also the most neglected, headache disorder. Curr Opin Neurol 19:305–309

Bendtsen L, Jensen R (2009) Tension-type headache. Neurol Clin 27:525–535

Bendtsen L, Jensen R, Olesen J (1996) A non-selective (amitriptyline), but not a selective (citalopram), serotonin reuptake inhibitor is effective in the prophylactic treatment of chronic tension-type headache. J Neurol Neurosurg Psychiatry 61:285–290

Bendtsen L, Buchgreitz L, Ashina S, Jensen R (2007) Combination of low-dose mirtazapine and ibuprofen for prophylaxis of chronic tension-type headache. Eur J Neurol 14:187–193

Bendtsen L, Evers S, Linde M, Mitsikostas DD, Sandrini G, Schoenen J (2010) EFNS guideline on the treatment of tension-type headache – Report of an EFNS task force. Eur J Neurol 17:1318–1325

Bigal ME, Lipton RB (2009) Overuse of acute migraine medications and migraine chronification. Curr Pain Headache Rep 13:301–307

Boline PD, Kassak K, Bronfort G, Nelson C, Anderson AV (1995) Spinal manipulation vs. amitriptyline for the treatment of chronic tension-type headaches: a randomized clinical trial. J Manipulative Physiol Ther 18:148–154

Bove G, Nilsson N (1998) Spinal manipulation in the treatment of episodic tension-type headache: a randomized controlled trial. J Am Med Assoc 280:1576–1579

Brennum J, Brinck T, Schriver L, Wanscher B, Soelberg SP, Tfelt-Hansen P, Olesen J (1996) Sumatriptan has no clinically relevant effect in the treatment of episodic tension-type headache. Eur J Neurol 3:23–28

Bronfort G, Nilsson N, Haas M, Evans R, Goldsmith CH, Assendelft WJ, Bouter LM (2004) Non-invasive physical treatments for chronic/recurrent headache. Cochrane Database Syst Rev 3:CD001878

Cady RK, Gutterman D, Saiers JA, Beach ME (1997) Responsiveness of non-IHS migraine and tension-type headache to sumatriptan. Cephalalgia 17:588–590

Cathcart S, Petkov J, Winefield AH, Lushington K, Rolan P (2010) Central mechanisms of stress-induced headache. Cephalalgia 30(3):285–295

Davis MA, Kononowech RW, Rolin SA, Spierings EL (2008) Acupuncture for tension-type headache: a meta-analysis of randomized, controlled trials. J Pain 9:667–677

Fogelholm R, Murros K (1992) Tizanidine in chronic tension-type headache: a placebo controlled double-blind cross-over study. Headache 32:509–513

Fricton J, Velly A, Ouyang W, Look JO (2009) Does exercise therapy improve headache? A systematic review with meta-analysis. Curr Pain Headache Rep 13:413–419

Fumal A, Schoenen J (2008) Tension-type headache: current research and clinical management. Lancet Neurol 7:70–83

Graff-Radford SB, Canavan DW (2005) Headache attributed to orofacial/temporomandibular pathology. In: Olesen J, Goadsby PJ, Ramadan N, Tfelt-Hansen P, Welch KM (eds) The Headaches. Lippincott Williams & Wilkins, Philadelphia, pp 1029–1035

Headache Classification Subcommittee of the International Headache Society (2004) The international classification of headache disorders: 2nd edition. Cephalalgia 24(Suppl 1):1–160

Holroyd KA, Nash JM, Pingel JD, Cordingley GE, Jerome A (1991) A comparison of pharmacological (amitriptyline HCL) and nonpharmacological (cognitive-behavioral) therapies for chronic tension headaches. J Consult Clin Psychol 59:387–393

Holroyd KA, O'Donnell FJ, Stensland M, Lipchik GL, Cordingley GE, Carlson BW (2001) Management of chronic tension-type headache with tricyclic antidepressant medication, stress management therapy, and their combination: a randomized controlled trial. J Am Med Assoc 285:2208–2215

Holroyd KA, Martin PR, Nash JM (2005) Psychological treatments of tension-type headache. In: Olesen J,

Goadsby PJ, Ramadan N, Tfelt-Hansen P, Welch KM (eds) The Headaches. Lippincott Williams & Wilkins, Philadelphia, pp 711–719

Hoyt WH, Shaffer F, Bard DA, Benesler JS, Blankenhorn GD, Gray JH, Hartman WT, Hughes LC (1979) Osteopathic manipulation in the treatment of muscle-contraction headache. J Am Osteopath Assoc 78:322–325

Jensen R, Roth JM (2005) Physiotherapy of tension-type headaches. In: Olesen J, Goadsby PJ, Ramadan N, Tfelt-Hansen P, Welch KM (eds) The Headaches. Lippincott Williams & Wilkins, Philadelphia, pp 721–726

Katsarava Z, Jensen R (2007) Medication-overuse headache: where are we now? Curr Opin Neurol 20:326–330

Lampl C, Marecek S, May A, Bendtsen L (2006) A prospective, open-label, long-term study of the efficacy and tolerability of topiramate in the prophylaxis of chronic tension-type headache. Cephalalgia 26:1203–1208

Langemark M, Olesen J (1987) Effervescent ASA versus solid ASA in the treatment of tension headache. A double-blind, placebo controlled study. Headache 27:90–95

Langemark M, Loldrup D, Bech P, Olesen J (1990) Clomipramine and mianserin in the treatment of chronic tension headache. A double-blind, controlled study. Headache 30:118–121

Langman MJ, Weil J, Wainwright P, Lawson DH, Rawlins MD, Logan RF, Murphy M, Vessey MP, Colin-Jones DG (1994) Risks of bleeding peptic ulcer associated with individual non-steroidal anti-inflammatory drugs. Lancet 343:1075–1078

Leinisch-Dahlke E, Jurgens T, Bogdahn U, Jakob W, May A (2005) Greater occipital nerve block is ineffective in chronic tension type headache. Cephalalgia 25:704–708

Linde K, Allais G, Brinkhaus B, Manheimer E, Vickers A, White AR (2009) Acupuncture for tension-type headache. Cochrane Database Syst Rev 21(1):CD007587

Lindelof K, Bendtsen L (2009) Memantine for prophylaxis of chronic tension-type headache–a double-blind, randomized, crossover clinical trial. Cephalalgia 29:314–321

Lipton RB, Cady RK, Stewart WF, Wilks K, Hall C (2002) Diagnostic lessons from the spectrum study. Neurology 58:S27–S31

Lyngberg AC, Rasmussen BK, Jorgensen T, Jensen R (2005) Prognosis of migraine and tension-type headache: a population-based follow-up study. Neurology 65:580–585

Martin PR, MacLeod C (2009) Behavioral management of headache triggers: Avoidance of triggers is an inadequate strategy. Clin Psychol Rev 29:483–495

Mehlisch DR, Weaver M, Fladung B (1998) Ketoprofen, acetaminophen, and placebo in the treatment of tension headache. Headache 38:579–589

Mitsikostas DD, Gatzonis S, Thomas A, Ilias A (1997) Buspirone vs amitriptyline in the treatment of chronic tension-type headache. Acta Neurol Scand 96:247–251

Murros K, Kataja M, Hedman C, Havanka H, Sako E, Farkkila M, Peltola J, Keranen T (2000) Modified-release formulation of tizanidine in chronic tension-type headache. Headache 40:633–637

Nash JM, Thebarge RW (2006) Understanding psychological stress, its biological processes, and impact on primary headache. Headache 46:1377–1386

Nestoriuc Y, Rief W, Martin A (2008) Meta-analysis of biofeedback for tension-type headache: efficacy, specificity, and treatment moderators. J Consult Clin Psychol 76:379–396

Olesen J, Bousser MG, Diener HC, Dodick D, First M, Goadsby PJ, Gobel H, Lainez MJ, Lance JW, Lipton RB, Nappi G, Sakai F, Schoenen J, Silberstein SD, Steiner TJ (2006) New appendix criteria open for a broader concept of chronic migraine. Cephalalgia 26:742–746

Prior MJ, Cooper KM, May LG, Bowen DL (2002) Efficacy and safety of acetaminophen and naproxen in the treatment of tension-type headache. A randomized, double-blind, placebo-controlled trial. Cephalalgia 22:740–748

Rasmussen BK, Jensen R, Schroll M, Olesen J (1992) Interrelations between migraine and tension-type headache in the general population. Arch Neurol 49:914–918

Russell MB, Rasmussen BK, Brennum J, Iversen HK, Jensen R, Olesen J (1992) Presentation of a new instrument: the diagnostic headache diary. Cephalalgia 12:369–374

Scher AI, Lipton RB, Stewart WF, Bigal M (2010) Patterns of medication use by chronic and episodic headache sufferers in the general population: results from the frequent headache epidemiology study. Cephalalgia 30:321–328

Silver N (2008) Headache (chronic tension-type). Clin Evidence, pp 1–21

Singh NN, Misra S (2002) Sertraline in chronic tension-type headache. J Assoc Physicians India 50:873–878

Steiner TJ, Lange R (1998) Ketoprofen (25 mg) in the symptomatic treatment of episodic tension-type headache: double-blind placebo-controlled comparison with acetaminophen (1000 mg). Cephalalgia 18:38–43

Steiner TJ, Lange R, Voelker M (2003a) Aspirin in episodic tension-type headache: placebo-controlled dose-ranging comparison with paracetamol. Cephalalgia 23:59–66

Steiner TJ, Lange R, Voelker M (2003b) Aspirin in episodic tension-type headache: placebo-controlled dose-ranging comparison with paracetamol. Cephalalgia 23:59–66

Stovner LJ, Hagen K, Jensen R, Katsarava Z, Lipton R, Scher A, Steiner T, Zwart JA (2007) The global burden of headache: a documentation of headache prevalence and disability worldwide. Cephalalgia 27:193–210

Torelli P, Jensen R, Olesen J (2004) Physiotherapy for tension-type headache: a controlled study. Cephalalgia 24:29–36

Ulrich V, Russell MB, Jensen R, Olesen J (1996) A comparison of tension-type headache in migraineurs and in non-migraineurs: a population-based study. Pain 67:501–506

van Ettekoven H, Lucas C (2006) Efficacy of physiotherapy including a craniocervical training programme for tension-type headache; a randomized clinical trial. Cephalalgia 26:983–991

van Gerven JM, Schoemaker RC, Jacobs LD, Reints A, Ouwersloot-van der Meij MJ, Hoedemaker HG, Cohen AF (1996) Self-medication of a single headache episode with ketoprofen, ibuprofen or placebo, home-monitored with an electronic patient diary. Br J Clin Pharmacol 42:475–481

Verhagen AP, Damen L, Berger MY, Passchier J, Merlijn V, Koes BW (2006) Is any one analgesic superior for episodic tension-type headache? J Fam Pract 55:1064–1072

Verhagen AP, Damen L, Berger MY, Passchier J, Koes BW (2009) Behavioral treatments of chronic tension-type headache in adults: are they beneficial? CNS Neurosci Ther 15:183–205

Von Graffenried B, Nuesch E (1980) Non-migrainous headache for the evaluation of oral analgesics. Br J Clin Pharmacol 10(Suppl 2):225S–231S

Zissis N, Harmoussi S, Vlaikidis N, Mitsikostas D, Thomaidis T, Georgiadis G, Karageorgiou K (2007) A randomized, double-blind, placebo-controlled study of venlafaxine XR in outpatients with tension-type headache. Cephalalgia 27:315–324

22 What to Tell Patients About Tension-Type Headache

Timothy J. Steiner[1,2] · Paolo Martelletti[3]
[1]Norwegian University of Science and Technology, Trondheim, Norway
[2]Faculty of Medicine, Imperial College London, London, UK
[3]School of Health Sciences, Sapienza University of Rome, Rome, Italy

Parts of this contribution have also been published as part of a Springer Open Choice article which is freely available at springerlink.com – DOI 10.1007/s10194-007-0428-1

Paolo Martelletti, Timothy J. Steiner (eds.), *Handbook of Headache*, DOI 10.1007/978-88-470-1700-9_22,
© Lifting The Burden 2011

Abstract: Headache disorders are real – they are not just in the mind.

This chapter summarizes information suitable for communication to patients with tension-type headache on types, symptoms, causes, and treatment strategies. The information is aimed at helping them to understand their headache, their diagnosis and their treatment, and to work with their health-care provider in a way that will get best results for them.

Introduction

Tension-type headache is the common sort of headache that nearly everyone has occasionally. Although never serious, it can make it difficult to carry on entirely as normal. In a few people, it becomes bothersome enough to need medical attention, usually because it has become frequent.

Who Gets Tension-Type Headache?

Tension-type headache affects most people from time to time, but women more than men. It also affects children.

What Are the Different Types of Tension-Type Headache?

Episodic tension-type headache is often referred to as "normal" or "ordinary" headache. It happens in attacks (*episodes*) that last for anything from half an hour to several days. The frequency of these varies widely between people, and in individual people over time.

In about three people in every 100, tension-type headache happens on more days than not. This is *chronic tension-type headache*, which is one of the chronic daily headache syndromes. In some cases, tension-type headache is always present – it may ease but never goes completely. This type of headache can be quite disabling and distressing.

What Are the Symptoms of Tension-Type Headache?

Usually, tension-type headache is described as a squeezing or pressure, like a tight band around the head or a cap that is too tight. It tends to be on both sides of the head, and often spreads down to or up from the neck. The pain is usually moderate or mild, but it can be severe enough to prevent everyday activities. Generally, there are no other symptoms, although some people with tension-type headache dislike bright lights or loud noises, and may not feel like eating much.

What Causes Tension-Type Headache?

Tension-type headache is generally thought of as a headache affecting or arising from muscles and their connections. Its causes appear to be many and varied. However, there are some factors that are more important than others:

Emotional tension: this can be anxiety, or stress.
Physical tension in the muscles of the scalp and neck: this may be caused by poor posture, for
    example when working at a computer, or by lifting a heavy object incorrectly.

What Can I Do to Help Myself?

Relax. Taking a break, having a massage or a warm bath, going for a walk, or taking exercise to get you away from the normal routine may help.

Cope with stress. If you have a stressful job, or are faced with a stressful situation that you cannot avoid, try breathing and relaxation exercises to prevent a possible headache. There are many audiotapes to guide you in these exercises.

Take regular exercise. Tension-type headache is more common in people who do not take much exercise compared with those who do. Try walking wherever possible or take stairs rather than the lift, so that exercise becomes a routine part of your life.

Treat depression. If you feel that you are depressed more often than not, it is important to ask for medical advice and get effective treatment.

Keep a Diary

Diary cards can record a lot of relevant information about your headaches – how often you get them, when they happen, how long they last, and what your symptoms are. They are valuable in helping with diagnosis, identifying trigger factors, and assessing how well treatments work.

Take Painkillers if Needed ...

Simple painkillers such as aspirin or ibuprofen usually work well in episodic tension-type headache. Paracetamol is less effective but suits some people.

... But Not Too Often

Medication only treats the symptoms of tension-type headache. This is perfectly acceptable if you do not get many. To manage frequent headache over the long term, it is better to try to treat the cause.

Always carefully follow the instructions that come with your medication. In particular, do not take painkillers too often because you can give yourself a worse headache from the treatment. This is called *medication-overuse headache.* To avoid this happening, never take medication to treat headache *regularly* on more than 2 or 3 days a week.

What Other Treatments Are There?

If you have frequent episodic tension-type headache, or more so if you have chronic tension-type headache, painkillers are not the answer. They will only make things worse over time. So-called prophylactic medications are an option. Unlike painkillers, you *should* take these every day because they work in a wholly different way. Their purpose is to make you less prone to headache and so prevent headache from even starting.

Your doctor or nurse can advise on the choice of medicines available and their likely side effects. Most were first developed for quite different conditions, so do not be surprised if you are offered a medication described as treatment for depression or epilepsy, or as a muscle relaxant. This is *not* why you are taking it. These medications work in tension-type headache too, as they do in other painful conditions.

If you are taking one of these, do follow the instructions carefully. Research has shown that a very common reason for this type of medication not working is that patients forget to take it.

Because posture sometimes plays a role in tension-type headache, and because of the muscles involved, your doctor or nurse may suggest physiotherapy to the head and neck. This can help some people greatly.

Other nondrug approaches include transcutaneous electrical nerve stimulation (TENS) (which is a treatment for pain), relaxation therapy including biofeedback or yoga, and acupuncture. These are not suitable for everybody, do not work for everyone, and are not available everywhere. Again, your doctor or nurse will give you advice.

Will These Treatments Work?

If the cause is identified and treated, episodic tension-type headache rarely continues to be a problem. Very often, it improves on its own, or the cause goes away, and no further treatment is needed.

For some people, especially with chronic tension-type headache, these treatments do not help or only partially help. If all else fails, you may be referred to a pain clinic that uses a wider range of treatments.

Do I Need Any Tests?

There are no tests to confirm the diagnosis of tension-type headache. This is based on your description of the headaches and the lack of any abnormal findings when you are examined. Be sure to describe your symptoms carefully. Also tell your doctor how many painkillers or other medications you are taking for your headaches, and how often you are taking them.

A brain scan is unlikely to help. If your doctor is at all unsure about the diagnosis, he or she may ask for tests to rule out other causes of headaches, but these are not often needed. If your doctor does not ask for any, it means they will not help to give you the best treatment.

Acknowledgment

The text of this chapter is taken from a leaflet prepared by *Lifting The Burden: the Global Campaign Against Headache*. It was drafted by a small writing group, revised following review by an international panel whose principal responsibility was to ensure worldwide cross-cultural relevance and, finally, checked for ease of comprehension by the Campaign for Plain English. The leaflet is endorsed by the World Health Organization and has been published in *Journal of Headache and Pain* (2007).

References

Lifting The Burden. The Global Campaign to Reduce the Burden of Headache Worldwide (2007) Information for people affected by tension-type headache. J Headache Pain 8(Suppl 1):S30–S31

Part 7

Cluster Headache and Other Trigeminal Autonomic Cephalalgias

23 How Cluster Headache and Other Trigeminal Autonomic Cephalalgias Present

Henrik Winther Schytz[1] · *Cristina Tassorelli*[2] · *Messoud Ashina*[1]
[1]Glostrup Hospital, University of Copenhagen, Glostrup, Copenhagen, Denmark
[2]University Consortium for Adaptive Disorders and Head Pain (UCADH), University of Pavia, Pavia, Italy

Paolo Martelletti, Timothy J. Steiner (eds.), *Handbook of Headache*, DOI 10.1007/978-88-470-1700-9_23,
© Lifting The Burden 2011

Abstract: The trigeminal autonomic cephalalgias (TACs) comprise of cluster headache (CH), paroxysmal hemicrania (PH), and short-lasting unilateral neuralgiform headache attacks with conjunctival injection and tearing (SUNCT). The TACs consist of severe headache attacks accompanied by prominent oculocephalic autonomic features. The TACs occur in both episodic and chronic forms, in which the episodic form is most frequent in CH compared to the predominance of chronic PH and chronic SUNCT. The three TACs can be differentiated from each other according to their attack duration, attack frequency, and therapeutic treatment response. CH has the longest duration of attacks with the lowest daily frequency. PH has an intermediate attack duration and frequency, whereas SUNCT has the shortest attack duration and highest daily attack frequency. CH is much more prevalent than PH and SUNCT, and is also characterized with more frequent nocturnal attacks as well as annual periodicity. CH may be triggered by alcohol and nitroglycerin during a cluster period. In contrast to CH and PH, SUNCT is very often triggered by cutaneous stimuli. A successful response oxygen treatment points to the CH diagnosis, a successful indomethacin-test strongly indicate PH, whereas negative responses following both treatments is likely to be seen in typical SUNCT patients.

Introduction

Cluster headache (CH), paroxysmal hemicrania (PH), and short-lasting unilateral neuralgiform headache attacks with conjunctival injection and tearing (SUNCT) are primary headaches with unilateral pain recently classified as trigeminal autonomic cephalalgias (TACs) (IHS 2004) (❷ *Table 23.1*). TACs can be very disabling conditions with a major impact on the patient's quality of life (May et al. 2006). TACs are accompanied by prominent oculocephalic autonomic features (mostly parasympathetic in nature), other primary headaches, such as migraine and hemicrania continua, may be accompanied by mild autonomic features. CH and PH exist in *an episodic form* characterized by attacks that recur in periods lasting 7 days to 1 year separated by pain-free periods lasting 1 month or longer, but also *a chronic form* occurring for more than 1 year or with short remissions lasting less than 1 month (IHS 2004). The 3 TAC entities can be differentiated from each other according to their attack duration, attack frequency, and therapeutic treatment response.

Established Knowledge

Cluster Headache

Epidemiology

CH is the most common TAC with a reported prevalence ranging from 0.06% to 0.3% (Tonon et al. 2002; Sjaastad and Bakketeig 2003; Torelli et al. 2005; Ekbom et al. 2006; Katsarava et al. 2007). CH mainly affects men with a female to male ratio of about 1:3 (Bahra et al. 2002; Ekbom et al. 2002), even though the number of female cluster headache patients seems to have increased over the years (Ekbom et al. 2002). In men with episodic and chronic CH and women with episodic CH, there is an onset peak at 29–30 years of age. In women, particularly

◻ Table 23.1

Diagnostic criteria for trigeminal autonomic cephalalgias from the International Classification of Headache Disorders (IHS 2004)

Cluster headache
• At least five attacks of severe or very severe unilateral orbital, supraorbital, or temporal pain lasting 15–180 min if untreated
• Headache accompanied by at least one of the following:
– Ipsilateral conjunctival infection or lacrimation
– Ipsilateral nasal congestion or rhinorrhea
– Ipsilateral eyelid edema
– Ipsilateral forehead and facial sweating
– Ipsilateral miosis or ptosis
– A sense of restlessness or agitation
• Attacks have a frequency from one every other day to eight per day
• Not attributed to another disorder
Paroxysmal hemicrania
• At least 20 attacks of headache of severe, unilateral orbital, supraorbital, or temporal pain that lasts 2–30 min
• Headache associated with at least one of the following signs:
– Ipsilateral conjunctival injection or lacrimation
– Ipsilateral nasal congestion or rhinorrhea
– Ipsilateral eyelid edema
– Ipsilateral forehead or facial sweating
– Ipsilateral miosis or ptosis
• Attack frequency of more than five headaches daily for more than one half of the time, although periods with lower frequency may occur
• Attacks are completely prevented by therapeutic doses of indomethacin
• Not attributed to another disorder
SUNCT
• 20 attacks of unilateral orbital, supraorbital, or temporal stabbing or pulsating pain lasting 5–240 s
• Pain is accompanied by ipsilateral conjunctival injection and lacrimation
• Attacks occur with a frequency from 3 to 200 per day
• Not attributed to another disorder

SUNCT short-lasting unilateral neuralgiform headache attacks with conjunctival injection and tearing

the chronic cases, there is a more even distribution of the age at onset across life and relatively more chronic cases after 50 (Ekbom et al. 2002). Interestingly, CH patients are often smokers (85% men and 60% women) and consume more alcohol than the background population (Black et al. 2006). However, there exist no correlation between withdrawal from alcoholic drinks or smoking and changes in the course of CH, even though giving up drinking might favor the onset of remission period in some cases (Black et al. 2006).

Periodicity

One remarkable and fascinating aspect of CH is its periodic pattern, with attacks often occurring at almost the same time every day (Ekbom 1970). Besides the circadian (certain times of day) periodicity, episodic CH can also show a circannual (certain seasons of the year) periodicity (Kudrow 1980; Russell 1981). A well-known feature of CH is that 51% of cluster attacks occur during sleep, with a peak frequency from 4 to 10 AM (Russell 1981). These nocturnal circadian attacks occur during both REM (rapid eye movement) and non-REM sleep periods (Kudrow et al. 1984). Circannual cluster periods have been shown to peak in February and June, which may be related to peaks in the minimum and maximum light hours of the day (Kudrow 1980, 1987).

Attack Characteristics

Typically, a cluster headache attack rapidly increases within 10 min (Torelli and Manzoni 2003) to an excruciating pain, which usually lasts between 70 and 160 min, but may range from 15 min to 3 h (Bahra et al. 2002; IHS 2004). During an attack, the site of pain is predominantly retro-orbital (92%) and temporal (70%) (Bahra et al. 2002). Thus, the pain is predominantly located in areas under the distribution of the first division of the trigeminal nerve. However, the pain might be experienced over a wide area including the forehead, jaw, cheek, upper and lower teeth, and, less commonly, the ear, nose, neck, shoulder (Bahra et al. 2002). Pain is strictly unilateral, indeed only 1% of patients experience a shift of the pain during an attack. However, it must be noted that 18% of CH subjects have reported pain side shift within one cluster period and from one period to the other (Bahra et al. 2002). The pain during cluster headache attacks is extremely intense, boring, pressing, or burning pain (Torelli and Manzoni 2005) and is described as one of the worst known pain experience (Blau 1993). CH patients are restless in up to 93% of cases (Bahra et al. 2002), which therefore has been considered a sensitive and specific parameter of CH. During attacks, patients tend to walk around, sit (or kneel), rock, and clutch the affected side of the head (Blau 1993). Patients may also, in order to alleviate or cope with the excruciating pain, rub their head, apply cold substances to the site of pain, or seek a dark room (Russell 1981).

During the active periods, CH attacks tend to recur several times per day (Bahra et al. 2002), but a high variability exists and therefore the criterion regarding attacks frequency of the IHS classification allows from one every second day to eight per day (IHS 2004). The "volcano" effect of episodic CH is well known, in which attacks are substantially shorter and less severe in the beginning and end of a cluster period than in the middle (Kudrow 1980). Interictal pain has also been reported in up to 50% during active cluster periods (Marmura et al. 2010). Episodic CH is the most frequent form of CH, whereas chronic CH occurs in 10–15% of cases (IHS 2004). However, CH may transform from the episodic to the chronic form (Torelli and Manzoni 2002), even though chronic CH may also occur de novo (primary) (Torelli et al. 2000). Most CH patients experience one cluster period per year lasting a mean of 9 weeks (Bahra et al. 2002), and it has been documented that 67% of CH patients have remissions lasting 1 year or less and 81% have remissions lasting 2 years or less (Kudrow 1980). CH, and likely the other TACs, may remain unrecognized due to a diagnostic delay with a median time between the first episode and the diagnosis of up to 3 years (Van Vliet et al. 2003).

Autonomic Symptoms

During a CH attack, the most frequent autonomic symptom is lacrimation (91%), followed by conjunctival injection (77%), nasal congestion (75%), ptosis or eyelid swelling (74%), and rhinorrhea (72%) (Bahra et al. 2002). Sweating seems to occur only in a minority of attacks (26%) and is difficult to assess clinically (Sjaastad et al. 1981). It has been reported that 3% of patients lack autonomic symptoms (Ekbom 1990), but this can still lead to a CH diagnosis, if a sense of restlessness and agitation is present during a CH attack (IHS 2004).

General Symptoms

Nausea, photophobia, and phonophobia, can be present in CH patients. In a large cohort, 50% of cluster patients reported nausea during an acute attack, and a similar percentage reported at least one episode of photophobia (56%) and phonophobia (43%), which remarkably could be lateralized (Bahra et al. 2002). Moreover, 6% of CH patients have reported typical migraine aura with their cluster headache, in which 36% had a personal history of migraine (Silberstein et al. 2000; Bahra et al. 2002).

Premonitory and Prodromal Symptoms

It has been reported that 8% of CH patients have premonitory symptoms from 1 day to 8 weeks before the onset of a cluster period, which can consist of changes in skin sensation, paresthesia, lethargy, and euphoria (Blau and Engel 1998). More frequently (61% of cases), CH patients are reported to experience prodromal symptoms only minutes before pain, such as mood alterations and sensations (tingling, pulsation) in the area of subsequent pain (Blau and Engel 1998). Thus, the identification of prodromal symptoms in a CH patient might be important for establishing early treatment of an attack.

Neurological Examination

Neurological examination of a CH patient may reveal mild ptosis and miosis on the side of the head, especially during or immediately following the attack, and from time to time impaired trigeminal sensation, although the latter will trigger a search for a lesion. Ipsilateral tenderness of the carotid artery, periorbital swelling, and congestion of the conjunctiva are also noted. During a cluster period, a mild, partial Horner syndrome ipsilateral to the pain is often present.

Triggers

CH attacks may be triggered by alcohol, nitroglycerin, and histamine during cluster periods (Ekbom 1968; Black et al. 2006).

Therapeutic Treatment Response

CH is the only primary headache responding to oxygen therapy. Inhaled oxygen at 100%, 12 L/min, delivered by non-rebreathing face mask at symptom is more likely to result in being pain-free at 15 min than compared to placebo (high-flow air) (78% versus 20%) (Cohen et al. 2009). In addition, CH attacks respond promptly, within 15 min, to 6 mg subcutaneous for a median of 96% of attacks treated (Ekbom et al. 1995). Verapamil in a daily dose of 240–960 mg is the drug of first choice in the prophylaxis of episodic and chronic cluster headache (Evers 2010), whereas chronic CH patients may also respond to prophylactic treatment with lithium (Halker et al. 2010). Controlled trials comparing verapamil and lithium with placebo show efficacy of both substances, with a more rapid action of verapamil (Evers 2010). Treatment of the TACs will be presented in detail in ❷ Chap. 25 Treatment of Cluster Headache and Other Trigeminal Autonomic Cephalalgias.

Paroxysmal Hemicrania

Epidemiology

PH is a rare condition with a prevalence estimated to be about 0.02% (Antonaci and Sjaastad 1989) and compromise only 3–6% of all TACs (May et al. 2006). The female to male ratio in PH has been reported to be 2.4:1 (Antonaci and Sjaastad 1989), which is in contrast to the male preponderance in CH. The mean age of onset is reported to be 37 years with a wide range from 5 to 68 (Cittadini et al. 2008). So far no evidence of genetic etiology exists in PH.

Attack Characteristics

The pain during PH attacks is very severe and most frequently described as sharp (51% of cases) and stabbing (49%), although throbbing (32%) and other qualities have been reported (Cittadini et al. 2008). The pain is usually located in the temporal region and orbital region (77% of cases), but also in the retro-orbital region (61%) (Cittadini et al. 2008). It occurs less frequently in other areas of the head and neck (Cittadini et al. 2008). Unilaterality of pain is a defining criteria of PH and found in 97% of cases (Cittadini et al. 2008). The mean length of the PH attacks is 17 min, and even though the IHS criterion regarding the length of attacks identifies a range between 2 and 30 min, more than half of the patients have the longest attacks lasting more than 30 min (Cittadini et al. 2008). The mean attack frequency per day is 11 with a range of 2–50 per day (Cittadini et al. 2008). As agitation is considered a hallmark of CH, it is interesting that 80% of PH patients are found to be agitated or restless (Cittadini et al. 2008). Furthermore, up to 58% of patients are reported to have mild interictal background, which can make differentiation from hemicrania continua difficult, but is usually attributed to co-occurrence of migraine, medication overuse (Cittadini et al. 2008).

In contrast to CH, PH patients do *not* appear to have any circadian or circannual periodicity (Cittadini et al. 2008). PH may show a chronic and an episodic pattern, but in contrast to CH, most PH patients (80%) suffer from the chronic form (Antonaci and Sjaastad 1989). In episodic PH, the duration of the headache phase ranges from 2 weeks to 5 months, with remission phases from 1 to 36 months (Newman and Lipton 1997).

Autonomic Symptoms

Lacrimation is the most frequent autonomic feature (87% of cases) during attacks, followed by conjunctival injection (68%), rhinorrhea (58%), nasal congestion (55%), ptosis (55%), eyelid edema (42%), forehead and facial sweating (32%), and miosis (10%). In addition, facial flushing is reported by 55% of patients (Cittadini et al. 2008).

General Symptoms

Up to 39% of PH patients report nausea and/or vomiting during the attacks (Cittadini et al. 2008). Furthermore, 65% of the patients have phonophobia, which is unilateral in 25% of cases (Cittadini et al. 2008). Photophobia is present in 65% of patients, being unilateral in 40% of cases (Cittadini et al. 2008). Interestingly, more than half of the PH patients have a personal history of migraine (Cittadini et al. 2008).

Neurologic Examination

Neurologic examination of a PH patient is most often normal after the cessation of an attack, even though trigeminal sensation might be impaired in some patients (Cittadini et al. 2008).

Triggers

PH attacks are not easily triggered, but stress (26%), nitroglycerin (25%), exercise (23%), alcohol (19%), and neck movement (19%) represent the most frequent known triggers (Antonaci and Sjaastad 1989; Cittadini et al. 2008).

Therapeutic Treatment Response

The IHS criteria require an absolute response to indomethacin in PH (IHS 2004) and therefore an INDO-test is a valid diagnostic tool, as CH and SUNCT are not responsive to this test (Antonaci et al. 2003; Cohen 2007). To rule out incomplete response, an INDO-test should be used in a dose of $\geq$150 mg daily orally or rectally, or $\geq$100 mg by injection, but for maintenance, smaller doses are often sufficient (IHS 2004). Furthermore, PH patients usually show *no* response to oxygen therapy or triptans, in contrast to CH patients (Cittadini et al. 2008).

SUNCT (Short-Lasting Unilateral Neuralgiform Headache Attacks with Conjunctival Injection and Tearing)

Epidemiology

The prevalence of SUNCT is unknown, but the low number of reported cases suggests that it is very rare. In 2006, the National Hospital for Neurology and Neurosurgery in the UK had collected 43 SUNCT cases, which were referred from all over the UK with a population of 59.6 million (Cohen et al. 2006). The female to male ratio has been reported to range 1:1.3–2 (Matharu et al. 2003; Cohen et al. 2006). The mean age at onset of SUNCT has been reported to be 48 (range = 19–75) (Cohen et al. 2006). There is only one reported case in the literature of a family history of SUNCT (Gantenbein and Goadsby 2005).

Attack Characteristics

SUNCT patients present with attacks that appear in one or more of the following three patterns: single stabs, a group of stabs, or a long attack with a "sawtooth" pattern of stabs in which the pain never returns to baseline (Cohen et al. 2006). Mean duration of attack seems to depend on the attack pattern with single stabs lasting 58 s, group of stabs 390 s and "sawtooth" stabs 1,270 s (Cohen 2007). Thus, some attacks appear to be longer than the diagnostic criteria for SUNCT (IHS 2004). The mean attack frequency per day is 57, but it may range from 2 to 600 (Cohen 2007).

Most patients describe the pain during attack as stab-like (67%), but some also describe it as an electric shock, with sharp or shooting quality (Cohen et al. 2006). The majority of SUNCT patients (67%) experience pain located in the eye, but it may also be located in the retro-orbital region (56%), forehead region (37%), or even in other regions of the face (Cohen et al. 2006). One patient in a series of 43 patients has been reported to have atypical bilateral attacks (Cohen et al. 2006). Up to 62% of SUNCT patients are agitated during the attacks (Cohen et al. 2006); therefore, agitation appears to be a general feature of all the TACs. SUNCT patients might have interparoxysmal pain after attacks, especially when having a personal or family history of migraine (Cohen et al. 2006). SUNCT can occur at any time of the day, and unlike cluster headache, it does not show any striking circadian rhythm; only 7% of SUNCT sufferers have nocturnal episodes (Cohen et al. 2006). However, 40% of SUNCT patients have attacks that occur during sleep or wakefulness (Cohen et al. 2006), but this might be triggered by naturally occurring cutaneous stimuli in the face. SUNCT patients might have seasonal variations of their attacks (Irimia et al. 2008b).

The International Headache Classification did not identify an episodic and a chronic form for SUNCT (IHS 2004); however, a recent prospective study conducted on 43 SUNCT patients shows that 30% of them had an episodic SUNCT (Cohen et al. 2006) and that some SUNCT patients might switch from an episodic form into a secondary chronic SUNCT (Cohen et al. 2006).

Autonomic Symptoms

Besides the obligate ipsilateral conjunctival injection and lacrimation associated with SUNCT attacks, 53% of patients show ipsilateral rhinorrhea, 51% ipsilateral ptosis, and 40% nasal blockage (Cohen et al. 2006).

General Symptoms

Nausea, vomiting, photophobia, and phonophobia are not normally associated with SUNCT, although they can be present, especially in patients with a previous or family history of migraine, reported in about half of SUNCT patients (Cohen et al. 2006). The photophobia and phonophobia are usually ipsilateral in SUNCT, as compared to bilateral in migraine (Irimia et al. 2008a).

Neurological Examination

Neurologic examination is often normal in SUNCT patients during and between attacks, except for the documented autonomic signs, which quickly abate when the attack ends. Yet, in a cohort of patients, 30% of SUNCT had abnormal examinations; generally these were sensory abnormalities at the site of attacks, either reduction of sensation or hyperesthesia to pinprick (Cohen et al. 2006). It is important to note that although SUNCT is by definition an idiopathic disorder, patients can present with symptomatic SUNCT caused by various intracranial abnormalities (Cohen et al. 2006) and therefore neuroimaging is very important in order to exclude secondary causes of SUNCT.

Triggers

Most SUNCT patients (74%) report triggerability of attacks from cutaneous stimuli such as touching the face, cold wind on the face, chewing, talking, or other stimuli such as movement of the neck or bright lights (Cohen et al. 2006).

Therapeutic Treatment Response

Interestingly, it has been reported that intravenous lidocaine seems highly effective for short-term prevention, although the effects can last up to 6 months after infusion (Cohen 2007). Lamotrigine up to 400 mg daily has also shown potential as a possible preventive treatment for SUNCT (Cohen et al. 2006). In addition, topiramate and gabapentin have also been suggested to be useful in the treatment of SUNCT (Goadsby et al. 2010).

Differential Diagnosis of Trigeminal Autonomic Cephalalgias

The three TACs can be differentiated from each other according to their attack duration, attack frequency, and therapeutic treatment response (❷ *Table 23.2*). Yet, there is an overlap in attack duration (❷ *Fig. 23.1*) as well as frequency between the three TACs. Furthermore, both SUNCT and PH might have longer attacks than presently stated in the IHS criteria. To differentiate between the TACs, it is necessary to compare all aspects of each headache spectrum to reach a conclusive diagnosis. It is also important to notice that there are case stories of patients with coexisting CH and PH (Shah and Prakash 2009).

There are certain characteristics that are helpful when differentiating between the three TACs. CH has the longest duration of attacks with the lowest daily frequency. PH has an intermediate attack duration and frequency, whereas SUNCT has the shortest attack duration and highest daily attack frequency. Both CH and SUNCT have a male preponderance in contrast to PH, even though this might be of little help in a daily clinical situation. In CH,

◻ Table 23.2
Characteristics of trigeminal autonomic cephalalgias

	Cluster headache	Paroxysmal hemicrania	SUNCT
Prevalence	0.06–0.3%	0.02%	Very rare
Sex ratio F/M	1:3	2.4:1	1:1.3–2
Mean age at onset	29	37	48
Attack duration (mean)	15–180 min (70–160 min)	2–30 min (17 min)	5 s to 4 min (58 s)
Attack frequency (mean)	1–8 day (5)	5–40 day (11)	3–200 day (59)
Chronic/episodic	Episodic (85%)	Chronic (80%)	Chronic (70%)
Pain quality	Boring, pressing, burning	Sharp, stabbing, throbbing	Stabbing, electric shock, sharp
Pain location	Retro-orbital, temporal	Temporal, orbital	Eye, retro-orbital
Triggers	Alcohol, nitroglycerin	Usually not triggered	Cutaneous stimuli
Autonomic features	Yes	Yes	Yes (CI & T)
Migrainers features	Yes	Yes	No
Indomethacin effects	–	++	–
Abortive treatment	Oxygen Sumatriptan s.c.	Indomethacin	Lidocain i.v.
Prophylactic treatment	Verapamil lithium	–	Lidocain i.v. Lamotrigine

SUNCT short-lasting unilateral neuralgiform headache attacks with conjunctival injection and tearing, *s.c.* subcutaneous, *i.v.* intravenous, *CI* conjunctival injection, *T* tearing

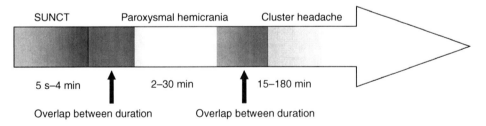

◻ Fig. 23.1
Overlap between attack duration in trigeminal autonomic cephalalgias. The duration of each trigeminal autonomic cephalalgia is specified by the International Classification of Headache Disorders (IHS 2004). *SUNCT* short-lasting unilateral neuralgiform headache attacks with conjunctival injection and tearing (Adapted from Leone and Bussone 2009)

the episodic form is most frequent compared to the predominance of chronic PH and chronic SUNCT. CH also seems to have an earlier age onset compared to PH and SUNCT, although the age variation is large. CH is much more prevalent than PH and SUNCT, and is also characterized with more frequent nocturnal attacks as well as annual periodicity. CH may be triggered by alcohol and nitroglycerin during a cluster period, whereas PH is not very easily triggered.

In contrast to CH and PH, SUNCT is very often triggered by cutaneous stimuli. In all TACs, the pain intensity is severe to very severe and patients are often agitated, even though it is less frequent in SUNCT as compared to CH. CH pain is often located retro-orbitally, whereas SUNCT pain is more often reported in the eye. General symptoms are usually most prominent amongst CH and PH patients as compared to SUNCT. A headache patient might present with a spectrum of head pain symptoms, which do not allow the headache to be classified into one particular TAC entity. In such a case, therapeutic medication trials can be most helpful in establishing a diagnosis. Especially an indomethacin-test and/or oxygen treatment would be highly important as diagnostic tools. Ideally, successful oxygen treatment would point to CH, whereas a successful indomethacin-test would strongly indicate PH, and negative responses following both treatments is likely to be seen in typical SUNCT patients.

Almost half of TAC patients have a history of migraine. For this reason, a headache patient might well have migraine attacks coexistent with their TAC. Furthermore, migraine attacks can resemble TAC features, since 27–73% of migraine patients have been reported to show autonomic symptoms, such as rhinorrhea, lacrimation, and flushing during attacks (Gupta and Bhatia 2007; Obermann et al. 2007). Yet, differentiation of migraine from PH and SUNCT is usually not a diagnostic problem considering that the latter two present with very short attacks of pain associated with prominent autonomic features. CH can be distinguished from migraine due to cluster periods with shorter and often nocturnal attacks associated with agitation – a migraine patient will typically prefer to lie still in bed instead of pacing around as typically seen during a CH attack. Lateralization of photophobia and phonophobia might be helpful in establishing a diagnosis, as these are more prominent features in TACs and relatively uncommon in migraine (Irimia et al. 2008a). Therapeutic intervention might also be helpful, even though a positive treatment response to sumatriptan and indomethacin is expected during a genuine migraine attack (Mett and Tfelt-Hansen 2008).

Trigeminal neuralgia (TN) is a unilateral disorder characterized by brief electric shock–like pains (IHS 2004), which can be challenging to differentiate from SUNCT. Both syndromes are short lasting, might have a high frequency of attacks, can be precipitated by cutaneous stimuli and have a usual onset during middle or old age. However, TN affects the first division of the trigeminal nerve in <5% of cases (IHS 2004), which is the region that most often affects SUNCT patients. TN also often has very short attack duration, less than 5 s, compared to SUNCT. In contrast to SUNCT, TN patients usually have a refractory period, following a painful attack, in which pain cannot be triggered. TN patients can have autonomic symptoms, but these are rare compared to the prominent autonomic symptoms in SUNCT (Matharu et al. 2003). Finally, TN has a female preponderance, which is the opposite in SUNCT (Manzoni and Torelli 2005; Cohen et al. 2006).

There are other primary headaches that might resemble TACs. Primary stabbing headache consists of a single stab or a series of stabs in the distribution of the first division of the trigeminal nerve, which can be misinterpreted as SUNCT (IHS 2004). However, the stabbing attacks last only a few seconds and there are usually no autonomic symptoms. Hemicrania continua is an indomethacin-responsive primary headache with autonomic symptoms characterized by daily and continuous pain without pain-free intervals (IHS 2004). The continuous pain is moderate, but might show exacerbations of severe pain. Thus, hemicrania continua differs from PH because of the continuous pain, and from migraine due to the absolute response on therapeutic doses of endomethacin (IHS 2004). Patients presenting with symptoms resembling CH and other TACs might have intracranial abnormalities causing these pain syndromes. Thus, neuroimaging is an essential part of diagnosing the TACs correctly.

Current Research

With the exeption of CH, the TACs were first officially classified by the International Headache Society in 2004 and based on their low frequency in the general population, there is an ongoing demand for research exploring the epidemiology and symptomatology of these disorders. As an example, short-lasting unilateral neuralgiform headache attacks with cranial autonomic symptoms (SUNA) are classified in the appendix of the ICHD-II (IHS 2004). SUNCT might be a subform of SUNA, which could become established as a TAC in the future headache classification. However, SUNA has rarely been reported (Cohen et al. 2006) and might need to be described in more detail before becoming validated as a TAC in the future classification of headache. An emerging interest in the clinical presentation of the TACs is the lateralization of symptoms (Goadsby et al. 2010). Thus, when present, photophobia and phonophobia are usually ipsilateral in SUNCT (Cohen et al. 2006) and PH (Cittadini et al. 2008), as compared to bilateral in migraine. Furthermore, the cranial autonomic symptoms in CH are also more likely to be lateralized in comparison to migraine patients where symptoms are more often bilateral (Lai et al. 2009). Interestingly, neuroimaging studies have shown hypothalamic activation ipsilateral to the pain in CH; ipsilateral, contralateral, bilateral, or absent in SUNCT; and contralateral in PH (Leone and Bussone 2009). Based on the neuroimaging findings of TAC patients, deep brain stimulation (DBS) has been explored as a possible novel treatment approach. Recently, a prospective crossover, double-blind, multicenter study assessed the efficacy of unilateral hypothalamic DBS in 11 patients with severe refractory chronic CH (Fontaine et al. 2010). Randomized phase findings of this study did not support the efficacy of DBS in refractory CCH, but open phase findings suggested long-term efficacy in more than 50% patients (Fontaine et al. 2010). Furthermore, DBS has also been successfully reported in some patients with PH and SUNCT (Leone and Bussone 2009). Percutaneous radiofrequency ablation of the sphenopalatine ganglion has also been attempted as treatment strategy as the parasympathetic nervous system is likely to be activated during cluster headache attacks. This strategy has been shown to be effective in reducing attack frequency in chronic cluster headache (Narouze et al. 2009). The importance of the parasympathetic nervous system was recently explored in a novel animal model of cluster headache (Akerman et al. 2009). The study demonstrated how oxygen can act specifically on parasympathetic nerve projections to the cranial vasculature to inhibit both evoked trigeminovascular activation and activation of the autonomic pathway, which might occur during cluster headache attacks. Thus, current research on pathophysiology and treatment are all linked to the anatomy and clinical presentation of the TAC, which needs to be explored further in future studies.

References

Akerman S, Holland PR et al (2009) Oxygen inhibits neuronal activation in the trigeminocervical complex after stimulation of trigeminal autonomic reflex, but not during direct dural activation of trigeminal afferents. Headache 49: 1131–1143

Antonaci F, Sjaastad O (1989) Chronic paroxysmal hemicrania (CPH): a review of the clinical manifestations. Headache 29(10):648–656

Antonaci F, Costa A et al (2003) Parenteral indomethacin (the INDOTEST) in cluster headache. Cephalalgia 23(3):193–196

Bahra A, May A et al (2002) Cluster headache: a prospective clinical study with diagnostic implications. Neurology 58(3):354–361

Black DF, Bordini CA et al (2006) Symptomatology of cluster headaches. In: The headaches. Lippincott Williams & Wilkins, Philadelphia, pp 789–796

Blau JN (1993) Behaviour during a cluster headache. Lancet 342(8873):723–725

Blau JN, Engel HO (1998) Premonitory and prodromal symptoms in cluster headache. Cephalalgia 18(2):91–93, discussion 71-2

Cittadini E, Matharu MS et al (2008) Paroxysmal hemicrania: a prospective clinical study of 31 cases. Brain 131(Pt 4):1142–1155

Cohen AS (2007) Short-lasting unilateral neuralgiform headache attacks with conjunctival injection and tearing. Cephalalgia 27(7):824–832

Cohen AS, Matharu MS et al (2006) Short-lasting unilateral neuralgiform headache attacks with conjunctival injection and tearing (SUNCT) or cranial autonomic features (SUNA) – a prospective clinical study of SUNCT and SUNA. Brain 129(Pt 10): 2746–2760

Cohen AS, Burns B et al (2009) High-flow oxygen for treatment of cluster headache. J Am Med Assoc 302(22):2451–2457

Ekbom K (1968) Nitrolglycerin as a provocative agent in cluster headache. Arch Neurol 19(5):487–493

Ekbom K (1970) A clinical comparison of cluster headache and migraine. Acta Neurol Scand 46(Suppl 41): 1–48

Ekbom K (1990) Evaluation of clinical criteria for cluster headache with special reference to the classification of the International Headache Society. Cephalalgia 10(4):195–197

Ekbom K, Krabbe A et al (1995) Cluster headache attacks treated for up to three months with subcutaneous sumatriptan (6 mg). Sumatriptan Cluster Headache Long-term Study Group. Cephalalgia 15(3):230–236.

Ekbom K, Svensson DA et al (2002) Age at onset and sex ratio in cluster headache: observations over three decades. Cephalalgia 22(2):94–100

Ekbom K, Svensson DA et al (2006) Lifetime prevalence and concordance risk of cluster headache in the Swedish twin population. Neurology 67(5):798–803

Evers S (2010) Pharmacotherapy of cluster headache. Expert Opin Pharmacother 11(13):1–7

Fontaine D, Lazorthes Y et al (2010) Safety and efficacy of deep brain stimulation in refractory cluster headache: a randomized placebo-controlled double-blind trial followed by a 1-year open extension. J Headache Pain 11:23–31

Gantenbein AR, Goadsby PJ (2005) Familial SUNCT. Cephalalgia 25(6):457–459

Goadsby PJ, Cittadini A et al (2010) Trigeminal autonomic cephalalgias: paroxysmal hemicrania, SUNCT/SUNA, and hemicrania continua. Semin Neurol 30(2):186–191

Gupta R, Bhatia MS (2007) A report of cranial autonomic symptoms in migraineurs. Cephalalgia 27(1):22–28

Halker R, Vargas B et al (2010) Cluster headache: diagnosis and treatment. Semin Neurol 30(2):175–185

IHS (2004) The international classification of headache disorders, 2nd edition. Cephalalgia 24(Suppl 1): 9–160

Irimia P, Cittadini E et al (2008a) Unilateral photophobia or phonophobia in migraine compared with trigeminal autonomic cephalalgias. Cephalalgia 28(6):626–630

Irimia P, Gallego-Perez Larraya J et al (2008b) Seasonal periodicity in SUNCT syndrome. Cephalalgia 28(1):94–96

Katsarava Z, Obermann M et al (2007) Prevalence of cluster headache in a population-based sample in Germany. Cephalalgia 27(9):1014–1019

Kudrow L (ed) (1980) Cluster headache, mechanism and management. Oxford University Press, New York

Kudrow L (1987) The cyclic relationship of natural illumination to cluster period frequency. Cephalalgia 7(Suppl 6):76–78

Kudrow L, McGinty DJ et al (1984) Sleep apnea in cluster headache. Cephalalgia 4(1):33–38

Lai TH, Fuh JL et al (2009) Cranial autonomic symptoms in migraine: characteristics and comparison with cluster headache. J Neurol Neurosurg Psychiatry 80(10):1116–1119

Leone M, Bussone G (2009) Pathophysiology of trigeminal autonomic cephalalgias. Lancet Neurol 8(8):755–764

Manzoni GC, Torelli P (2005) Epidemiology of typical and atypical craniofacial neuralgias. Neurol Sci 26(Suppl 2):s65–s67

Marmura MJ, Pello SJ et al (2010) Interictal pain in cluster headache. Cephalalgia 30(12):1531–1534. Published online

Matharu MS, Cohen AS et al (2003) Short-lasting unilateral neuralgiform headache with conjunctival injection and tearing syndrome: a review. Curr Pain Headache Rep 7(4):308–318

May A, Leone M et al (2006) EFNS guidelines on the treatment of cluster headache and other trigeminal-autonomic cephalalgias. Eur J Neurol 13(10): 1066–1077

Mett A, Tfelt-Hansen P (2008) Acute migraine therapy: recent evidence from randomized comparative trials. Curr Opin Neurol 21(3):331–337

Narouze S, Kapural L et al (2009) Sphenopalatine ganglion radiofrequency ablation for the management of chronic cluster headache. Headache 49(4): 571–577

Newman LC, Lipton RB (1997) Paroxysmal hemicranias. In: Goadsby PJ, Silberstein SD (eds) Headache. Butterworth-Heinemann, Boston, pp 243–250

Obermann M, Yoon MS et al (2007) Prevalence of trigeminal autonomic symptoms in migraine: a population-based study. Cephalalgia 27(6):504–509

Russell D (1981) Cluster headache: severity and temporal profiles of attacks and patient activity prior to and during attacks. Cephalalgia 1(4):209–216

Shah ND, Prakash S (2009) Coexistence of cluster headache and paroxysmal hemicrania: does it exist? A case report and literature review. J Headache Pain 10(3):219–223

Silberstein SD, Niknam R et al (2000) Cluster headache with aura. Neurology 54(1):219–221

Sjaastad O, Bakketeig LS (2003) Cluster headache prevalence. Vaga study of headache epidemiology. Cephalalgia 23(7):528–533

Sjaastad O, Saunte C et al (1981) Cluster headache. The sweating pattern during spontaneous attacks. Cephalalgia 1(4):233–244

Tonon C, Guttmann S et al (2002) Prevalence and incidence of cluster headache in the Republic of San Marino. Neurology 58(9):1407–1409

Torelli P, Manzoni GC (2002) What predicts evolution from episodic to chronic cluster headache? Curr Pain Headache Rep 6(1):65–70

Torelli P, Manzoni GC (2003) Pain and behaviour in cluster headache. A prospective study and review of the literature. Funct Neurol 18(4):205–210

Torelli P, Manzoni GC (2005) Behavior during cluster headache. Curr Pain Headache Rep 9(2):113–119

Torelli P, Cologno D et al (2000) Primary and secondary chronic cluster headache: two separate entities? Cephalalgia 20(9):826–829

Torelli P, Beghi E et al (2005) Cluster headache prevalence in the Italian general population. Neurology 64(3):469–474

Van Vliet JA, Eekers PJE et al (2003) Features involved in the diagnostic delay of cluster headache. J Neurol Neurosurg Psychiatry 74:1123–1125

24 Mechanisms of Cluster Headache and Other Trigeminal Autonomic Cephalalgias

Sanjay Prakash[1] · Jakob Møller Hansen[2]
[1]Medical College & SSG Hospital, Baroda, Gujarat, India
[2]Glostrup Hospital, University of Copenhagen, Glostrup, Copenhagen, Denmark

Paolo Martelletti, Timothy J. Steiner (eds.), *Handbook of Headache*, DOI 10.1007/978-88-470-1700-9_24,
© Lifting The Burden 2011

Abstract: The trigeminal autonomic cephalalgias (TACs) are a group of primary headache disorders characterized by paroxysmal unilateral head pain that occurs in association with ipsilateral cranial autonomic features. The TACs comprises cluster headache, paroxysmal hemicrania, short-lasting unilateral neuralgiform headache attacks with conjunctival injection and tearing (SUNCT), and short-lasting unilateral neuralgiform headache attacks with cranial autonomic symptoms (SUNA).

The TACs differ in attack duration and frequency as well as the response to therapy. However, there are considerable clinical and therapeutic overlaps among the TACs and it has been hypothesized that all TACs may have a common pathophysiology. Both peripheral and central mechanisms are involved in generation of attacks and trigeminovascular-nociceptive pathways, including trigeminal autonomic reflex are the final pathways for the manifestations of these disorders. The periodicity of TAC attacks, endocrinal abnormalities, and hypothalamic activation suggest that the hypothalamus may play a key role in the pathogenesis of TACs. A number of hypothalamic nuclei and circuits have been suggested for the abnormalities of nociceptive, autonomic, and neuroendocrine functions of TACs, including orexinergic, somatostatinergic, serotoninergic, and opioidergic pathways. The interrelations of these circuits and their relations with the trigeminal autonomic reflex are still to be determined. Dysfunctions in the hypothalamus and its circuits may facilitate inputs on the trigeminovascular system and lead to the various TAC symptoms. Secondary TACs may result from a range of other disorders.

Introduction

The trigeminal autonomic cephalalgias (TACs) are a group of primary headache disorders characterized by paroxysmal unilateral head pain that occurs in association with ipsilateral cranial autonomic features (IHS 2004). These autonomic features include redness (conjunctival injection) and tearing (lacrimation), one-sided nasal congestion or discharge (rhinorrhea), forehead and facial sweating, constriction of a pupil (miosis), as well as drooping (ptosis) and swelling of an eyelid (edema) (IHS 2004).

The TACs comprises four separate disorders: cluster headache (CH), paroxysmal hemicrania (PH), short-lasting unilateral neuralgiform headache attacks with conjunctival injection and tearing (SUNCT), and short-lasting unilateral neuralgiform headache attacks with cranial autonomic symptoms (SUNA) (❷ *Table 24.1*).

CH was probably first described in detail in 1641 by Nicolaas Tulp (Koehler 1993). However, both PH (Sjaastad and Dale 1974) and SUNCT (Sjaastad et al. 1978, 1989) are newly described entities, and SUNA was presented in the appendix of the ICHD-II (IHS 2004). Only a few cases of SUNCT and SUNA are described in the literature (Cohen 2007), therefore any similarities or dissimilarities should be judged very cautiously. From a mechanistic point of view, the pathophysiology of the TACs is likely to be related to other primary headaches, such as migraine, due to the trigeminal distribution of the pain.

The TACs differ in attack duration and frequency as well as the response to therapy (IHS 2004). A recent review (Leone and Bussone 2009), however, suggests that a significant overlap exists among the TACs in relation to attack duration and frequency (❷ *Fig. 24.1*).

Proper randomized controlled trials (level of evidence I) in TACs have only been conducted in cluster headache, but considerable overlap might exist in treatment responses among the TACs. A response to indomethacin is a cardinal feature for a diagnosis of PH (Cittadini et al. 2008), but a recent review (Prakash et al. 2010) suggests that even CH patients may show

Table 24.1

Overview of the trigeminal autonomic cephalalgias (TACs).

	Prevalence/ 1-year incidence	Debut (years)	Male/ female	Attack frequency	Duration	Pain sensation	Treatment	References
Cluster headache	124/ 100,000/ and 53/ 100,000	20–40	4:1	1–8/day	15–180 min	Severe or very severe unilateral orbital, supraorbital, and/or temporal. Often nightly attacks	Subcutaneous sumatriptan and high-flow inhaled oxygen	(Fischera et al. 2008; Cohen et al. 2009)
Paroxysmal hemicrania	0.5/1,000 and 0.1/ 100,000	34	1:3	>5/day Up to 2–40 attacks/day	2–30 min	Unilateral, always affects the same side, often oculo-fronto-temporal	Absolute effectiveness of indomethacin	(Sjaastad et al. 1980; Antonaci and Sjaastad 1989; IHS 2004; Koopman et al. 2009)
SUNCT	6.6/ 100,000/ and 1.2/ 100,000	50	2:1	1–200/day	5–250 s	Unilateral orbital, supraorbital, or temporal stabbing or pulsating. Attacks are much briefer than in any other TAC	Difficult. Lamotrigene, topiramate, and gabapentin might be helpful	(Goadsby and Lipton 1997; Matharu et al. 2003; Cohen et al. 2006b; Williams and Broadley 2008)
SUNA	6.6/100,000 and 1.2/ 100,000	50	1:2	≥1/day for more than half of the time	2 s–10 min	Unilateral orbital, supraorbital, or temporal stabbing or pulsating. No refractory period follows attacks triggered from trigger areas	Difficult. Lamotrigene, topiramate, and gabapentin might be helpful	(IHS 2004; Cohen et al. 2006b; Williams and Broadley 2008)

SUNCT short-lasting unilateral neuralgiform headache attacks with conjunctival injection and tearing, *SUNA* short-lasting unilateral neuralgiform headache attacks with cranial autonomic symptoms

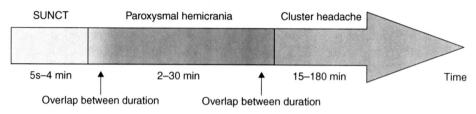

◻ Fig. 24.1

Overlap between attack duration in trigeminal autonomic cephalalgias. The duration of the trigeminal autonomic cephalalgia as specified by the International Classification of Headache Disorders (IHS 2004). *SUNCT* short-lasting unilateral neuralgiform headache attacks with conjunctival injection and tearing (Reproduced with permissions from Leone and Bussone 2009)

a response to indomethacin, though the response may not be as immediate as found in PH and larger doses of indomethacin might be needed in CH.

Verapamil and topiramate (drugs for CH prophylaxis) may be effective in PH and SUNCT (Shabbir and McAbee 1994; Matharu et al. 2002; Narbone et al. 2005; Camarda et al. 2008). Hypothalamic stimulation may have an effect on all three types of TACs (Leone and Bussone 2009). The lack of response to oxygen in PH and SUNCT may be because the duration of attacks are too brief to have any significant effect.

The typical circadian and circannual periodicity of CH attacks are usually not described in relation to PH and SUNCT. This could be because of the chronic nature of PH and SUNCT, as periodicity (especially circannual) cannot be defined even in a chronic variety of CH, especially chronic CH without any remission period. The periodicity of CH generally becomes less evident after a few years (Dodick et al. 2000). Predictability of nocturnal attack onset was noted only in about 70% of patients with CH. The predictability for day attack was 41% for episodic CH and 25% for chronic CH (Bahra et al. 2002). Nevertheless, seasonal variation has been reported even with episodic PH (Sio 2004) and SUNA (Baldacci et al. 2009).

Most of the pathophysiological studies on TACs have been done in CH. The literature is relatively sparse on PH, SUNCT, and SUNA. However, because of the considerable clinical and therapeutic overlaps among the TACs, it can be hypothesized that all three TACs would share a common pathophysiology.

Established Knowledge

Genetic Predisposition

To date, no molecular genetic clues have been identified for TACs but a number of studies suggest a genetic predisposition for CH (Russell et al. 1995a; Leone et al. 2001). In a study by El Amrani et al., all first-degree relatives of cluster headache patients were directly interviewed by a physician, and the population relative risk was estimated at 17.6 (10.2–24.9) (95% CI) (El Amrani et al. 2002). Several transmission patterns have been suggested for familial CH, including autosomal dominant inheritance pattern with low penetrance (Russell et al. 1995b), but autosomal recessive or multifactorial pattern has also been suggested in a few families (De Simone et al. 2003; Russell 2004). Genetic factors might affect age at onset of familial CH in women (Torelli and Manzoni 2003). Identification of genes for cluster headache is likely to be difficult because most families reported have few affected members and genetic heterogeneity is likely (Russell 2004).

There are only a few case reports of familial PH (Cohen et al. 2006a) or SUNCT (Gantenbein and Goadsby 2005) and so far no genetic predisposition has been suggested.

Central Mechanisms

Clinical Evidences

Cluster headache shows a typical circadian and circannual periodicity (Pringsheim 2002). Nightly attacks, with severe pain causing awakening during rapid eye movement (Dexter and Weitzman 1970), point toward the involvement of the hypothalamus, especially suprachiasmatic nucleus (SCN) (Overeem et al. 2002).

A typical behavior (restlessness) during attacks of CH also indicates brain dysfunction, especially hypothalamus (Torelli and Manzoni 2005). The presence of marked cranial autonomic features in the TACs suggests disinhibition of trigeminal autonomic reflex by the hypothalamus. The trigeminal autonomic reflex (TAR) accounts for some of the autonomic symptoms of TACs (❷ Fig. 24.2). This reflex pathway consists of a brainstem connection between the trigeminal nerve and facial parasympathetic outflow (Goadsby and Lipton 1997).

Biochemical Evidences

Based on its integrative role in rhythm regulation of the autonomic nervous system, the hypothalamus could be importantly involved in TAC pathogenesis (Medina et al. 1979). A number of neuroendocrinological observations support this hypothesis. Melatonin, a pineal hormone, is a marker of circadian rhythms (Mirick et al. 2008) and during cluster periods the 24-h plasma melatonin level is reduced, and alterations in the timing of peak and trough levels are observed (Chazot et al. 1984; Waldenlind et al. 1987). This suggests involvement of the hypothalamus–pineal gland connection (Stillman and Spears 2008; Waldenlind and Bussone 2006). However, reduced melatonin levels are probably not direct disease causative, as melatonin as adjunctive therapy did not improve the clinical outcome (Pringsheim et al. 2002).

The circadian production of cortisol, ACTH, and growth hormone is also altered in CH (Meyer et al. 2007). The reduced response of cortisol to the ovine corticotrophin-releasing hormone and insulin-induced hypoglycemia both in cluster periods and the remission phases indicate abnormality in the hypothalamic–pituitary–adrenal (HPA) axis. The reduced response of cortisol to m-chlorophenylpiperazine (5-HT1A/2 C agonist) further suggests serotoninergic dysfunction in the hypothalamus (Stillman and Spears 2008; Waldenlind and Bussone 2006).

Low testosterone levels with a phase shift of the morning peak have been noted in both episodic and chronic CH (Facchinetti et al. 1986). A reduced TSH response to TRH test has been observed in one study (Bussone et al. 1988). The levels of norepinephrine (NE) and its metabolites were reduced in plasma and cerebrospinal fluid in a study and a significant

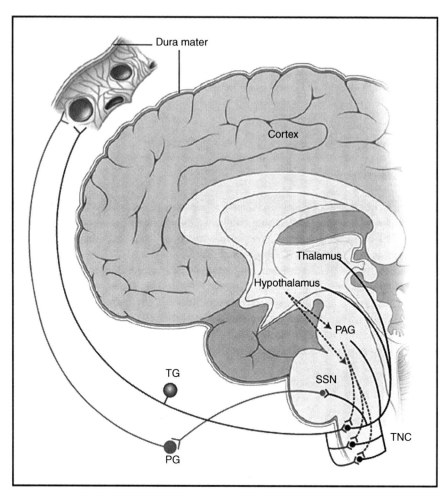

◘ Fig. 24.2
Trigeminal autonomic reflex. Stimulation of the trigeminovascular pathways results in a rebound activation of the cranial parasympathetic outflow, which may account for some of the autonomic symptoms in cluster headache and migraine. The trigeminal nucleus caudalis sends ascending nociceptive projections to the brainstem and higher structures, including the periaqueductal gray and hypothalamus, and in turn receives descending orexinergic modulatory influences from these structures. *PAG* periaqueductal gray, *PG* pterygopalatine ganglion, *SSN* superior salivatory nucleus, *TG* trigeminal ganglion, *TNC* trigeminal nucleus caudalis (Reproduced with permissions from Holland and Goadsby 2009)

correlation was noted between plasma NE levels and individual clinical attack of CH. All these changes have been suggested to be central in origin. A few immunological observations suggest a role in cluster headache for certain lymphocyte subpopulations, certain cytokines, lymphocyte, β-endorphin, and the human leukocyte antigen (HLA) system.

Most of these observations were, however, not corroborated in other studies (Waldenlind and Bussone 2006; Stillman and Spears 2008).

Neuroradiological Evidences

Neuroimaging abnormalities have been reported in all TACs (May and Goadsby 2006). Most studies, however, have been done in CH patients. Neuroimaging modalities for CH and other TACs include functional (functional MRI), structural (morphometry), and biochemical (magnetic resonance spectroscopy) modalities (DaSilva et al. 2007; Matharu and May 2008).

A PET study, done in four nitroglycerine-triggered cluster attacks, showed activation in the structure of the pain neuromatrix, especially in the anterior cingulate cortex and the temporal cortex (Hsieh et al. 1996). Subsequent PET studies also revealed activation of the ipsilateral posterior-inferior hypothalamic gray matter (May et al. 2000).

Structure neuroimaging, using voxel-based morphometry (May et al. 1999), have shown an increase in volume of the post-hypothalamic gray matter in patients with CH. The area of structural abnormality is almost identical to the area of activation observed during an attack in the PET study. A few earlier studies failed to demonstrate hypothalamic activation in patients with spontaneous and glyceryl trinitrate–induced migraine (Weiller et al. 1995; Cao et al. 2002; Afridi et al. 2005a, b) and hypothalamic activation was considered specific for CH. In a recent study of spontaneous attacks of migraine without aura, activation was reported in the midbrain, pons, and hypothalamus (Denuelle et al. 2007).

PET study in patients with PH (Matharu et al. 2006) has demonstrated activation of contralateral posterior hypothalamus, ventral midbrain, red nucleus, and substantia nigra. The activation pattern in neuroimaging studies of SUNCT is highly variable (Cohen 2007). In a BOLD contrast–magnetic resonance imaging study of patients with SUNCT, hypothalamic activation ipsilateral to the pain, similar to CH, was reported. In other functional study, there was hypothalamic activation bilaterally in five and contralaterally (like PH) in two out of the nine patients with SUNCT. Two SUNCT patients had ipsilateral negative activation. In a recent observation (Auer et al. 2009), strong brainstem activation without the activation of the hypothalamus (like migraine) was noted during the pain attacks.

Although, abnormalities were noted in multiple neuronal structures in CH and other TACs in the neuroimaging, the findings were more consistent in the hypothalamus and the inferior posterior gray matter. This may explain the autonomic and circadian features of these disorders, as well as the pain characteristics (Da Silva et al. 2007).

Electrophysiological Evidences

Electrophysiological data suggest that central disinhibition of the trigeminal nociceptive system is important in CH (van Vliet et al. 2003). The impairment of the pain control system might even be associated with periodic failure of the mechanisms involved in the organization of biological rhythms (Nappi et al. 2002).

A significant abnormality in auditory-evoked potentials, suggesting impairment in the central transmission, was noted in a few studies in CH patients. Impairment in visually evoked event-related potentials (ERPs) and abnormalities in cognitive processing via visually evoked ERPs have also been observed in other studies (Holle et al. 2009).

Antonaci et al. reported that PH patients had reduced pain thresholds, reduced corneal reflex thresholds, and normal blink reflexes (Antonaci et al. 1994). Another electrophysiological study compared visually evoked event-related potentials in CH patients with PH and controls and found no changes in visually evoked ERPs in patients with PH (Evers et al. 1997). All these observations are supportive of higher brain abnormalities in CH patients.

Therapeutic Evidences

Proper randomized controlled trials (level of evidence I) have only been conducted in cluster headache, where both oxygen treatment and triptans have shown efficacy (Sumatriptan Cluster Headache Study Group 1991; Cittadini et al. 2006; Cohen et al. 2009). A Cochrane review reported that zolmitriptan and sumatriptan are effective in the acute treatment of cluster headaches (Law et al. 2010), while another systematic review reported only weak evidence for hyperbaric and normobaric oxygen therapy; but this was based on only four small trials (Bennett et al. 2008).

Each TAC shows responsiveness to different treatments (Lenaerts 2008) that suggest different pathophysiological mechanisms. Some overlap, however, have been described.

A positive treatment response to indomethacin is diagnostic for paroxysmal hemicrania (IHS 2004), but CH patients may also respond favorably (Prakash et al. 2010). Sumatriptan is an effective drug for aborting cluster headache attacks (Sumatriptan Cluster Headache Study Group 1991) and possibly in PH (Pascual and Quijano 1998). Sumatriptan was effective in terminating CH attacks even after resection of the trigeminal nerve (Matharu and Goadsby 2002). Stimulation of 5-HT1B/D receptors in the ventrolateral periaqueductal gray matter decreases the excitability of neurons in the trigeminal nucleus caudalis (Bartsch et al. 2004a), and in CH and other primary headache disorders, sumatriptan impairs GH, prolactin, and ACTH secretion (Rainero et al. 2001; Pinessi et al. 2003), suggesting a central site of action for sumatriptan.

Lithium and verapamil, the first-line preventive therapy for CH (Leone et al. 2009), are also known to have central effects. Lithium is known to accumulate in the hypothalamus. A few observations have demonstrated an increased activity of the cerebral serotonergic neurons by the Lithium. Verapamil can modulate the central neurons via interactions with muscarinic, serotoninergic, and dopaminergic receptors (Bussone 2008).

Deep brain stimulation (DBS) of posterior hypothalamus in drug-resistant chronic CH also improves the structure and quality of sleep (Vetrugno et al. 2007). Hypothalamic stimulation can improve both chronic CH (Leone et al. 2001), SUNCT (Leone et al. 2005), and PH (Walcott et al. 2009); for a review see Goadsby (2007).

These observations suggest that the pain and other features of CH probably directly arise from the hypothalamus. However, continuous stimulation for few weeks or months is essential to produce benefit. Acute stimulation is unable to prevent ongoing CH attacks (Leone et al. 2006). These suggest a possibility of complex mechanisms in relieving headache by hypothalamic stimulation. This may involve the resetting of a complex circuit including brain structures additional to the trigeminal system, hypothalamus, and connections between them.

Recently, the less invasive technique of occipital nerve stimulation (ONS) has shown promise in drug-refractory chronic cluster headache. In a prospective pilot study ONS was found effective in the highly problematic patient group with drug-resistant chronic cluster headache (Magis et al. 2007). The authors suggested that the reason for the time lag of almost 2 months between implantation and significant clinical improvement was due to slow neuromodulatory processes at the level of upper brain stem or diencephalic centers.

A similar study on intractable chronic cluster headache reported improvement in 10 of 14 patients (Burns et al. 2009).

Relief by vagus nerve stimulation (VNS) in drug-resistant chronic CH is another indicator of central mechanism. VNS has the capability to influence various areas of the brain, including hypothalamus and other regions of the pain neuromatrix (Broggi et al. 2009).

Peripheral Mechanisms

For more than 40 years, CH was considered as a vascular headache, suggesting vasodilatation of cranial vasculature as the main mechanism for the generation of headache. The characteristic pulsating pain and the relief by vasoconstrictor agents support involvement of vascular factors. Stretching of the trigeminal nerve endings surrounding the internal carotid artery were suggested as the source of pain in CH patients. Vasodilatation of intracranial vessels ipsilateral to pain has been demonstrated in a few observations (Lance and Goadsby 2005). An MRA study on neurovascular mechanisms of trigeminal sensation, however, suggested that the pain drives changes in vessel caliber in migraine and cluster headache, not vice versa (May et al. 2001). The same group performed a highly interesting PET study in cluster patients, and reported that the dilatation of cranial vessels observed in spontaneous attacks could also be induced by GTN and capsaicin injection. They therefore suggested that vasodilatation is not specific to any particular headache syndrome but generic to cranial neurovascular activation, probably mediated by the trigemino-parasympathetic reflex (May et al. 2000).

Increased concentrations of calcitonin gene-related peptide and vasoactive intestinal polypeptide in the jugular vein during attacks of CH (Goadsby and Edvinsson 1994) and PH (Goadsby and Edvinsson 1996) suggest a possibility of trigeminovascular involvement.

The sterile inflammation of the cavernous sinus is another proposed peripheral mechanism for the genesis of pain in CH. This assumption is based on findings of inflammation on orbital phlebography. These orbital phlebographies showed ipsilateral narrowing of the superior ophthalmic vein and a partial occlusion of the cavernous sinus suggestive of a venous vasculitis (Hannerz 1991). Increased activity in the areas of cavernous sinus was demonstrated in a few patients with CH by single-photon emission computerized tomography (SPECT) scanning. Moreover, significantly elevated cytokine interleukin-2 (IL-2) has been reported during active periods of CH. IL-2 is known to activate the hypothalamus (Empl et al. 2003). A response to steroid in aborting CH further supported inflammation theory (Shapiro 2005). However, raised IL-2 and a response to steroid may not be specific for inflammation of the orbit and inflammatory process may be even in central neuronal structures.

The efficacy of sumatriptan during attacks is supposed to be because of its action on 5-HT1D and 5-HT1B receptors at trigeminal nerve endings and on the walls of vessels. The improvement of pain after surgical lesions of the nerve further supports a peripheral hypothesis. Narouze et al. (2009) suggested that sphenopalatine ganglion radiofrequency ablation might be an effective modality of treatment for patients with intractable chronic cluster headaches. Sphenopalatine ganglion block has also been suggested as an alternative in drug-resistant PH (Morelli et al. 2010). Jarrar et al. (2003) demonstrated trigeminal nerve section as an effective treatment with acceptable morbidity for a carefully selected group of patients.

Secondary TACs may provide important evidence to support a role for peripheral structures in the TAC pathophysiology because the clinical features of secondary TACs are almost similar to that of primary forms. It has been suggested that the pain mechanism in secondary

TACs may be related to direct irritation of the pain-sensitive structures and subsequent activation of trigeminal nerve endings in those structures (Favier et al. 2007). The improvement of symptoms after surgical removal of these lesions is another indirect indication for a role of peripheral structures in the pathogenesis of primary CH (Bigal et al. 2003).

However, many conflicting observations or opinions emerged against peripheral mechanisms. Vasodilation is not specific for CH and it is noted in other headache disorders and even in experimental forehead pain (May et al. 2001). Moreover, CH attacks may occur even if vasodilation is prevented by trigeminal nerve sectioning. This suggests, although indirectly, a central dysfunction in the generation of pain in patients with CH. However, to lose all peripheral input, transection of cervical afferents, in addition to transection of trigeminal nerve, is needed.

A response to sumatriptan in aborting an attack even after resection of trigeminal nerve further questions the role of peripheral structure in the pathogenesis of CH (Matharu and Goadsby 2002). The peripheral theory fails to explain many characteristic features of CH and other TACs such as: circadian and circannual periodicity of CH, gender differences among TACs, different responses to therapy, and behavioral abnormalities during an attack in CH and PH.

Interrelations Between Central and Peripheral Mechanisms

The hypothalamus probably plays a major role in the pathophysiology of TACs. However, it is not clear whether the hypothalamus is itself the generator of TACs or whether it is activated in response to a generator situated elsewhere. Even the pathways associated with the hypothalamus for the generation of attacks are not well described. Trigeminal nerve stimulation resulting in cranial outflow has been demonstrated in a few experimental pain studies. Some degree of cranial autonomic symptomatology is a normal physiological response to cranial nociceptive stimuli and cranial autonomic features may be a part of other headache disorders. The distinction between TACs and other headache syndromes is the degree of cranial autonomic activation (Goadsby et al. 2001). The marked cranial autonomic features of TACs may be caused by a central disinhibition of the trigeminal autonomic reflex (TAR) by the hypothalamus, possibly through direct hypothalamic-trigeminal connections (Malick et al. 2000).

Current Research

The understanding of the pathophysiology of primary headache syndromes, including the trigeminal autonomic cephalalgias, has improved tremendously in recent years. Still lacking, however, are good animal models as well as validated human models to enhance our understanding of TAC pathogenesis.

In CH patients, certain polymorphism of the hypocretin receptor 2 gene (HCRTR2) leads to a significantly higher risk of developing CH (OR 1.58–1.75), as reported in a meta-analysis (Rainero et al. 2007). Rainero et al. (2010) have reported a significant association between alcohol dehydrogenase (ADH) 4 gene and CH, an interesting observation, as alcohol is a well-known trigger of attacks in many CH patients (Evans and Schürks 2009).

The molecular basis of CH is yet to be determined. Case control analyses of the calcium channel gene (CACNA1A), the nitric oxide synthase genes (NOS1, NOS2A, and NOS3), and the clock gene have revealed no allelic association (Russell 2004; Rainero et al. 2005). Mitochondrial mutations demonstrated in a few patients are probably chance findings, as it could not be confirmed in the larger case series. A few case reports of concordant monozygotic twin pairs have been reported in the literature (Russell 2004). However, in a Swedish twin population survey, twin concordance was very low. These observations suggest the importance of both genetic and environmental factors for the development of CH (Ekbom et al. 2006).

Abnormalities suggestive of permanent hypothalamic dysfunction have been reported in a recent proton magnetic resonance spectroscopy (^{1}H-MRS) study (Matharu and May 2008). The reduced NAA/Cr and Cho/Cr were significant in episodic CH in comparison with controls and migraine patients (Wang et al. 2006) and reduced NAA/Cr was also noted in both episodic and chronic CH (Lodi et al. 2006).

A few recent observations and hypothesis have been made to determine the pathways and mechanisms responsible for the hypothalamic dysfunctions. The proposed mechanisms or pathways influencing the hypothalamus (and finally TAR and clinical features of the TACs) include the orexinergic, somatostatinergic, and opioidergic pathways.

The orexinergic system has emerged as a main pathway to influence the hypothalamus (Holland and Goadsby 2009). The orexins (A and B), also named hypocretin 1 and 2, are neuropeptides that are mainly synthesized in neurons within and around the lateral and posterior hypothalamus. The orexin-containing neurons project to multiple neuronal systems (Peyron et al. 1998).

The evidence for a role of the orexinergic system in the modulation of CH and other headache disorders is increasing. The widespread projections of the orexinergic system have led to its implication in a variety of functions including nociceptive processing and autonomic and neuroendocrine functions (Holland and Goadsby 2009). Activation of the orexin A receptor elicits an antinociceptive effect, whereas orexin B receptor activation elicits a pronociceptive effect. Injection of orexin A into the posterior hypothalamus resulted in decrease of A- and C-fiber responses to dural stimulation as well as spontaneous activity. However, injection of orexin B elicited increased response to dural stimulation in of A- and C-fiber responses and resulted in increased spontaneous activity. Responses to facial thermal stimulation were also different with both the orexins (decreased with orexin A and increased with orexin B) (Bartsch et al. 2004b). In another experimental animal study, orexin A inhibits both central and peripheral pathways whereas orexin B facilitates central transmission.

In the hypothalamus, orexin projections are found in a number of nuclei, including the suprachiasmatic nucleus (SCN) (Abrahamson et al. 2001). SCN is the main neural oscillator for several circadian and seasonal rhythms of many episodic syndromes. Recently, Brown et al. (2008) suggested that orexins can act directly on many SCN neurons to regulate their firing rate and it may alter SCN neurophysiology and the transmission of information through the SCN to other CNS regions. Orexins also modulate neuroendocrine functions and recent observations suggest that the orexin system could modulate all the neuroendocrine axes (Lopez et al. 2010). It has also been suggested that they can modulate the autonomic nervous system.

The role of melatonin or the pineal gland in CH and other headache disorders is explained by opioidergic dysfunction and other abnormalities (Matharu and May 2008). A recent observation indicates that orexins can modulate even pineal gland and melatonin production (Appelbaum et al. 2009). Neurons containing hypocretin are also related to serotonergic system (Domínguez et al. 2010). Serotonergic nerve endings in the hypothalamus mainly originate from the rostral group of raphe nuclei in the midbrain, the dorsal and median raphe nuclei. Serotonergic input hyperpolarized orexin neurons via the 5-HT1A receptor.

This mechanism has been implicated in the regulation of sleep–wakefulness states. However, it may have role even in CH and other primary headache disorders. Somatostatin, another hypothalamic neuropeptide, is known to modulate neuroendocrine, autonomic, and metabolic functions. Manipulation of the posterior hypothalamic somatostatin receptors modulates trigeminal nociceptive transmission (Holland and Goadsby 2009). Orexins are also known to modulate somatostatin neurons. Octreotide, a somatostatin analog, is effective in the abortive treatment of acute cluster headache (Matharu et al. 2004). Therefore, a possibility of an interaction between somatostatin fibers and TAR exists.

In conclusion, the evidences support a role of the hypothalamus and TAR for the generation of pain in CH and other TACs. A number of hypothalamic circuits have been suggested for the abnormalities of nociceptive, autonomic, and neuroendocrine functions. These circuits may be orexinergic, somatostatinergic, serotoninergic, and opioidergic. The interrelations of these circuits are still to be determined. Orexinergic innervation was, however, found in cell groups of all these fibers/circuits. Therefore, the orexinergic fibers seem to modulate the functions of all the circuits.

A dysfunction in the hypothalamus and its circuits may result in destabilization of various inputs on the trigeminovascular system (including central disinhibition of TAR) leading to various symptoms of TACs. However, in secondary TACs peripheral components may be predominant and initiating factors for the generation of pain and other symptoms (Favier et al. 2007; Leone and Bussone 2009).

References

Abrahamson EE, Leak RK, Moore RY (2001) The suprachiasmatic nucleus projects to posterior hypothalamic arousal systems. NeuroReport 12:435–440

Afridi SK, Giffin NJ, Kaube H et al (2005a) A positron emission tomography study in spontaneous migraine. Arch Neurol 62:1270–1275

Afridi SK, Matharu MS, Lee L et al (2005b) A PET study exploring the laterality of brainstem activation in migraine using glyceryl trinitrate. Brain 128:932–939

Antonaci F, Sjaastad O (1989) Chronic paroxysmal hemicrania (CPH): a review of the clinical manifestations. Headache 29:648–656

Antonaci F, Sandrini G, Danilov A, Sand T (1994) Neurophysiological studies in chronic paroxysmal hemicrania and hemicrania continua. Headache 34:479–483

Appelbaum L, Wang GX, Maro GS, Mori R, Tovin A, Marin W, Yokogawa T, Kawakami K, Smith SJ, Gothilf Y, Mignot E, Mourrain P (2009) Sleep-wake regulation and hypocretin-melatonin interaction in zebrafish. Proc Natl Acad Sci USA 106(51):21942–21947

Auer T, Janszky J, Schwarcz A, Dóczi T, Trauninger A, Alkonyi B, Komoly S, Pfund Z (2009) Attack-related brainstem activation in a patient with SUNCT syndrome: an ictal fMRI study. Headache 49:909–912

Bahra A, May A, Goadsby PJ (2002) Cluster headache: a prospective clinical study with diagnostic implications. Neurology 58:354–361

Baldacci F, Nuti A, Lucetti C, Cafforio G, Morelli N, Orlandi G, Bonuccelli U (2009) SUNA syndrome with seasonal pattern. Headache 49:912–914

Bartsch T, Knight YE, Goadsby PJ (2004a) Activation of 5-HT(1B/1D) receptor in the periaqueductal gray inhibits nociception. Ann Neurol 56:371–381

Bartsch T, Levy MJ, Knight YE, Goadsby PJ (2004b) Differential modulation of nociceptive dural input to (hypocretin) orexin A and B receptor activation in the posterior hypothalamic area. Pain 109:367–378

Bennett MH, French C, Schnabel A, Wasiak J, Kranke P (2008) Normobaric and hyperbaric oxygen therapy for migraine and cluster headache. Cochrane Database Syst Rev July 16(3):CD005219

Bigal ME, Rapoport AM, Camel M (2003) Cluster headache as a manifestation of intracranial inflammatory myofibroblastic tumour: a case report with pathophysiological considerations. Cephalalgia 23:124–128

Broggi G, Messina G, Franzini A (2009) Cluster headache and TACs: rationale for central and peripheral neuromodulation. Neurol Sci 30(Suppl 1):S75–S79

Brown TM, Coogan AN, Cutler DJ, Hughes AT, Piggins HD (2008) Electrophysiological actions of orexins on rat suprachiasmatic neurons in vitro. Neurosci Lett 448:273–278

Burns B, Watkins L, Goadsby PJ (2009) Treatment of intractable chronic cluster headache by occipital nerve stimulation in 14 patients. Neurology 72:341–345

Bussone G (2008) Cluster headache: from treatment to pathophysiology. Neurol Sci 29:S1–S6

Bussone G, Frediani F, Leone M, Grazzi L, Lamperti E, Boiardi A (1988) TRH test in cluster headache. Headache 28:462–464

Camarda C, Camarda R, Monastero R (2008) Chronic paroxysmal hemicrania and hemicrania continua responding to topiramate: two case reports. Clin Neurol Neurosurg 110:88–91

Cao Y, Aurora SK, Nagesh V, Patel SC, Welch KMA (2002) Functional MRI-BOLD of brainstem structures during visually triggered migraine. Neurology 59:72–78

Chazot G, Claustrat B, Brun J, Jordan D, Sassolas G, Schott B (1984) A chronobiological study of melatonin, cortisol growth hormone and prolactin secretion in cluster headache. Cephalalgia 4:213–220

Cittadini E, May A et al (2006) Effectiveness of intranasal zolmitriptan in acute cluster headache: a randomized, placebo-controlled, double-blind crossover study. Arch Neurol 63(11):1537–1542

Cittadini E, Matharu MS et al (2008) Paroxysmal hemicrania: a prospective clinical study of 31 cases. Brain 131(Pt 4):1142–1155

Cohen AS (2007) Short-lasting unilateral neuralgiform headache attacks with conjunctival injection and tearing. Cephalalgia 27:824–832

Cohen AS, Matharu MS, Goadsby PJ (2006a) Paroxysmal hemicrania in a family. Cephalalgia 26:486–488

Cohen AS, Matharu MS, Goadsby PJ (2006b) Short-lasting unilateral neuralgiform headache attacks with conjunctival injection and tearing (SUNCT) or cranial autonomic features (SUNA)–a prospective clinical study of SUNCT and SUNA. Brain 129:2746–2760

Cohen AS, Burns B, Goadsby PJ (2009) High-flow oxygen for treatment of cluster headache: a randomized trial. JAMA 302:2451–2457

Da Silva AF, Goadsby PJ, Borsook D (2007) Cluster headache: a review of neuroimaging findings. Curr Pain Headache Rep 11:131–136

De Simone R, Fiorillo C, Bonuso S, Castaldo G (2003) A cluster headache family with possible autosomal recessive inheritance. Neurology 26;61(4):578–579

Denuelle M, Fabre N, Payoux P, Chollet F, Geraud G (2007) Hypothalamic activation in spontaneous migraine attacks. Headache 47:1418–1426

Dexter JD, Weitzman ED (1970) The relationship of nocturnal headaches to sleep stage patterns. Neurology 20:513–518

Dodick DW, Rozen TD, Goadsby PJ, Silberstein SD (2000) Cluster headache. Cephalalgia 20:787–803

Domínguez L, Morona R, Joven A, González A, López JM (2010) Immunohistochemical localization of orexins (hypocretins) in the brain of reptiles and its relation to monoaminergic systems. J Chem Neuroanat 39:20–34

Ekbom K, Svensson DA, Pedersen NL, Waldenlind E (2006) Lifetime prevalence and concordance risk of cluster headache in the Swedish twin population. Neurology 67:798–803

El Amrani M, Ducros A, Boulan P, Aidi S, Crassard I, Visy JM, Tournier-Lasserve E, Bousser MG (2002) Familial cluster headache: a series of 186 index patients. Headache 42:974–977

Empl M, Fordeneuther S, Schwarz M, Müller N, Straube A (2003) Soluble interleukin- 2 receptors increase during active periods of clustermheadache. Headache 43:63–68

Evans RW, Schürks M (2009) Alcohol and cluster headaches. Headache 49:126–129

Evers S, Bauer B, Suhr B, Husstedt BIW, Grotemeyer KH (1997) Cognitive processing in primary headache: a study on event-related potentials. Neurology 48:108–113

Facchinetti F, Nappi G, Cicoli C, Micieli G, Ruspa M, Bono G, Genazzani AR (1986) Reduced testosterone levels in cluster headache: a stress-related phenomenon? Cephalalgia 6:29–34

Favier I, van Vliet JA, Roon KI, Witteveen RJW, Verschuuren JJGM, Ferrari MD, Haan J (2007) Trigeminal autonomic cephalgias due to structural lesions: a review of 31 cases. Arch Neurol 64:25–31

Fischera M, Marziniak M, Gralow I, Evers S (2008) The incidence and prevalence of cluster headache: a meta-analysis of population-based studies. Cephalalgia 28:614–618

Gantenbein A, Goadsby PJ (2005) Familial SUNCT. Cephalalgia 25:457–459

Goadsby PJ (2007) Neuromodulatory approaches to the treatment of trigeminal autonomic cephalalgias. Acta Neurochir Suppl 97:99–110

Goadsby PJ, Edvinsson L (1994) Human in vivo evidence for trigeminovascular activation in cluster headache. Neuropeptide changes and effects of acute attacks therapies. Brain 117:427–434

Goadsby PJ, Edvinsson L (1996) Neuropeptide changes in a case of chronic paroxysmal hemicrania—evidence for trigemino-parasympathetic activation. Cephalalgia 16:448–450

Goadsby PJ, Lipton RB (1997) A review of paroxysmal hemicranias, SUNCT syndrome and other shortlasting headaches with autonomic feature, including new cases. Brain 120:193–209

Goadsby PJ, Matharu MS, Boes CJ (2001) SUNCT syndrome or trigeminal neuralgia with lacrimation. Cephalalgia 21:82–83

Hannerz J (1991) Orbital phlebography and signs of inflammation in episodic and chronic cluster headache. Headache 31:540–542

Holland PR, Goadsby PJ (2009) Cluster headache, hypothalamus, and orexin. Curr Pain Headache Rep 13:147–154

Holle D, Obermann M, Katsarava Z (2009) The electrophysiology of cluster headache. Curr Pain Headache Rep 13:155–159

Hsieh JC, Hannerz J, Ingvar M (1996) Right-lateralised central processing for pain of nitroglycerin-induced cluster headache. Pain 67:59–68

IHS Headache Classification Subcommittee of the International Headache Society (2004) The international classification of headache disorders, 2nd edn. Cephalalgia 24(Suppl 1):1–160

Jarrar RG, Black DF, Dodick DW, Davis DH (2003) Outcome of trigeminal nerve section in the treatment of chronic cluster headache. Neurology 60:1360–1362

Koehler PJ (1993) Prevalence of headache in Tulp's observations medicae (1641) with a description of cluster headache. Cephalalgia 13:318–320

Koopman JS, Dieleman JP et al (2009) Incidence of facial pain in the general population. Pain 147(1–3):122–127

Lance JM, Goadsby PJ (2005) Mechanism and management of headache, 7th edn. Butterworth-Heinemann, Philadelphia, pp 195–252

Law S, Derry S et al (2010) Triptans for acute cluster headache. Cochrane Database Syst Rev 14 Apr (4): CD008042

Lenaerts ME (2008) Update on the therapy of the trigeminal autonomic cephalalgias. Curr Treat Options Neurol 10:30–35

Leone M, Bussone G (2009) Pathophysiology of trigeminal autonomic cephalalgias. Lancet Neurol 8:755–764

Leone M, Russell MB, Rigamonti A, Attanasio A, Grazzi L, D'Amico D, Usai S, Bussone G (2001a) Increased familial risk of cluster headache. Neurology 56:1233–1236

Leone M, Franzini A, Bussone G (2001b) Stereotactic stimulation of posterior hypothalamic gray matter in a patient with intractable cluster headache. N Engl J Med 345:1428–1429

Leone M, Franzini A, D'Andrea G, Broggi G, Casucci G, Bussone G (2005) Deep brain stimulation to relieve drug-resistant SUNCT. Ann Neurol 57:924–927

Leone M, Franzini A, Broggi G, Mea E, Proietti Cecchini A, Bussone G (2006) Acute hypothalamic stimulation and ongoing cluster headache attacks. Neurology 67:1844–1845

Leone M, Franzini A et al (2009) Cluster headache: pharmacological treatment and neurostimulation. Nat Clin Pract Neurol 5(3):153–162

Lodi R, Pierangeli G, Tonon C et al (2006) Study of hypothalamic metabolism in cluster headache by proton MR spectroscopy. Neurology 66:1264–1266

Lopez M, Tena-Sempere M, Dieguez C (2010) Cross-talk between orexins (hypocretins) and the neuroendocrine axes (hypothalamic-pituitary axes). Front Neuroendocrinol 31(2):113–127

Magis D, Allena M, Bolla M, De Pasqua V, Remacle JM, Schoenen J (2007) Occipital nerve stimulation for drug-resistant chronic cluster headache: a prospective pilot study. Lancet Neurol 6:314–321

Malick A, Strassman RM, Burstein R (2000) Trigemino-hypothalamic and reticulohypothalamic tract neurons in the upper cervical spinal cord and caudal medulla of the rat. J Neurophysiol 84(4): 2078–2112

Matharu MS, Goadsby PJ (2002) Persistence of attacks of cluster headache after trigeminal nerve root section. Brain 125:976–984

Matharu M, May A (2008) Functional and structural neuroimaging in trigeminal autonomic cephalalgias. Curr Pain Headache Rep 12:132–137

Matharu MS, Boes CJ, Goadsby PJ (2002) SUNCT syndrome: prolonged attacks, refractoriness and response to topiramate. Neurology 58:1307

Matharu MS, Cohen AS, Boes CJ, Goadsby PJ (2003) Short-lasting unilateral neuralgiform headache with conjunctival injection and tearing syndrome: a review. Curr Pain Headache Rep 7:308–318

Matharu MS, Levy MJ, Meeran K, Goadsby PJ (2004) Subcutaneous octreotide in cluster headache: randomized placebo-controlled double-blind crossover study. Ann Neurol 56:588–594

Matharu MS, Cohen AS, Frackowiak RS, Goadsby PJ (2006) Posterior hypothalamic activation in paroxysmal hemicrania. Ann Neurol 59:535–545

May A, Goadsby PJ (2006) Neuroimaging in trigeminal autonomic cephalalgias. In: Olesen J, Goadsby PJ, Ramadan NM, Tfelt-Hansen P, Welch KMA (eds) The headaches, 3rd edn. Lippincott Williams & Wilkins, Philadelphia, pp 775–782

May A, Ashburner J, Büchel C, McGonigle DJ, Friston KJ, Frackowiak RS, Goadsby PJ (1999) Correlation between structural and functional changes in brain in an idiopathic headache syndrome. Nat Med 5:836–838

May A, Bahra A, Buchel C, Frackowiak RSJ, Goadsby PJ (2000) PET and MRA findings in cluster headache and MRA in experimental pain. Neurology 55:1328–1335

May A, Buchel C, Turner R, Goadsby PJ (2001) Magnetic resonance angiography in facial and other pain: neurovascular mechanisms of trigeminal sensation. J Cereb Blood Flow Metab 21:1171–1176

Medina JL, Diamond S, Fareed J (1979) The nature of cluster headache. Headache 19:309–322

Meyer EL, Marcus C, Waldenlind E (2007) Nocturnal secretion of growth hormone, noradrenaline, cortisol and insulin in cluster headache remission. Cephalalgia 27:363–367

Mirick DK, Davis S (2008) Melatonin as a biomarker of circadian dysregulation. Cancer Epidemiol Biomark Prev 17:3306–3313

Morelli N, Mancuso M, Felisati G, Lozza P, Maccari A, Cafforio G, Gori S, Murri L, Guidetti D (2010) Does sphenopalatine endoscopic ganglion block have an effect in paroxysmal hemicrania? A case report. Cephalalgia 30(3):365–367

Nappi G, Sandrini G, Alfonsi E, Cecchini AP, Micieli G, Moglia A (2002) Impaired circadian rhythmicity of nociceptive reflex threshold in cluster headache. Headache 42:125–131

Narbone MC, Gangemi S, Abbate M (2005) A case of SUNCT syndrome responsive to verapamil. Cephalalgia 25:476–478

Narouze S, Kapural L, Casanova J, Mekhail N (2009) Sphenopalatine ganglion radiofrequency ablation for the management of chronic cluster headache. Headache 49:571–577

Overeem S, van Vliet JA, Lammers GJ, Zitman FG, Swaab DF, Ferrari MD (2002) The hypothalamus in episodic brain disorders. Lancet Neurol 1:437–444

Pascual J, Quijano J (1998) A case of chronic paroxysmal hemicrania responding to subcutaneous sumatriptan. J Neurol Neurosurg Psychiatry 65:407

Peyron C, Tighe DK, van den Pol AN, de Lecea L, Heller HC, Sutcliffe JG, Kilduff TS (1998) Neurons containing hypocretin (orexin) project to multiple neuronal systems. J Neurosci 18:9996–10015

Pinessi L, Rainero I, Valfrè W, Lo Giudice R, Ferrero M, Rivoiro C, Arvat E, Gianotti L, Del Rizzo P, Limone P (2003) Abnormal 5-HT1D receptor function in cluster headache: a neuroendocrine study with sumatriptan. Cephalalgia 23(5):354–360

Prakash S, Shah ND, Chavda BV (2010) Cluster headache responsive to indomethacin: case reports and a critical review of the literature. Cephalalgia 30:975–982

Pringsheim T (2002) Cluster headache: evidence for a disorder of circadian rhythm and hypothalamic function. Can J Neurol Sci 29:33–40

Pringsheim T, Magnoux E, Dobson CF, Hamel E, Aubé M (2002) Melatonin as adjunctive therapy in the prophylaxis of cluster headache: a pilot study. Headache 42:787–792

Rainero I, Valfrè W, Savi L et al (2001) Neuroendocrine effects of subcutaneous sumatriptan in patients with migraine. J Endocrinol Invest 24:310–314

Rainero I, Rivoiro C, Gallone S, Valfrè W, Ferrero M, Angilella G, Rubino E, De Martino P, Savi L,

Lo Giudice R, Pinessi L (2005) Lack of association between the 3092 T → C clock gene polymorphism and cluster headache. Cephalalgia 25:1078–1081

Rainero I, Rubino E, Valfrè W, Gallone S, De Martino P, Zampella E, Pinessi L (2007) Association between the G1246A polymorphism of the hypocretin receptor 2 gene and cluster headache: a meta-analysis. J Headache Pain 8:152–156

Rainero I, Rubino E, Gallone S, Fenoglio P, Negro E, De Martino P, Savi L, Pinessi L (2010) Cluster headache is associated with the alcohol dehydrogenase 4 (ADH4) gene. Headache 50:92–98

Russell MB (2004) Epidemiology and genetics of cluster headache. Lancet Neurol 3:279–283

Russell MB, Andersson PG, Thomsen LL (1995a) Familial occurrence of cluster headache. J Neurol Neurosurg Psychiatry 58:341–343

Russell MB, Andersson PG, Thomsen LL, Iselius L (1995b) Cluster headache is an autosomal dominant inherited disorder in some families. A complex segregation analysis. J Med Genet 32:954–956

Shabbir N, McAbee G (1994) Adolescent chronic paroxysmal hemicrania responsive to verapamil monotherapy. Headache 34:209–210

Shapiro RE (2005) Corticosteroid treatment in cluster headache: fvidence, rationale, and practice. Curr Pain Headache Rep 9:126–131

Sio HC (2004) Seasonal episodic paroxysmal hemicrania responding to cyclooxygenase-2 inhibitors. Cephalalgia 24:414–415

Sjaastad O, Dale I (1974) Evidence for a new (?), treatable headache entity. Headache 14:105–108

Sjaastad O, Russell D, Hørven I et al (1978) Multiple neuralgiform unilateral headache attacks associated with conjunctival injection and appearing in clusters: a nosological problem [abstract]. Proceedings of the Scandinavian Migraine Society. p 31

Sjaastad O, Apfelbaum R, Caskey W, Christoffersen B, Diamond S, Graham J, Green M, Hørven I, Lund-Roland L, Medina J, Rogado S, Stein H (1980) Chronic paroxysmal hemicrania (CPH). The clinical manifestations. A review. Ups J Med Sci Suppl 31:27–33

Sjaastad O, Saunte C, Salvesen R, Fredriksen TA, Seim A, Røe OD, Fostad K, Løbben OP, Zhao JM (1989) Shortlasting unilateral neuralgiform headache attacks with conjunctival injection, tearing, sweating, and rhinorrhea. Cephalalgia 9:147–156

Stillman M, Spears R (2008) Endocrinology of cluster headache: potential for therapeutic manipulation. Curr Pain Headache Rep 12:138–144

Sumatriptan Cluster Headache Study Group (1991) Treatment of acute cluster headache with sumatriptan. The Sumatriptan Cluster Headache Study Group. N Engl J Med 325:322–326

Torelli P, Manzoni GC (2003) Clinical observations on familial cluster headache. Neurol Sci 24:61–64

Torelli P, Manzoni GC (2005) Behavior during cluster headache. Curr Pain Headache Rep 9:113–119

van Vliet JA, Vein AA, Le Cessie S, Ferrari MD, van Dijk JG, Dutch RUSSH Research Group (2003) Impairment of trigeminal sensory pathways in cluster headache. Cephalalgia 23:414–419

Vetrugno R, Pierangeli G, Leone M, Bussone G, Franzini A, Brogli G, D'Angelo R, Cortelli P, Montagna P (2007) Effect on sleep of posterior hypothalamus stimulation in cluster headache. Headache 47:1085–1090

Walcott BP, Bamber NI, Anderson DE (2009) Successful treatment of chronic paroxysmal hemicrania with posterior hypothalamic stimulation: technical case report. Neurosurgery 65:E997

Waldenlind E, Bussone G (2006) Biochemistry, circannual and circadian rhythms, endocrinology, and immunology of cluster headaches. In: Olesen J, Goadsby PJ, Ramadan NM, Tfelt-Hansen P, Welch KMA (eds) The headaches, 3rd edn. Lippincott Williams & Wilkins, Philadelphia, pp 755–766

Waldenlind E, Gustafsson SA, Ekbom K, Wetterberg L (1987) Circadian secretion of cortisol and melatonin in cluster headache during active cluster periods and remission. J Neurol Neurosurg Psychiatry 50:207–213

Wang SJ, Lirng JF, Fuh JL, Chen JJ (2006) Reduction in hypothalamic 1 H-MRS metabolite ratios in patients with cluster headache. J Neurol Neurosurg Psychiatry 77:622–625

Weiller C, May A, Limmroth V et al (1995) Brainstem activation in spontaneous human migraine attacks. Nat Med 1:658–660

Williams MH, Broadley SA (2008) SUNCT and SUNA: clinical features and medical treatment. J Clin Neurosci 15:526–534

25 Treatment of Cluster Headache and Other Trigeminal Autonomic Cephalalgias

Peer Carsten Tfelt-Hansen[1] · *Shireen Qureshi*[2] · *Paolo Martelletti*[3]
[1]Glostrup Hospital, University of Copenhagen, Glostrup, Copenhagen, Denmark
[2]Saudi Aramco, Dhahran Health Center, Dhahran, Saudi Arabia
[3]School of Health Sciences, Sapienza University of Rome, Rome, Italy

Paolo Martelletti, Timothy J. Steiner (eds.), *Handbook of Headache*, DOI 10.1007/978-88-470-1700-9_25,
Lifting The Burden 2011

Abstract: Cluster headache is one of a group of primary headache disorders (trigeminal autonomic cephalalgias) of uncertain mechanism that are characterized by frequently recurring, short-lasting but extremely severe headache. Involvement of the suprachiasmatic nucleus of the hypothalamus, the biological clock, has been correlated to clinical features and abnormalities of circadian rhythm seen in cluster headaches. It probably affects about 1/1,000 adults with characteristically recognizable features at ratio of 5:1 in men to women.

Symptomatic acute treatments include triptans and inhalational oxygen. A wide range of preventative medication is considered depending on the length of cluster attacks, not by whether the patient has episodic or chronic form. Refractory drug-resistant chronic cluster headache is the unique form eligible for surgical choices.

Introduction

The prevalence of cluster headache is 1/1,000 with a sex ratio of 5:1 (M:F). Thus most doctors will rarely be confronted with patients with cluster headache. The clinical picture is, however, so typical that diagnosis can be made by taking the history (see ❷ Chap. 23). Cluster headache should be classified as episodic (85%) and chronic (15%) cluster headache because the choice of preventive drug depends on the cluster headache sub-form. In contrast, the acute attack treatment, triptans and oxygen, is the same for both sub-forms. Cluster headache may have up to eight attacks and patients are limited to two doses of triptans per day. Thus, generally, the emphasis should be on preventive drug treatment.

Established Knowledge

Cluster Headache Attack Treatment

Sumatriptan

Subcutaneous sumatriptan is the most effective, as well as expensive among acute treatments. In a randomized, double-blind, placebo-controlled trial, sumatriptan 6 mg subcutaneous has been shown to be effective compared to placebo after 15 min from administration (74% vs 26%) (The Sumatriptan Cluster Headache Study Group 1991). Administration of sumatriptan is also possible through nasal spray, although less effective. Intranasal sumatriptan 20 mg is effective at 30 min from administration, compared to placebo (57% vs 26%) (van Diet JA et al. 2003). The use of triptans is limited at two administrations per day.

Zolmitriptan

Intranasal zolmitriptan is the only other triptan which proved to be effective in acute treatment. In a randomized, placebo-controlled trial, zolmitriptan 10 mg was superior to placebo after 30 min from administration (62% vs 21%) (Cittadini et al. 2006; Hedlund et al. 2009).

Oxygen

Inhalation of high-flow oxygen is a safe and effective treatment to abort cluster headache attacks. In a randomized trial, high-flow oxygen at 100% for 15 min at rate of 7–12 l/min from attack beginning resulted statistically superior to placebo (air) (Cohen et al. 2009; Fogan 1985). The great advantage of oxygen relies in the absence of adverse events, the possibility to combine it with different therapies, and in the fact that inhalation can be repeated more times during the day.

Miscellanea

Locally applied lidocaine drops nasally at dose of 1 ml of 4% lidocaine repeated once after 15 min was proven effective. Sphenopalatine ganglion blockade with cocaine or lidocaine temporarily relieves pain. Octreotide, a somatostatin receptor agonist, showed in a proof study a better response when compared with placebo (May et al. 2006).

Preventive Treatment of Cluster Headache

The introduction in a single patient of preventative treatments depends on length of the attack and frequency of the attacks.

Verapamil

Verapamil has proven prophylactic efficacy in episodic cluster headache (Leone et al. 2000). In this placebo-controlled randomized clinical trial, verapamil was used in a dose of 360 mg daily and this dose should generally be the starting dose after a normal ECG has been demonstrated. The dose can be increased, depending on effect and adverse events, by 80 mg each week or 2. ECG and BP should be controlled before each increase in dose. The usual maximal daily dose is 720 mg (Francis et al. 2010).

The most common adverse events are constipation, dizziness, distal edema, hypotension, fatigue, and bradycardia (Leone and Rapaport 2006). β-Blockers should not be given together with verapamil.

Lithium

Lithium, being effective in mania, was introduced in the treatment of cluster headache because of the episodic and chronobiological nature of this disorder (Ekbom 1977, 1981; Kudrow 1977). Lithium is, however, generally most effective in chronic cluster headache. The drug should be started in a dose of 600 mg daily and the plasma level of lithium should be measured after10 days. The dose can if necessary be increased with 300 mg for each dose step. There is no therapeutic range for therapy in cluster headache but plasma levels of lithium of 0.6–0.8 mmol/l should be aimed at. The adverse events of lithium are postural tremor, insomnia, nausea, slurred speech, and blurred vision. Psychiatric side effects are common as well as the long-term side effect of hypothyroidism and diabetes insipidus.

Corticosteroids

Corticosteroids are rapidly effective drugs for cluster headache (Leone and Rapaport 2006). Prednisolone is given in a maximum dose of 60 mg once daily. Every second or third day the dose is tapered by 10 mg down to zero. The drugs should generally not be used in chronic cluster headache.

Methysergide

Clinical experiences from over 50 years from its introduction by Federigo Sicuteri in cluster headache (Sicuteri 1959) indicate that methysergide is a rather effective drug in this disorder. The dose used should be slowly titrated and varies from 1 to 2 mg thrice daily. The adverse events are nausea, dizziness, abdominal pain, and peripheral edema (Leone and Rapaport 2006). Methysergide is not in general use due to its adverse events with prolonged use: retroperitonal, pleural, and cardiac fibrosis. Methysergide is most appropriate for patients with short cluster periods (less than 4 months) (Francis et al. 2010).

Ergotamine Tartrate

Ergotamine tartrate 2 mg orally taken at bed time can be used in an attempt to prevent nocturnal attacks of cluster headache attacks (Tfelt-Hansen, personal observation). Ergotamine tartrate can be used for extended periods without problems (Leone and Rapaport 2006).

Topiramate

In open studies, topiramate has been somewhat effective in doses up 200 mg/day (Leone and Rapaport 2006). The most important adverse events are somnolence and cognitive symptoms.

Valproate

Valproate, in doses of 1,000 to 2,000 mg, is a tertiary drug in migraine prevention. Open studies indicated 54–74% responding patients. There is, however, one negative placebo-controlled study in mostly episodic cluster headache patients ($n = 96$) (El Amrani et al. 2002). The placebo-response was 62%, most likely due to spontaneous remission (El Amrani et al. 2002).

Pizotifen

Pizotifen was moderately but statistically significant effective in one placebo-controlled trial (Ekbom 1969). It can be used in one dose before retiring of 1.5–3 mg. The main adverse events are sedation and weight gain.

Melatonin

Melatonin in an evening dose of 10 mg resulted in less attacks than placebo in a pilot study (Leone et al. 1996).

Miscellanea

Not so rarely combinations of preventive drugs are used in chronic cluster headache. The basis is in most cases verapamil to which is added lithium, ergotamine, or methysergide.

Greater Occipital Nerve Blockade

Injections of local anesthetics plus corticosteroids (up to 120 mg of methylprednisolone) around the greater occipital nerve (GON) on the side of the attack can be used. In one placebo-controlled study, the procedure caused remission in 11/13 patients whereas placebo was not effective in any of the ten patients (Ambrosini et al. 2005). The GON blockade is usually effective for 4 weeks or more (Ambrosini et al. 2005).

Current Research

Treatment of Cluster Headache

Surgery is a last-resort measure in treatment-resistant cluster headache. Hypothalamic stimulation and stimulation of GON can be effective in medical treatment–resistant chronic cluster headache patients (Burns et al. 2007; Magis et al. 2007) (see ❷ Chap. 26).

Forty percent of patients with cluster headache reported improvement after radiofrequency lesion of the ipsilateral sphenopalatine ganglion.

Other procedures including radiofrequency thermocoagulation of trigeminal ganglion and gamma knife radiosurgery have been suggested.

Treatment of Other Trigeminal Autonomic Cepahalgias (TACs)

Paroxysmal hemicrania (PH) is highly sensitive to indomethacin at a daily dosage of 100–225 mg. Other NSAIDs or sumatriptan or oxygen showed limited or null efficacy in PH treatment. Short-lasting Unilateral Neuralgiform headache with Conjunctival injection and Tearing (SUNCT) syndrome showed to be sensitive to treatment with lamotrigine (400 mg), topiramate, gabapentin, intravenous lidocaine, or phenytoin (May et al. 2006). However, the rarity of these forms renders very difficult the organizations of a large series of clinical trials.

References

Ambrosini A, Vandenhede M, Rossi P, Aloj F, Sauli E, Pierelli F et al (2005) Suboccipital injection with a mixture of rapid- and long-acting steroids in cluster headache: a double-blind, placebo-controlled study. Pain 118:92–96

Burns B, Watkins L, Goadsby PJ (2007) Treatment of medically intractable cluster headache by occipital nerve stimulation: long-term follow-up of eight patients. Lancet 369:1099–1106

Cittadini E, May A, Straub A et al (2006) Effectiveness of intranasal zolmitriptan in acute cluster headache: a randomized, placebo-controlled double-blind crossover study. Arch Neurol 63: 1537–1542

Cohen AS, Burns B, Goadsby PJ (2009) High-flow oxygen for treatment of cluster headache: a randomized trial. JAMA 302:2451–2457

Ekbom K (1969) Prophylactic treatment of cluster headache with a new serotonin antagonist, BC 105. Acta Neurol Scand 45:601–610

Ekbom K (1977) Lithium in the treatment of chonic cluster headache. Headache 17:39–40

Ekbom K (1981) Lithium for cluster headache: review of the literature and preliminary results of long-term treatment. Headache 21:132–139

El Amrani M, Massiou H, Bousser MG (2002) A negative trial of sodium valproate in cluster headache: methodological issues. Cephalalgia 22:205–208

Fogan L (1985) Treatment of cluster headache. A double-blind comparison of oxygen v air inhalation. Arch Neurol 42:362–363

Francis GJ, Becker WJ, Pringsheim TM (2010) Acute and preventive pharamcologic treatment of cluster headache. Neurology 75:463–473

Hedlund C, Rapoport A, Dodick D, Goadsby PJ (2009) Zolmitriptan nasal spray in the acute treatment of cluster headache: a meta-analysis of two studies. Headache 49:1315–1323

Kudrow L (1977) Lithium prophylaxis for chronic cluster headache. Headache 17:15–18

Leone M, D'Amico D, Frediani F, Moschiano F, Grazzi L, Attanasio A et al (2000) Verapamil in the prophylaxis of episodic cluster headache: a double-blind study versus placebo. Neurology 54:1382–1385

Leone M, D'Amico D, Moschiano F, Fraschini F, Bussone G (1996) Melatonin versus placebo in the prophylaxis of cluster headache: a double-blind pilot study with parallel groups. Cephalalgia 16:494–496

Leone M, Rapaport A (2006) Preventive and surgical management of cluster headache. In: Olesen J, Goadsby PJ, Ramadan NM, Tfelt-Hansen P, Welch KMA (eds) The headaches, 3rd edn. Lippincott Williams & Wilkins, Philadelphia, pp 809–814

Magis D, Allena M, Bolla M, DePasqua V, Remacle JM, Schoenen J (2007) Occipital nerve stimulation for drug-resistant chronic cluster headache: a prospective pilot study. Lancet Neurol 6:314–321

May A, Leone M, Afra J, Linde M, Sandor PS, Evers S et al (2006) EFNS guidelines on the treatment of cluster headache and other trigeminal-autonomic cephalalgias. Eur J Neurol 13:1066–1077

Sicuteri F (1959) Prophylactic and therapeutic properties of 1-methyllysergic acid butanolamide in migraine. Int Arch Allergy 15:300–307

The Sumatriptan Cluster Headache Study Group (1991) Treatment of acute cluster headache with sumatriptan. N Engl J Med 325:353–354

van Diet JA, Bahra A, Martin V et al (2003) Intranasal sumatriptan in cluster headache: randomized, placebo- controlled, double-blind study. Neurology 60:630–633

26 Surgical Interventions for Cluster Headache, Including Implanted Stimulators

Koen Paemeleire[1] · *Paolo Martelletti*[2]
[1]Ghent University Hospital, Ghent, Belgium
[2]School of Health Sciences, Sapienza University of Rome, Rome, Italy

Paolo Martelletti, Timothy J. Steiner (eds.), *Handbook of Headache*, DOI 10.1007/978-88-470-1700-9_26,
© Lifting The Burden 2011

Abstract: Refractory cluster headache (rCH) is one of the most devastating conditions known to man. Historically, only destructive procedures were available for these desperate patients in which all drug therapies failed. The surgical interventions were aimed at the sensory trigeminal nerve, including the trigeminal sensory root, Gasserian ganglion, and supra- or infraorbital nerves; or the autonomic pathways involved in cluster headache (CH), including the nervus intermedius, nervus petrosus major, and sphenopalatine ganglion. Especially, trigeminal destructive procedures are associated with potential serious long-term consequences such as anesthesia dolorosa, as well as corneal anesthesia and ulceration. The surgical management of rCH is changing drastically with the advent of neuromodulatory techniques, such as occipital nerve stimulation and hypothalamic deep brain stimulation. These techniques were developed based on the physiology of the trigeminocervical complex and on evidence for a hypothalamic generator in CH, respectively. The potential therapeutic effect of each technique should be carefully balanced against known potential long-term consequences, knowing that long-term data on the rate of recurrence of CH after a procedure are generally lacking. No conclusive recommendations can be formulated at present, but we will suggest some guidelines toward implementing surgical interventions for rCH in clinical practice. We will briefly touch upon greater occipital nerve block as a transitional treatment.

Established Knowledge

Introduction

There is no universally accepted definition of refractory cluster headache (rCH) at present and there is no set of criteria in the International Classification of Headache Disorders second edition (ICHD-II). There is a great need to develop the concept, as a percentage of chronic cluster headache (CH) patients and episodic CH patients with frequent cluster bouts are refractory to medical treatment indeed, or have contraindications, intolerance, and resistance to drugs used in CH prevention. It is estimated that drugs are ineffective in about 10–20% of chronic CH patients (May 2005), but we are lacking formal epidemiological data. For these patients surgical procedures are available, as a last resort when the pharmacological options have been fully exploited. However, with the recent surge of data on occipital nerve stimulation, one can envision that this minimally invasive technique may be used earlier in the course of the disorder if further controlled studies confirm the efficacy and safety.

The rationale for available surgical treatments in rCH is based on the three basic aspects of CH pathophysiology: strictly unilateral distribution head pain, cranial autonomic features, and chronobiology pointing at the hypothalamus. Surgical approaches, including destructive procedures and neuromodulatory procedures are summarized in ❷ *Table 26.1*. Many of these techniques have been abandoned today.

There are a few important aspects when considering and evaluating surgical procedures for rCH:

1. It has been shown that a good proportion of chronic cluster patients eventually go into remission spontaneously (Manzoni et al. 1991). This is illustrated by 9 out of 12 cluster patients that were chronic for at least 2 years and went into remission while on a waiting list

◘ Table 26.1

Surgical procedures for refractory cluster headache

A. Neuromodulatory procedures	Occipital nerve stimulation
	Hypothalamic deep brain stimulation
	Vagus nerve stimulation
	Supraorbital nerve stimulation
	Cervical epidural neurostimulation
B. Destructive procedures	Sectioning of the trigeminal sensory root
	Radiofrequency trigeminal rhizotomy
	Alcohol injection in supra- or infraorbital nerves
	Alcohol or glycerol injection in/around the Gasserian ganglion
	Balloon compression of the Gasserian ganglion
	Gamma knife radiosurgery of the trigeminal nerve root entry zone
	Microvascular decompression of the trigeminal nerve ± section or decompression of the nervus intermedius
	Sphenopalatine ganglion resection or radiofrequency treatment
	Nervus intermedius section or decompression
	Microvascular decompression of the facial nerve
	Nervus petrosus major section or neurectomy
	Medullary trigeminal tractotomy

for hypothalamic deep brain stimulation (DBS) in the context of a clinical trial (Schoenen et al. 2005). Changes in drug therapy were only made in some of them.

2. Attacks may switch sides after an intervention even if the patient has always experienced strictly unilateral attacks (Jarrar et al. 2003; Magis et al. 2007).

3. There are well-documented cases of persistence of rCH after complete trigeminal root section, indicating that CH may be generated primarily from within the brain (Matharu and Goadsby 2002).

4. Long-term follow-up of destructive procedures is generally limited, but recurrence of CH in responders may be seen in the short term (Morgenlander and Wilkins 1990).

5. Most studies on surgical interventions are retrospective and observational. There is only one randomized placebo-controlled double-blind trial in the domain of neuromodulation (Fontaine et al. 2010).

6. Because of the severity of the pain, the placebo response in CH has been considered to be small. However upon review of the available data, the placebo response appeared to be of the same magnitude as that seen in migraine studies (Nilsson Remahl et al. 2003).

7. Because of the unbearable nature of chronic CH, higher percentages of adverse events and lower percentages of responders have been allowed to accept a therapy as worthwhile (Dodick 2005).

Greater Occipital Nerve Blockade

The results of greater occipital nerve (GON) block ipsilateral to the pain were first described in 1985 in CH (Anthony 1985). Some open-label and uncontrolled studies (Peres et al. 2002; Afridi et al. 2006) and a double-blind placebo-controlled trial (Ambrosini et al. 2005) now support the efficacy of GON block. A mixture of the local anesthetic lidocaine and a corticosteroid, such as betamethasone (Ambrosini et al. 2005), triamcinolone (Peres et al. 2002), and methylprednisolone (Afridi et al. 2006), is generally injected. The efficacy of the injection does not seem to be related to the lidocaine in the solution, but rather to the corticosteroid (Anthony 1985; Ambrosini et al. 2005). Hence, the term "block" is a bit confusing as none of the patients reported marked occipital numbness in the placebo-controlled study (Ambrosini et al. 2005). It is not ruled out that the (main) effect of the corticosteroid injection in the suboccipital region is systemic, although intramuscular injections were ineffective in one study (Anthony 1987) and higher doses are generally needed for systemic administration (Ambrosini et al. 2005). A double-blind trial comparing suboccipital and intramuscular injections of the same mixture is awaited to further verify a specific effect. At present, GON block is an interesting option as a single suboccipital injection completely suppressed CH attacks in more than 80% of CH patients in the double-blind placebo-controlled study, and the effect was maintained for at least 4 weeks in the majority of them (Ambrosini et al. 2005). As such, GON blockade is merely a transitional treatment to bridge time to a long-term treatment.

Destructive Procedures

Destructive procedures have historically been the only long-term option. Sectioning of the sensory trigeminal root should, however, now be considered as a very last resort for a desperate patient indeed, as it is associated with significant and permanent long-term morbidity, including anesthesia dolorosa and corneal anesthesia (Jarrar et al. 2003). Strict ophthalmological follow-up is necessary to avoid corneal ulceration. Furthermore, the long-term success rate of sensory trigeminal root section is far from guaranteed (Morgenlander and Wilkins 1990; Matharu and Goadsby 2002) and CH attacks may develop on the contralateral side (Jarrar et al. 2003). Complete trigeminal sensory root sectioning seems to be more effective than partial sectioning (Kirkpatrick et al. 1993). Other destructive procedures targeting (part of) the trigeminal nerve include retrogasserian glycerol injection (Ekbom et al. 1987; Hassenbusch et al. 1991; Pieper et al. 2000), radiofrequency trigeminal rhizotomy (Onofrio and Campbell 1986; Mathew and Hurt 1988; Taha and Tew 1995), trigeminal ganglion balloon compression (Constantoyannis et al. 2008), and alcohol injections of the supra- and infraorbital nerves (Dodick 2005). Discouraging results have been reported with medullary trigeminal tractotomy (Sweet 1988). Percutaneous radiofrequency trigeminal rhizotomy at one point in time was the most frequently performed procedure (Campbell 2000), and is still performed in many centers today. However, it does not figure in a recent evidence-based clinical practice algorithm for interventional management of CH (van Kleef et al. 2009).

Gamma knife radiosurgery of the trigeminal nerve root entry zone has been reported in five chronic CH patients with negligible short-term and long-term sequelae (Ford et al. 1998). Unfortunately later reports did not corroborate the initial enthusiasm as many failures were reported as well as sequelae (Donnet et al. 2005; McClelland et al. 2007). In a prospective open trial of gamma knife treatment for rCH, a low rate of pain cessation and a significant number of trigeminal nerve injuries, including deafferentiation pain, were observed at 1-year follow-up (Donnet et al. 2005). The authors of the prospective trial judged the radiosurgery a less attractive procedure because of the low rate of pain cessation in conjunction with significant morbidity.

Microvascular decompression of the trigeminal nerve with or without microvascular decompression or sectioning of the nervus intermedius was reported to be effective in chronic CH in a single series of 28 patients treated between 1974 and 1996 and with an average follow-up of 5.3 years (Lovely et al. 1998). The rationale for the combined approach was to treat both the pain, mediated by the trigeminal system, as well as the autonomic symptoms, thought to be mediated by the nervus intermedius. There was no morbidity from nervus intermedius sectioning and there were no instances of trigeminal neuropathy. Complications included infection, cerebrospinal fluid leak, and postoperative headache requiring a lumbar puncture. Substantial long-term relief was provided in almost half the patients as nine patients had at least 90% improvement and five at least 50% improvement. These procedures carry the risk of cerebellopontine angle surgery and require an experienced neurosurgical team. Furthermore findings of vascular compression were consistent at operation, but could be detected with advanced MRI techniques nowadays. Further experience with this combined approach is needed (Dodick 2005).

Autonomic pathways have been interrupted specifically too to treat rCH, especially cranial parasympathetic fibers, originating from the superior salivatory nucleus, and sequentially traversing the nervus intermedius (which leaves the brainstem as part of the facial nerve), nervus petrosus major, and sphenopalatine ganglion to provide innervation to the lacrimal gland. Percutaneous radiofrequency ablation of the sphenopalatine ganglion is performed in many centers, but the evidence base is rather poor. The parasympathetic sphenopalatine ganglion is located in the sphenopalatine fossa, close to the maxillary nerve and the internal maxillary artery, and can be targeted via an infrazygomatic approach or via the lateral nasal wall (Felisati et al. 2006). In the most recent published series of 15 patients, the mean attack frequency improved from 17 attacks/week to 8 attacks per week at 18 months follow-up (Narouze et al. 2009). Two patients developed episodic CH on the contralateral side but reported complete relief of their usual unilateral CHs. Only three patients remained headache free and off medications for the duration of follow-up (between 18 and 24 months). An earlier study reported on complete pain relief in 3 out of 10 chronic cluster patients after radiofrequency lesioning of the sphenopalatine ganglion, but no relief was found in 4 patients with an average follow-up of 24 months (Sanders and Zuurmond 1997). Another study with 20 patients reported on good results, which were always temporary (Felisati et al. 2006). Radiofrequency lesioning of the sphenopalatine ganglion can result in postoperative epistaxis, cheek hemorrhage, a lesion of the maxillary nerve, and hypesthesia of the palate (Sanders and Zuurmond 1997; Narouze et al. 2009). Total destruction of the sphenopalatine ganglion could result in eye dryness (Meyer et al. 1970), but the radiofrequency treatment now only aims at a partial lesion of the ganglion (van Kleef et al. 2009). Pulsed radiofrequency is perhaps safer, but data on its efficacy in CH are lacking at present. In a recent review, radiofrequency treatment of the sphenopalatine ganglion was put forward as the interventional treatment of choice for rCH (van Kleef et al. 2009). Small series exist on other procedures directed at the autonomic pathways, including nervus intermedius section (Rowed 1990), facial nerve decompression (Solomon and Apfelbaum 1986), and nervus petrosus major section (Denecke 1977).

Neuromodulatory Procedures

There has been considerable progress in neurostimulation approaches, both central and peripheral, in the treatment of primary headache disorders, including chronic CH (Magis and Schoenen 2008; Bartsch et al. 2009).

Central neuromodulation emerged as a result of functional neuroimaging, revealing activation in the ipsilateral posteroinferior hypothalamus during spontaneous and nitroglycerin-induced CH attacks (May et al. 1998; Sprenger et al. 2004). The first case treated with hypothalamic DBS was reported in 2001 in a chronic CH patient who had previously undergone ablative trigeminal surgery (Leone et al. 2001). Hypothalamic DBS has since been performed at several institutions and has been shown to be effective and relatively safe in the management of chronic rCH (Bartsch et al. 2009; Grover et al. 2009; Sillay et al. 2009). Nevertheless clear failures have been reported too (Pinsker et al. 2008). On review of the open-label data in 2009, 36 (71%) out of 55 patients (71%) were improved with hypothalamic DBS, including 25 patients (46%) that became completely headache free (Bartsch et al. 2009). A preliminary analysis indicates that hypothalamic DBS is associated with a marked reduction of direct costs of drug-resistant chronic CH (Leone et al. 2009).The assessment of efficacy of hypothalamic DBS for chronic CH was limited to open studies until 2009. However, in 2010 the first randomized placebo-controlled double-blind trial of unilateral hypothalamic DBS in 11 chronic rCH patients was published (Fontaine et al. 2010). During a randomized phase of 1 month active and sham stimulation were compared and no significant difference was observed between active and sham stimulation. The randomized phase was followed by a 1-year open phase during which every patient received effective hypothalamic DBS. At the end of the 1 year open phase, 6 out of 11 had responded to chronic stimulation of which 3 were completely pain free. Even though the randomized phase did not support the efficacy of hypothalamic DBS for chronic CH, the open phase data corroborated previous open studies. This suggests hypothalamic DBS acts via slow neuromodulatory processes (Ambrosini and Schoenen 2010). In order to obtain level I evidence for hypothalamic DBS in chronic CH, additional controlled studies with a longer randomized phase are required. Hypothalamic DBS is not devoid of potential serious adverse events. Infection, transient loss of consciousness, micturition syncopes, transient ischemic attack, asymptomatic third ventricular hemorrhage, panic attack, and even death due to intracerebral hemorrhage along the lead tract have been reported (Franzini et al. 2003; Schoenen et al. 2005; Fontaine et al. 2010). Many authors advocate the use of ONS prior to hypothalamic DBS when considering a neuromodulation procedure (Ambrosini 2007; Leone et al. 2008; Bartsch et al. 2009; Burns et al. 2009). Criteria have been proposed to select chronic CH patients that are suitable candidates for DBS (Leone et al. 2004).

Occipital nerve stimulation (ONS) was originally described in the treatment of occipital neuralgia (Weiner and Reed 1999), but it is a promising modality of treatment for chronic rCH based on both retrospective and prospective data. Peripheral nerve stimulation is a minimally invasive and reversible procedure. The rationale to apply ONS in CH is based on the concept of a trigeminocervical complex (TCC). Physiological studies in animals have pointed at convergence of trigeminal (trigeminal nucleus caudalis) and upper cervical (dorsal horns C1–C3) nociceptive information, and thus a loss of spatial specificity at the level of the second-order neurons of what is collectively called the TCC (Bartsch and Goadsby 2003). The concept of a TCC is furthermore supported by human experimental evidence (Piovesan et al. 2001; Busch et al. 2006). This functional continuum between occipital and trigeminal nociceptive input is important to understand how occipital neurostimulation could be effective in CH, characterized by activation of the trigeminovascular system. A stimulator is implanted under local or general anesthesia at the level of the occipitocervical junction, such that stimulation causes slight paresthesia in the distribution of the occipital nerves. The technique is however far from standardized as many technical variations have been described (Paemeleire and Bartsch 2010). In chronic CH results have been variable, as at least 50% improvement was noted in about 1/3 and 2/3 of patients respectively in the two largest case series, one prospective on 8 patients and one retrospective on 14 patients (Magis et al. 2007; Burns et al. 2009). The delay to clinical efficacy is variable and in the prospective study, a delay of 2 months or more between implantation and significant clinical improvement was noted, which suggests that ONS acts via slow neuromodulatory processes in chronic CH and argues against a 1-month trial period that is often part of the procedure and may be required for reimbursement (Magis et al. 2007). ONS is a safe technique and so far not a single neurological deficit has been reported with the technique. However, there is a consistent need for frequent reinterventions (including for battery replacement and lead migration) and some unpleasant local side effects may arise (including discomfort, shock-like sensation, neck stiffness, muscle spasm, and lead tip erosion). Some have opted for immediate bilateral ONS implantation after reports of contralateral development of cluster attacks in patients who described side locked attacks before implantation (Burns et al. 2009).

A beneficial effect of high cervical epidural neurostimulation has been reported in a single case of chronic CH (Wolter et al. 2008). A good result with vagus nerve stimulation was reported in two chronic CH patients (Mauskop 2005) and in one additional patient who had initially improved after hypothalamic DBS (Franzini et al. 2009). A beneficial outcome of supraorbital nerve stimulation has been reported in a single patient (Narouze and Kapural 2007). The numbers are too small to allow any conclusion. Whether these neurostimulation methods have a place in the management of chronic rCH patients remains to be determined (Magis and Schoenen 2008).

State of the Art

GON blockade with (a mixture of lidocaine and) corticosteroid is an interesting transitional treatment as it may suppress CH attacks for a few weeks in the majority of CH patients.

As the effectiveness of many surgical interventions, including radiofrequency treatment of the sphenopalatine ganglion, ONS, and hypothalamic DBS, only stems from uncontrolled studies, no conclusive evidence is available yet. Recommendations should not be solely based on therapeutic effect. The potential effect of a technique should be closely balanced against the burden and risk of the procedure. The surgical management of rCH is changing rapidly with the development of neuromodulation techniques.

In 2006, the European Federation of Neurological Societies (EFNS) has published guidelines on the treatment of CH, including general recommendations on surgical procedures (May et al. 2006). The EFNS warns for the lack of reliable long-term data on the outcome of surgical procedures, especially as some procedures may be associated with serious complications. The EFNS proposes that surgical procedures are not indicated in most CH patients, but that patients with intractable chronic CH should be referred to centers with expertise in both destructive and neuromodulatory procedures to be offered all reasonable alternatives before a definitive procedure is conducted.

Radiofrequency treatment of the sphenopalatine ganglion appears to be reasonably safe with open-label evidence supporting its use, and has recently been suggested as a first-line treatment (van Kleef et al. 2009), although some experts have almost abandoned destructive procedures in favor of neuromodulation techniques (Matharu and Goadsby 2008).

ONS has not achieved as high proportion of pain-free patients as DBS, but several centers now first offer the less invasive treatment of these two (Grover et al. 2009).The level of evidence supporting ONS is equal to that of radiofrequency treatment of the sphenopalatine ganglion according to a recent review (van Kleef et al. 2009). ONS is a safe technique but revisions are often necessary. The potential of ONS should be further explored in experienced centers, preferably in the context of clinical trials. Hypothalamic DBS should be left to experienced centers. A controlled trial of hypothalamic DBS with a longer blinded phase is needed to further support its usefulness.

Given the severity of CH, which may drive patients to suicidal ideations (Rothrock 2006), more aggressive and destructive procedures may be opted for. Patients should, however, be fully informed about the potential long-term consequences.

Finally, local reimbursement issues and available expertise may dictate the surgical treatment strategy in rCH, rather than the science supporting the available techniques.

Current Research

At present the therapeutic potential, the mechanisms of action, as well as the optimal technique of neurostimulation procedures is being further explored.

Occipital Nerve Stimulation

Most often electrodes typically used for spinal cord stimulation are employed for ONS. Bilateral electrodes can be inserted through a single midline incision, and connected to an implantable impulse generator in the subclavicular, abdominal, or gluteal area. Reinterventions are frequent and may be due to lead fracture, lead migration (which may occur in up to 100% of patients at 3-year follow-up, depending on the technique) and need for battery replacement (Schwedt et al. 2007; Bartsch et al. 2009). A recent development is the Bion device. It is a rechargeable mini-neurostimulator with a cylindrical shape, a length of 27 and 3 mm in diameter. It can easily be implanted adjacent to the GON. If bilateral ONS is required, a device must be implanted both on the left and on the right side (Trentman et al. 2009). Optimal stimulation parameters for ONS, such as pulse width, amplitude, and frequency, are determined by trial and error, but systematic study has begun with the Bion device (Trentman et al. 2009).

Hypothalamic DBS

The hypothalamic target for DBS in chronic CH was chosen on the basis of neuroimaging studies revealing structural and functional abnormalities in the posterior part of the hypothalamus (Bartsch et al. 2009). The target reported by the Milan group in commissural coordinates is 2 mm lateral to the midline, 5 mm inferior to the axial plane containing anterior and posterior commissures, and 3 mm posterior to the midcommissural point (Franzini et al. 2003). It has been argued that this target is posterior to the hypothalamus or rather in the border zone between posterior hypothalamus, anterior periventricular gray matter, and inferior thalamus (Sillay et al. 2009). Using probabilistic tractography, the functional connectivity of this target has been explored with highly consistent connections with the reticular nucleus and cerebellum (Owen et al. 2007). $H_2^{15}O$-positron emission tomography data argue against an unspecific anti-nociceptive effect or pure inhibition of hypothalamic activity, and rather suggest modulation of the pain matrix (May 2008).

References

Afridi SK, Shields KG, Bhola R, Goadsby PJ (2006) Greater occipital nerve injection in primary headache syndromes – prolonged effects from a single injection. Pain 122:126–129

Ambrosini A (2007) Occipital nerve stimulation for intractable cluster headache. Lancet 369:1063–1065

Ambrosini A, Schoenen J (2010) Commentary on Fontaine et al.: "Safety and efficacy of deep brain stimulation in refractory cluster headache: a randomized placebo-controlled double-blind trial followed by a 1-year open extension". J Headache Pain 11:21–22

Ambrosini A, Vandenheede M, Rossi P, Aloj F, Sauli E, Pierelli F, Schoenen J (2005) Suboccipital injection with a mixture of rapid- and long-acting steroids in cluster headache: a double-blind placebo-controlled study. Pain 118:92–96

Anthony M (1985) Arrest of attacks of cluster headache by local steroid injection of the occipital nerve. In: Rose FC (ed) Migraine: clinical and research advances. Karger, London, pp 169–173

Anthony M (1987) The role of the occipital nerve in unilateral headache. In: Advances in headache research. Proceedings of the sixth international migraine symposium 1986, London. John Libbey & Co Ltd, London, pp 257–262

Bartsch T, Goadsby PJ (2003) The trigeminocervical complex and migraine: current concepts and synthesis. Curr Pain Headache Rep 7:371–376

Bartsch T, Paemeleire K, Goadsby PJ (2009) Neurostimulation approaches to primary headache disorders. Curr Opin Neurol 22:262–268

Burns B, Watkins L, Goadsby PJ (2009) Treatment of intractable chronic cluster headache by occipital nerve stimulation in 14 patients. Neurology 72:341–345

Busch V, Jakob W, Juergens T, Schulte-Mattler W, Kaube H, May A (2006) Functional connectivity between trigeminal and occipital nerves revealed by occipital nerve blockade and nociceptive blink reflexes. Cephalalgia 26:50–55

Campbell JK (2000) Surgical and ablative management of cluster headache. In: Olesen J, Goadsby PJ (eds) Cluster headache and related conditions. Oxford University Press, Oxford, pp 264–270

Constantoyannis C, Kagadis G, Chroni E (2008) Percutaneous balloon compression for trigeminal neuralgias and autonomic cephalalgia. Headache 48: 130–134

Denecke HJ (1977) Greater petrosal nerve surgery in long-term cluster headache (author's transl). HNO 25:48–50

Dodick DW (2005) Chronic cluster headache. In: Goadsby PJ, Silberstein SD, Dodick DW (eds) Chronic daily headache for clinicians. BC Decker, London, pp 65–80

Donnet A, Valade D, Regis J (2005) Gamma knife treatment for refractory cluster headache: prospective open trial. J Neurol Neurosurg Psychiatry 76: 218–221

Ekbom K, Lindgren L, Nilsson BY, Hardebo JE, Waldenlind E (1987) Retro-Gasserian glycerol injection in the treatment of chronic cluster headache. Cephalalgia 7:21–27

Felisati G, Arnone F, Lozza P, Leone M, Curone M, Bussone G (2006) Sphenopalatine endoscopic ganglion block: a revision of a traditional technique for cluster headache. Laryngoscope 116:1447–1450

Fontaine D, LaMertens P, Blond S, Geraud G, Fabre N, Navez M, Lucas C, Dubois F, Gonfrier S, Paq Zorthes Y, Uis P, Lanteri-Minet M (2010) Safety and efficacy of deep brain stimulation in refractory cluster headache: a randomized placebo-controlled double-blind trial followed by a 1-year open extension. J Headache Pain 11:23–31

Ford RG, Ford KT, Swaid S, Young P, Jennelle R (1998) Gamma knife treatment of refractory cluster headache. Headache 38:3–9

Franzini A, Ferroli P, Leone M, Broggi G (2003) Stimulation of the posterior hypothalamus for treatment of chronic intractable cluster headaches: first reported series. Neurosurgery 52:1095–1099

Franzini A, Messina G, Leone M, Cecchini AP, Broggi G, Bussone G (2009) Feasibility of simultaneous vagal nerve and deep brain stimulation in chronic cluster headache: case report and considerations. Neurol Sci 30(Suppl 1):S137–S139

Grover PJ, Pereira EA, Green AL, Brittain JS, Owen SL, Schweder P, Kringelbach ML, Davies PT, Aziz TZ

(2009) Deep brain stimulation for cluster headache. J Clin Neurosci 16:861–866

Hassenbusch SJ, Kunkel RS, Kosmorsky GS, Covington EC, Pillay PK (1991) Trigeminal cisternal injection of glycerol for treatment of chronic intractable cluster headaches. Neurosurgery 29:504–508

Jarrar RG, Black DF, Dodick DW, Davis DH (2003) Outcome of trigeminal nerve section in the treatment of chronic cluster headache. Neurology 60:1360–1362

Kirkpatrick PJ, O'Brien MD, MacCabe JJ (1993) Trigeminal nerve section for chronic migrainous neuralgia. Br J Neurosurg 7:483–490

Leone M, Franzini A, Bussone G (2001) Stereotactic stimulation of posterior hypothalamic gray matter in a patient with intractable cluster headache. N Engl J Med 345:1428–1429

Leone M, May A, Franzini A, Broggi G, Dodick D, Rapoport A, Goadsby PJ, Schoenen J, Bonavita V, Bussone G (2004) Deep brain stimulation for intractable chronic cluster headache: proposals for patient selection. Cephalalgia 24:934–937

Leone M, Proietti Cecchini A, Franzini A, Broggi G, Cortelli P, Montagna P, May A, Juergens T, Cordella R, Carella F, Bussone G (2008) Lessons from 8 years' experience of hypothalamic stimulation in cluster headache. Cephalalgia 28:787–797

Leone M, Franzini A, Cecchini AP, Mea E, Broggi G, Bussone G (2009) Costs of hypothalamic stimulation in chronic drug-resistant cluster headache: preliminary data. Neurol Sci 30(Suppl 1):S43–S47

Lovely TJ, Kotsiakis X, Jannetta PJ (1998) The surgical management of chronic cluster headache. Headache 38:590–594

Magis D, Schoenen J (2008) Neurostimulation in chronic cluster headache. Curr Pain Headache Rep 12:145–153

Magis D, Allena M, Bolla M, De Pasqua V, Remacle JM, Schoenen J (2007) Occipital nerve stimulation for drug-resistant chronic cluster headache: a prospective pilot study. Lancet Neurol 6:314–321

Manzoni GC, Micieli G, Granella F, Tassorelli C, Zanferrari C, Cacallini (1991) A cluster headache – course over ten years in 189 patients. Cephalalgia 11:169–174

Matharu MS, Goadsby PJ (2002) Persistence of attacks of cluster headache after trigeminal nerve root section. Brain 125:976–984

Matharu M, Goadsby PJ (2008) Trigeminal autonomic cephalalgias: diagnosis and management. In: Silberstein SD, Lipton RB, Dodick DW (eds) Wolff's headache. Oxford University Press, Oxford, pp 379–430

Mathew NT, Hurt W (1988) Percutaneous radiofrequency trigeminal gangliorhizolysis in intractable cluster headache. Headache 28:328–331

Mauskop A (2005) Vagus nerve stimulation relieves chronic refractory migraine and cluster headaches. Cephalalgia 25:82–86

May A (2005) Cluster headache: pathogenesis, diagnosis, and management. Lancet 366:843–855

May A (2008) Hypothalamic deep-brain stimulation: target and potential mechanism for the treatment of cluster headache. Cephalalgia 28:799–803

May A, Bahra A, Buchel C, Frackowiak RS, Goadsby PJ (1998) Hypothalamic activation in cluster headache attacks. Lancet 352:275–278

May A, Leone M, Afra J, Linde M, Sandor PS, Evers S (2006) EFNS guidelines on the treatment of cluster headache and other trigeminal-autonomic cephalalgias. Eur J Neurol 3:1066–1077

McClelland S III, Barnett GH, Neyman G, Suh JH (2007) Repeat trigeminal nerve radiosurgery for refractory cluster headache fails to provide long-term pain relief. Headache 47:298–300

Meyer JS, Binns PM, Ericsson AD, Vulpe M (1970) Sphenopalatine gangionectomy for cluster headache. Arch Otolaryngol 92:475–484

Morgenlander JC, Wilkins RH (1990) Surgical treatment of cluster headache. J Neurosurg 72:866–871

Narouze SN, Kapural L (2007) Supraorbital nerve electric stimulation for the treatment of intractable chronic cluster headache: a case report. Headache 47:1100–1102

Narouze S, Kapural L, Casanova J, Mekhail N (2009) Sphenopalatine ganglion radiofrequency ablation for the management of chronic cluster headache. Headache 49:571–577

Nilsson Remahl AI, Laudon Meyer E, Cordonnier C, Goadsby PJ (2003) Placebo response in cluster headache trials: a review. Cephalalgia 23:504–510

Onofrio BM, Campbell JK (1986) Surgical treatment of chronic cluster headache. Mayo Clin Proc 61:537–544

Owen SL, Green AL, Davies P, Stein JF, Aziz TZ, Behrens T, Voets NL, Johansen-Berg H (2007) Connectivity of an effective hypothalamic surgical target for cluster headache. J Clin Neurosci 14:955–960

Paemeleire K, Bartsch T (2010) Occipital nerve stimulation for headache disorders. Neurotherapeutics 7(2):213–219

Peres MF, Stiles MA, Siow HC, Rozen TD, Young WB, Silberstein SD (2002) Greater occipital nerve blockade for cluster headache. Cephalalgia 22:520–522

Pieper DR, Dickerson J, Hassenbusch SJ (2000) Percutaneous retrogasserian glycerol rhizolysis for treatment of chronic intractable cluster headaches: long-term results. Neurosurgery 46:363–368

Pinsker MO, Bartsch T, Falk D, Volkmann J, Herzog J, Steigerwald F, Diener HC, Deuschl G, Mehdorn M (2008) Failure of deep brain stimulation of the posterior inferior hypothalamus in chronic cluster headache – report of two cases and review of the literature. Zentralbl Neurochir 69:76–79

Piovesan EJ, Kowacs PA, Tatsui CE, Lange MC, Ribas LC, Wenneck LC (2001) Referred pain after painful stimulation of the greater occipital nerve in humans: evidence of convergence of cervical afferences on trigeminal nuclei. Cephalalgia 21:107–109

Rothrock J (2006) Cluster: a potentially lethal headache disorder. Headache 46:327

Rowed DW (1990) Chronic cluster headache managed by nervus intermedius section. Headache 30:401–406

Sanders M, Zuurmond WW (1997) Efficacy of sphenopalatine ganglion blockade in 66 patients suffering from cluster headache: a 12- to 70-month follow-up evaluation. J Neurosurg 87:876–880

Schoenen J, Di Clemente L, Vandenheede M, Fumal A, De Pasqua V, Mouchamps M, Remacle JM, de Noordhout AM (2005) Hypothalamic stimulation in chronic cluster headache: a pilot study of efficacy and mode of action. Brain 128:940–947

Schwedt TJ, Dodick DW, Hentz J, Trentman TL, Zimmerman RS (2007) Occipital nerve stimulation for chronic headache – long-term safety and efficacy. Cephalalgia 27:153–157

Sillay KA, Sani S, Starr PA (2009) Deep brain stimulation for medically intractable cluster headache. Neurobiol Dis 38(3):361–368

Solomon S, Apfelbaum RI (1986) Surgical decompression of the facial nerve in the treatment of chronic cluster headache. Arch Neurol 43:479–482

Sprenger T, Boecker H, Tolle TR, Bussone G, May A, Leone M (2004) Specific hypothalamic activation during a spontaneous cluster headache attack. Neurology 62:516–517

Sweet WH (1988) Surgical treatment of chronic cluster headache. Headache 28:669–670

Taha JM, Tew JM Jr (1995) Long-term results of radiofrequency rhizotomy in the treatment of cluster headache. Headache 35:193–196

Trentman TL, Rosenfeld DM, Vargas BB, Schwedt TJ, Zimmerman RS, Dodick DW (2009) Greater occipital nerve stimulation via the Bion microstimulator: implantation technique and stimulation parameters. Clinical trial: NCT00205894. Pain Physician 12:621–628

van Kleef M, Lataster A, Narouze S, Mekhail N, Geurts JW, van Zundert J (2009) Evidence-based interventional pain medicine according to clinical diagnoses. 2. Cluster headache. Pain Pract 9:435–442

Weiner R, Reed K (1999) Peripheral neurostimulation for control of intractable occipital neuralgia. Neuromodulation 2:217–222

Wolter T, Kaube H, Mohadjer M (2008) High cervical epidural neurostimulation for cluster headache: case report and review of the literature. Cephalalgia 28:1091–1094

27 What to Tell Patients About Cluster Headache

Timothy J. Steiner[1,2] · *Paolo Martelletti*[3]
[1]Norwegian University of Science and Technology, Trondheim, Norway
[2]Faculty of Medicine, Imperial College London, London, UK
[3]School of Health Sciences, Sapienza University of Rome, Rome, Italy

Parts of this contribution have also been published as part of a Springer Open Choice article which is freely available at springerlink.com – DOI 10.1007/s10194-007-0428-1

Paolo Martelletti, Timothy J. Steiner (eds.), *Handbook of Headache*, DOI 10.1007/978-88-470-1700-9_27,
· Lifting The Burden 2011

Abstract: Headache disorders are real – they are not just in the mind.

This chapter summarizes information suitable for communication to cluster headache patients on types, symptoms, causes, triggers, and treatment strategies. The information is aimed at helping them to understand their headache, their diagnosis, and their treatment, and to work with their health-care provider in a way that will get best results for them.

Introduction

Cluster headache is the name given to short-lasting attacks of very severe one-sided head pain, usually in or around the eye. These usually start without warning, one or more times every day, generally at the same times each day or during the night. Quite often, the first one will wake the person up an hour or so after falling asleep.

Cluster headache is sometimes said to be a type of migraine, but this is not so. It is a quite distinct headache and needs different treatment from migraine.

Who Gets Cluster Headache?

Cluster headache is not common. It affects up to three in every 1,000 people. Men are five times more likely than women to have cluster headache, which makes it unusual among headache disorders. The first attack is likely to happen between the ages of 20 and 40, but cluster headache can start at any age.

What Are the Different Types of Cluster Headache?

Episodic cluster headache is more common. This type happens daily for limited periods (*episodes*) and then stops, a feature giving rise to the term "cluster." Usually these periods last from 6 to 12 weeks, but they can end after 2 weeks or go on for anything up to 6 months. They tend to come at about the same time each year, often spring or autumn, but some people have two or three episodes every year and others have gaps of two or more years between episodes.

In between, people with episodic cluster headache have no symptoms of the condition at all.

Chronic cluster headache, which accounts for about one in ten cases of cluster headache, does not stop. Daily or near-daily attacks continue year after year without a break.

Episodic cluster headache can turn into chronic cluster headache, and vice versa.

What Are the Symptoms of Cluster Headache?

There are a highly recognizable group of symptoms. Most importantly, cluster headache is excruciatingly painful. The pain is strictly one-sided and always on the same side (although in episodic cluster headache it can switch sides from one episode to another). It is in, around, or behind the eye and described as searing, knife-like, or boring. It becomes worse very quickly, reaching full force within 5–10 min, and when untreated lasts between 15 min and 3 hours (most commonly between 30 and 60 min). In marked contrast to migraine, during which most people want to lie down and keep as quiet as possible, cluster headache causes agitation. People with this condition cannot keep still – they will pace around or rock violently backwards and forwards, even going outside.

Also, the eye on the painful side becomes red and waters and the eyelid may droop. The nostril feels blocked, or runs. The other side of the head is completely unaffected.

What Causes Cluster Headache?

Despite a great deal of medical research into the cause of cluster headache, it is still not known. Much interest centers on the timing of attacks, which appears to link to circadian rhythms (the biological clock). Recent research has highlighted changes in a part of the brain known as the hypothalamus, the area that controls the body clock.

Many people with cluster headache are or have been heavy smokers. How this may contribute to causing cluster headache, if it does, is not known. Stopping smoking is always a good thing for health reasons, but it rarely has any effect on the condition.

What Are the Triggers?

So-called triggers set off a headache attack. Alcohol, even a small amount, may trigger an attack of cluster headache during a cluster episode but not at other times. We do not understand how this happens. There do not appear to be other common trigger factors.

Do I Need Any Tests?

Because of its set of symptoms, cluster headache is easy to recognize. There are no tests to confirm the diagnosis, which is based on your description of the headaches and other symptoms and the lack of any abnormal findings when your doctor examines you. Therefore, it is very important to describe your symptoms carefully.

If your doctor is not sure about the diagnosis, tests including a brain scan may be carried out to rule out other causes of headaches. However, these are not often needed. If your doctor does not ask for a brain scan, it means that it will not help to give you the best treatment.

What Treatments Are There?

There are a number of treatments for cluster headache that often work well. They all need a doctor's prescription. The most usual treatments for the attack are 100% oxygen, which needs a cylinder, high-flow regulator, and mask from a supplier, or an injected drug called sumatriptan, which you can give to yourself using a special injection device.

Preventative medications are the best treatments for most people with cluster headache. You take these every day for the length of the cluster episode to stop the headaches returning. They are effective, but you do need rather close medical supervision, often with blood tests, because of the possible side effects. You may be referred to a specialist for this. The referral should be urgent because, if you have this condition, we know you are suffering greatly.

What if These Do Not Work?

There are a range of preventative medications. If one does not work very well, another may. Sometimes, two or more are used together.

What Can I Do to Help Myself?

Ordinary painkillers do not work – they take too long, and the headache will usually have run its course before they take effect. For effective treatment, you will need to ask for medical help. Do this at the start of a cluster episode, as treatment appears to be more successful when started then.

Keep a Diary

You can use diary cards to record a lot of relevant information about your headaches – how often you get them, when they happen, how long they last, and what your symptoms are. They are valuable in helping with diagnosis, identifying trigger factors, and assessing how well treatments work.

Will My Cluster Headache Get Better?

Cluster headache may return for many years. However, it seems to improve in later life for most people, particularly those with chronic cluster headache.

Acknowledgment

The text of this chapter is taken from a leaflet prepared by *Lifting The Burden: The Global Campaign Against Headache*. It was drafted by a small writing group, revised following review by an international panel whose principal responsibility was to ensure worldwide cross-cultural relevance, and, finally, checked for ease of comprehension by the Campaign for Plain English. The leaflet is endorsed by the World Health Organization and has been published in *Journal of Headache and Pain* (2007).

References

Lifting The Burden. The Global Campaign to Reduce the Burden of Headache Worldwide (2007) Information for people affected by cluster headache. J Headache Pain 8(Suppl 1):S32–S33

Part 8

Other Primary Headache Disorders

28 New Daily Persistent Headache, Hemicrania Continua, Primary Stabbing Headache, Hypnic Headache, Nummular Headache

Stefan Evers[1] · *Juan A. Pareja*[2]
[1]University of Münster, Münster, Germany
[2]Hospital Quirón Madrid, Madrid, Spain

Paolo Martelletti, Timothy J. Steiner (eds.), *Handbook of Headache*, DOI 10.1007/978-88-470-1700-9_28,
© Lifting The Burden 2011

Abstract: In section 4 of the International Headache Society classification, a group of miscellaneous idiopathic headache disorders is described. Among these, new daily persistent headache, hemicrania continua, primary stabbing headache, and hypnic headache can be found. In addition, nummular headache is defined as an idiopathic headache; however, it is only described in the research section of the classification. The typical clinical features, the epidemiology, and the management of these headaches are described. Most of them do not require specific treatment and are, at least in part, responsive to indomethacin. Symptomatic causes of these headache features have to be ruled out by brain scanning and other procedures. In detail, new daily persistent headache is mostly refractory to any kind of treatment, although antidepressants and anticonvulsants are tried. Hemicrania continua shows an absolute response to indomethacin, but an alternative treatment could be greater occipital nerve stimulation. Primary stabbing headache is also often responsive to indomethacin, in many cases patients do not really suffer from this headache disorder. Hypnic headache can be treated by a cup of strong coffee before going to bed or by lithium. Nummular headache is responsive to anticonvulsants in some cases.

New Daily Persistent Headache

Description

New daily persistent headache (NDPH) has first been integrated in the revised version of the IHS classification in 2004 (see ❷ *Table 28.1*). The differentiation from chronic tension-type headache is very difficult and still debated. NDPH is an acute or subacute (within 3 days) beginning headache which is present from this time on continuously every day. The semiology of this headache resembles that of chronic tension-type headache, sometimes it can have migrainous features. This means that this headache is bilateral, mostly not pulsating, more dull and of mild-to-moderate intensity; mild phonophobia, photophobia, and/or nausea can be accompanying symptoms, up to 60% of the patients report such symptoms (Silberstein et al. 1994; Goadsby and Boes 2002; Li and Rozen 2002).

An obligatory predisposition is that the patients remember the acute or subacute onset of the headache and that no episodic headache with increasing frequency had been present before the onset of the new chronic headache.

Experimental studies or models of this headache type are not available. Some authors report on a postinfectious occurrence. Already in the first description of this headache disorder, an association with viral infection has been reported (Vanast 1986). Later case reports and small case series have repeatedly presented patients with this headache type and a positive and high titer for Epstein-Barr virus antibodies (Diaz-Mitoma et al. 1987; Evans 2003; Li and Rozen 2002; Mack 2004). In a large case series on children ($n = 175$) with chronic headache, 40 children with an acute onset have been identified. Of these children, 43% showed an onset of headache during an infection which was in half of the sufferers an Epstein-Barr virus infection (Mack 2004).

Prevalence

According to population-based studies, about 3–5% of the population suffer from chronic headache (i.e., more than 15 days per month). Of these patients, 2–3% suffer from

◘ Table 28.1
International Headache Society criteria of new daily persistent headache

A. Headache for >3 months fulfilling the criteria B–D
B. Headache is daily and unremitting from onset or from <3 days from onset
C. At least two of the following pain characteristics:
1. Bilateral location
2. Pressing/tightening (non-pulsating) quality
3. Mild or moderate intensity
4. Not aggravated by routine physical activity such as walking or climbing stairs
D. Both of the following:
1. No more than one of photophobia, phonophobia, or mild nausea
2. Neither moderate or severe nausea or vomiting
E. Not attributed to another disorder

chronic tension-type headache with a preponderance of the female sex (2–1). About 2% have a chronic migraine and about 0.2% have an NDPH or very rarely a hemicrania continua (Lainez and Monzon 2001; Lanteri-Minet et al. 2003). In an Indian study from the year 2003, 1.5% of all patients with chronic headache had an NDPH (Chakravarty 2003). Very recently, the population-based 1-year prevalence in adults in Norway was found to be 0.03% (Grande et al. 2009).

For this chronic headache type, an equal sex ratio (Takase et al. 2004) or a mild preponderance of women has been described (Evans 2003; Li and Rozen 2002). The age at onset shows two peaks: one between the age of 10 and 30 and one between the age of 50 and 60. Thirty to 40% of the patients have other primary headaches in their prior history (Li and Rozen 2002; Takase et al. 2004). It is possible that another peak of the age at onset lies in childhood (Mack 2004).

Diagnosis

The diagnosis of NDPH is based on the criteria of the IHS (see ❷ *Table 28.1*). Other disorders with a subacute onset of continuous headache such as pseudotumor cerebri, sinus thrombosis, benign intracranial hypotension, or chronic meningitis have to be excluded. An overuse of analgesics or migraine drugs contradicts to the diagnosis of new daily persistent headache.

Management

Evidence-based treatment recommendations have not been published for this headache type. According to an expert consensus, it is agreed that the treatment of this specific headache type is very difficult (Evans and Rozen 2001; Goadsby and Boes 2002; Takase et al. 2004). The basic therapy of this headache disorder should be chosen according to the primary features. If the headache is more migraine-like, a treatment with valproic acid (900 mg per day) has been recommended, if the headache is more like a tension-type headache, tricyclic antidepressants (e.g., amitriptyline up to 150 mg per day) should be given (Goadsby and Boes 2002;

Rozen 2003b). A specific treatment strategy with an initial centrally acting muscle-relaxing drug, then a tricyclic antidepressant, then a selective serotonin reuptake inhibitor, and finally an antiepileptic drug resulted in a relief of more than 50% of headache days in about 25% of the patients (Takase et al. 2004). There are no observations on the long-term course of this headache disorder. In a former study, it has been assumed that about 30% of the patients are free of headache after 3 months and about 80% after 24 months (Vanast 1986). This observation has not been confirmed by other authors (Evans and Rozen 2001; Goadsby and Boes 2002; Takase et al. 2004). Normally, this headache disorder shows a refractoy course with a duration of at least 40 months in more than 50% of the sufferers (Takase et al. 2004).

Complications and Prognosis

Complications and the long-term prognosis of this headache type are not known. However, patients should be informed that this headache type, although benign in nature, is difficult to treat and can persist for decades without complete relief by pain management.

Hemicrania Continua

Description

Hemicrania continua (HC) was described by Sjaastad and Spierings (1984) as a syndrome characterized by a unilateral, moderate, fluctuating, continuous headache, absolutely responsive to indomethacin.

The headache is strictly unilateral, without side shift though rare bilateral cases (Pasquier et al. 1987; Trucco et al. 1992) and unilateral, side-shifting attacks (Newman et al. 1992; Matharu et al. 2006) have been described. The pain predominates in the anterior region of the head though any part of the head can be affected (Bordini et al. 1991). The pain typically fluctuates from mild to moderate intensity, and is mostly reported as dull, aching, or pressing in character (Sjaastad and Spierings 1984; Pareja et al. 2001a, b; Bordini et al. 1991; Newman et al. 1994). Precipitating mechanisms – at least noticeable ones – are as a rule lacking in HC.

The temporal pattern is mostly chronic and continuous although some patients have an episodic or remitting forms. Documented transition from the remitting to the chronic stage has been reported (Sjaastad and Spierings 1984; Bordini et al. 1991; Newman et al. 1994; Peres et al. 2001). There is one case report of a patient who became episodic following a chronic onset (Pareja 1995).

In the majority of patients, exacerbations of severe pain are superimposed on the continuous baseline pain. These exacerbations can last from 20 min to several days. During exacerbations, the pain may be accompanied by a variable combination of ipsilateral autonomic features (❯ Table 28.2) commonly lacrimation and conjunctival injection, but also ipsilateral ocular discomfort and nasal stuffiness may occur. When present, all these accompaniments seem to have a modest dimension, at least as compared with other unilateral headaches such as cluster headache and paroxysmal hemicrania (Bordini et al. 1991). Indeed, photophobia, phonophobia, nausea, and vomiting may also be present during exacerbations. In a considerable number of patients primary stabbing headaches occur, predominantly during the exacerbations (Peres et al. 2001).

☐ Table 28.2

International Headache Society criteria of hemicrania continua

A. Headache for >3 months fulfilling criteria B–D
B. All of the following characteristics:
1. Unilateral pain without side shift
2. Daily and continuous, without pain-free periods
3. Moderate intensity, but with exacerbations of severe pain
C. At least one of the following autonomic features occurs during exacerbations and ipsilateral to the side of pain:
1. Conjunctival injection and/or lacrimation
2. Nasal congestion and/or rhinorrhea
3. Ptosis and/or miosis
D. Complete response to therapeutic doses of indomethacin
E. Not attributed to another disorder

The pathophysiology of HC is largely unknown. The exploration of forehead sweating (Antonaci 1991), pupillometry (Antonaci and Sjaastad 1992) and pain pressure threshold (Antonaci et al. 1992) has not yielded any evidence of gross impairment in HC. The same trend was observed using pericranial nerve blockade (Antonaci et al. 1997) and sumatriptan response (Antonaci et al. 1998a).

A PET study reported significant activation of the contralateral posterior hypothalamus and ipsilateral dorsal rostral pons in association with the headache of HC. These areas corresponded with those active in cluster headache and migraine, respectively. In addition, there was activation of the ipsilateral ventrolateral midbrain, which extended over the red nucleus and the substantia nigra, and bilateral pontomedullary junction (Matharu et al. 2004). PET studies in one HC patient lacking autonomic features documented activation of the dorsal pons and absence of activation in the hypothalamus (Irimia et al. 2009). The data suggest that HC is driven centrally and may support the clinical similarities to other primary headaches, though its pathophysiology may be completely unique.

Prevalence

Although an epidemiological survey has never been performed, HC is regarded as a rare syndrome. However, the condition may have been underdiagnosed or underreported and may be more common than earlier appreciated (Peres et al. 2001). The disorder has a female preponderance (sex ratio of 2.4:1) and a mean age of onset of 28 years (range: 5–67 years) (Peres et al. 2001).

Diagnosis

The diagnosis is made on the basis of clinical history, neurological examination, and a therapeutic trial of indomethacin (Pareja et al. 2001a, b). HC patients respond dramatically, within 24 h, and many in less than 8 h, to a standard oral dose of 75–150 mg daily of indomethacin (Pareja and Sjaastad 1996). If administered intramuscularly, 50–100 mg ("indotest"), the response should be expected within 1–2 h (Antonaci et al. 1998b).

There have been several reports of HC-like pictures concurrent with other disorders possibly indicating secondary HC forms. A patient with a C_7 root irritation due to a disk herniation has been noted to aggravate the condition (Sjaastad and Antonaci 1995). A patient with HIV developed HC, though whether this was causal is unclear (Brilla et al. 1998). A case of a mesenchymal tumor in the sphenoid bone has also been reported in which the response to indomethacin faded after 2 months (Antonaci and Sjaastad 1992). Eight cases of post-traumatic HC have been reported although the temporal relationship of the trauma to the onset of HC is very variable (Lay and Newman 1999). Moreover, one patient with brain infarction (Valença et al. 2007), two patients with carotid dissection (Rogalewski and Evers 2005; Ashkenazi et al. 2007), one patient with pineal cyst (Peres et al. 2004), one patient with pituitary tumor (Levy et al. 2005), a postpartum case (Spitz and Peres 2004) and two patients with lung cancer (Eross et al. 2002; Evans 2007) have also been reported.

Considering the possibility of HC-like pictures, an MRI of the brain is a reasonable screening investigation to exclude secondary causes. Moreover, one should at least be highly aware of two potentially dangerous situations: (1) continuously high indomethacin requirement and (2) decreasing indomethacin effect.

Management

The treatment of HC is prophylactic. HC has a prompt and enduring response to indomethacin. Typical fluctuation of pain exists, and patients need to modify the dose accordingly, dosages ranging between 25 mg every 2 days and 250 mg daily (Sjaastad and Spierings 1984; Bordini et al. 1991; Newman et al. 1994; Pareja et al. 2001a, b, c; Peres et al. 2001). Indomethacin provides only a remission, not a cure. Skipping or delaying doses may result in the recurrence of the headache.

No other drug is consistently effective in HC. Virtually all nonsteroidal anti-inflammatory drugs have been tried in HC and – in equipotent doses – not one showed the extraordinary effect provided by indomethacin. Other drugs reported to be partially or completely effective, usually in isolated cases, include ibuprofen (Newman et al. 1994; Kumar and Bordiuk 1991), piroxicam beta-cyclodextrin (Trucco et al. 1992; Sjaastad and Antonaci 1995), naproxen (Bordini et al. 1991), aspirin (Espada et al. 1999), rofecoxib (Peres and Zuckerman 2000), paracetamol with caffeine (Bordini et al. 1991); melatonin (Rozen 2006; Spears 2006) and topiramate (Matharu et al. 2006; Brighina et al. 2007; Camarda et al. 2008). In one patient with HC associated with ipsilateral trochleodynia, separate treatments with indomethacin and trochlear injection of corticosteroids were absolutely effective in controlling both ocular and head pain (Cuadrado et al. 2010a).

The use of anesthetic and corticosteroid injections around the greater occipital nerve homolateral to the pain may provide a transitory relief in some HC patients (Afridi et al. 2006). In HC patients who are unable to tolerate indomethacin treatment or when it is contraindicated, occipital nerve stimulation may be a therapeutic alternative (Schwedt et al. 2006, 2007; Cohen et al. 2007; Burns et al. 2008). Preliminary results indicate that such a therapy is rather satisfactory though its efficacy is lesser than the one obtained with indomethacin.

Complications and Prognosis

HC appears to be a chronic condition in most patients though several cases have been reported in whom indomethacin could be discontinued and the patients remained pain free (Newman et al. 1994; Espada et al. 1999).

HC patients may expect sustained efficacy of indomethacin treatment without developing tachyphylaxis, though between a quarter to half develop gastrointestinal side effects (Newman et al. 1994; Pareja et al. 2001c). Concurrent treatment with gastric mucosa protective agents should be considered as patients are expected to require long-term treatment.

Indomethacin does not seem to alter the condition in the long term, though in one reported patient indomethacin seemed to satisfactorily modify the natural history of HC (Rozen 2009). Of note is that a significant proportion of patients can decrease the dose of indomethacin required to maintain a pain-free state (Pareja et al. 2001c).

Primary Stabbing Headache

Description

Primary stabbing headache (PSH) is characterized by transient, cephalic, ultrashort stabs of pain. The disorder was described by Lansche in 1964 under "ophthalmodynia periodica." Later on, Sjaastad et al. (1979) described "jabs and jolts syndrome" and, lastly, Raskin and Schwartz (1980) described "icepick-like headache." The clinical features in the various descriptions are so similar that they probably refer to the same syndrome that is now officially named PSH in the International Classification of Headache Disorders (ICHD, see ❷ *Table 28.3*).

PSH attacks are generally characterized by moderate-to-severe jabbing/stabbing pain, lasting from a fraction of a second to 3 s (Pareja et al. 1996; Sjaastad et al. 2001). Occasional attacks might last up to 5–10 s (Pareja et al. 1996; Sjaastad et al. 2001; Dangond and Spierings 1993). The mean duration of attacks has been estimated at 2.2 s (Pareja et al. 1996) and 1.4 s (Piovesan et al. 2001), respectively. Attack frequency is generally low, with one or a few attacks per day. At maximum, there could be 100–300 attacks per day (Sjaastad et al. 2002). Rarely, accumulations may occur, even attaining a *status* pattern lasting 1 week (Martins et al. 1995). Most patients exhibit a sporadic pattern, with an erratic, unpredictable alternation between symptomatic and non-symptomatic periods (Pareja et al. 1996). PSH is a diurnal disorder, with nocturnal attacks seldom reported.

❏ Table 28.3

International Headache Society criteria of primary stabbing headache

A. Head pain occurring as a single stab or a series of stabs and fulfilling criteria B–D
B. Exclusively or predominantly felt in the distribution of the first division of the trigeminal nerve (orbit, temple, and parietal area)
C. Stabs last for up to a few seconds and recur with irregular frequency ranging from one to many per day
D. No accompanying symptoms
E. Not attributed to another disorder

The paroxysms generally occur spontaneously. Some patients, nevertheless, have the impression that some attacks could be provoked by neck movements, cough, abdominal strain, and touching the hair (Sjaastad et al. 2002). Occasionally, bright light, emotional stress, and postural changes have also been reported to trigger attacks (Raskin and Schwartz 1980; Pareja et al. 1996).

Paroxysms almost invariably are unilateral, and are predominantly felt in the distribution of the first division (V-1) of the trigeminal nerve. Temporal and fronto-ocular areas are most frequently affected. Although attacks may recur in the same area, the stabs tend to move from one area to another, in either the same or the opposite hemicranium. Synchronous stabs in both halves of the head may also occur, and these can be either symmetric or asymmetric (Pareja et al. 1996; Sjaastad et al. 2003).

Jabs may be accompanied by a shock-like feeling and even by head movement – "jolts" – or vocalization (Sjaastad et al. 2002). On rare occasions, conjunctival hemorrhage (Pareja et al. 1996) and monocular vision loss (Zacaria et al. 2000) have been described as associated features.

PSH may concur, synchronously or independently, with other primary headaches, and frequently sharing the same symptomatic area. Migraine is the most frequently associated headache (Lansche 1964; Raskin and Schwartz 1980; Pareja et al. 1996; Sjaastad and Bakketeig 2006) but also tension-type headache (Drumond and Lance 1984), cluster headache (Lance and Anthony 1971; Ekbom 1975), paroxysmal hemicrania (Sjaastad et al. 1979), SUNCT (Pareja and Sjaastad 1994), cervicogenic headache (Fredriksen et al. 1987), hemicrania continua (Sjaastad and Spierings 1984), and supraorbital neuralgia (Sjaastad et al. 2004; Pareja and Caminero 2006) may concur with PSH. Contrary to what is the case in adults, in childhood it is usually not associated with other headaches (Soriani et al. 1996; Fusco et al. 2003; Vieira et al. 2006).

In PSH the lack of topographic organization with multifocal, rather chaotic, localizations may reflect a shifting origin of paroxysms, probably elicited in single fibers of the pericranial nerves, mostly of the first trigeminal branch. In fact, the pain is felt superficially, and the profile of the single attack is spikelike, both features pointing to a peripheral origin of attacks. Even in peripheral sensory disorders, the origin of the process may be anywhere alongside the sensory unit, but with a distal perception of signs and symptoms. Loss of control from supraspinal sensitive centers may liberate the sensory units thus producing "sensitive twitches" (Pareja and Sjaastad 2010) that could be perceived as stabbing or jabbing pain.

Prevalence

PSH is a frequent complaint. In two populations studies, the prevalence of PSH was found to be 2% (Rasmussen 1995) and 0.2% (Monteiro 1995). In a large epidemiological study of headache (The Vågå study), a prevalence of ultrashort paroxysms of 35.2% with a female preponderance (female/male ratio of 1.49), and a mean age of onset of 28 years (range: 5–65 years), was found (Sjaastad et al. 2001). A prevalence of the same magnitude was found in a sample of Brazilian migraineurs (Piovesan et al. 2001).

Diagnosis

PSH is considered a primary headache. Therefore, diagnosis is entirely based upon assessment of the clinical features and distinction from other similar headaches. The typical spatial and temporal development of the symptoms provides a safe basis for the diagnosis (❷ Table 28.3).

When PSH is strictly and permanently localized to one area, an underlying structural lesion or dysfunction should be ruled out. Similar symptoms as in PSH have been described in some patients with documented intracranial structural lesions or ocular conditions such as meningioma (Mascellino et al. 2001), pituitary adenoma (Levy et al. 2003), cerebrovascular diseases (Pareja et al. 1996; Piovesan et al. 2001), cranial and ocular trauma, ophthalmic herpes zoster (Pareja et al. 1996), and giant cell arteritis (Raskin and Schwartz 1980).

Management

Treatment is rarely necessary. With frequent attacks, drug therapy may possibly be indicated. Indomethacin, 75–150 mg, daily, seemed to be of some avail (Mathew 1981; Pareja et al. 1999) in that one third seemed to get complete relief, whereas another third showed a partial response. Celecoxib (Piovesan et al. 2002), nifedipine (Jacome 2001), melatonin (Rozen 2003a), and gabapentin (França et al. 2004) have been reported as effective in isolated cases/small series of patients.

Complications and Prognosis

The long-term course is invariably benign and no complications are to be expected.

Hypnic Headache

Description

Hypnic headache has been described for the first time in 1988 (Raskin 1988) and has been integrated into the IHS classification in 2004. In this entity, almost every night (at least every week) a headache attack occurs during sleep. These attacks typically begin always at the same time after sleep onset. This is why this headache has also been called clockwise headache. For all published cases of hypnic headache, a meta-analysis has been performed (Evers and Goadsby 2003b). According to this meta-analysis, the headache is regularly bilateral and frontotemporal or diffuse, it is of moderate intensity and lasts 30 min to 3 h. There are no accompanying autonomous or vegetative symptoms. Rarely, a second headache attack can occur in the same night. This headache normally starts after the age of 50, the mean age at onset is 63 with a broad range of 36–83. The course is chronic, only about 20% of the patients show spontaneous remission. The most severe problem of this headache is the impaired quality of life due to the disturbed sleep.

The exact pathophysiology is unknown. Polysomnographic studies could show that the headache frequently occurs during the first REM-sleep phase (Dodick 2000; Evers et al. 2003a; Pinesi et al. 2003). An association between REM-sleep phases and the onset of attacks is also known for cluster headache (Dexter and Weitzman 1970; Nobre et al. 2003; Pfaffenrath et al. 1986) and – less impressive – for migraine (Dodick et al. 2003). Probably, these headache types result from a dysfunction of the central pain-controlling systems in the brain stem during REM sleep.

Prevalence

The population-based prevalence of this headache is unknown. In two case series, hypnic headache represented about 0.1 of all patients in a tertiary headache clinic (Dodick et al. 1998; Evers and Goadsby 2003b). Women are about two times more often affected than men. There is no comorbidity known, neither with other idiopathic headaches nor with psychiatric or internal diseases.

Diagnosis

The diagnosis of hypnic headache is strictly according to the IHS criteria (see ❯ *Table 28.4*). If the diagnostic criteria are completely fulfilled, no further diagnostic procedures are recommended. In any uncertain cases, an MRI brain scan should be performed. For the differential diagnosis of sleep-related disorders, a polysomnography is necessary.

Management

Hypnic headache often requires no treatment if it occurs infrequently (i.e., less than three times per week) and if there is no impairment of the quality of life. Often, it is sufficient to inform the patients about the harmless nature of the headache. Controlled studies for drug treatment are not available. According to a meta-analysis, the first step of treatment should be a trial of strong coffee or oral caffeine (Evers and Goadsby 2003b). About 50% of the sufferers show a remission of the nightly attack if they drink a strong coffee before going to sleep.

If caffeine is not effective, a drug prophylaxis can be given. Drug of first choice is lithium in a dose of 150–600 mg per day. Lithium should be dosed according to the plasma level (0.6–1.2 mmol/l). Controls of the thyroid and renal functions are necessary. About 75% of the patients taking lithium report good or very good efficacy. Drugs of second choice are indomethacin (100–150 mg per day) and flunarizine (10 mg in the evening). Prophylactic inhalation of oxygen during the night, beta-blockers, and antidepressants have been ineffective in the majority of cases.

◻ Table 28.4
International Headache Society criteria of hypnic headache

A. Dull headache fulfilling criteria B–D
B. Develops only during sleep, and awakens patient
C. At least two of the following characteristics:
1. Occurs >15 times per month
2. Lasts >15 min after waking
3. First occurs after age of 50
D. No autonomic symptoms and not more than one of nausea, photophobia, or phonophobia
E. Not attributed to another disorder

There are nearly no reports on the acute treatment of hypnic headache attacks. A moderate efficacy in aborting the attacks has only been reported for acetylsalicylic acid.

Complications and Prognosis

Complications of hypnic headache are not known. Also, the prognosis of hypnic headache is not known. There are episodic and chronic courses making it useful to stop treatment from time to time and see whether it is still needed.

Nummular Headache

Description

Nummular headache (NH) is a well-defined clinical picture characterized by local pain that is exclusively felt in a round or elliptical area of the head, typically 1–6 cm in diameter in the absence of underlying lesion. NH was described by Pareja et al. in 2002 and was subsequently included in the appendix of the ICHD in 2004.

Although any region of the head may be affected, the parietal area, particularly the most convex part (*tuber parietale*), is the common localization of NH. The pain remains confined to the same symptomatic area which does not change in shape or size with time. A bifocal localization has recently been described (Cuadrado et al. 2009). The pain intensity is generally low to moderate, though some patients experience severe pain (Pareja et al. 2004; Barriga et al. 2004; Dach et al. 2006; Trucco et al. 2006; Grosberg et al. 2007; Pareja et al. 2008; Kraya and Gaul 2008). Lancinating exacerbations, lasting from several seconds to minutes, or 2 h may superimpose the baseline pain, or may occasionally be the prevailing pain profile (Ruscheweyh et al. 2010). Autonomic accompaniments and precipitating mechanisms are typically lacking. Exacerbations may be spontaneous or provoked by mechanical stimuli (e.g., touching, combing hair) in the symptomatic area.

The temporal pattern is chronic in two thirds and episodic in one third. Pseudoremissions may be observed when the pain reaches a very low grade or only discomfort (not pain) is reported. At times, discomfort may prevail but also true remissions can ensue. Either during symptomatic periods or interictally the affected area may show a variable combination of symptoms and signs of sensory dysfunction, such as hypoesthesia, paresthesia, dysesthesia, or tenderness (Pareja et al. 2002, 2004). In addition, a minority of patients may develop trophic changes such as a patch of skin depression, hair loss, reddish color, and local increased temperature (Pareja et al. 2008). Skin biopsies were performed in three patients with trophic changes, and were not specific for any particular dermatological disease.

Size and shape of the symptomatic area along with signs and symptoms of local sensory dysfunction suggests a neuralgia of a terminal branch of a pericranial nerve. However, two features militate against such a concept: (1) anesthetic block of the symptomatic area is usually of no avail and (2) the occasional topography with an elliptical symptomatic area divided in half by the midline. Trophic changes together with pain and sensory disturbances could represent a restricted form of complex regional pain syndrome. This should be taken as a possible evolution of the underlying morbid process of NH. However, at this stage of development, the source of NH is unclear. Therefore, we prefer to provisionally consider NH as an *epicrania*, that is, an "in situ" headache probably stemming from epicranial tissues, that is, internal and external layers of the skull, and all the layers of the scalp, including epicranial nerves and arteries (Pareja et al. 2003).

The confinement of pain and sensory symptoms to a small cranial area apparently reflects a nongeneralized and rather limited disorder. In fact, there is some evidence supporting this hypothesis. For instance, NH patients did not show increased pericranial tenderness to palpation when compared to healthy control subjects (Fernández-de-las-Peñas et al. 2007). Furthermore, evidence of increased mechanical pain sensitivity (lower pressure pain thresholds, PPT) restricted to the symptomatic area in NH has been found (Fernández-de-las Peñas et al. 2006). Finally, patients with NH show similar topographical pressure pain sensitivity maps of the head when compared to healthy controls, with local decrease of PPT levels restricted to the symptomatic zone in comparison with the non-symptomatic symmetrical point (Cuadrado et al. 2010b).

The clinical observations do not suggest a psychogenic origin of NH, since the majority of patients with NH have no previous diagnoses of another psychopathological disease (Pareja et al. 2004). NH is not associated with depression and anxiety, since patients with NH showed similar mood states to those of healthy controls (Fernández-de-las Peñas et al. 2009). Furthermore, in NH patients, neither depressive symptoms nor anxiety levels were related to headache clinical parameters.

Prevalence

Eight years after the first description, more than 120 NH patients have been reported but population epidemiological data are still lacking. According to the data at hand, the female to male ratio is 1.8:1 and the mean age of onset is 43 years (range 6–79). In a hospital-based series, an incidence of 6.4/100,000 person-years was estimated (Pareja et al. 2004). In an outpatient neurological service, NH represented 0.25% of all consultations, and 1.25% of the consultations because of headache (Guerrero et al. 2007). Those figures are probably an underestimate because not all patients suffering from NH are referred to a hospital.

Diagnosis

Diagnosis of NH is clinical (❷ *Table 28.5*). Neuroimaging studies, such as skull x-ray, CT scan, or MRI of the head, are systematically normal.

◻ Table 28.5
International Headache Society criteria of nummular headache

A. Mild to moderate head pain fulfilling criteria B and C
B. Pain is felt exclusively in a rounded or elliptical area typically 2–6 cm in diameter
C. Pain is chronic and either continuous or interrupted by spontaneous remissions lasting weeks to months
D. No attributed to another disorder

Although NH is mostly regarded as a primary disorder, various focal headaches with a nummular pattern have been related to local lesions of the scalp (García Pastor et al. 2002), the skull (Álvaro et al. 2009), or the adjacent intracranial structures (Guillem et al. 2007, 2009).

Management

In many patients, treatment is not necessary and simple reassurance is adequate. In patients with low to moderate pain, regular analgesics may suffice. In cases with persistent, moderate to intense pain and lack of response to analgesics, a preventive therapy with neuromodulators may be indicated. In such instances, gabapentin (300–900 mg daily) (Evans and Pareja 2005; Trucco 2007) proved to be effective in a substantial number of patients. Alternatively, tricyclic antidepressants rendered satisfactory results in a small series of NH patients (Grosberg et al. 2007).

Botulinum toxin type A, 10 Units injected in the symptomatic area (Seo and Park 2005) or 25 Units injected in several points distributed in both the symptomatic and surrounding areas (Mathew et al. 2008), was useful. It is worth mentioning that anesthetic block of the symptomatic area has been tried extensively and was generally of no avail.

Complications and Prognosis

Because NH is a recently described syndrome, there is a paucity of literature on its natural history and long-term prognosis. The available evidence suggests that it is a benign condition that may spontaneously remit.

References

Afridi SK, Shields KG, Bhola R, Goadsby PJ (2006) Greater occipital nerve injection in primary headache syndromes: prolonged effects from a single injection. Pain 122:126–129

Álvaro LC, García JM, Areitio E (2009) Nummular headache: a series with symptomatic and primary cases. Cephalalgia 29:379–383

Antonaci F (1991) The sweating pattern in "hemicrania continua". Funct Neurol 6:371–375

Antonaci F, Sjaastad O (1992) Hemicrania continua: a possible symptomatic case, due to mesenchymal tumor. Funct Neurol 7:471–474

Antonaci F, Bovim G, Fasano ML, Bonamico L, Shen JM (1992) Pain thresholds in humans. A study with pressure algometer. Funct Neurol 7:283–288

Antonaci F, Pareja JA, Caminero AB, Sjaastad O (1997) Chronic paroxysmal hemicrania and hemicrania continua: anaesthetic blockades of pericranial nerves. Funct Neurol 12:11–15

Antonaci F, Pareja JA, Caminero AB, Sjaastad O (1998a) CPH and hemicrania continua: lack of efficacy of sumatriptan. Headache 38:197–200

Antonaci F, Pareja JA, Caminero AB, Sjaastad O (1998b) Chronic paroxysmal hemicrania and hemicrania continua. Parenteral indomethacin: the 'indotest'. Headache 38:122–128

Ashkenazi A, Abbas MA, Sharma DK, Silberstein SD (2007) Hemicrania continua-like headache associated with internal carotid artery dissection may respond to indomethacin. Headache 47:127–130

Barriga FJ, Hernández T, Pardo J (2004) Cefalea numular: serie prospectiva de 20 nuevos casos. Neurologia 19:541, abstract

Bordini C, Antonaci F, Stovner LJ, Schrader H, Sjaastad O (1991) "Hemicrania continua": a clinical review. Headache 31:20–26

Brighina F, Palermo A, Cosentino G, Fierro B (2007) Prophylaxis of hemicrania continua: two new cases effectively treated with topiramate. Headache 47:441–443

Brilla R, Evers S, Sörös P, Husstedt IW (1998) Hemicrania continua in an HIV-infected outpatient. Cephalalgia 18:287–288

Burns B, Watkins L, Goadsby PJ (2008) Treatment of hemicrania continua by occipital nerve stimulation with a bion device: long-term follow-uo of a cross over study. Lancet Neurol 7:1001–1012

Camarda C, Camarda R, Monastero R (2008) Chronic paroxysmal hemicrania and hemicrania continua responding to topiramate. Two case reports. Clin Neurol Neurosurg 110:88–91

Chakravarty A (2003) Chronic daily headaches: clinical profile in Indian patients. Cephalalgia 23:348–353

Cohen AS, Matharu MS, Goadsby PJ (2007) Trigeminal autonomic cephalalgia. Current and future treatments. Headache 47:951–962

Cuadrado ML, Valle B, Fernández de las Peñas C, Barriga FJ, Pareja JA (2009) Bifocal nummular headache: the first three cases. Cephalalgia 29:583–586

Cuadrado M, Porta-Etessam J, Pareja JA, Matías-Guiu J (2010a) Hemicrania continua responsive to trochlear injection of corticosteroids. Cephalalgia 30:373–374

Cuadrado ML, Valle B, Fernández-de-las-Peñas C (2010b) Pressure pain sensitivity of the head in patients with nummular headache: a cartographic study. Cephalalgia 30(2):200–206

Dach F, Speciali J, Eckeli A, Rodrigues GG, Bordini CA (2006) Nummular headache: three new cases. Cephalalgia 26:1234–1237

Dangond T, Spierings ELH (1993) Idiopathic stabbing headaches lasting a few seconds. Headache 33:257–258

Dexter JD, Weitzman ED (1970) The relationship of nocturnal headaches to sleep stage patterns. Neurology 20:513–518

Diaz-Mitoma F, Vanast WJ, Tyrrell DL (1987) Increased frequency of Epstein-Barr virus excretion in patients with new daily persistent headaches. Lancet i:411–415

Dodick DW (2000) Polysomnography in hypnic headache syndrome. Headache 40:748–752

Dodick DW, Mosek AC, Campbell JK (1998) The hypnic ("alarm clock") headache syndrome. Cephalalgia 18:152–156

Dodick DW, Eross E, Parish JM (2003) Clinical, anatomical, and physiological relationship between sleep and headache. Headache 43:282–292

Drummond PD, Lance JW (1984) Neurovascular disturbances in headache patients. Clin Exp Neurol 20:93–99

Ekbom K (1975) Some observations on pain in cluster headache. Headache 14:219–225

Eross EJ, Swanson JW, Dodick DW (2002) Hemicrania continua: an indomethacin-responsive case with an underlying malignant etiology. Headache 42:527–529

Espada F, Escalza I, Morales-Asín F, Nasas I, Iñiguez C, Mauri JA (1999) Hemicrania continua: nine new cases. Cephalalgia 19:442

Evans RW (2003) New daily persistent headache. Curr Pain Headache Rep 7:303–307

Evans RW (2007) Hemicrania continua-like headache due to nonmetastatic lung cancer: a vagal cephalalgia. Headache 47:1349–1351

Evans R, Pareja JA (2005) Nummular headache. Headache 45:164–165

Evans RW, Rozen TD (2001) Etiology and treatment of new daily persistent headache. Headache 41:830–832

Evers S, Goadsby PJ (2003b) Hypnic headache. Clinical features, pathophysiology, and treatment. Neurology 60:905–910

Evers S, Rahmann A, Schwaag S, Lüdemann P, Husstedt IW (2003a) Hypnic headache - the first German cases including polysomnography. Cephalalgia 23:20–23

Fernández-de-las Peñas C, Cuadrado ML, Barriga FJ, Pareja JA (2006) Local decrease of pressure pain threshold in nummular headache. Headache 46:1195–1198

Fernández-de-las-Peñas C, Peñacoba-Puente C, López-López A, Valle B, Cuadrado ML, Barriga FJ, Pareja JA (2009) Depression and anxiety are not related to nummular headache. J Headache Pain 10:441–445

Fernández-de-las-Peñas C, Cuadrado ML, Barriga FJ, Pareja JA (2007) Pericranial tenderness is not related to nummular headache. Cephalalgia 27:182–186

França MC Jr, Costa ALC, Maciel JA Jr (2004) Gabapentin-responsive idiopathic stabbing headache. Cephalalgia 24:993–996

Fredriksen TA, Hovdal H, Sjaastad O (1987) "Cervicogenic headache": clinical manifestations. Cephalalgia 7:147–160

Fusco C, Pisani F, Faienza C (2003) Idiopathic stabbing headache: clinical characteristics of children and adolescents. Brain Dev 25:237–240

García-Pastor A, Guillem-Mesado A, Salinero-Paniagua J, Giménez-Roldán S (2002) Fusiform aneurysm of the scalp: an unusual cause of focal headache in Marfan syndrome. Headache 42:908–910

Goadsby PJ, Boes C (2002) New daily persistent headache. J Neurol Neurosurg Psychiat 72(Suppl 2): ii6–ii9

Grande RB, Aaseth K, Lundqvist C, Russell MB (2009) Prevalence of new daily persistent headache in the general population. The Akershus study of chronic headache. Cephalalgia 29:1149–1155

Grosberg BM, Solomon S, Lipton RB (2007) Nummular headache. Curr Pain Headache Rep 11:310–312

Guerrero AL, Martín-Polo J, Tejero MA, Gutiérrez F, Iglesias F, Sánchez-Barranco F (2007) Representación de la cefalea numular en una consulta general de neurología. Neurologia 22:716, Abstract

Guillem A, Barriga FJ, Giménez-Roldán S (2007) Nummular headache secondary to an intracranial mass lesion. Cephalalgia 27:943–944

Guillem A, Barriga FJ, Giménez-Roldán S (2009) Nummular headache associated to arachnoid cysts. J Headache Pain 10:215–217

Irimia P, Arbizu J, Prieto E, Fernández-Torrón R, Martínez-Vila E (2009) Activation of the brainstem but not of the hypothalamus in hemicrania continua without autonomic symptoms. Cephalalgia 29: 974–979

Jacome DE (2001) Exploding head syndrome and idiopathic stabbing headache relieved by nifedipine. Cephalalgia 21:617–618

Kraya T, Gaul C (2008) Münzkopfschmerz: eine bislang wenig bekannte Kopfschmerzkrankung. Nervenarzt 79:202–205

Kumar KL, Bordiuk JD (1991) Hemicrania continua: a therapeutic dilemma. Headache 31:345

Láinez MJ, Monzon MJ (2001) Chronic daily headache. Curr Neurol Neurosci Rep 1:118–124

Lance JW, Anthony M (1971) Migrainous neuralgia or cluster headache? J Neurol Sci 13:401–414

Lansche RK (1964) Ophthalmodynia periodica. Headache 4:247–249

Lanteri-Minet M, Auray JP, El Hasnaoui A, Dartigues JF, Duru G, Henry P, Lucas C, Pradalier A, Chazot G, Gaudin AF (2003) Prevalence and description of chronic daily headache in the general population in France. Pain 102:143–149

Lay CL, Newman LC (1999) Postraumatic hemicrania continua. Headache 39:275–279

Levy MJ, Matharu MS, Goadsby PJ (2003) Prolactinomas, dopamine agonists and headache: two case reports. Eur J Neurol 10:169–171

Levy MJ, Matharu MS, Meeran K, Powell M, Goadsby PJ (2005) The clinical characteristics of headache in patients with pituitary tumours. Brain 128: 1921–1930

Li D, Rozen TD (2002) The clinical characterisation of new daily persistent headache. Cephalalgia 22: 66–69

Mack KJ (2004) What incites new daily persistent headache in children? Pediatr Neurol 31:122–125

Martins IP, Parreira E, Costa I (1995) Extratrigeminal icepick status. Headache 35:107–110

Mascellino AM, Lay CL, Newman LC (2001) Stabbing headache as the presenting manifestation of intracranial meningioma: a report of two patients. Headache 41:599–601

Matharu MS, Cohen AS, McGonigle DJ, Wrd N, Frackowiak RSJ, Goadsby PJ (2004) Posterior hypothalamic and brainstem activation in hemicrania continua. Headache 44:747–761

Matharu MS, Bradbury P, Swash M (2006) Hemicrania continua: side alternation and response to topiramate. Cephalalgia 26:341–344

Mathew NT (1981) Indomethacin responsive headache syndromes. Headache 21:147–150

Mathew NT, Kailasam J, Meadors L (2008) Botulinum toxin type A for the treatment of nummular headache: four case studies. Headache 48:442–447

Monteiro JM (1995) Cefaleias. Estudio epidemiologico e clinico de uma população urbana. MD Thesis, Porto

Newman LC, Lipton RB, Russell M, Solomon S (1992) Hemicrania continua: attacks may alternate sides. Headache 32:237–238

Newman LC, Lipton RB, Solomon S (1994) Hemicrania continua: ten new cases and a review of the literature. Neurology 44:2111–2114

Nobre ME, Filho PF, Dominici M (2003) Cluster headache associated with sleep apnoea. Cephalalgia 23:276–279

Pareja JA (1995) Hemicrania continua: remitting stage evolved from the chronic form. Headache 35: 161–162

Pareja JA, Caminero AB (2006) Supraorbital neuralgia. Curr Pain Headache Rep 10:302–305

Pareja JA, Sjaastad O (1994) SUNCT syndrome in the female. Headache 34:217–220

Pareja JA, Sjaastad O (1996) Chronic paroxysmal hemicrania and hemicrania continua. Interval between indomethacin administration and response. Headache 36:20–23

Pareja JA, Sjaastad O (2010) Primary stabbing headache. In: Nappi G, Moskowitz MA (eds) Handbook of clinical neurology, vol 97, Headache (3 rd series). Elsevier BV, Amsterdam, pp 445–449

Pareja JA, Ruiz J, de Isla C, Al-Sabbah H, Espejo J (1996) Idiopathic stabbing headache (jabs and jolts syndrome). Cephalalgia 16:93–96

Pareja JA, Kruszewski P, Caminero AB (1999) SUNCT syndrome versus idiopathic stabbing headache (jabs and jolts syndrome). Cephalalgia 19(Suppl 25):46–48

Pareja JA, Vincent M, Antonaci F, Sjaastad O (2001a) Hemicrania continua. Diagnostic criteria and nosologic status. Cephalalgia 21:874–877

Pareja JA, Antonaci F, Vincent M (2001b) The hemicrania continua diagnosis. Cephalalgia 21:940–946

Pareja JA, Caminero AB, Franco E, Casado JL, Pascual J, Sánchez del Río M (2001c) Dose, efficacy and tolerability of long-term indomethacin treatment of chronic paroxysmal hemicrania and hemicrania continua. Cephalalgia 21:906–910

Pareja JA, Caminero AB, Serra J, Barriga FJ, Dobato JL, Barón M, Vela L, Sánchez del Río M (2002) Numular headache: a coin-shaped cephalgia. Neurology 58:1678–1679

Pareja JA, Pareja J, Yangüela J (2003) Nummular headache, trochleitis, supraorbital neuralgia, and other epicranial headaches and neuralgias: the epicranias. J Headache Pain 4:125–131

Pareja JA, Pareja J, Barriga FJ, Barón M, Dobato JL, Pardo J, Sánchez C, Vela L (2004) Nummular headache. A prospective series of 14 new cases. Headache 44:611–614

Pareja JA, Cuadrado ML, Fernández de las Peñas C, Nieto C, Sols M, Pinedo M (2008) Nummular headache with trophic changes inside the painful area. Cephalalgia 28:186–190

Pasquier F, Leys D, Petit H (1987) Hemicrania continua: the first bilateral case. Cephalalgia 7:169–170

Peres MFP, Zuckerman E (2000) Hemicrania continua responsive to rofecoxib. Cephalalgia 20:130–131

Peres MFP, Silberstein SD, Nahmias S, Sechter AL, Youssef I, Rozen TED (2001) Hemicrania continua is not that rare. Neurology 57:948–951

Peres MF, Zuckerman E, Porto PP, Brandt RA (2004) Headaches and pineal cyst: a (more than) coincidental relationship? Headache 44:929–930

Pfaffenrath V, Pollmann W, Ruther E, Lund R, Hajak G (1986) Onset of nocturnal attacks of chronic cluster headache in relation to sleep stages. Acta Neurol Scand 73:403–407

Pinesi L, Rainero I, Cicolin A, Zibetti M, Gentile S, Mutani R (2003) Hypnic headache syndrome: association of the attacks with REM sleep. Cephalalgia 23:150–154

Piovesan EJ, Kowacs P, Lange M, Pachecs C, Piovesan L, Werneck L (2001) Prevalencia e caracteristicas de cefaleia idiopatica em punhaladas em uma população de migranoses. Arq Neuropsychiatr 59:201–225

Piovesan EJ, Zuckerman E, Kowacs PA, Werneck LC (2002) COX-2 inhibitor for the treatment of idiopathic stabbing headache secondary to cerebrovascular diseases. Cephalalgia 22:197–200

Raskin NH (1988) The hypnic headache syndrome. Headache 28:534–536

Raskin NH, Schwartz RK (1980) Icepick-like pain. Neurology 3:203–205

Rasmussen BK (1995) Epidemiology of headache. Cephalalgia 15:45–68

Rogalewski A, Evers S (2005) Symptomatic hemicrania continua after internal carotid dissection. Headache 45:167–169

Rozen TD (2003a) Melatonin as treatment for idiopathic stabbing headache. Neurology 61:865–866

Rozen TD (2003b) New daily persistent headache. Curr Pain Headache Rep 7:218–223

Rozen TD (2006) Melatonin responsive hemicrania continua. Headache 46:1203–1204

Rozen TD (2009) Can indomethacin act as a disease modifying agent in hemicrania continua? A supportive clinical case. Headache 49:759–761

Ruscheweyh R, Buchheister A, Gregor N, Jung A, Evers S (2010) Nummular headache: six new cases and lancinating pain attacks as possible manifestation. Cephalalgia 30(2):249–53

Schwedt T, Dodick D, Trentman T, Zimmerman R (2006) Occipital nerve stimulation for chronic cluster headache and hemicrania continua: pain relief and persistence of autonomic featues. Cephalalgia 26:1025–1027

Schwedt T, Dodick D, Hentz J, Trentman T, Zimmerman R (2007) Occipital nerve stimulation for chronic headache. Long term safety and efficacy. Cephalalgia 27:153–157

Seo MW, Park SH (2005) Botulinum toxin treatment in nummular headache. Cephalalgia 25:991, Abstract

Silberstein SD, Lipton RB, Solomon S, Mathew NT (1994) Classification of daily and near daily headaches: proposed revisions to the IHS-criteria. Headache 34:1–7

Sjaastad O, Antonaci F (1995) A piroxicam derivative partly effective in chronic paroxysmal hemicrania and hemicrania continua. Headache 35:549–550

Sjaastad O, Bakketeig LS (2006) Migraine with aura: visual disturbances and interrelationship with the pain phase. J Headache Pain 7:127–135

Sjaastad O, Spierings ELH (1984) Hemicrania continua: another headache absolutely responsive to indomethacin. Cephalalgia 4:65–70

Sjaastad O, Egge K, Horven I, Kayed K, Lund-Roland L, Russell D, Slordahl Conradi I (1979) Chronic paroxysmal hemicrania. Mechanical precipitation of attacks. Headache 19:31–36

Sjaastad O, Pettersen H, Bakketeig LS (2001) The Vågå study; epidemiology of headache I: The prevalence of ultrashort paroxysms. Cephalalgia 21:207–215

Sjaastad O, Pettersen H, Bakketeig LS (2002) The Vågå study of headache epidemiology II. jabs: clinical manifestations. Acta Neurol Scand 105:25–31

Sjaastad O, Pettersen H, Bakketeig LS (2003) Extracephalic jabs/idiopathic stabs. Vågå study of headache epidemiology. Cephalalgia 23:50–54

Sjaastad O, Petersen HC, Bakketeig LS (2004) Supraorbital neuralgia. Vågå study of headache epidemiology. Cephalalgia 25:296–304

Soriani S, Battistella PA, Arnaldi C, De Cralo L, Cernetti R, Corra S, Tosato G (1996) Juvenile idiopathic stabbing headache. Headache 36:565–567

Spears RC (2006) Hemicrania continua. A case in which a patient experienced complete relief on melatonin. Headache 46:524–527

Spitz M, Peres MF (2004) Hemicrania continua postpartum. Cephalalgia 24:603–604

Takase Y, Nakano M, Tatsumi C, Matsuyama T (2004) Clinical features, effectiveness of drug-based treatment, and prognosis of new daily persistent headache (NDPH): 30 cases in Japan. Cephalalgia 24:955–959

Trucco M (2007) Nummular headache: another headache treated with gabapentine. J Headache Pain 8:137–138

Trucco M, Antonaci F, Sandrini G (1992) Hemicrania continua: a case responsive to piroxicam-beta-cyclodextrin. Headache 19:442

Trucco M, Mainardi F, Perego G, Zanchin G (2006) Nummular headache: first Italian case and therapeutic proposal. Cephalalgia 26:354–356

Valença MM, Andrade-Valença LP, da Silva WF, Dodick DW (2007) Hemicrania continua secondary to an ipsilateral brainstem lesion. Headache 47: 438–441

Vanast WJ (1986) New daily persistent headaches definition of a benign syndrome. Headache 26:318

Vieira JP, Salgueiro AB, Alfaro M (2006) Short-lasting headaches in children. Cephalalgia 26:1220–1224

Zacaria A, Graber M, Davis P (2000) Idiopathic stabbing headache associated with monocular vision loss. Arch Neurol 57:745–746

29 Headache Associated with Sexual Activity

Carlos Alberto Bordini[1] · *Dominique Valade*[2]
[1]Clínica Neurológica Batatais, Batatais, SP, Brazil
[2]Lariboisière Hospital, Paris, France

Paolo Martelletti, Timothy J. Steiner (eds.), *Handbook of Headache*, DOI 10.1007/978-88-470-1700-9_29,
© Lifting The Burden 2011

Abstract: Two entities are currently identified: headache occurring before orgasm and headache occurring during orgasm. *Primary headache associated with sexual activity* is more frequent in men than women (mean age: 40), and is more frequent in migraineurs. Preorgasmic headache is typically a bilateral pain, predominant in the occipital and cervical regions. It is described as a dull ache that increases progressively, typically intensifying as sexual excitement increases, and lasting a couple of hours to several days. This type of headache might be caused by an excessive tightening of the head and neck muscles during sexual activity. Orgasmic headache is the most common variety of sex headache. It usually gives no warning, as in thunderclap headache. Its duration is highly variable (from few minutes to 3 h, usually, but can last up to 48 h). This type of headache is usually isolated, but accompanying symptoms such as nausea, emesis, phonophobia, or photophobia can be found. Practically, this headache must be considered as a thunderclap headache. At first manifestation, a subarachnoid hemorrhage must be ruled out as a priority, and then other medical conditions, as preruptured aneurysm, arterial dissection (carotid, vertebral, or intracranial dissection), diffuse segmental vasoconstriction, bout of hypertension, and CSF hypotension. Once all conditions from the list above have been ruled out, the headache is considered as primary. It is essential to reassure the patient, and propose first nonmedicinal approaches (relaxation, biofeedback, even though scientific evidences are poor for such treatments). If necessary, beta-blockers (propranolol) or calcium-channel inhibitors (diltiazem) can be proposed. Taking indomethacin 30 min before sex could also be helpful.

Established Knowledge

Introduction

The headaches associated with sexual activity (HSA) appear in item 4, in ICHD-II (Headache Classification Committee of the International Headache Society 2004) "Other primary headaches," whose short description is "Headache precipitated by sexual activity, usually starting as a dull bilateral ache as sexual excitement increases and suddenly becoming intense at orgasm, in the absence of any intracranial disorder." The diagnostic criteria are seen in ❷ *Table 29.1.* The item C (Not attributed to another disorder) seems to be of paramount importance for the headache to be classified as "Primary," since many neurological conditions may be brought up by sexual activity. In the latter, "if a new headache occurs for the first time in close temporal relation to another disorder that is a known cause of headache, this headache is coded according to the causative disorder as a secondary headache."

The previously used terms were benign sex headache, benign vascular sexual headache. The term "coital cephalalgia" was abandoned because the headache may also be precipitated by masturbation and during nocturnal emissions; by similar reason orgasmic headache is now a subitem in the ICHD-II because HSA may occur without orgasm (Newman et al. 2008).

Epidemiology

There are scant data on the prevalence of primary HSA (PHAS) in the general population. In one population-based epidemiological survey, the lifetime prevalence for HSA was 1% (Rasmussen and Olesen 1992), even though in cohort studies of headache clinics, it is estimated that patients with HSA account for up to 1.3% (Frese et al. 2003a). Males are more frequently affected than females (Lance 1976).

Clinical Features

Primary headaches associated with sexual activity (PHSA) are separated in preorgasmic and orgasmic headaches (❯ *Table 29.1*)

Preorgasmic headaches are bilateral and can be reduced by deliberate muscle relaxation and resemble tension-type headache; usually there is a dull ache in the head and neck. They represent about 20% of all PHSA (Newman et al. 2008). Orgasmic headaches account for about 75% of cases. They begin abruptly at the moment of orgasm and are excruciatingly severe, localized in frontal areas or generalized. The pain quality is explosive or throbbing, and typically lasts from 1 min to 3 h. About 50% of PHSA patients also have migraine (Silbert et al. 1991). In the first edition of ICHD (Headache Classification Committee of the International Headache Society 1988) a postural type was also described. This seems to be the least common type affecting approximately 5% of sufferers. It worsens with standing or sitting and is relieved if the sufferer lies down. It may be caused by a spontaneous tear in the dura mater developing during sexual activity. In ICHD-II, this rare headache subtype is classified as headaches attributed to spontaneous (or idiopathic) low CSF pressure, because it is, probably, due to CSF leakage.

According to an analysis of 51 patients (Frese et al. 2003a) the following features were observed. Mean age at onset is about 35 years; type 1 (preorgasmic) occurred in 22%, while type 2 (orgasmic) occurred in 78%. Two thirds of patients had their headaches in a bout, that is, at least two attacks occurring in at least 50% of sexual activities for at least 2 weeks and then none despite continuing sexual activities. The bouts lasted from 2 days to 18 months (mean 3.2 ± weeks). The number of attacks within a bout ranged from 2 to 50. One third of patients did not display the "bout pattern," instead they suffer PHSA for long periods without remission. In these latter patients, most have infrequent attacks (<20% of sexual activity), but 20% of them suffered PHSA during nearly every sexual activity. The mean duration of attacks was 30 min; in 86% of patients the severe pain lasted less than 4 h. Nausea, vomiting, and dizziness occurred in some cases but were rare. There seem to exist some differences between the clinical features of type 1 and type 2 PHSA (❯ *Table 29.2*).

◘ Table 29.1

Primary headache associated with sexual activity

Description: Headache precipitated by sexual activity, usually starting as a dull bilateral ache as sexual excitement increases and suddenly becoming intense at orgasm, in the absence of any intracranial disorder
Preorgasmic headache
A. Dull ache in the head and neck associated with awareness of neck and/or jaw muscle contraction and fulfilling criterion B
B. Occurs during sexual activity and increases with sexual excitement
C. Not attributed to another disorder
Orgasmic headache
A. Sudden severe ("explosive") headache meeting criterion B
B. Occurs at orgasm
C. Not attributed to another disorder[a]

[a]On first onset of orgasmic headache it is mandatory to exclude conditions such as subarachnoid hemorrhage and arterial dissection

☐ **Table 29.2**

Some differences of clinical features between type 1 and type 2 of headaches attributed to sexual activity

	Type 1	Type 2
Sex ratio (female: male)	2:9 (1:4.5)	11:29 (1:2.6)
Occipital/diffuse localization	82%	75%
Throbbing quality	36%	50%
Arterial hypertension	27%	15%
Comorbid migraine	9%	30%
Comorbid exertional headache	9%	35%
Comorbid tension-type headache	55%	43%

About 40% of patients can terminate the headache by stopping the sexual activity and 51% of patients report they can ease the headache by taking a more passive role during sexual activity. In type 2 PHSA, the onset time is exactly at orgasm or up 5 s before it (Evers and Lance 2006).

One point that we must have in mind is that the diagnosis of PHSA is predicated upon the exclusion of secondary causes as subarachnoid hemorrhage (SAH), arterial dissection and lesions of the posterior fossa (Newman et al. 2008), CSF pathways, and cervical spine.

Pathophysiology

The exact mechanism is not known. Due to the nature of the headache, it has been suggested that type 1 is related to muscle contraction or tension-type headache (Lance 1992; Pascual et al. 1996). Due to the similarity to exertional headache, it has been postulated that an increase in intracranial pressure due to a Valsalva maneuver during coitus might play a role in PHSA (Calandre et al. 1996). An interesting study on cognitive processing was performed in patients with the explosive subtype of headache associated with sexual activity (HSA type 2) (Frese et al. 2003b). The most important finding of this study is that patients with PHSA type 2 have a loss of cognitive habituation as measured by visual event-related potentials (ERP). This characteristic is shared with migraine patients. According to the authors, such abnormality points to a dysfunction in cortical information processing similar to the abnormal information processing seen in migraine, which is an interictal cortical dysfunction probably due to inadequate control by the so-called state-setting, chemically addressed pathways originating in the brainstem.

On the other hand, a clinical comparison between type 1 and type 2 and experimental data have not given any evidence that these are pathophysiologically distinct disorders (Frese et al. 2003a).

Diagnosis

First of all, the diagnosis of PHSA requires the exclusion of conditions such as SAH, and arterial dissection in the first episode. It is known (Lundberg and Osterman 1974) that SAH occurs during sexual activity in about 4–12% of all cases and cerebral or brainstem infarction at the time of orgasm has been reported (Lance 1992; Lasoasa 2003). Signs that could indicate a serious underlying condition are: vomiting; decreased level of consciousness; meningism; visual, sensory, or motor disturbances; and severe headache persisting beyond 24 h. In the presence of such disturbances a neurological examination and CT scan of the brain are mandatory. If there is a possibility of SAH and if the CT scan is normal, a lumbar puncture has to be performed. Arterial dissection should be excluded by ultrasound examination or magnetic resonance angiography.

Prognosis

The prognosis is good. In general the condition only appears during a period of time and disappears without treatment. In few patients the headache can occur for long periods, sometimes for years.

Management

If the diagnosis is PHSA, the first attitude is reassurance for the patient and his or her partner. To advice that the course of the condition is limited in time, the headaches recur during several sexual encounters over a period of time and never return again, but also inform that the course may be unpredictable; some patients experience them from time to time throughout their lifetime.

It has been reported that when patients resume sexual activity within days after an attack, the headache may recur (Porter and Jancovik 1981); so advising the patients to refrain from sex for a week after an attack might be prudent. For patients with the preorgasmic subtype, it may be useful to stop the sexual activity as soon as the headache begins or to assume a more passive role.

Pharmacotherapy: indomethacin 50–100 mg taken 30–60 min before sexual activity (Newman et al. 2008), or naratriptan 2.5 mg taken 2 h before may be useful as short-term prophylaxis (Pascual et al. 1996; Kumar and Reuler 1993). The acute treatment for an attack that has already begun is, in general, worthless but can be tried with triptans or NSAIDs (Frese et al. 2003a). For patients with longer lasting bouts or with frequent attacks, propranolol in doses from 40 to 240 mg/day is reported to be effective (Porter and Jancovik 1981), but there is one report about the failure of this treatment (Evans and Pascual 2000).

Current Research

What is usually found concerning headache and sexual activity are papers from third care sets, either suggesting to foster patients to tell doctors about this kind of illness in order to gather more knowledge on the topic, or articles depicting headaches associated with sexual activity with numerous neurological conditions such as *amaurosis fugax*, central nervous system angiitis, and stroke.

Some articles explore other aspects of the relationship between sexual activity and migraine; they may deserve some attention and will be shortly discussed.

Houle et al. (Houle et al. 2006) studied the relationship between migraine and self-reported sexual desire. It was found that migraineurs had higher scores as measured by a sexual interview inventory than patients suffering from tension-type headache. Authors suggest that migraine and sex are at least partially modulated by serotonin (5-HT), and that migraineurs might have chronically low systemic 5-HT. As sexual desire also has been linked to serotonin levels, authors make the hypothesis that migraine and sexual desire are both modulated by similar serotonergic phenomena.

Moreover, sometimes, patients report relief that orgasm may even bring relief or suppression of a migraine attack (Couch 2001). Couch and Bearss (Couch and Bearss 1990) carried out a study in which 83 women were questioned as to whether they had sexual intercourse during headache; 57 of them indicated they had; 10 (17.5%) patients reported they were pain free if they get an orgasm; and 28 (30%) reported some relief. Authors call attention to the fact that the "pain-free" response is twice the pain-free response of approximately 9% reported for placebo in most studies. Almost half of those who employed this nondrug therapy received some degree of relief. It would appear that orgasm is significantly less effective than triptans or DHE, but when effective, the onset of relief is faster than with parenteral sumatriptan.

As for possible underlying mechanisms for such effect, authors looked for an interesting article on basic science (Caba et al. 1998) where it was shown that stimulation of the posterior vagina in rats will produce an analgesic effect. The authors postulate that this is a physiologic reflex related to the birth process to produce pain relief when the cervix and pelvic outlet are stretched. Couch and Bearss suggest that such reflex might play a role for the relief of migraine by orgasms.

Conclusions

The relationship between sexual activity and headache is complex; usually sexual activity may provoke headache. In such situations the existence of structural lesions must be ruled out. The increased sexual desire in migraineurs and that orgasm may abort a migraine attack may point us to a new and challenging field of research, and we may finish quoting Evers and Lance (Evers and Lance 2006): "Headache attributed to sexual activity can be very frightening, and explanation, counseling, and reassurance can be the most important therapeutic approaches. Widespread knowledge about the existence and nature of this headache disorder will improve medical care and help patients to confide their complaints to their doctors."

References

Caba M, Komisaruk BR, Beyer C (1998) Analgesic synergism between AP5 (an NMDA receptor antagonist) and vaginocervical stimulation in the rat. Pharmacol Biochem Behav 61:45–48

Calandre L, Hernandez-Lain A, Lopes-Valdez E (1996) Benign Valsalva's maneuver headache: an MRI study of six cases. Headache 36:251–253

Couch JR (2001) Orgasm headache. Headache 41:512–514

Couch J, Bearss C (1990) Relief of migraine with sexual intercourse. Headache 30:302

Evans RW, Pascual J (2000) Orgasmic headache: clinical diagnosis and treatment. Headache 40:491–494

Evers S, Lance JW (2006) In primary headache attributed to sexual activity. In: Olesen J, Goadsby PJ, Ramadan NM et al (eds) The headaches, 3rd edn. Lippincott Williams & Wilkins, Philadelphia, pp 841–846

Frese A, Eikermann A, Frese K et al (2003a) Headache associated with sexual activity. Demography, clinical features and comorbidity. Neurology 61: 796–800

Frese A, Frese K, Ringelstein EB, Husstedt I-W, Evers S (2003b) Cognitive processing in headache associated with sexual activity. Cephalalgia 23:545–551

Headache Classification Committee of the International Headache Society (2004) The international classification of headache disorders, 2nd edn. Cephalalgia 24(Suppl 1):9–160

Headache Classification Committee of the International Headache Society (1998) Classification and diagnostic criteria for headache disorders, cranial neuralgias and facial pain. Cephalalgia 8(Suppl 7):1–96

Houle TT, Dhingra LK et al (2006) Not tonight, I have a headache? Headache 46:983–990

Kumar KL, Reuler JB (1993) Uncommon headaches: diagnosis and treatment. J Gen Int Med 8:333–341

Lance JW (1976) Headaches related to sexual activity. J Neurol Neurosurg Psychiatry 39:1226–1230

Lance JW (1992) Benign coital headache. Cephalalgia 12:339

Lasoasa DS (2003) Not so benign sexual headache. Headache 34:808

Lundberg PO, Osterman PO (1974) The benign and malignant forms of orgasmic cephalalgia. Headache 14:164–165

Newman LC, Grosberg BM, Dodick DW (2008) Other primary headaches. In: Silberstein SD, Lipton RDe, Dodick DW (eds) Wolff's headache and other head pain, 8th edn. Oxford University Press, New York, pp 431–447

Pascual J, Iglesias F, Oterino A et al (1996) Exertional and sexual headaches: an analysis of 72 benign and symptomatic cases. Neurology 46:1520–1524

Porter M, Jancovik J (1981) Benign coital cephalalgia: differential diagnosis and treatment. Arch Neurol 38:710–712

Rasmussen BK, Olesen J (1992) Symptomatic and non symptomatic headaches in a general population. Neurology 42:1225–1231

Silbert PL, Edis RH, Stewart-Wynn EGG, Gubbay SS (1991) Benign vascular sexual headache and exertional headache: inter-relationships and long term prognosis. J Neurol Neurosurg Psychiat 54:417–421

Part 9

Headache That Has Become Difficult to Treat

30 Headache Occurring on More Days Than Not

Christina Sun-Edelstein[1] · *Alan Rapoport*[2,3]
[1]Centre for Clinical Neurosciences and Neurological Research,
St Vincent's Hospital, Melbourne, Australia
[2]The David Geffen School of Medicine at UCLA, Los Angeles, CA, USA
[3]The New England Center for Headache, Stamford, CT, USA

Paolo Martelletti, Timothy J. Steiner (eds.), *Handbook of Headache*, DOI 10.1007/978-88-470-1700-9_30,
© Lifting The Burden 2011

Abstract: The term "chronic daily headache" (CDH) is commonly used to refer to primary headache that occurs on at least 15 days per month (more days than not). CDH is common, and associated with social, behavioral, and occupational disability. In recent years, the concept of disease modification has been applied to migraine, with an emphasis on the identification of factors that might prevent disease progression. The early recognition of high-risk patients and the utilization of a multidisciplinary treatment plan while headaches are still in the episodic phase appear to be critical aspects in preventing or minimizing progression and resultant disability. In this chapter, risk factors for CDH will be reviewed and principles of preventing headache chronification, including the initiation of preventive medication and behavioral treatment, the recognition of medication overuse, and the implementation of lifestyle modifications, will be discussed. Areas of ongoing research will also be addressed.

Established Knowledge

Introduction

The term "chronic daily headache" (CDH) is descriptive rather than diagnostic, commonly used to refer to primary headache that occurs on at least 15 days per month (more days than not). CDH can be of short duration, lasting less than 4 h (including chronic cluster headache, chronic paroxysmal hemicrania, and hypnic headache), or long duration, lasting for 4 or more hours per day. Though long-duration CDH comprises chronic migraine, chronic tension-type headache, hemicrania continua, and new daily persistent headache, the majority of CDH sufferers in the general population have chronic migraine or chronic tension-type headache (Castillo et al. 1999; Scher et al. 1998).

CDH often evolves from episodic headaches, in particular, episodic migraine. Though most people with episodic migraine do not transform into chronic migraine sufferers, a significant subgroup does experience chronification and worsening. According to population-based studies, approximately 3% of people with episodic migraine transform into chronic migraine in a typical year (Scher et al. 2003a). Epidemiological studies (Scher et al. 1998; Stovner et al. 2007; Lipton et al. 2007) have estimated that CDH affects approximately 3–4% of the world's population, and 1–2% of children and adolescents. CDH is associated with significant impairment and disability, and is less responsive to acute and preventive treatments than episodic migraine.

Headache transformation is often gradual (Bigal and Lipton 2009), evolving from low-frequency to high-frequency episodic migraine and then into a chronic pattern. However, this process is not necessarily irreversible, as spontaneous or treatment-induced remissions are possible (Bigal and Lipton 2008a). Given the detrimental impact on patient quality of life caused by CDH, it is imperative for physicians to identify those patients who are susceptible to its development and initiate a treatment plan to prevent its onset. In addition to traditional headache management, which involves acute and preventive headache medications, an understanding of CDH risk factors, comorbid disorders, and the lifestyle modifications that can preclude disease progression is critical when considering the prevention of this disorder (Bigal and Lipton 2006b).

Risk Factors for the Development of CDH

Several modifiable and non-modifiable risk factors for the development of CDH have been identified.

Non-Modifiable Risk Factors

With regard to non-modifiable demographic variables, CDH appears to be more common in women, Caucasians, and people with less education and lower socioeconomic status. Low socioeconomic status is also associated with a poorer prognosis. Married people were shown to have a lower risk of CDH and better prognosis at follow-up in a prospective study (Scher et al. 2003a) when compared to those who were not currently married (single, widowed, divorced, or separated). Though pediatric data is limited, there appears to be a higher prevalence in adolescent girls than boys.

Modifiable Risk Factors

Modifiable risk factors include medication overuse, attack frequency, obesity, snoring and sleep disturbances, comorbid pain conditions, head or neck injury, psychiatric comorbidities and major life events, and possibly smoking and caffeine consumption (Scher et al. 2008a; Wang et al. 2000).

Medication Overuse

The overuse of acute medication, now referred to as "medication overuse headache" (MOH), is one of the most important risk factors for CDH, and has thus received a substantial degree of attention in the headache literature. Population-based studies have indicated that medication overuse is present in about 30% of people with CDH, and over 80% of patients in headache subspecialty centers have MOH (Mathew 1990a; Rapoport et al. 1996; Dodick 2002; Bigal et al. 2004; Katsarava et al. 2004; Scher et al. 2008a). In a study that followed 532 consecutive patients with episodic migraine over the course of 1 year, the risk of developing chronic headache was 19 times higher in patients with medication overuse compared to those without medication overuse (Katsarava et al. 2004). Though the pathophysiology of MOH is not fully understood, it likely involves the sensitization of central pain pathways (Cupini and Calabresi 2005) and the up-regulation of the pro-nociceptive 5-HT(2A) receptor (Supornsilpchai et al. 2010).

MOH has been defined by the second edition of the International Classification of Headache Disorders as a headache that is present on at least 15 days per month, and has developed or markedly worsened during a period of at least 3 months during which one or more drugs used for acute and/or symptomatic treatment of headache have been taken on more than 10 days per month (or 15 days per month in the case of simple analgesics). Though the criteria also require a 2-month withdrawal period before the diagnosis of MOH can be made, a proposed revision (Olesen et al. 2006) eliminated that requirement. This revision to the MOH criteria still resides in the appendix and has not yet been incorporated into the body of the ICHD-II, and therefore there is some controversy as to whether or not it is official. In an effort to eliminate the confusion and streamline diagnostic and research efforts, it is our strong opinion that these changes should be adopted immediately.

MOH occurs only in patients with a prior history of headaches. Though migraineurs appear to be most susceptible to the development of MOH, it can also occur in patients with chronic tension-type headache (CTTH), hemicrania continua, posttraumatic headache, and new daily persistent headache (Bahra et al. 2003). In these patients, the daily or near-daily use of simple analgesics (i.e., acetaminophen), combination analgesics (i.e., simple analgesics combined with caffeine, butalbital, or codeine), opioids, ergotamine tartrate, or triptans, either alone or in combination, results in the transformation from episodic to chronic headaches. Patients with cluster headache seem less susceptible and the drug dihydroergotamine rarely causes MOH in our experience. The association between migraine progression and barbiturate or opiate exposure appears to be particularly strong, in that the critical frequency may be as low as 5 and 8 days per month, respectively (Bigal and Lipton 2008c). These drugs have been described as accelerating disease progression (Chan and Holford 2001). In contrast, anti-inflammatory medications may be protective in patients with less than 10 headache days per month at baseline, but can induce migraine progression in those with a higher headache frequency (Bigal and Lipton 2008c).

During the period of transformation, patients usually report an increase in headache frequency and a change in headache quality. A daily, dull, annoying, featureless headache that often persists throughout the day emerges, and increasing doses of acute care medications are usually needed, at more frequent intervals, to alleviate the pain. Superimposed on the daily headache are exacerbations typical of the original headache disorder (often migraine), which can occur several times per week or several times per month.

This topic is discussed in more detail later in this chapter, and in ❷ Chap. 50.

Attack Frequency

Baseline headache frequency is another important risk factor for migraine chronification, and this risk increases in a nonlinear manner as headache frequency increases (Castillo et al. 1999; Scher et al. 2003a). While a baseline headache frequency of <3 per month has been associated with a low risk of transformation, the risk increases rapidly for higher frequencies (Scher et al. 2003a). Though increased attack frequency may be a consequence of headache chronification, it may also contribute to the progression of migraine by triggering the process of central sensitization and lowering the threshold for pain (Welch et al. 2001).

Obesity

The association between obesity and migraine progression has been shown in several studies. One study showed that the relative odds of CDH in obese individuals (body mass index [BMI] >/= 30) were five times higher than in people of normal weight (Scher et al. 2003a). BMI is also associated with attack frequency in migraineurs (Bigal et al. 2006) and is a stronger risk factor for chronic migraine than chronic tension-type headache (Bigal and Lipton 2006a). A recent review (Peterlin et al. 2010) concluded that the prevalence of CDH is increased in those with TBO (total body obesity), that TBO is associated with an increased risk of transforming from episodic to chronic daily headache, and that abdominal obesity may be associated with CDH.

Snoring and Sleep Disturbances

The association between snoring and sleep disturbances and CDH persists independent of variables that are known to be associated with sleep disorders, such as male gender, obesity, and increased age (Scher et al. 2003b; Wiendels et al. 2006). In the Copenhagen Male Study (Jennum et al. 1994), a large cross-sectional study of 3,323 Danish men, an odds ratio (OR) of 1.5 (95% CI 1.3, 1.8, $p < 0.0001$) for headache among self-reported snorers was reported, and this association was almost doubled in the presence of chronic daily headache. Another population-based case-control study found that CDH sufferers were more likely to be habitual or daily snorers compared to controls (Scher et al. 2003b).

Comorbid Pain Conditions

People with migraine or frequent headache are more likely to have comorbid pain conditions, especially related to musculoskeletal pain or arthritis, when compared to those without headache (Scher et al. 2006). A Norwegian population survey also found that headache sufferers were more likely to report musculoskeletal symptoms when compared with non-sufferers and that the strength of the association increased with increasing headache frequency (Hagen et al. 2002). There also appears to be a stronger association between headache and pain areas closer to the head, such as the neck and shoulders, as compared to areas in the lower quadrants of the body (Hasvold and Johnsen 1993; Boardman et al. 2005).

Head or Neck Injury

The data on this topic is sparse but there is some evidence that head or neck injury is a risk factor for CDH. In a population study (Couch et al. 2007), head or neck injury was a greater CDH risk factor for men than women, and did not necessarily have a close temporal relationship to the onset of chronic headache. The risk of CDH was increased in those with lifetime injuries to the head or neck, even if those injuries occurred long before the onset of CDH. In addition, the severity of the injury was not obviously related to CDH. However, other studies on persistent headache as a consequence of head and neck injury found contrary results (Obelieneiene et al. 1998; Mickeviciene et al. 2002; Mickeviciene et al. 2004; Schrader et al. 2006).

Psychiatric Comorbidities and Stressful Life Events

A bidirectional relationship between chronic pain conditions and psychiatric disorders such as depression and anxiety has been well demonstrated (McWilliams et al. 2004), and psychosocial variables play a significant role in the development of chronic disability in these syndromes. Among CDH patients, mood disorders are comorbid conditions in over half the population (Dodick 2006), and chronic migraineurs are more likely to have depression and anxiety relative to patients with chronic tension-type headache (Zwart et al. 2003). In addition, chronic migraine has been found to be more common in women with major depressive disorder (Karakurum et al. 2004). The obesity variable also affects this relationship. Not only has obesity been found to be associated with depression and anxiety, obese migraineurs with depression are more likely to have higher headache frequency and headache-related disability compared to normal-weight migraineurs without depression (Tietjen et al. 2007).

Stressful life events, including moves, death of family or friends, changes in marital status, and ongoing stressful life events, have been recognized as risk factors for CDH in clinic-based and other selected populations (Scher et al. 2008a). A population-based study (Scher et al. 2008b) also showed that compared with episodic headache controls, subjects with frequent headache had more major life changes during the year before or the same year, with the odds of frequent headaches increasing with each antecedent life event.

Childhood Maltreatment

In a paper assessing the relationship between different types of childhood abuse and migraine characteristics in a multicenter headache clinic population (Tietjen et al. 2010), physical abuse, emotional abuse, and emotional neglect were reported to be possible risk factors for the development of chronic headache, including transformed migraine. This association appeared to be independent of depression and anxiety, which are linked to both childhood abuse and CDH. Furthermore, emotional abuse was associated with severe headache-related disability, allodynia, and an earlier onset of migraine.

Smoking

One population-based study (Wiendels et al. 2006) showed that chronic headaches were associated with smoking. Though the authors had speculated that smokers were more likely to overuse medications due to a tendency toward substance use, smoking rates did not differ between medication overusers and non-overusers. However, since the age of smoking onset was not documented, it was not clear whether smoking is merely a secondary phenomenon.

Caffeine Consumption

The relationship between caffeine consumption and CDH is as yet unclear. Though abrupt caffeine withdrawal in people with CDH (or even episodic migraine) is associated with rebound headache, the role of caffeine in increasing the risk of developing chronic headaches is not as clear. One case-control study (Scher et al. 2004) showed that although current caffeine intake was not related to CDH, pre-CDH use was a modest risk factor, especially for women, subjects younger than 40 years, and those with chronic episodic (as opposed to chronic continuous) headache. However, a large population-based study (Wiendels et al. 2006) showed no significant relationship between current caffeine intake and CDH. A better understanding of caffeine as a CDH risk factor is of great interest given the widespread consumption of caffeinated beverages as well as the use of caffeine-containing medications for the acute treatment of headaches.

Preventive Treatment

Initiating Preventive Treatment

The American Migraine Prevalence and Prevention Study (AMPP) demonstrated that preventive treatment is underutilized, in that only 12.4% of respondents in this population-based study were using preventive treatment, though 38.8% were potentially candidates for it (Lipton et al. 2007). Many patients, even those with frequent headaches, are reluctant to start preventive medication because of the daily regimen and potential adverse events. However, delaying preventive treatment often results in the frequent use of acute care medications and the subsequent development of MOH and increased headache frequency. Furthermore, there appears to be a critical period during which preventive medications are most effective, as patients with frequent (over 15 days per month) but not daily headaches have been shown to have more improvement with prevention than those with daily headaches (Rothrock et al. 1994).

Recent guidelines (Dodick and Silberstein 2007) recommended the initiation of preventive treatment in the following scenarios:

- More than one attack per week
- Acute medication consumption >2 days per week
- Acute medication is contraindicated, not tolerated, or ineffective
- Patient preference
- Uncommon migraine conditions (i.e., hemiplegic migraine)

Others have suggested that preventive treatment be started even earlier, when headache frequency is ≥2 per month (Evers et al. 2009). However, the authors believe this is too aggressive a plan for many patients. We also believe there is a close association between frequency and degree of disability in helping to decide on whether or not to use prevention. One bad migraine attack per month, if it lasts 2–3 days, causes a lot of disability, and does not respond well to acute care treatment, may require preventive therapy. Quality of life and work or school performances are other factors to be considered when considering headache prevention. Although there is no clear-cut evidence regarding the optimal duration of preventive treatment, some authors have recommended at least 6 months of good headache control prior to considering a gradual taper and potential discontinuation of migraine prophylaxis in patients with less frequent migraine attacks, fewer years of migraine, and fewer comorbid conditions. At least 12 months of good control has been advised for those with a longer migraine history, chronic migraine, and multiple comorbid conditions (Evans et al. 2004). Short- or long-term rational combination therapy has also been recommended in escalating episodic migraine, chronic migraine, refractory migraine, and status migrainosus (Peterlin et al. 2008). There is also some evidence that preventive treatments may continue to have a beneficial effect in some patients even after the medication has been discontinued (Wober et al. 1991; Rothrock and Mandizibal 2000).

Information on specific preventive medications is detailed in the headache-specific chapters (❯ Chaps. 17, ❯ 21, ❯ 25, ❯ 28).

Early Intervention in Children and Adolescents

A recent review (Charles et al. 2009) demonstrated several significant trends in chronic headache. First, children and adolescents who were treated early in the disease with targeted therapy had brisker responses to treatment, less disability, and a better prognosis. Second, many adults with chronic, refractory migraine had onset of headaches in childhood or adolescence, and were not treated appropriately. Third, there appears to be a window of opportunity early in the course childhood or adolescent migraine during which treatment can have a disease-modifying effect and thus halt the progression of pain and disability. As such, comprehensive acute care and preventive treatment in children, adolescents, and young adults may improve long-term outcome.

Given the recent epidemiological evidence suggesting that chronic daily headache in children and adolescents has increased over the past few decades (Linder 2005), and that 46% of adult migraineurs report that symptoms started before age 20, there is compelling reason to treat migraine early, aggressively, and comprehensively in the course of the disease in order to minimize long-term disability (Charles et al. 2009). This includes public awareness programs, risk factor modification, pharmacological therapy (which may include rational combination therapy in severe cases), and behavioral treatment (Charles et al. 2009).

Acute Care Medications

There has been some speculation that the intermittent use of triptans in the acute treatment of migraine may confer a protective, disease-modifying effect. While this has not been formally studied, a long-term effect might be inferred when one considers the cumulative effect, over the lifetime of a migraineur, of shorter attacks, improved cognition, and decreased anxiety associated with effective treatment. In addition, triptans can abort headache pain prior to the development of central sensitization, as manifest by cutaneous allodynia

(Burstein et al. 2004). The judicious use of triptans may therefore potentially improve overall function and delay progression to disability (Loder and Biondi 2003). However, until long-term trials are conducted, the cumulative benefit of triptans is only theoretical. Some would speculate that aggressive use of triptans could lead to medication overuse headache and an increase in frequency of attacks.

Medication Overuse Headache: Recognition and Treatment

The recognition of frequent acute care medication usage is critical in preventing the development of chronic daily headache that results from medication overuse. MOH, once it occurs, is particularly challenging to treat. Furthermore, patients who are actively overusing symptomatic drugs are often refractory to treatment with preventive medications (Mathew et al. 1990b, Limmroth et al. 2002)

Patient education and the complete cessation and subsequent withdrawal of the offending drug are the foundations of MOH treatment. Medication withdrawal may be extremely difficult given the psychological and physical dependence on the drug or drugs (Calabresi and Cupini 2005). Furthermore, a severe withdrawal headache and other withdrawal symptoms (i.e., nausea, vomiting, tachycardia, sleep disturbances, and anxiety) usually occur. These withdrawal symptoms may last up to 14 days, or even longer (Katsarava et al. 2001). Patients frequently report prior failed attempts at medication discontinuation and therefore express skepticism, and at times refusal, about trying once again.

Many medications have been used to treat withdrawal symptoms, including analgesics, antiemetics, sedatives, central muscle relaxants, neuroleptics, antidepressants (amitriptyline), antiepileptics (valproate, topiramate), intravenous dihydroergotamine, subcutaneous sumatriptan, oral triptans, steroids, oxygen, and electric stimulation. However, no evidence-based recommendations can be made regarding the most effective withdrawal therapy (Rossi et al. 2009). Patients who overuse opiates, barbiturates, or benzodiazepines may be particularly difficult to treat and often require inpatient treatment for detoxification. Hospital admission may also be considered for those with significant psychiatric and/or medical comorbidities or prior failures at withdrawal.

Behavioral Treatments

Behavioral treatments, which were introduced nearly 40 years ago, have been increasingly recognized as useful tools in all headache management, but especially for CDH. The US Headache Consortium recommendations for behavioral treatment of migraine include Grade A evidence that relaxation training, thermal biofeedback combined with relaxation training, electromyographic biofeedback, and cognitive-behavioral therapy may be considered as treatment options for the prevention of migraine. There is Grade B evidence for behavioral therapy combined with preventive drug therapy to achieve added clinical improvement for migraine (Campbell et al. 2000).

A review of meta-analyses and evidence-based reviews of behavioral treatments (Andrasik 2007) showed that relaxation, biofeedback, and cognitive therapy result in significant decreases in headache activity of up to 60%. Furthermore, not only do behavioral treatments produce benefits similar to those resulting from traditional pharmacological treatments, combining behavioral and pharmacological treatments can increase overall effectiveness. Studies have also shown that these effects persist over time, for periods of up to 7 years posttreatment (Blanchard 1992), even in the absence of contact with a therapist (Andrasik et al. 1984). Our experience is that most patients with frequent headaches need ongoing contact with a headache-knowledgeable physician to do well.

However, certain types of headache, including chronic daily headache and medication overuse headache, appear to be especially difficult to treat with behavioral interventions (Andrasik 2003). Initiation of behavioral treatments should therefore be initiated early in the course of the disease, as a means of preventing episodic headaches from progressing to chronic patterns. Children and adolescents may particularly benefit from these interventions in that they provide strategies for coping with pain at an early age. In addition, using an integrated approach that combines medication and behavioral therapy can be helpful in alleviating pain and reinforcing patient motivation to maintain clinical improvements (Andrasik 2007; Andrasik et al. 2009). While frequent treatment sessions with a therapist may be costly, meta-analyses have supported the efficacy of limited-contact or home-based behavioral treatments (Andrasik 2007).

Lifestyle Modifications

The treatment of both episodic and chronic headaches should encompass both lifestyle modifications as well as pharmacologic therapy. Ideally, the implementation of lifestyle modifications pertaining to sleep hygiene, exercise, and nutrition should take place prior to the development of CDH, and can indeed be used as a form of prevention. Some of these topics are discussed in more detail in ❷ Chap. 8.

Dietary Modifications
Patients frequently ask for dietary advice as part of their headache treatment plan. They should initially be advised to keep a headache and food diary so as to identify potential food triggers. Frequently reported dietary triggers include alcohol, chocolate, cheese, nitrates and nitrites, caffeine, and monosodium glutamate. While the data supporting the role of these substances as headache triggers is controversial (with the exception of alcohol and caffeine), the evidence suggests that subsets of migraineurs may be sensitive to them (Martin and Behbehani 2001). We find that most migraineurs have their own particular collection of triggers that often affect them by triggering an attack, some of them usually food triggers. Skipping or delaying meals can also trigger headaches. In patients whose headaches appear to be triggered by delayed food intake, midmorning and midafternoon snacks might also be recommended.

Sleep Hygiene
Up to 52% of migraineurs report that sleep disturbances trigger headaches (Robbins 1994; Scharff et al. 1995), and sleep disorders are a well-documented risk factor for the chronification of migraine. Though the relationship between migraine and sleep has not been fully elucidated, it may involve an interaction between sleep-related structures such as the suprachiasmatic nucleus and the medial preoptic nucleus, release of orexins from the hypothalamus, and structures involved in pain modulation, such as the noradrenergic neurons in the locus coeruleus and the serotoninergic neurons in the dorsal raphe (after Martin and Behbehani 2001).

Though it is also unclear whether headaches instigate sleep disturbances or vice versa, some evidence suggests that improving sleep hygiene can improve migraine headaches and possibly revert transformed migraines to episodic patterns (Calhoun and Ford 2007). The evaluation of patients with frequent migraine attacks should therefore include a sleep history, and on occasion a polysomnogram, and education about sleep hygiene. Aspects of good sleep hygiene include consistent bedtimes that allow 8 h in bed, elimination of TV, reading, and music in bed, visualization techniques to shorten the time to sleep onset, eating dinner at least 4 h before bedtime, limiting fluids and exercise within 2 h of bedtime and the discontinuation of any naps during the day.

Exercise

Exercise, particularly aerobic exercise, is often recommended as part of a multidisciplinary approach in the treatment of headache. The physiological mechanism underlying the beneficial effect of exercise on headaches is not well understood but may involve the secretion of encephalin and endorphins (Genazzani et al. 1984; Koseoglu et al. 2003), nitric oxide production (Narin and Pinar 2003), or endothelial protection via decreased levels of plasma norepinephrine, vasoconstrictor prostanoids, and free radicals (Higashi et al. 1999; Varin et al. 1999). At present, there are no clear-cut guidelines for headache sufferers in terms of optimal frequency, intensity, and duration of exercise. In addition, exercise may exacerbate headaches and was reported to be a headache trigger in up to 22% of migraineurs in a recent study (Kelman 2007). To better delineate exercise parameters for headache sufferers, one group recently showed that a moderate-intensity level aerobic training program consisting of three 40-min sessions per week over 12 weeks was well tolerated, with no increases in migraines and with some patients reporting that headaches and quality of life had improved (Varkey et al. 2009).

Though exercise is frequently promoted as part of the multidisciplinary management of headaches, the evidence supporting its benefit in reducing headaches is based primarily on anecdotal reports and observational studies. A recent review (Busch and Gaul 2008) of the available studies and case reports on the therapeutic effect of exercise in the treatment of migraine found that methodological problems limited most of the studies. The authors thus concluded that more studies are necessary before exercise can be recommended based on evidence-based medicine (EBM) criteria, and suggested that future trials aim to quantify and clarify the analgesic effect of exercise in migraine using randomized controlled methods. We believe that exercise may help migraineurs as long as it does not worsen their headaches. Besides, it is probably important for promoting overall health and surely increases their general feeling of well-being. Therefore 20–40 min sessions of moderate aerobic exercise is often recommended up to five times a week for our patients who can tolerate it. For those that cannot, we recommend starting at a very low level of exercise and building that up gradually. It is often the patients that say they cannot tolerate any level of exercise that need it the most, in our experience.

Current Research

One of the primary goals in the area of headache research is the development of biomarkers of disease activity, which can then be used to monitor disease progression. As such, the prevention of disease progression has become a leading goal in the treatment of headache patients. Currently, disease progression and treatment efficacy are measured by monitoring headache frequency and severity, and resultant disability (occupational, social, and behavioral). However, growing evidence suggests that headache frequency and severity are correlated not only with disability but permanent central nervous system structural damage. Migraine progression may be accompanied by anatomical changes manifest by brain lesions and functional changes such as the development of allodynia.

Neuroimaging Findings in CDH

Radiographic findings such as subclinical posterior circulation strokes and diffuse white matter lesions have led to speculation that migraine may be a progressive brain disease, and that MRI findings may be an indicator of cumulative brain insults resulting from frequent attacks (Lipton and Pan 2004). Imaging studies have shown that elevated iron levels in the periaqueductal gray matter were increased in proportion to disease duration in patients with migraine and chronic daily headache, indicating that iron deposition may represent progressive neuronal damage resulting from repeated migraine episodes (Welch et al. 2001). An increase in white matter lesions has also been associated with an increase in headache frequency (Kruit et al. 2004). Studies of visual function in migraineurs suggest that cerebral ischemia during episodes of migraine with aura may cause subtle neuronal damage to the primary visual cortex (Khalil et al. 2000). In the future, some of these forms of CNS structural and functional change may be used as biomarkers to monitor disease progression.

Allodynia and CDH

Early recognition of cutaneous allodynia may also play an important role in the prevention of headache chronicity. Allodynia, which refers to the perception of pain from nonpainful stimuli on normal skin, has recently been described as a putative risk factor for migraine progression (Bigal and Lipton 2008a). Cutaneous allodynia, which develops in two-thirds of migraine patients, is a manifestation of central sensitization, and may be considered a form of attack progression (Burstein et al. 2000; Yarmitsky et al. 2003). Repeated episodes of central sensitization have been associated with permanent neuronal damage, non-response to treatment, and disease progression (Burstein et al. 2000; Burstein et al. 2004).

The prevalence of cutaneous allodynia has been shown to be significantly higher in chronic migraine than in episodic migraine, and is higher in both of these groups when compared with other headaches (Lipton et al. 2008). The development of cutaneous alloydynia appears to be influenced by several risk factors. Non-modifiable risk factors include male sex, African-American race, and decreased educational level, while modifiable risk factors include obesity, depression, and high attack frequency. Other variables associated with the development of cutaneous allodynia include high pain intensity and high levels of headache-related disability (Bigal et al. 2008). Central sensitization is also more likely to develop in migraineurs with a long history of the disorder and high attack frequency (Mathew et al. 2004).

Identification and Modification of Risk Factors

The identification of risk factors associated with the chronification of migraine should also be a priority in headache research; an understanding of these risk factors lends insight into the mechanisms and pathophysiology of headache and also provides the groundwork for treatments and interventions intended to modify disease progression (Bigal and Lipton 2008b). Putative risk factors currently under investigation include cutaneous allodynia, pro-inflammatory states, prothrombotic states, and specific genes (Bigal and Lipton 2009). In addition, better prognostic markers and methods to monitor patients during the early stages of headache are needed (Loder and Biondi 2003).

Conclusions

The cornerstones of CDH prevention are risk factor assessment and modification, early recognition of frequent acute care medication usage, and the implementation of a multidisciplinary approach that includes lifestyle modifications, behavioral treatment, and traditional medical therapy, while headaches are still episodic. Risk factor modification may include the use of behavioral and pharmacologic treatments to decrease attack frequency, weight loss and the maintenance of a lower BMI, recognizing and avoiding medication overuse, treating sleep disturbances, and screening for psychiatric comorbidities. The early use of preventive medications and the judicious use of acute care medications such as triptans are also likely to be important treatment strategies in the prevention of headache chronification. Though we currently rely on clinical information to determine treatment efficacy and disease progression, the future development of biomarkers of disease activity may broaden the extent to which disease modification can be achieved.

References

Andrasik F (2003) Behavioral treatment approaches to chronic headache. Neurol Sci 24(Suppl 2):S80–S85

Andrasik F (2007) What does the evidence show? Efficacy of behavioural treatments for recurrent headaches in adults. Neurol Sci 28:S70–S77

Andrasik F, Blanchard EB, Neff DF, Rodichok LD (1984) Biofeedback and relaxation training for chronic headache: a controlled comparison of booster treatments and regular contacts for long-term maintenance. J Consult Clin Psychol 52:609–615

Andrasik F, Buse DC, Grazzi L (2009) Behavioral medicine for migraine and medication overuse headache. Curr Pain Headache Rep 13:241–248

Bahra A, Walsh M, Menon S et al (2003) Does chronic daily headache arise de novo in association with regular use of analgesic? Headache 43:179–180

Bigal ME, Ashina S, Burstein R et al (2008) Prevalence and characteristics of allodynia in headache sufferers: a population study. Neurology 70:1525–1533

Bigal ME, Rapoport AM, Sheftell FD, Tepper SJ, Lipton RB (2004) Transformed migraine and medication overuse in a tertiary headache centre- clinical characteristics and treatment outcomes. Cephalalgia 24:483–490

Bigal ME, Liberman JN, Lipton RB (2006) Obesity and migraine: a population study. Neurology 66: 545–550

Bigal ME, Lipton RB (2006a) Obesity is a risk factor for transformed migraine but not chronic tension-type headache. Neurology 67:252–257

Bigal ME, Lipton RB (2006b) Modifiable risk factors for migraine progression (or for chronic daily headaches): clinical lessons. Headache 46(Suppl 3): S144–S146

Bigal ME, Lipton RB (2008a) Clinical course in migraine: conceptualizing migraine transformation. Neurology 71:848–855

Bigal ME, Lipton RB (2008b) The prognosis of migraine. Curr Opin Neurol 21:301–308

Bigal ME, Lipton RB (2008c) Excessive acute migraine medication use and migraine progression. Neurology 71:1821–1828

Bigal ME, Lipton RB (2009) What predicts the change from episodic to chronic migraine? Curr Opin Neurol 22:269–276

Blanchard EB (1992) Psychological treatment of benign headache disorders. J Consult Clin Psychol 60: 537–551

Boardman HF, Thomas E, Millson DS, Croft PR (2005) Psychological, sleep, lifestyle, and comorbid associations with headache. Headache 45:657–669

Burstein R, Cutrer MF, Yarmitsky D (2000) The development of cutaneous allodynia during a migraine attack: clinical evidence for the sequential recruitment of spinal and supraspinal nociceptive neurons in migraine. Brain 123:1703–1709

Burstein R, Collins B, Jakubowski M (2004) Defeating migraine pain with triptans: a race against the development of cutaneous allodynia. Ann Neurol 55:19–26

Busch V, Gaul C (2008) Exercise in migraine therapy – is there any evidence for efficacy? A critical review. Headache 48:890–899

Calabresi P, Cupini LM (2005) Medication-overuse headache: similarities with drug addiction. Trends Pharmacol Sci 26:62–68

Calhoun AH, Ford S (2007) Behavioral sleep modification may revert transformed migraine to episodic migraine. Headache 47:1178–1183

Campbell JK, Penzien DB, Wall EM (2000) Evidence-based guidelines for migraine headaches: behavioral and physical treatments. Retrieved from http://www.aan.com/. Accessed 1 Feb 2010

Castillo J, Munoz P, Giitera V, Pascual J (1999) Kaplan Award 1998: epidemiology of chronic daily headache in the general population. Headache 39:190–196

Chan PL, Holford NH (2001) Drug treatment effects on disease progression. Annu Rev Pharmacol Toxicol 41:625–659

Charles JA, Peterlin BL, Rapoport AM, Linder SL, Kabbouche MA, Sheftell FD (2009) Favorable outcome of early treatment of new onset child and adolescent migraine-implications for disease modification. J Headache Pain 10:227–233

Couch JR, Lipton RB, Stewart WF, Scher AI (2007) Head or neck injury increases the risk of chronic daily headache: a population-based study. Neurology 69:1169–1177

Cupini LM, Calabresi P (2005) Medication-overuse headache: pathophysiological insights. J Headache Pain 6:199–202

Dodick DW (2002) Debate: analgesic overuse is a cause, not consequence, of chronic daily headache analgesic overuse is not a cause of chronic daily headache. Headache 42:547–554

Dodick DW (2006) Chronic daily headache. N Engl J Med 354:158–165

Dodick DW, Silberstein SD (2007) Migraine prevention. Pract Neurol 7:383–393

Evans RW, Loder E, Biondi DM (2004) When can successful migraine prophylaxis be discontinued? Headache 44:1040–1042

Evers S, Afra J, Frese A et al (2009) EFNS guideline on the drug treatment of migraine-revised report of an EFNS task force. Eur J Neurol 16:968–981

Genazzani AR, Nappi G, Facchinetti F, Micieli G, Petraglia F, Bono G et al (1984) Progressive impairment of CSF β-EP levels in migraine sufferers. Pain 18:127–133

Hagen K, Einarsen C, Zwart JA et al (2002) The co-occurrence of headache and musculoskeletal symptoms amongst 51050 adults in Norway. Eur J Neurol 9:527–533

Hasvold T, Johnsen R (1993) Headache and neck or shoulder pain – frequent and disabling complaints in the general population. Scand J Prim Health Care 11:219–224

Higashi Y, Sasaki S et al (1999) Clinical abstracts: vascular disease. Mod Med 67:30

Jennum P, Hein HO, Suadicani P, Gyntelberg F (1994) Headache and cognitive dysfunctions in snorers. A cross-sectional study of 3323 men aged 54–74 years: the Copenhagen Male Study. Arch Neurol 51:937–942

Karakurum B, Soylu O, Karatas M et al (2004) Personality, depression, and anxiety as risk factors for chronic migraine. Int J Neurosci 114:1391–1399

Katsarava Z, Fritsche G, Muessig M, Diener HC, Limmroth V (2001) Clinical features of withdrawal headache following overuse of triptans and other headache drugs. Neurology 57:1694–1698

Katsarava Z, Schneeweiss S, Kurth T et al (2004) Incidence and predictors for chronicity of headache in patients with episodic migraine. Neurology 62:788–790

Kelman L (2007) The triggers or precipitants of the acute migraine attack. Cephalalgia 27:394–402

Khalil NM, Legg NJ, Anderson DJ (2000) Long term decline of P100 amplitude in migraine with aura. J Neurol Neursurg Psychiatry 69:507–511

Koseoglu E, Akboyrz A, Soyeur A, Ersoy AO (2003) Aerobic exercise and plasma beta endorphin levels in patients with migrainous headache without aura. Cephalalgia 23:972–976

Kruit MC, Van Buchem MA, Hofman PAM et al (2004) Migraine as a risk factor for subclinical brain lesions. JAMA 291:427–434

Limmroth V, Katsarava Z, Fritsche G et al (2002) Features of medication overuse headache following overuse of different acute headache drugs. Neurology 59:1011–1014

Linder SL (2005) Do children and adolescents have chornic daily headache? Yes! Curr Pain Headache Rep 9:358–362

Lipton RB, Pan J (2004) Is migraine a progressive brain disease? JAMA 291:493–494

Lipton RB, Bigal ME, Diamond M, Freitag F, Reed ML, Diamond M, Freitag F, Reed ML, Stewart WF, AMPP

Advisory Group (2007) Migraine prevalence, disease burden, and the need for preventive therapy. Neurology 68:343–349

Lipton RB, Bigal ME, Ashina S et al (2008) Cutaneous allodynia in the migraine population. Ann Neurol 63:148–158

Loder E, Biondi D (2003) Disease modification in migraine: a concept that has come of age? Headache 43:135–143

Martin VT, Behbehani MM (2001) Toward a rational understanding of migraine trigger factors. Med Clin North Am 85:911–941

Mathew NT (1990) Drug-induced headache. Neurol Clin 8:903–912

Mathew NT, Kurman R, Perez F (1990) Drug induced refractory headache – clinical features and management. Headache 30:634–638

Mathew NT, Kailasam J, Seifert T (2004) Clinical recognition of allodynia in migraine. Neurology 63:848–852

McWilliams LA, Goodwin RD, Cox BJ (2004) Depression and anxiety associated with three pain condition: results from a nationally representative sample. Pain 111:77–83

Mickeviciene D, Schrader H, Nestvold K et al (2002) A controlled historical cohort study on the post-concussion syncrome. Eur J Neurol 9:581–587

Mickeviciene D, Schrader H, Obelieniene D et al (2004) A controlled prospective inception cohort study on the post-concussion syndrome outside the medico-legal context. Eur J Neurol 11:411–419

Narin SO, Pinar L (2003) The effects of exercise and exercise-related changes in blood nitric oxide level on migraine headache. Clin Rehabil 17:624–630

Obelieneiene D, Bovim G, Scharder H et al (1998) Headache after whiplash: a historical cohort study outside the medico-legal context. Cephalalgia 18:559–564

Olesen J, Bousser MG, Diener HC, Dodick D, First M, Goadsby PJ, Gobel H, Lainez MJ, Lance JW, Lipton RB, Nappi G, Sakai F, Schoenen J, Silberstein SD, Steiner TJ (2006) Headache Classification Committee: new appendix criteria open for a broader concept of chronic migraine. Cephalalgia 26:742–746

Peterlin BL, Calhoun A, Siegel S, Mathew N (2008) Rational combination therapy in refractory migraine. Headache 48:805–819

Peterlin BL, Rapoport AM, Kurth T (2010) Migraine and obesity: epidemiology, mechanisms, and implications. Headache 50(4):631–648

Rapoport A, Stang ZP, Gutterman DL et al (1996) Analgesic rebound headache in clinical practice: data from a physician survey. Headache 36:14–19

Robbins L (1994) Precipitating factors in migraine: a retrospective review of 494 patients. Headache 34:214–216

Rossi P, Jensen R, Nappi G, Allena M, The COMOESTAS Consortium (2009) A narrative review on the management of medication overuse headache: the steep road from experience to evidence. J Headache Pain 10:407–417

Rothrock JF, Kelly NM, Brody ML, Golbeck A (1994) A differential response to treatment with divalproex sodium in patients with intractable headache. Cephalalgia 14:241–244

Rothrock JF, Mendizabal JE (2000) An analysis of the "carry-over effect" following successful short-term treatment of transformed migraine with divalproex sodium. Headache 40:17–19

Scharff L, Turk DC, Marcus DA (1995) Triggers of headache episodes and coping responses of headache diagnostic groups. Headache 35:397–403

Scher AI, Stewart WF, Liberman J, Lipton RB (1998) Prevalence of frequent headache in a population sample. Headache 38:497–506

Scher AI, Stewart WF, Ricci JA, Lipton RB (2003a) Factors associated with the onset and remission of chronic daily headache in a population-based study. Pain 106:81–89

Scher AI, Lipton RB, Stewart WF (2003b) Habitual snoring as a risk factor for chronic daily headache. Neurology 60:1366–1368

Scher AI, Stewart WF, Lipton RB (2004) Caffeine as a risk factor for chronic daily headache: a population-based study. Neurology 63:2022–2027

Scher AI, Stewart WF, Lipton RB (2006) The comorbidity of headache with other pain syndromes. Headache 46:1416–1423

Scher AI, Midgette LA, Lipton RB (2008a) Risk factors for headache chronification. Headache 48:16–25

Scher AI, Stewart WF, Buse D et al (2008b) Major life changes before and after the onset of chronic daily headache: a population-based study. Cephalalgia 28:868–876

Schrader H, Stovner LJ, Obelieniene D et al (2006) Examination of the diagnostic validity of "headache attributed to whiplash injury": a controlled, prospective study. Eur J Neurol 13:1226–1232

Stovner L, Hagen K, Jensen R et al (2007) The global burden of headache: a documentation of headache prevalence and disability worldwide. Cephalalgia 27:193–210

Supornsilpchai W, le Grand SM, Srikiatkhachorn A (2010) Involvement of pro-nociceptive 5-HT(2A) receptor in the pathogenesis of medication-overuse headache. Headache 50(2):185–197

Tietjen GE, Brandes JL, Peterlin BL et al (2010) Childhood maltreatment and migraine (part II). Emotional abuse as a risk factor for headache chronification. Headache 50:32–41

Tietjen GE, Peterlin BL, Brandes JL et al (2007) Depression and anxiety-effect on the migraine-obesity relationship. Headache 47:866–875

Varin R, Mulder P, Richard V, Tamion F (1999) Exercise improves flow-mediated vasodilatation of skeletal muscle arteries in rats with chronic heart failure: role of nitric oxide, prostanoids, and oxidant stress. Circulation 99:2951–2957

Varkey E, Cider A, Carlsson J, Linde M (2009) A study to evaluate the feasibility of an aerobic exercise program in patients with migraine. Headache 49:563–570

Wang SJ, Fuh JL, Lu SR et al (2000) Chronic daily headache in Chinese elderly: prevalence, risk factors and biannual follow-up. Neurology 54:314–319

Welch KMA, Nagesh V, Aurora SK, Gelman N (2001) Periaqueductal gray matter dysfunction in migraine: cause or the burden of illness? Headache 41:629–637

Wiendels NJ, Neven AK, Rosendaal FR et al (2006) Chronic frequent headache in the general population: prevalence and associated factors. Cephalalgia 26:1434–1442

Wober C, Wober-Bingol C, Koch G, Wessely P (1991) Long-term results of migraine prophylaxis with flunarizine and beta-blockers. Cephalalgia 11:251–256

Yarmitsky D, Goor-Aryeh I, Bajwa ZH et al (2003) 2003 Wolff Award: possible parasympathetic contributions to peripheral and central sensitization during migraine. Headache 43:704–714

Zwart JA, Dyb G, Hagen K et al (2003) Depression and anxiety disorders associated with headache frequency The Nord-Trondelag Health Study. Eur J Neurol 10:147–152

31 Mechanisms of Chronic Migraine

Sheena K. Aurora[1] · *Ninan T. Mathew*[2]
[1]Swedish Neurosciences Institute, Seattle, WA, USA
[2]Houston Headache Clinic, Houston, TX, USA

Paolo Martelletti, Timothy J. Steiner (eds.), *Handbook of Headache*, DOI 10.1007/978-88-470-1700-9_31,
© Lifting The Burden 2011

Abstract: Chronic migraine typically evolves from episodic migraine over months to years in susceptible individuals. Headaches increase in frequency over time, becoming less intense but more disabling and less responsive to treatment. The results of electrophysiological and functional imaging studies indicate that chronic migraine is associated with abnormalities in the brain stem that may be progressive. Additionally, chronic migraine is associated with a greater degree of impairment in cortical processing of sensory stimuli than is episodic migraine, perhaps due to a more pervasive or persistent cortical hyperexcitability. These findings fit with the model of migraine as a spectrum disorder, in which the clinical and pathophysiological features of migraine may progress over time. This progression is postulated to result from changes in nociceptive thresholds and ensuing central sensitization caused by recurrent migraine in susceptible individuals, for whom a variety of risk factors have been described. This may lead to changes in baseline neurologic function between episodes of headache, evident not only in electrophysiological and functional imaging studies, but also as an increase in depression, anxiety, nonhead pain, fatigue, gastrointestinal disorders, and other somatic complaints that may occur after years of episodic migraine. From the current research and migraine models, a conceptualization of chronic migraine is emerging in which relatively permanent and pervasive central changes have occurred that warrant novel and tolerable treatments. This model also implies that prevention of chronic migraine is an important goal in the management of episodic migraine, particularly in individuals who exhibit risk factors for chronic transformation.

Established Knowledge

Migraine is a debilitating primary headache disorder that is ranked by the World Health Organization as 19th among all causes of years lived with disability (WHO 2007). Since there are no biological markers for migraine, the diagnosis is based on clinical history. Episodic migraine is characterized by recurrent headaches that last 4–72 h, with pain typically described as unilateral, pulsating, moderate or severe, aggravated by routine physical activity, and associated with nausea and/or photophobia and phonophobia. The diagnosis of chronic migraine is made when headaches occur on at least 15 days/month, where at least half meet criteria outlined for episodic migraine or are treated with an acute migraine-specific medication (ergotamine or triptans) (International Headache Society 2007; Bigal et al. 2007; The International Classification of Headache Disorders 2004).

Although at the time of this writing no genetic mutations have been identified in chronic migraine, important advances in the pathogenesis and pathophysiology of migraine have been made over the past several decades. A persistent finding has been the lack of structural abnormalities (Wang et al. 2001), which has led to a focus on functional alterations in the brain. In several variants of familial hemiplegic migraine, mutations have been identified in genes that code for P/Q type calcium channels (CACNA1A) or sodium-potassium pumps (ATP1A2) (Ophoff et al. 1996; De Fusco et al. 2003). These mutations may result in increased synaptic concentrations of glutamate, leading to neuronal hyperexcitability (Ophoff et al. 1996) and subsequent cortical spreading depression (Goadsby 2007). Cortical spreading depression is likely the basis for migraine aura, as evidenced by both animal and human studies (Goadsby 2007; Lauritzen 1994). Although the link between cortical spreading depression and migraine *pain* is not definitely established, the ability of selected preventive medications to inhibit this phenomenon in the laboratory has suggested that inhibition of cortical spreading depression may provide a model system in which to test future pharmacotherapies.

Functional imaging and neurophysiological studies continue to provide insight into the pathophysiology of migraine. These techniques include positron emission tomography (PET), perfusion-weighted imaging, magnetoencephalography (MEG), functional magnetic resonance imaging (fMRI), and blood oxygenation level-dependent (BOLD)-fMRI. Using BOLD-fMRI, changes consistent with cortical spreading depression have been observed, beginning in the extrastriate cortex and progressing to the occipital cortex during spontaneous visual aura in several migraineurs (Hadjikhani et al. 2001). These results are supported by a controlled study using MEG in which visually triggered aura was associated with MEG-direct current shifts typical of those observed during cortical spreading depression (Bowyer et al. 2001). PET techniques have been used to examine brain regions that are activated by migraine pain, although exact anatomical localization is not possible. Using this technique, a 1995 study reported activity in the dorsal raphe nuclei, periaqueductal gray (PAG), and locus coeruleus during spontaneous migraine (Weiller et al. 1995). Subsequent studies using fMRI, which allows more precise anatomical localization, have identified activity in the red nucleus and substantia nigra during spontaneous migraine-related visual aura and visually triggered migraine (Welch et al. 1998; Cao et al. 2002). Although these areas are best known for their roles in motor function, they are also involved in sensory processing and pain (Chudler and Dong 1995; Brown et al. 1997; Iadarola et al. 1998).

The majority of functional studies have been directed at understanding the pathophysiology of aura and episodic migraine. However, it is also critical to investigate chronic migraine because it is frequently refractory to treatment and is extremely disabling. Individuals with chronic migraine exhibit disability scores that are nearly twice as high as those with episodic migraine and miss significantly more work, school, housework, and social/leisure activities (Bigal et al. 2003). Chronic migraine typically evolves from episodic migraine and is frequently associated with acute pain medication overuse (Bigal et al. 2003). Over a period of months or years, episodic headaches increase in frequency and decrease in overall intensity and the headache pattern includes fewer typical migraines (Bigal et al. 2005a; Bigal et al. 2005b). It is of interest to determine how the differences between episodic and chronic migraine are manifested in cortical and brainstem neurophysiology. In the following section, we examine the findings of neurophysiological and imaging studies that have attempted to differentiate episodic and chronic migraine with the goal of understanding the functional correlates of chronic migraine in the brain. We then consider these findings in the context of models designed to explain the evolution of episodic migraine into chronic migraine.

Current Research

Magnetic Suppression of Perceptual Accuracy

Magnetic suppression of perceptual accuracy (MPSA) is a test that examines the effects of transcranial magnetic stimulation on visual perception. This technique has been used as an index of cortical excitability in migraine (Aurora et al. 2005). In the MPSA test, individuals are shown a series of three letters (trigrams) flashed briefly on a computer screen. Each trigram is followed by an interval that varies from 40 to 190 ms, at which time a single magnetic pulse is delivered to the occipital skull via a stimulation coil.

In normal participants, MPSA profiles show a U-shaped function, in which the accuracy of reporting the letters is good at short (40 ms) and long (190 ms) intervals, but no better than chance for mid-range (100 ms) intervals. In contrast, individuals with migraine show a flattened function, whereby perceptual accuracy is relatively maintained at the 100 ms and other mid-range intervals (Aurora et al. 2005; Aurora et al. 2007). Perceptual accuracy differences are also evident between those with episodic and chronic migraine. In chronic migraine, the accuracy of letter reporting is not measurably influenced by transcranial stimulation of the visual cortex at any of the intervals from 40 to 190 ms (Aurora et al. 2005; Aurora et al. 2007). In episodic migraine, the accuracy of letter reporting is decreased at the mid-range intervals and most pronounced at the 100 ms interval, but not as much as in normal individuals. Thus, there appears to be a continuum of cortical excitability in migraineurs, with episodic migraine associated with more cortical excitability than controls, but chronic migraine associated with yet a greater degree of cortical excitability than either episodic migraine or controls (Aurora et al. 2005).

The neural basis for suppression of perceptual accuracy in the MSPA test is believed to be the preferential activation of inhibitory neurons by a high-intensity transcranial magnetic stimulus at the 100 ms time point (Moliadze et al. 2003). In patients with migraine, it may be more difficult to suppress perception at the mid-range intervals because of increased baseline cortical excitability, which may be caused by impaired intracortical inhibitory mechanisms (Mulleners et al. 2001). The greater degree of suppression observed in chronic migraine compared with episodic migraine may be due to a more pervasive or persistent cortical hyperexcitability.

Functional Imaging Techniques

Functional imaging techniques have been used to determine the activity of various brain regions in individuals with migraine, either during or between attacks. We used PET to examine cerebral glucose metabolism (a marker of cellular activity) in 10 individuals with chronic migraine (Aurora et al. 2007). These individuals were subjected to brain scans during the interictal period using (Bigal et al. 2003) F-fluorodeoxygluose (FDG) PET (Aurora et al. 2007). We found increased cerebral metabolism in the pons and right temporal cortex and decreased metabolism in several areas bilaterally in the medial frontal, parietal, and somato-sensory cortices, as well as bilaterally in the caudate nuclei. These findings may suggest that normal inhibitory capacity of the cortex is reduced in chronic migraine (Aurora et al. 2007).

Several studies have examined cerebral activation in episodic migraine (Weiller et al. 1995; Afridi et al. 2005). In a PET study, increased blood flow was noted in the cingulate, auditory, and visual association cortices and in the brain stem during the migraine (Weiller et al. 1995). However, following injection of the acute migraine medication sumatriptan, which induced complete relief from headache and phono- and photophobia, only the brain stem remained activated. In a subsequent PET study of evoked migraine, activation of the pons (a brainstem structure) was noted both during and following an attack, compared to the pre-migraine baseline (Afridi et al. 2005). However, other structures, including the anterior cingulate, bilateral insula, bilateral cerebellar hemispheres, prefrontal cortex, and putamen, were active during the migrainous attack but not after it was fully controlled with sumatriptan. This study also found that the side of the pons that was activated corresponded to the laterality of the migraines. Thus, these authors suggest that lateralization of pain in migraine may be due to lateralized dysfunction of the brain, as manifested in the dorsal pons (Afridi et al. 2005). However, to our knowledge, no one has identified activation of the pons in episodic migraine between attacks and chronic migraineurs during attacks. High-resolution MRI was used to map iron homeostasis as an indicator of brain. Our group has compared the activation of brainstem nuclei in episodic and chronic migraine (Welch et al. 2001). In this study, we examined episodic migraineurs function; measures included the relaxation rates R2, R2', and R2*. Results showed a significant increase in R2' and R2* values in the periaqueductal gray of both migraine groups compared with the control group, but no difference between the episodic and chronic migraine groups. We found positive correlations between duration of illness and R2' for both migraine groups. In the red nucleus and substantia nigra, the chronic migraine group showed a significant decrease in R2' and R2* values compared with the episodic migraine and control groups (Welch et al. 2001). From these data, we concluded that iron homeostasis in the periaqueductal gray is persistently and progressively impaired in migraineurs, which may be caused by repeated migraine attacks.

Summary of Electrophysiological and Functional Imaging Findings

Taken together, these findings suggest that certain features of brain dysfunction may be persistently manifest in individuals with chronic migraine, but only during and/or following attacks in those with episodic migraine. In the MRSA test, those with episodic migraine show an intermediate level of failure to suppress the perceptual images when the magnetic stimulus is applied 100 ms after the visual stimulus, whereas those with chronic migraine show near complete failure to suppress these images. Similarly, selected brain regions such as the pons may be overactive *during* an attack in episodic migraine, but may be continuously overactive in chronic migraine. The significant decreases in the MRI values R2' and R2* in the substantia nigra and red nucleus noted in chronic migraine are probably attributable to hyperoxia associated with head pain during an attack and thus may be more frequent in chronic migraine (Welch et al. 2001). All individuals with chronic migraine in the MRI study were experiencing headache at the time of the scan, whereas all of the episodic migraineurs were between headaches (Welch et al. 2001). Thus, the electrophysiological and functional imaging evidence suggests a spectrum of migraine in which changes observed in episodic migraine are more pronounced than those in chronic migraine.

Current Models of Migraine

As initially suggested by Mathew in 1982 (Mathew et al. 1982), migraine is currently conceptualized as a continuum or spectrum disorder, in which episodic migraine may or may not evolve into chronic migraine (Bigal and Lipton 2008; Cady et al. 2004). Approximately 3% of individuals with episodic migraine progress to chronic migraine over the course of a year (Bigal and Lipton 2008). The clinical evolution appears to occur gradually over months or years, with some individuals progressing from infrequent attacks (2–104 headache days/year) to frequent episodic attacks (105–179 headache days/year), to chronic migraine (Bigal and Lipton 2008). However, the transition is not always toward greater headache frequency, but may also manifest as a transition to a more episodic pattern of headaches (Bigal and Lipton 2008; Scher et al. 2008).

Despite the spectrum conceptualization of migraine, important distinctions between episodic and chronic migraine exist. The burden of chronic migraine is substantially greater than that of episodic migraine, as evidenced by disability scores (Bigal et al. 2003), ability to work and engage in everyday activities (Bigal et al. 2003), and emergency department visits (Freitag et al. 2005). Additionally, treatment of chronic migraine is frequently unsuccessful and no therapies are currently approved by the US Food and Drug Administration for this condition. Furthermore, pharmacotherapies currently used for the treatment of chronic migraine are typically accompanied by intolerable side effects (Goadsby 2005). Because of these distinctions, as well as the pathophysiological differences noted below and the functional correlates observed in electrophysiological and imaging studies, it is critical to focus on chronic migraine as unique condition, even though its relationship to episodic migraine – primarily as a predisposing condition – is acknowledged.

A number of studies have attempted to define the factors associated with the progression of episodic to chronic migraine. Nonmodifiable risk factors include female sex, lower socioeconomic status, and marital status (unmarried associated with higher risk) (Scher et al. 2008). Modifiable risk factors for progression include obesity, snoring, other pain syndromes, previous neck or head injury, stressful life events, caffeine intake, and acute headache medication use (Scher et al. 2008). Sleep disorders, psychopathology (especially anxiety and depression), and gastrointestinal disorders also occur more frequently in those with chronic migraine than those with episodic migraine (Scher et al. 2008; Penzien et al. 2008; Ferrari et al. 2007).

Two recent models of migraine incorporate neurological changes as a central tenet of migraine progression (Bigal and Lipton 2008; Cady et al. 2004). Bigal and Lipton (2008) postulate that physiological progression of migraine may be indicated by changes in nociceptive thresholds and pain pathways (allodynia and central sensitization). These authors also note that anatomical progression of migraine may be evident as stroke, white matter lesions, or lesions outside the brain (Bigal and Lipton 2008). Cady et al. (2004) emphasize the changes in baseline neurologic function between episodes of headache. These authors note that depression, anxiety, nonhead pain, fatigue, gastrointestinal disorders, and other somatic complaints that occur after years of episodic migraine may serve as an indicator of chronic transformation (Cady et al. 2004). In support of these models, chronic migraine has been associated with altered cortical processing of pain (de Tommaso et al. 2005), frontal lobe dysfunction (Mongini et al. 2005), and vascular malformation in the brain stem (Obermann et al. 2006).

A related finding in migraine research that may have implications for chronification is the observation of cutaneous allodynia. Burstein and colleagues reported that 79% of 44 individuals with migraine seen at a medical center demonstrated a pain response to non-noxious stimuli during a migraine attack (Burstein et al. 2000). Later studies confirmed this finding and noted its occurrence in individuals with episodic as well as chronic migraine (Bigal and Lipton 2006; Lovati et al. 2007; Cooke et al. 2007). One study found that individuals who met the criteria for episodic migraine with aura or chronic migraine showed a higher frequency of cutaneous allodynia than episodic migraineurs without aura (Lovati et al. 2007); another study reported a tendency of chronic migraineurs to have more severe cutaneous allodynia than episodic migraineurs, although the study did not appear to separate migraineurs with and without aura (Bigal and Lipton 2008).

Cutaneous allodynia in migraine is believed to represent sensitization of second-order brainstem trigeminal neurons (Burstein et al. 2000), referred to as central sensitization. It has been suggested that chronic migraine may be due to the chronic sensitization of central pain pathways caused by repeated attacks of migraine (Bigal and Lipton 2008; Cooke et al. 2007). Cutaneous allodynia has been associated with refractoriness to triptans (Burstein and Jakubowski 2004) and chronic migraineurs frequently do not obtain adequate relief from triptans. However, cutaneous allodynia has also been described in episodic migraine. It will be important to determine the prevalence of cutaneous allodynia in the general population of episodic migraineurs, as opposed to the clinical population that has been studied to date, as the latter may exhibit more severe or frequent migraines that lead them into professional consultation. Another possibility is that chronic migraineurs exhibit more persistent or severe central sensitization than those with episodic migraine. One study found that several individuals with transformed migraine who were tested on headache-free days exhibited cutaneous allodynia on those days as well as their headache days (Cooke et al. 2007). Another study found that 29% of individuals with chronic migraine exhibited severe cutaneous allodynia, in contrast to 20% of individuals with episodic migraine (Bigal and Lipton 2008). These findings may indicate a more persistent or pervasive central sensitization in chronic migraine. Coupled with observations of lower pain thresholds in chronic migraine than episodic migraine (Kitaj and Klink 2005) and abnormal cortical processing of cutaneous nociceptive input (de Tommaso et al. 2005; de Tommaso et al. 2003), these results support the pathophysiological progression of migraine that involves disruption of central pain mechanisms.

Implications

The clinical, neurological, and functional studies of chronic migraine are increasingly suggestive of a pathophysiological state in which the brain exhibits enduring and pervasive alterations, in contrast to the intermittent changes noted in episodic migraine during attacks. As such, chronic migraine is characterized by neurological alterations that are evident even in the absence of headache – as the baseline condition – or as more extreme or severe changes. Given the disability associated with chronic migraine and the substantial interference of this condition with everyday activities, it is critically important to understand and attempt to prevent chronification and also to also devise effective, tolerable treatments.

Given the differences noted between episodic and chronic migraine in central pain processing, treatments are likely to differ – a concept supported by clinical experience. With episodic migraine, abortive medications such as the triptans are often effective. The potential for chronification suggests that the frequency of headaches should be closely monitored in patients with risk factors for progression, with the goal of preventing the development of chronic migraine (Lipton and Bigal 2008). For patients who have already developed chronic migraine, novel treatments that do not force patients to choose between pain relief and serious side effects must be sought (Goadsby 2005). Investigations into the efficacy of these treatments are complicated by a number of factors (Lipton and Bigal 2008); however, rigorous clinical studies are essential for establishing efficacy and comparing different treatments. As research continues to progress in these areas, the unique entity of chronic migraine is increasingly recognized as a critical target for effective intervention that has the potential to substantially reduce patient suffering.

References

Afridi SK, Matharu MS, Lee L et al (2005) A PET study exploring the laterality of brainstem activation in migraine using glyceryl trinitrate. Brain 128(Pt 4):932–939

Aurora SK, Barrodale PM, Tipton RL, Khodavirdi A (2007) Brainstem dysfunction in chronic migraine as evidenced by neurophysiological and positron emission tomography studies. Headache 47(7):996–1003, discussion 1004–1007

Aurora SK, Barrodale P, Chronicle EP, Mulleners WM (2005) Cortical inhibition is reduced in chronic and episodic migraine and demonstrates a spectrum of illness. Headache 45(5):546–552

Bigal ME, Lipton RB (2008) Concepts and mechanisms of migraine chronification. Headache 48(1):7–15

Bigal M, Rapoport A, Sheftell F, Tepper S, Lipton R (2007) The International Classification of Headache Disorders revised criteria for chronic migraine-field testing in a headache specialty clinic. Cephalalgia 27:230–234

Bigal ME, Rapoport AM, Lipton RB, Tepper SJ, Sheftell FD (2003) Assessment of migraine disability using the migraine disability assessment (MIDAS) questionnaire: a comparison of chronic migraine with episodic migraine. Headache 43(4):336–342

Bigal ME, Rapoport AM, Sheftell FD, Tepper SJ, Lipton RB (2005a) Chronic migraine is an earlier stage of transformed migraine in adults. Neurology 65(10):1556–1561

Bigal ME, Sheftell FD, Tepper SJ, Rapoport AM, Lipton RB (2005b) Migraine days decline with duration of illness in adolescents with transformed migraine. Cephalalgia 25(7):482–487

Bowyer SM, Aurora KS, Moran JE, Tepley N, Welch KM (2001) Magnetoencephalographic fields from patients with spontaneous and induced migraine aura. Ann Neurol 50(5):582–587

Brown LL, Schneider JS, Lidsky TI (1997) Sensory and cognitive functions of the basal ganglia. Curr Opin Neurobiol 7(2):157–163

Burstein R, Jakubowski M (2004) Analgesic triptan action in an animal model of intracranial pain: a race against the development of central sensitization. Ann Neurol 55(1):27–36

Burstein R, Yarnitsky D, Goor-Aryeh I, Ransil BJ, Bajwa ZH (2000) An association between migraine and cutaneous allodynia. Ann Neurol 47(5):614–624

Cady RK, Schreiber CP, Farmer KU (2004) Understanding the patient with migraine: the evolution from episodic headache to chronic neurologic disease. A proposed classification of patients with headache. Headache 44(5):426–435

Cao Y, Aurora SK, Nagesh V, Patel SC, Welch KM (2002) Functional MRI-BOLD of brainstem structures during visually triggered migraine. Neurology 59(1):72–78

Chudler EH, Dong WK (1995) The role of the basal ganglia in nociception and pain. Pain 60(1):3–38

Cooke L, Eliasziw M, Becker WJ (2007) Cutaneous allodynia in transformed migraine patients. Headache 47(4):531–539

De Fusco M, Marconi R, Silvestri L et al (2003) Haploinsufficiency of ATP1A2 encoding the Na+/K+ pump alpha2 subunit associated with familial hemiplegic migraine type 2. Nat Genet 33(2):192–196

de Tommaso M, Valeriani M, Guido M et al (2003) Abnormal brain processing of cutaneous pain in patients with chronic migraine. Pain 101(1–2):25–32

de Tommaso M, Losito L, Difruscolo O, Libro G, Guido M, Livrea P (2005) Changes in cortical processing of pain in chronic migraine. Headache 45(9):1208–1218

Ferrari A, Leone S, Vergoni AV et al (2007) Similarities and differences between chronic migraine and episodic migraine. Headache 47(1):65–72

Freitag FG, Kozma CM, Slaton T, Osterhaus JT, Barron R (2005) Characterization and prediction of emergency department use in chronic daily headache patients. Headache 45(7):891–898

Goadsby PJ (2005) Advances in the understanding of headache. Br Med Bull 73–74:83–92

Goadsby PJ (2007) Recent advances in understanding migraine mechanisms, molecules and therapeutics. Trends Mol Med 13(1):39–44

Hadjikhani N, Sanchez Del Rio M, Wu O et al (2001) Mechanisms of migraine aura revealed by functional MRI in human visual cortex. Proc Natl Acad Sci USA 98(8):4687–4692

Headache Classification Subcommittee of the International Headache Society (2004) The International Classification of Headache Disorders: 2nd edition. Cephalalgia 24(Suppl 1):9–160

Iadarola MJ, Berman KF, Zeffiro TA et al (1998) Neural activation during acute capsaicin-evoked pain and allodynia assessed with PET. Brain 121(Pt 5):931–947

International Headache Society (2007) IHS classification ICDH II. Migraine. Available at: http://ihs-classification.org/en/02_klassifikation/02_teil1/01.01.00_migraine.html. Accessed 3 Dec 2007

Kitaj MB, Klink M (2005) Pain thresholds in daily transformed migraine versus episodic migraine headache patients. Headache 45(8):992–998

Lauritzen M (1994) Pathophysiology of the migraine aura. The spreading depression theory. Brain 117(Pt 1):199–210

Lipton RB, Bigal ME (2008) Looking to the future: research designs for study of headache disease progression. Headache 48(1):58–66

Lovati C, D'Amico D, Rosa S et al (2007) Allodynia in different forms of migraine. Neurol Sci 28(Suppl 2):S220–S221

Mathew NT, Stubits E, Nigam MP (1982) Transformation of episodic migraine into daily headache: analysis of factors. Headache 22(2):66–68

Moliadze V, Zhao Y, Eysel U, Funke K (2003) Effect of transcranial magnetic stimulation on single-unit activity in the cat primary visual cortex. J Physiol 553(Pt 2):665–679

Mongini F, Keller R, Deregibus A, Barbalonga E, Mongini T (2005) Frontal lobe dysfunction in patients with chronic migraine: a clinical-neuropsychological study. Psychiatry Res 133(1):101–106

Mulleners WM, Chronicle EP, Palmer JE, Koehler PJ, Vredeveld JW (2001) Suppression of perception in migraine: evidence for reduced inhibition in the visual cortex. Neurology 56(2):178–183

Obermann M, Gizewski ER, Limmroth V, Diener HC, Katsarava Z (2006) Symptomatic migraine and pontine vascular malformation: evidence for a key role of the brainstem in the pathophysiology of chronic migraine. Cephalalgia 26(6):763–766

Ophoff RA, Terwindt GM, Vergouwe MN et al (1996) Familial hemiplegic migraine and episodic ataxia type-2 are caused by mutations in the Ca2+ channel gene CACNL1A4. Cell 87(3):543–552

Penzien DB, Rains JC, Lipton RB (2008) Introduction to the special series on the chronification of headache: mechanisms, risk factors, and behavioral strategies aimed at primary and secondary prevention of chronic headache. Headache 48(1):5–6

Scher AI, Midgette LA, Lipton RB (2008) Risk factors for headache chronification. Headache 48(1):16–25

Wang HZ, Simonson TM, Greco WR, Yuh WT (2001) Brain MR imaging in the evaluation of chronic headache in patients without other neurologic symptoms. Acad Radiol 8(5):405–408

Weiller C, May A, Limmroth V et al (1995) Brain stem activation in spontaneous human migraine attacks. Nat Med 1(7):658–660

Welch KM, Nagesh V, Aurora SK, Gelman N (2001) Periaqueductal gray matter dysfunction in migraine: cause or the burden of illness? Headache 41(7):629–637

Welch KM, Cao Y, Aurora S, Wiggins G, Vikingstad EM (1998) MRI of the occipital cortex, red nucleus, and substantia nigra during visual aura of migraine. Neurology 51(5):1465–1469

World Health Organization (WHO) (2007) Headache disorders. Available at: http://www.who.int/mediacentre/factsheets/fs277/en/. Accessed 3 Dec 2007

32 Medical Interventions for Migraine That Has Become Difficult to Treat

Paolo Martelletti · Andrea Negro
School of Health Sciences, Sapienza University of Rome, Rome, Italy

Paolo Martelletti, Timothy J. Steiner (eds.), *Handbook of Headache*, DOI 10.1007/978-88-470-1700-9_32,
© Lifting The Burden 2011

Abstract: Migraine is an episodic painful disorder which can gradually chronify, and is among the most common neurological diseases in clinical practice. Such process is often accompanied by the appearance of acute drugs overuse. Chronic migraine (CM) constitutes migraine's natural evolution in its chronic form and involves headache frequency of 15 days/month, with features similar to those of migraine attacks. Migraine given by drugs overuse, defined by ICDH-II in 2004 (and revised in 2005) as MOH, represents a common and debilitating disorder, which can be defined as generation, perpetuation and persistence of intense chronic migraine caused by the frequent and excessive use of (symptomatic) drugs for at least 3 months, for a certain number of days per month, giving an immediate relief. Migraine's progression from an episodic to a chronic form is generally influenced by baseline headache frequency, inappropriate use of rescue self-medication, absence of referral to headache centers during the worsening period in terms of headache days frequency, as well as by lack of education in avoiding trigger factors or inadequate lifestyle rhythms (fasting, sleepiness). In MOH sufferers, the only treatment of choice is represented by drug withdrawal. Successful detoxification is necessary to ensure improvement in the headache status when treating patients who overuse acute medications. Possible therapeutic agents in CM re-prophylaxis after detoxification are OnabotulinumtoxinA and Topiramate. The future in relapse prevention of CM complicated by MOH consists in considering how drugs currently used, such as triptans and emerging therapies, present responsivity profiles related to well-defined genetic polymorphisms.

Established Knowledge

The Chronic Migraine Entity

Migraine is an episodic painful disorder which can gradually chronify, and is among the most common neurological diseases in clinical practice. Such process is often accompanied by the appearance of acute drugs overuse. Chronic migraine (CM) constitutes migraine's natural evolution in its chronic form and involves headache frequency of 15 days/month, with features similar to those of migraine attacks (Headache Classification Committee 2006). The prevalence rate of chronic migraine in general population is 2–4% (Stovner and Andree 2010). Overall, population studies estimate that patients who have low-frequency episodic migraine or high-frequency episodic migraine will transition to CM at the rate of about 2.5% per year (Lipton 2009). In 2006, criteria for definition of CM have been revised by the Headache Classification Committee. Such criteria implied the presence of attacks of headache (tension-type and/or migraine) occurring for over 15 days/month. Further criteria are adherence for 8 days/month to clinical features of migraine without aura (MO) as well as response to specific treatments for migraine (Silberstein et al. 2005). The *International Classification of Headache Disorders*, II version (ICHD-II) recognizes 24 types of chronic headache and states primary episodic headaches as chronic when attacks appear for more than 15 days per month, for at least 3 months (De Filippis et al. 2007). The condition described represents a subset of chronic daily headache (CDH), defined as the recurrence of headache for more than 15 days for month, for more than 3 months consecutively. At present, CM represents the most important challenge for tertiary headache centers, to which over 50% of patients refer for monitoring the chronicization process and its possible complication with medication overuse headache (MOH). MOH affects 1–1.4% of general population and about 30–50% of CM patients show multiple phases of acute drugs abuse evolving in MOH (Allena et al. 2009).

Migraine given by drugs overuse, defined by ICDH-II in 2004 (and revised in 2005) as MOH, represents a common and debilitating disorder, which can be defined as generation, perpetuation and persistence of intense chronic migraine caused by the frequent and excessive use of (symptomatic) drugs for at least 3 months, for a certain number of days per month, giving an immediate relief. MOH is associated with overuse of a combination of analgesics, barbiturates, opioids, Ergot alkaloids, aspirin, FANS, caffeine and triptans (Silberstein et al. 2005; De Filippis et al. 2006, 2007). All the drugs employed for headache treatment can cause MOH. In fact, the first definition for this particular headache form has been that of drug-induced headache in 1988. Such definition was later modified in order to emphasize the role of drugs abuse in the development of headache. Classification of abuse is related to the pharmaceutical class applied during acute treatment, namely, of 15 days/month for analgesics and nonsteroid anti-inflammatory drugs (NSAID), 10 days/month for mixed drugs (triptans, ergotamines, opioids, and NSAID) (Evers and Marziniak 2010). Because of easy availability and low expense, the greatest problem appears to be associated with barbiturate-containing combination analgesics and over-the-counter caffeine-containing combination analgesics. Even though triptans overuse headache is not encountered with great frequency, all triptans should be considered potential inducers of MOH (Smith and Stoneman 2004). MOH can be distinguished as simple (MOH Type I) or complex (MOH Type II). Simple cases involve relatively short-term drug overuse, relatively modest amounts of overused medications, minimal psychiatric contribution, and no history of relapse after drug withdrawal. In contrast, complex cases often present with multiple psychiatric comorbidities and a history of relapse (Lake 2006). Drug misure disables the activity of standard effective therapy and rapidly worsens migraine crises patterns (Rossi et al. 2009). Migraine's chronicization progression to CM and the subsequent appearance of MOH is realized through a period of time involving several months or years, during which an increase of attacks frequency occurs. Such escalation often produces a daily or almost daily pattern, with a more or less faded symptomatology according to cases. The trend results more clear and frequent in patients presenting comorbidities with migraine, such as psychiatric or cardio-cerebrovascular disorders (Bigal and Lipton 2009a; Pompili et al. 2009, 2010). Such trend is often associated with the increase of drug intake and subsequent abuse. In some cases, symptom history becomes less adherent to a classic migraine attack (Castillo et al. 1999; Stovner et al. 2006; Bigal and Lipton 2008a). Headache features differ from the original headache form since pain can vary according to severity and location. Furthermore, the assumption of previously effective medication could develop or worsen headache. Asthenia, nausea, anxiety or gastrointestinal problems are associated with pain symptomatology (Diener and Limmroth 2004). Although MOH and CM are associated, the causal path is controversial (MOH as a cause or consequence). There are several different theories regarding the etiology of MOH, including: (1) central sensitization from repetitive activation of nociceptive pathways; (2) a direct effect of the medication on the capacity of the brain to inhibit pain; (3) cellular adaptation in the brain; (4) a decrease in blood serotonin due to repetitive medication administration with alteration of serotonin receptors; and (5) changes in the periaqueductal gray matter (Cupini and Calabresi 2005).

Risk Factors and Chronicization of Migraine

In presence of CM's low prevalence, an extremely high disability grade has been ascertained which is caused by such chronic form. Therefore, special attention should be paid to both control and reduction of risk factors which might favor the migraine chronicization process and/or the outbreak of MOH (Scher et al. 2008; Buse et al. 2009a; Vargas and Dodick 2009). Among the risk factors for chronicization there are non-changeable agents such as demography, age, and socioeconomic status, as well as changeable factors, such as obesity and specific psychological patterns. In chronic patients the risk of abuse of pain killer medications increases up to 30% in general population, and to 80% in patients under treatment in specialist centers, 80% (Katsarava et al. 2004; Scher et al. 2008; Bigal and Lipton 2009b). Migraine's progression from an episodic to a chronic form is generally influenced by baseline headache frequency, inappropriate use of rescue self-medication, absence of referral to headache centers during the worsening period in terms of headache days frequency, as well as by lack of education in avoiding trigger factors or inadequate lifestyle rhythms (fasting, sleepiness). Cross-sectional data from the Frequent Headache Epidemiology study and the American Migraine Prevalence and Prevention study (AMPP) show that patients with chronic daily headaches have lower levels of education and household income (Lipton 2009). Among modifiable risk factors for chronicization are caffeine use/misuse (dietary and drug-containing caffeine), obesity and sleep disorders, such as snoring and sleep apnea (Bigal and Lipton 2009b). In a study conducted on 8,219 patients with Episodic Migraine (EM), as a part of the AMPP, the progression to chronic or transformed migraine (TM) had a rate of 2.5% per year, with an increased risk associated with any use of barbiturates and opiates, after adjusting for covariates, while triptans were not. NSAIDs were protective or inducers depending on the headache frequency (protective against transition to TM at low to moderate monthly headache days, associated with increased risk of transition to TM at high levels of monthly headache days) (Bigal et al. 2008). Regarding opioids's association with migraine progression, the critical dose of exposure is around 8 days per month, and the effect is more pronounced in men (Bigal and Lipton 2008b, 2009a). Barbiturates also induce migraine progression, and the effect is dose dependent (critical dose around 5 days of exposure per month) and more pronounced in women (Bigal and Lipton 2008b, 2009a). Triptans induce migraine progression only in those with high migraine frequency at baseline (<14 days per month), but not overall (Bigal and Lipton 2008b, 2009a). NSAIDs protect against migraine progression unless individuals have 10 or more headache days per month (when they become inducers, rather than protective). Finally, caffeine-containing over-the-counter products increase risk of progression (Bigal and Lipton 2008b, 2009a). The Severity of Dependence Scale (SDS) score has appear to be a significant predictor of medication overuse among chronic headache patients with sensitivity, specificity, positive and negative predictive values of 0.79, 0.84, 0.84, and 0.79, respectively, in men and 0.76, 0.77, 0.73, and 0.79 in women. Since the value of SDS for detecting medication overuse and dependency like behavior among people with chronic headache, it may be used to identify chronic headache patients who may benefit from detoxification (Lundqvist et al. 2010).

Withdrawal from Drug Abuse

In MOH sufferers, the only treatment of choice is represented by drug withdrawal. Successful detoxification is necessary to ensure improvement in the headache status when treating patients who overuse acute medications. Discontinuation of the acute medication can result in withdrawal headache, nausea, vomiting and sleep disturbances. Although there are no studies comparing gradual with abrupt interruption, the widespread opinion of expertise rulers is that abrupt interruption results more effective. Different procedures have been suggested for withdrawal, namely, at home, at the hospital, with or without the use of steroids, with re-prophylaxes performed immediately or at the end of the wash-out period. However, no final agreement has been reached except for withdrawal from abuse in order to reinstate the natural course of CM or high-frequency migraine (Hagen et al. 2010; Lovell and Marmura 2010; Rossi et al. 2010). Early introduction of preventive treatment without a previous detoxification program reduced total headache suffering more effectively compared with abrupt withdrawal (Hagen et al. 2009). A further step beyond drug interruption results upon smoothing symptoms following interruption, through pharmacological support. The detoxification period is based on the use of various classes of drugs, among which corticosteroids certainly are the most frequently employed. Oral prednisolone constitutes the most common treatment during detoxification; when compared with placebo, it reduces the duration of withdrawal headache (Krymchantowski and Barbosa 2000; Paemeleire et al. 2006; Obermann and Katsarava 2007; Pageler et al. 2008). Prednisolone administered orally the first 6 days after medication withdrawal has no effect on withdrawal headache in unselected patients with chronic daily headache and medication overuse, not reducing headache intensity during the same period (Bøe et al. 2007). A Brazilian study on 150 CM patients have shown that CM patients with moderate overuse of SM other than opioids may be detoxified on an outpatient basis regardless of the strategy adopted with regard to the use of regular drugs during the initial days of withdrawal, but prednisolone and naratriptan may be useful for reducing withdrawal symptoms and rescue medication consumption (Krymchantowski and Moreira 2003). A withdrawal and detoxification therapeutic regimen that obtained good results at 6 months of follow-up in a sample of patients suffering from probable CM and probable MOH during admission in eight Italian hospitals consisted in abrupt discontinuation of the overused drug and by a therapeutic protocol including i.v. hydration, dexamethasone, metoclopramide and benzodiazepines for 7–10 days. Prophylactic medication was started immediately after admission (Trucco et al. 2010). Data suggest that the patients affected by CDH and medication overuse benefit from withdrawal therapy performed during hospitalization (dexamethasone 4 mg i.v./day for 1 week, diazepam 6 mg/day for 10 days) plus prophylaxis with amitriptyline (from 10 to 20 mg/day) plus topiramate (from 50 to 100 mg/day) for at least 6 months. This combination seems a good pharmacological solution to reduce the risk of relapse (Valguarnera and Tanganelli 2010). In patients with migraine plus MOH and low medical needs, effective drug withdrawal may be obtained through the imparting of advice alone (Rossi et al. 2006). In the follow-up period, the primary goal is to outline an effective prophylaxis therapy. Therapeutic success, defined as a total absence of headache or headache frequency reduction over 50% in a period of time from 1 to 6 months, stands around 72–74% (De Filippis et al. 2006). Relapse percentages during the first year after withdrawal range between 22% and 44% (Katsarava et al. 2005; Farinelli et al. 2010; Trucco et al. 2010). Numerous factors (e.g., adverse effects, tolerability, cost, frequency of dosage, hesitancy to take daily medication, failure to complete treatment) negatively influence compliance with the preventive pharmacology for migraine prophylaxis (Cady and Schreiber 2008).

Re-Prophylaxis of Chronic Migraine

Possible therapeutic agents in CM re-prophylaxis after detoxification are OnabotulinumtoxinA and Topiramate (Farinelli et al. 2010). Both drugs have been approved for CM treatment in view of their well-defined resistance to previous prophylaxis drugs. OnabotulinumtoxinA is a substance obtained from the gram-positive anaerobic bacterium *Clostridium botulinum*. Its action occurs through the block of peripheral acetylcholine release at the level of peripheral cholinergic nerve endings (Simpson 1980). Traveling in the general vascular circulation, OnabotulinumtoxinA reaches the extracellular space. The mechanism through which OnabotulinumtoxinA exits from vasculature is unknown. At the level of neuromuscular injection, OnabotulinumtoxinA arrests spontaneous quantal release of acetylcholine via cleavage of SNAP-25 protein (synaptosomal protein with a molecular weight of 25 kDa), producing muscular relaxation. Such mechanism of action can generate both the botulism disorder and the use of OnabotulinumtoxinA as a therapeutic agent in clinical practice. Paralysis at muscular local level and reduced muscular contraction cannot explain alone OnabotulinumtoxinA's pain relief. This suggests indirect reduction on central sensitization by inhibition of peripheral sensitization of nociceptive fibers, by inhibiting the release of neuromediators such as glutamate and substance P or *c-fos* gene expression (Aoki 2003). A contribution of calcitonin gene-related peptide (CGRP) to migraine pathophysiology is suggested by a study of Durham et al. on cultures of trigeminal ganglia neurons incubated with toxin; this incubation has shown the reduction of secretory stimulation of CGRP neurotransmitter respect to control cultures (Durham et al. 2004). OnabotulinumtoxinA has been extensively used in our University-based Hospital during the last decade as pioneering off-label drug to treat drug-resistant CM patients (Farinelli et al. 2006). Recent evidence, from the PREEMPT clinical program (PREEMPT1; PREEMPT2; and Pooled PREEMPT), reports that 1,384 patients were randomized for a multicenter randomized placebo-controlled phase 3 trial. During a period of 24 weeks, two injections cycles were carried out. OnabotulinumtoxinA (155–195 U) or placebo were administered through the fixed site method. OnabotulinumtoxinA resulted remarkably more effective than a placebo in terms of frequency reduction during headache days (primary endpoint) as well as in the increase of health-related quality of life, which has been measured through a specific questionnaire. Adverse events proved to be mild and resolved without sequelae. The most frequent were neck pain (9.8%), and muscular weakness (5.2%) (Aurora et al. 2010; Diener et al. 2010; Dodick et al. 2010). Such studies will allow a profound change in the expectations of CM patients in terms of a definitive efficacious response to their medical needs. Subjects treated with OnabotulinumtoxinA showed improvements from baseline in measures of headache frequency, and improvements from baseline and in comparison with placebo treatment in headache impact and treatment satisfaction but did not differ from placebo-treated subjects in measures of headache frequency and severity (Cady and Schreiber 2008). A meta-analysis of eight randomized, double-blind, placebo-controlled trials considering 1,601 patients with a history of episodic migraine did not find significant clinical and statistical differences from placebo in lowering the frequency of migraine headaches (Shuhendler et al. 2009). Migraine patients often suffer greatly as a result of the adverse effects of the drugs used, showing fatigue, dizziness, reduced concentration, loss of appetite, weight gain, hair loss and changes in libido. These side effects are not known in association with OnabotulinumtoxinA (Göbel 2004). Last July 2010 botulinum toxin type A has been licensed by the Medicines and Healthcare Products Regulatory Agency (MHRA) in the UK for the prophylaxis of headaches in adults who have CM. This is the first license worldwide of botulinum toxin type A for this indication, and is also the first prophylactic (preventative) treatment to receive a specific license for patients with chronic migraine. In October 2010 also the US Food and Drug Administration approved Botox injection (OnabotulinumtoxinA) to prevent headaches in adult patients with chronic migraine.

The use of Topiramate in preventing migraine's chronicization process or in reverting consolidated CM is well known (Ruiz and Ferrandi 2009; Stovner et al. 2009). Topiramate is a sulfamate-substituted monosaccharide, presenting several mechanisms of molecular action such as effects inhibition of voltage-dependent channels of calcium and sodium, signal enhancement of $GABA_A$ receptors, modulation of glutamate-mediated neurotransmission and carbonic anhydrase inhibition. In migraine, such spectrum of actions could reduce nociceptive transmission at the central system level through trigeminovascular modulation and inhibition of the cortical spreading depression (Storer and Goadsby 2004; Akerman and Goadsby 2005). The usefulness of anticonvulsant agents such as Topiramate might consist in the block of voltage-dependent channels of calcium and sodium or in the ability to enhance the activity of $GABA_A$ receptors (Silberstein et al. 2004). In migraine, Topiramate acts by reducing nociceptive transmission at the central system level through trigeminovascular modulation and inhibition of the cortical spreading depression (Farinelli et al. 2009). A 26 week randomized double-blind placebo-controlled study have shown that migraine's preventative treatment with Topiramate at a dosage of 100 or 200 mg/day, but not 50 mg/day, is able to reduce the risk of transformation to a chronic form (Silberstein et al. 2004). Such progression risk is extremely high in a subset of patients with elevated migraine frequency and frequent acute medication intake. The most common adverse events (AEs) during Topiramate treatment were paresthesias (8%), cognitive symptoms (7.3%), fatigue (4.7%), insomnia (3.4%), nausea (2.3%), loss of appetite, anxiety, and dizziness (2.1%). Paresthesia, due to the inhibition of carbonic anhydrase, is the most common side effect although it does not constitute the main reason for therapy discontinuation. Cognitive symptoms are represented by concentration/attention as well as memory difficulties. The majority of AEs appears during the titration period, generally within 6 weeks. These data suggest that if patients do no present AEs by the end of such period, they will be safe from such events (Farinelli et al. 2009). In a randomized double-blind placebo-controlled trial, both Topiramate's efficacy and tolerance have been investigated in the prevention of CM, with a dose target of 100 mg per day. Topiramate considerably reduced the mean number of monthly headache days (primary endpoint) compared with placebo. In the subgroup of patients with drugs abuse, mostly triptans, Topiramate reduced significantly the mean number of monthly migraine days from baseline (Diener et al. 2007). In a randomized, double-blind placebo-controlled parallel group multicenter trial, Topiramate has been tested in the prevention of CM. Titration period was of 4 weeks with a maintenance period of 12 weeks and the final mean Topiramate maintenance was 86 mg/day. Topiramate proved to be effective in reducing migraine headache days and migraine headache days relative to baseline (Silberstein et al. 2007). Although from these studies Topiramate results well-tolerated, eventual adverse events are possible. Láinez et al. analyzed three large multicenter studies and found that therapy discontinuation occurred in 25% of patients administered with Topiramate and in 1% of patients treated with placebo. The majority of AEs appeared during the titration period, generally within 6 weeks. These data suggest that in case patients do no present AEs in such period, they will be safe from such events (Láinez et al. 2007). In conclusion, migraine's preventative treatment with Topiramate is able to reduce the risk of transformation into a chronic form. Such progression risk is extremely high in a subset of patients with elevated migraine frequency and frequent acute medication intake (Ruiz and Ferrandi 2009). Further confirmation on the validity of such therapeutic approach for CM results from a study comparing OnabotulinumtoxinA and Topiramate (Farinelli et al. 2009). The study reports no particular differences among treatments in terms of efficacy, but there is a significant difference for what concerns safety profiles, which is definitely in favor of OnabotulinumtoxinA. In fact, AEs due to Topiramate therapy result more often in abandoning the treatment itself (Stovner et al. 2009). In US claims database analyses involving >4,000 patients with migraine, Topiramate significantly reduced triptan use by up to 20% in the

12-month period after starting treatment. Reductions were also noted in the numbers of ED visits, diagnostic procedures, hospital admissions and migraine-related hospitalization days (Láinez 2009). A study conducted in a large series to assess prospectively the impact of prophylaxis on health-related quality of life (HRQOL), using the Short Form 36 (SF-36), and daily activities, using the Migraine Disability Assessment Score (MIDAS), indicates that migraine prophylaxis has the potential to reduce the global burden of migraine on individuals and society (D'Amico et al. 2006).

Education and Management During Migraine Chronicization Process

Several studies have shown that migraine substantially impairs a person's functions during attacks and diminishes HRQoL during and between attacks. Despite its impact, migraine remains underestimated, under diagnosed, and undertreated. The assessment of migraine-related impairment and the impact on the daily activities and HRQoL may be favored by tools as the 36-Item Short-Form Health Survey and the Headache Impact Test, and by improving communication during the office visit through active listening, use of open-ended questions, and use of the "ask-tell-ask" strategy can also help in assessing (Buse et al. 2009b). In some cases, MOH appears to belong to the spectrum of addictive behaviors. In clinical practice, behavioral management of MOH should be undertaken besides pharmacological management (Radat et al. 2008). Migraine has a significant burden on patients and families/cohabitants, being cause of not only reduced productivity and absences from work/school, but also decreased ability to participate in home/family life and social/leisure activities, and time missed from family/social occasions (MacGregor et al. 2004). Worry in expectation of the next migraine attack can have negative effects on the family and social lives and work productivity of patients with migraine. The benefits of preventive pharmacotherapy for migraine may be measured over time in terms of changes in the frequency of acute attacks, impact of acute treatment on headache recurrence within the next 24 h, and reduction in overall functional impairment (Freitag 2007). A disease management model based on a multidisciplinary team (neurologists and nurse practitioners) is appeared to improve individualized patient care, increase patient/provider rapport and communication through an educational class, and empower the patient to take control of their health care by utilizing shared decision making. This model has improved patient satisfaction and reduced overall health care utilization (Blumenfeld and Tischio 2003). An Italian pilot study on 26 patients with probable MOH (pMOH) have suggested that short-term psychodynamic psychotherapy in conjunction with drug withdrawal and prophylactic pharmacotherapy relieves headache symptoms in pMOH, reducing both long-term relapses and the burden of CM (Altieri et al. 2009). The importance of a migraine education is proved by the Mercy Migraine Management Program (MMMP), an educational program for physicians and patients. Patients participating in the MMMP reported improvements in their headache frequency as well as the cognitive and emotional aspects of headache management, especially among those with high amounts of worry about their headaches at the beginning of the program (Smith et al. 2010). A headache management program that appeared to improve the outcomes consisted of: (1) a class specifically designed to inform patients about headache types, triggers, and treatment options; (2) diagnosis and treatment by a professional especially trained in headache care (based on US Headache Consortium guidelines); and (3) proactive follow-up by a case manager (Matchar et al. 2008). A short information about the possible role of medication overuse in headache chronification is appeared to be a modified brief intervention which can improve chronic headache and medication overuse in the general population (Grande et al. 2010).

Current Research

Pharmacogenomic and Chronic Migraine

The future in relapse prevention of CM complicated by MOH consists in considering how drugs currently used, such as triptans and emerging therapies, present responsivity profiles related to well-defined genetic polymorphisms (Di Lorenzo et al. 2009; Mathew and Farhan 2009; Simmaco et al. 2009; Gentile et al. 2010a). The feasible diagnostic setting for a tailored treatment of CM based on the application of pharmacogenomics will allow us to predetermine the efficacy of single old and new drugs by avoiding abuse and chronicization due to non-responsivity of the abused drug (Gentile et al. 2010b).

Conclusions

The management of CM patients in re-prophylaxis after detoxification of abusers still appears complicated (Negro et al. 2010). Both Topiramate and OnabotulinumtoxinA can be considered safe as well as effective, therefore representing a treatment choice. Regarding abusers, the first step always consists in drug interruption. Only after detoxification a new prophylaxis therapy, which otherwise would result useless from the start, could be outlined. Furthermore, considering relapse frequency in chronic patients towards symptomatic drugs, future studies on those two prophylaxis therapies associated in the treatment of refractory patients after detoxification are appropriate (Rossi et al. 2009). The future in relapse prevention of CM complicated by MOH consists in considering how drugs currently used such as triptans and emerging therapies present responsivity profiles related to well-defined genetic polymorphisms (Di Lorenzo et al. 2009; Farinelli et al. 2009; Stovner et al. 2009; Gentile et al. 2010b). The feasible diagnostic setting for tailored treatment of CM based on the application of pharmacogenomics will allow us to predetermine the efficacy of single old and new drugs by avoiding abuse due to non-responsivity of the abused drug (Simmaco et al. 2009).

References

Akerman S, Goadsby PJ (2005) Topiramate inhibits cortical spreading depression in rat and cat: impact in migraine aura. NeuroReport 16:1383–1387

Allena M, Katsarava Z, Nappi G, the COMOESTAS Consortium (2009) From drug-induced headache to medication overuse headache. A short epidemiological review, with a focus on Latin American countries. J Headache Pain 10:71–76

Altieri M, Di Giambattista R, Di Clemente L, Fagiolo D, Tarolla E, Mercurio A, Vicenzini E, Tarsitani L, Lenzi GL, Biondi M, Di Piero V (2009) Combined pharmacological and short-term psychodynamic psychotherapy for probable medication overuse headache: a pilot study. Cephalalgia 29(3):293–299

Aoki KR (2003) Evidence for antinociceptive activity of botulinum toxin type A in pain management. Headache 43:S9–S15

Aurora SK, Dodick DW, Turkel CC, DeGryse RE, Silberstein SD, Lipton RB, Diener HC, Brin MF, on behalf of PREEMPT 1 Trial (2010) OnabotulinumtoxinA for treatment of chronic migraine: results from the double-blind, randomized, placebo-controlled phase of the PREEMPT 1 trial. Cephalalgia 30:793–803

Bigal ME, Lipton RB (2008a) Concepts and mechanisms of migraine chronification. Headache 48:7–15

Bigal ME, Lipton RB (2008b) Excessive acute migraine medication use and migraine progression. Neurology 71(22):1821–1828

Bigal ME, Lipton RB (2009a) Overuse of acute migraine medications and migraine chronification. Curr Pain Headache Rep 13(4):301–307

Bigal ME, Lipton RB (2009b) What predicts the change from episodic to chronic migraine? Curr Opin Neurol 22:269–276

Bigal ME, Serrano D, Buse D, Scher A, Stewart WF, Lipton RB (2008) Acute migraine medications and evolution from episodic to chronic migraine: a longitudinal population-based study. Headache 48(8):1157–1168

Blumenfeld A, Tischio M (2003) Center of excellence for headache care: group model at Kaiser Permanente. Headache 43(5):431–440

Bøe MG, Mygland A, Salvesen R (2007) Prednisolone does not reduce withdrawal headache: a randomized, double-blind study. Neurology 69(1):26–31

Buse DC, Marcia FT, Rupnow FT, Lipton RB (2009a) Assessing and managing all aspects of migraine: migraine attacks, migraine related functional impairment, common comorbidities, and quality of life. Mayo Clin Proc 84:422–435

Buse DC, Rupnow MF, Lipton RB (2009b) Assessing and managing all aspects of migraine: migraine attacks, migraine-related functional impairment, common comorbidities, and quality of life. Mayo Clin Proc 84(5):422–435

Cady R, Schreiber C (2008) Botulinum toxin type A as migraine preventive treatment in patients previously failing oral prophylactic treatment due to compliance issues. Headache 48(6):900–913

Castillo J, Muñoz P, Guitera V, Pascual J (1999) Kaplan award 1998: epidemiology of chronic daily headache in the general population. Headache 39:190–196

Cupini LM, Calabresi P (2005) Medication-overuse headache: pathophysiological insights. J Headache Pain 6(4):199–202

D'Amico D, Solari A, Usai S, Santoro P, Bernardoni P, Frediani F, De Marco R, Massetto N, Bussone G, Progetto Cefalee Lombardia Group (2006) Improvement in quality of life and activity limitations in migraine patients after prophylaxis. A prospective longitudinal multicentre study. Cephalalgia 26(6):691–696

De Filippis S, Salvatori E, Coloprisco G, Martelletti P (2006) Chronic daily headache: management and rehabilitation. Clin Ter 157(2):153–157

De Filippis S, Salvatori E, Farinelli I, Coloprisco G, Martelletti P (2007) Chronic daily headache and medication overuse headache: clinical read-outs and rehabilitation procedures. Clin Ter 158(4):343–347

Di Lorenzo C, Di Lorenzo G, Sances G et al (2009) Drug consumption in medication overuse headache is influenced by brain derived neurotrophic factor Val66Met polymorphism. J Headache Pain 10:349–355

Diener HC, Limmroth V (2004) Medication-overuse headache: a worldwide problem. Lancet Neurol 3:475–483

Diener HC, Bussone G, Van Oene JC et al (2007) Topiramate reduces headache days in chronic migraine: a randomized, double- blind, placebo-controlled study. Cephalalgia 27:814–823

Diener HC, Dodick DW, Aurora SK, Turkel CC, DeGryse RE, Lipton RB, Silberstein SD, Brin MF, on behalf of the PREEMPT 2 Chronic Migraine Study Group (2010) OnabotulinumtoxinA for treatment of chronic migraine: results from the double-blind, randomized, placebo-controlled phase of the PREEMPT 2 trial. Cephalalgia 30:804–814

Dodick DW, Turkel CC, DeGryse RE, Aurora SK, Silberstein SD, Lipton RB, Diener H-C, Brin MF, on behalf of the PREEMPT Chronic Migraine Study Group (2010) OnabotulinumtoxinA for treatment of chronic migraine: pooled a results from the doubleblind, randomized, placebo-controlled phases of the PREEMPT Clinical Program. Headache 50:921–936

Durham PL, Cady R, Cady R (2004) Regulation of calcitonin gene-related peptide secretion from trigeminal nerve cells by botulinum toxin type A: implications for migraine therapy. Headache 44:35–43

Evers S, Marziniak M (2010) Clinical features, pathophysiology, and treatment of medication overuse headache. Lancet Neurol 9:391–401

Farinelli I, Coloprisco G, De Filippis S, Martelletti P (2006) Long-term benefits of botulinum toxin type A (Botox) in chronic daily headache: a five-year long experience. J Headache Pain 7:407–412

Farinelli I, De Filippis S, Coloprisco G, Missori S, Martelletti P (2009) Future drugs for migraine. Int Emerg Med 4:367–373

Farinelli I, Dionisi I, Martelletti P (2010) Rehabilitating chronic migraine complicated by medication overuse headaches: how we can prevent migraine relapse? Int Emerg Med 6(1):23–28

Freitag FG (2007) The cycle of migraine: patients' quality of life during and between migraine attacks. Clin Ter 29(5):939–949

Gentile G, Borro M, Lala N, Missori S, Simmaco M, Martelletti P (2010a) Genetic polymorphisms related to efficacy and overuse of triptans in chronic migraine. J Headache Pain 11(5):431–435

Gentile G, Missori S, Borro M, Sebastianelli A, Simmaco M, Martelletti P (2010b) Frequencies of genetic polymorphisms related to triptans metabolism in chronic migraine. J Headache Pain 11:151–156

Göbel H (2004) Botulinum toxin in migraine prophylaxis. J Neurol 251(Suppl 1):I8–I11

Grande RB, Aaseth K, Benth JŠ, Lundqvist C, Russell MB (2010) Reduction in medication-overuse headache after short information. The Akershus study of chronic headache. Eur J Neurol 18:129–137

Hagen K, Albretsen C, Vilming ST, Salvesen R, Grønning M, Helde G, Gravdahl G, Zwart JA, Stovner LJ (2009) Management of medication overuse headache: 1-year randomized multicentre open-label trial. Cephalalgia 29(2):221–232

Hagen K, Jensen R, Bøe MG, Stovner LJ (2010) Medication overuse headache: a critical review of end points in recent followup studies. J Headache Pain 11(5):373–377

Headache Classification Committee, Olesen J, Bousser MG, Diener HC, Dodick D, First M, Goadsby PJ, Göbel H, Lainez MJ, Lance JW, Lipton RB, Nappi G, Sakai F, Schoenen J, Silberstein SD, Steiner TJ (2006) New appendix criteria open for a broader concept of chronic migraine. Cephalalgia 26: 742–746

Katsarava Z, Schneeweiss S, Kurth T et al (2004) Incidence and predictors for chronicity of headache in patients with episodic migraine. Neurology 62: 788–790

Katsarava Z, Muessig M, Dzagnidze A, Fritsche G, Diener HC, Limmroth V (2005) Medication overuse headache: rates and predictors for relapse in a 4-year prospective study. Cephalalgia 25:12–15

Krymchantowski AV, Barbosa JS (2000) Prednisone as initial treatment of analgesic-induced daily headache. Cephalalgia 20:107–113

Krymchantowski AV, Moreira PF (2003) Out-patient detoxification in chronic migraine: comparison of strategies. Cephalalgia 23(10):982–993

Láinez MJ (2009) The effect of migraine prophylaxis on migraine-related resource use and productivity. CNS Drugs 23(9):727–738

Láinez MJ, Freitag FG, Pfeil J, Ascher S, Olson WH, Schwalen S (2007) Time course of adverse events most commonly associated with topiramate for migraine prevention. Eur J Neurol 14:900–906

Lake AE 3rd (2006) Medication overuse headache: biobehavioral issues and solutions. Headache 46(Suppl 3): S88–S97

Lipton RB (2009) Tracing transformation: chronic migraine classification, progression, and epidemiology. Neurology 72(5 Suppl):S3–S7

Lovell BV, Marmura MJ (2010) New therapeutic developments in chronic migraine. Curr Opin Neurol 23:254–258

Lundqvist C, Benth JS, Grande RB, Aaseth K, Russell MB (2010) An adapted Severity of Dependence Scale is valid for the detection of medication overuse: the Akershus study of chronic headache. Eur J Neurol. doi:10.1111/j.1468-1331.2010.03202.x

MacGregor EA, Brandes J, Eikermann A, Giammarco R (2004) Impact of migraine on patients and their families: the Migraine and Zolmitriptan Evaluation (MAZE) survey– Phase III. Curr Med Res Opin 20(7):1143–1150

Matchar DB, Harpole L, Samsa GP, Jurgelski A, Lipton RB, Silberstein SD, Young W, Kori S, Blumenfeld A (2008) The headache management trial: a randomized study of coordinated care. Headache 48(9):1294–1310

Mathew NT, Farhan AJ (2009) A double-blind comparison of OnabotulinumtoxinA (BOTOX®) and Topiramate (TOPAMAX®) for the prophylactic treatment of chronic migraine: a pilot study. Headache 49:1466–1478

Negro A, D'Alonzo L, Martelletti P (2010) Chronic migraine: comorbidities, risk factors, and rehabilitation. Intern Emerg Med 5(Suppl 1):S13–S19

Obermann M, Katsarava Z (2007) Management of medication overuse headache. Expert Rev Neurother 7:1145–1155

Paemeleire K, Crevits L, Goadsby PJ, Kaube H (2006) Practical management of medication-overuse headache. Acta Neurol Belg 106:43–51

Pageler L, Katsarava Z, Diener HC, Limmroth V (2008) Prednisone versus placebo in withdrawal therapy following medication overuse headache. Cephalalgia 28:152–156

Pompili M, Di Cosimo D, Innamorati M, Lester D, Tatarelli R, Martelletti P (2009) Psychiatric comorbidity in patients with chronic daily headache and migraine: a selective overview including personality traits and suicide risk. J Headache Pain 10:283–290

Pompili M, Serafini G, Di Cosimo D, Innamorati M, Lester D, Forte D, Girardi N, De Filippis S, Tatarelli R, Martelletti P (2010) Psychiatric comorbidity and suicide risk in patients with chronic migraine. Neuropsychiatr Dis Treat 6:81–91

Radat F, Creac'h C, Guegan-Massardier E, Mick G, Guy N, Fabre N, Giraud P, Nachit-Ouinekh F, Lantéri-Minet M (2008) Behavioral dependence in patients with medication overuse headache: a cross-sectional study in consulting patients using the DSM-IV criteria. Headache 48(7):1026–1036

Rossi P, Di Lorenzo C, Faroni J, Cesarino F, Nappi G (2006) Advice alone vs. structured detoxification programmes for medication overuse headache: a prospective, randomized, open-label trial in transformed migraine patients with low medical needs. Cephalalgia 26(9): 1097–1105

Rossi P, Jensen R, Nappi G, Allena M, the COMOESTAS Consortium (2009) A narrative review on the management of medication overuse headache: the steep road from experience to evidence. J Headache Pain 10:407–417

Rossi P, Faroni JV, Nappi G (2010) Short-term effectiveness of simple advice as a withdrawal strategy in simple and complicated medication overuse headache. Eur J Neurol. doi:10.1111/j.1468- 1331.2010.03157

Ruiz L, Ferrandi D (2009) Topiramate in migraine progression. J Headache Pain 10:419–422

Scher AI, Midgette LA, Lipton RB (2008) Risk factors for headache chronification. Headache 48:16–25

Shuhendler AJ, Lee S, Siu M, Ondovcik S, Lam K, Alabdullatif A, Zhang X, Machado M, Einarson TR (2009) Efficacy of botulinum toxin type A for the prophylaxis of episodic migraine headaches: a meta-analysis of randomized, double-blind, placebo-controlled trials. Pharmacotherapy 29(7):784–791

Silberstein SD, Neto W, Schmitt J, Jacobs D et al (2004) Topiramate in migraine prevention: results of a large controlled trial. Arch Neurol 61:490–495

Silberstein S, Olesen J, Bousser MG et al (2005) The international classification of headache disorders, 2nd edn (ICHD-II). Revised of criteria for 8.2 medication-overuse headache. Cephalalgia 25:460–465

Silberstein SD, Lipton RB, Dodick DW et al (2007) Efficacy and safety of topiramate for the treatment of chronic migraine: a randomized, double-blind, placebo-controlled trial. Headache 47:170–180

Simmaco M, Borro M, Missori S, Martelletti P (2009) Pharmacogenomics in migraine: catching biomarkers for a predictable disease control. Expert Rev Neurother 9:1267–1269

Simpson LL (1980) Kinetic studies on the interaction between botulinum toxin type A and the cholinergic neuromuscular junction. J Pharmacol Exp Ther 213:504–508

Smith TR, Stoneman J (2004) Medication overuse headache from antimigraine therapy: clinical features, pathogenesis and management. Drugs 64(22):2503–2514

Smith TR, Nicholson RA, Banks JW (2010) Migraine education improves quality of life in a primary care setting. Headache 50(4):600–612

Storer RJ, Goadsby PJ (2004) Topiramate inhibits trigeminovascular neurons in the cat. Cephalalgia 24:1049–1056

Stovner LJ, Andree C (2010) Prevalence of headache in Europe: a review of the Eurolight project. J Headache Pain 11(4):289–299

Stovner LJ, Zwart JA, Hagen K, Terwindt GM, Pascual J (2006) Epidemiology of headache in Europe. Eur J Neurol 13:333–345

Stovner LJ, Tronvik E, Hagen K (2009) New drugs for migraine. J Headache Pain 10:395–406

Trucco M, Meineri P, Ruiz L, Gionco M, Gruppo Neurologico Ospedaliero Interregionale per lo Studio delle Cefalee" (Neurological Hospital Interregional Group for the Study of Headaches) (2010) Medication overuse headache: withdrawal and prophylactic therapeutic regimen. Headache 50(6):989–997

Valguarnera F, Tanganelli P (2010) The efficacy of withdrawal therapy in subjects with chronic daily headache and medication overuse following prophylaxis with topiramate and amitriptyline. Neurol Sci 31(Suppl 1):S175–S177

Vargas BB, Dodick DW (2009) The face of chronic migraine: epidemiology, demographics and treatment strategies. Neurol Clin 27:467–479

33 Psychological Interventions for Headache That Has Become Difficult to Treat

Donna Maria Coleston-Shields
Neurosciences Unit, University Hospital Coventry & Warwickshire, Coventry, UK

Paolo Martelletti, Timothy J. Steiner (eds.), *Handbook of Headache*, DOI 10.1007/978-88-470-1700-9_33,
© Lifting The Burden 2011

Abstract: While it may be argued that all headache patients could benefit from psychological pain management of some form, restricted access to psychology services or prohibitive waiting lists may mean that the headache clinician has to focus psychological efforts only when psychological difficulties are suspected and these factors may be making the headache harder to treat. An association between headache, migraine in particular, and depression has long been described. The task is to recognize and formally describe low mood and increased anxiety (using basic standardized assessments), and then to interpret such symptoms appropriately: do they represent a primary psychological disorder (clinical depression or anxiety) or are they instead a consequence of the experience of head pain? Especially if the former is the case, referral on to specialist psychology services may be necessary, but it may be possible for the headache clinician to recommend or make use of some basic psychological techniques, particularly those involving relaxation training, which when learned properly and used regularly can be impressively effective.

Essential Knowledge

The Longstanding Association Between Psychology and Headache

Much work on psychology and headache, especially early research, has involved the concept of a "headache personality type," making use of measurement tools such as the Minnesota Multiphasic Personality Inventory (MMPI and more recently, MMPI-2) (e.g., Andrasik et al. 1982). This research has had some limitations; there has been dispute in the literature as to what might constitute a psychological headache profile for a number of different headache types (e.g., Schnider et al. 1995; Vilming et al. 1997; De Fidio et al. 2000), and such an approach may have limitations in the therapeutic management of headache. Instead factors such as "catastrophization" and coping ability may be more useful clinically (Lucas et al. 2007).

In addition to the idea that psychology can affect headache, a body of literature has emerged that describes how psychology can be used to "fix" headache. Very early approaches involved the perspective of psychodynamic psychotherapy, focusing on underlying etiology "related to the repression of hostile aggressive impulses" (from Eisenbud 1937). From the 1970s onward, relaxation training became popular (e.g., Warner and Lance 1975). Many of these techniques remain in use now, and additionally, behavioral and cognitive behavioral therapy (CBT) can be adapted for use in pain management and with headache patients in particular. Originally developed for treatment of clinical anxiety and depression (Beck 1993), CBT has been shown to be particularly effective in managing headache, holding its own on comparison with pharmacological treatment (Holroyd et al. 2001; Kaushik et al. 2005) and possibly even facilitating a reduction in medication use (Zsombok et al. 2003).

Which Patients Might Benefit from Psychological Therapy?

Ideally, all headache patients should have access to some form of psychological input since psychological interventions are not only useful when there is concurrent psychopathology (clinical depression or anxiety), or when headache has become difficult to treat. Rather, they can be used to assist pain management for the majority of patients, given that the experience of many headaches is essentially a bio-psychological phenomenon, a perception of heightened pain (Wall 1999; Fulbright et al. 2001). This input does not need to be on a costly (both in terms of time and finance) one-to-one basis. Group management can be a useful alternative, and self-help guidance can be beneficial, with a number of popular texts in circulation (e.g., Duckro et al. 1999). In the Netherlands, migraine patients themselves have been trained to help fellow patients manage and even prevent headache (Mérelle et al. 2008a, b), and advancing technology has been used to provide behavioral headache self-management at a distance (Sorbi and van der Vaart 2010).

In reality, psychology services can be hard to find or may have prohibitive waiting lists, so that clinicians working with headache must use such a resource sparingly. Instead the emphasis must be on involving psychology only when psychological difficulties are suspected and when these factors may be making the headache harder to treat. An association between depression and migraine has long been postulated (e.g., Harvey and Hay 1984; Jenkinson 1990; Merskey 1992; Franchini et al. 2004), and while there continues to be debate as to the prevalence of low mood in headache patients, it is now generally accepted that the concurrence does indeed exist.

The difficulty for the headache clinician is in recognizing and formally describing low mood and increased anxiety levels, then in knowing how to interpret such symptoms if they are noted. It is probably too simplistic to say that if a patient is experiencing low mood, then they must be clinically depressed and this depression is somehow causative for or exacerbating the headache. The possibility that the headache is itself causing the low mood and increased anxiety must also be considered. For this reason, full assessment of psychological factors can be invaluable.

Assessing Psychological Need

Psychological assessment can ensure that clinical problems are described as fully as possible. For measurement of the headache itself, structured diaries can produce rich information on frequency, duration, severity, trigger factors (both physical and behavioral), patient responses to their headache (emotional, behavioral, and cognitive), lifestyle, "workstyle" (covering the concept of "presenteeism" when the patient attends work despite their headache and so fails to achieve much; Baskin and Weeks 2003), and possible secondary gains (perhaps a rarer phenomenon in pain than generally believed). Many basic examples exist (e.g., MacGregor and Jensen 2008; many available online also) which can be elaborated to include all or some of the above. If one has access to a psychologist, they will be useful in defining and redefining the headache diary for maximum data collection, and they will be able to distinguish what is "statistically significant" from what is "clinically significant."

Further, there are various standardized assessments used in the field of health (as opposed to clinical) psychology that, while not specific to headache, will formally measure a number of psychological factors that may be associated with headache, such as general health-related behaviors (e.g., Prohaska et al. 1985), specific pain motivated behaviors (e.g., Richards et al. 1982), coping styles (e.g., Carver et al. 1989; Carver 1997), and causal and control beliefs (e.g., Wallston et al. 1978). Coping and control beliefs link to the concept of "locus of control" (Baskin and Weeks 2003), an important factor for the headache clinician to consider as, whether a patient feels they have power to change their health status or not, may be a useful predictor of the success of treatment overall (e.g., Voils et al. 2005; Lucas et al. 2007).

For measurement of concurrent psychiatric illness, many standardized mental health assessments also exist. These include the Beck Depression Inventory (BDI) (Beck 1996) and Beck Anxiety Inventory (BAI) (Beck 1990), Schema Inventories (Young 1999), the General Health Questionnaire (GHQ) (Goldberg 1981), and the Hospital Anxiety Depression Scale (HADS) (Zigmond and Snaith 1983). While the BDI, BAI, and Schema Inventories may have potential for distinguishing whether low mood and anxiety are causal for or consequential to the headache, their administration and interpretation probably require specialist psychology knowledge as they link to specific psychotherapies (Beck 1993; Young 1999). The GHQ and HADS however, may be useful to headache clinicians as a first step in formally describing low mood and increased anxiety levels in their headache patients.

Overall, when assessing for psychological factors, it is important for the clinician to consider what it is that is being treated: are they treating the headache or are they attempting to treat a distinct psychological disorder? By using a suitable screening measure such as the GHQ or HADS, by discussing matters such as lifestyle, work, and to what extent the patient feels they can "beat" the headache (hinting at "locus of control"), the headache clinician will equip themselves with sufficient information to decide whether psychological input is necessary, and if it is, whether to refer on to specialist psychology services for treatment of a concurrent psychological disorder, or whether there is some form of psychological input they can recommend or provide themselves.

Psychological Therapy/Intervention

Psychological interventions for headache may be grouped as follows: relaxation training, therapies for migraine and tension-type headache, and therapy for chronic daily headache (CDH).

Relaxation therapies are suitable for use with most diagnoses of headache, and their administration does not necessarily require specialist psychology input; indeed, a number of self-help training methods exist. Relaxation therapies include controlled breathing (Kaushik et al. 2005), progressive muscular relaxation (PMR) and guided visualization (Duckro et al. 1999), and attention control training (ACT) (initially developed for sports training, Nideffer 1979). Different methods may better suit different headache diagnoses (e.g., tension-type headache may respond best to PMR) or be appropriate for different patient needs (e.g., ACT can be used in situations when one is required to be awake, alert, and totally aware of the environment, rather than withdrawn and quiet). Specifically designed for use with headache, the effectiveness of biofeedback based on "hand warming" has long been reported (e.g., Sargent et al. 1972, 1973; Daly et al. 1983), but this technique involves specialist equipment. Overall, relaxation techniques, when learned properly and used regularly, can be impressively effective.

For migraine and tension-type headache, adapted behavioral and cognitive behavioral management (Beck 1993; Holroyd et al. 2005; Holroyd and Drew 2006) may be required. The focus for the psychologist is on "monitoring" and "pacing." Considering monitoring, migraine and tension-type headache patients can be poor at tracking the course of their headache, often not paying attention to warning signs that could alert them and provide them with an opportunity to avoid the headache. Considering pacing, patients may push themselves to, for example, stay at work when they should be at home (presenteeism, referred to previously), or they may work harder when they return to the workplace after the headache; this latter feature may have to do with guilt about letting others down (rather than based in a personality trait). By encouraging patients to formally track and challenge their maladaptive behaviors and negative cognitions (thoughts) (e.g., Pryse-Phillips et al. 1998), their sense of coping and control may be increased, accompanied by an increase in mood and reduction in anxiety, and perhaps also a reduction in their experience of head pain.

With CDH, the approach is different as the patient may benefit from being discouraged from monitoring and checking behaviors. The psychologist may encourage them not to look for reassurance, not to monitor or check their symptoms, not to find out about their illness or related illnesses, and not to avoid anything that may be associated with the illness (based on Kuchemann and Sanders 2007). CDH may require a different approach because this diagnosis is often less acceptable to the patient: they may feel that it simply describes their symptoms and does not refer to cause; they may feel that they need to seek out the cause of their headache, and resentment can build toward the clinician who is only treating their head pain and who is not helping them to uncover what is truly wrong with them, a tumor perhaps. In this respect, CDH can be more challenging for the headache clinician to manage on their own psychologically.

Referring on to Specialist Psychology Services

If a headache clinician feels that specialist psychology input is necessary, they face the task of accessing an appropriate service. Pain management, to include headache, comes under the remit of health psychology as opposed to clinical psychology, since the latter is involved primarily with provision of mental health care. That said, headache may represent a special case given the fact that there is an association with low mood and increased anxiety; thus, if the headache clinician does not have access to a specific health psychology service, psychologists in either adult or older adult mental health services may be willing to accept referrals with negotiation as many will have experience of working across both mental and physical health fields.

Current Research

Psychological intervention for headache is literally moving into new areas. An interesting international perspective is developing as methods already used for some time are being applied to new populations, for example, in Korea (Kang et al. 2009); and in Japan, characteristics of mood disorders in headache have been studied with specific focus on medication-overuse headache (MOH) (Kaji and Hirata 2009). MOH is itself an interesting area for psychologists; as data emerge on psychological variables (e.g., Usai et al. 2009) it may be that psychological therapies for MOH are developed, perhaps based on existing interventions used in drug and alcohol addiction. Finally, identification of the genetic bases of comorbidity between mood disorders and migraine, specifically involving the serotonin transporter gene (Marino et al. 2009), could have implications for essential integration of psychological interventions with pharmacological headache therapies.

References

Andrasik F, Blanchard EB, Arena JG, Teders SJ, Teevan RC, Rodichock LD (1982) Psychological functioning in headache sufferers. Psychosom Med 44(2):171–182

Baskin SM, Weeks RE (2003) The biobehavioral treatment of headache. In: Moss D, McGrady A, Davies T, Wickramasekera I (eds) Handbook of mind-body medicine in primary care. Sage, Thousand Oaks, pp 205–222

Beck AT (1990) Beck anxiety inventory. The psychological corporation. Harcourt Brace & Company, San Antonio

Beck AT (1993) Cognitive therapy and the emotional disorders. Penguin, New York

Beck AT (1996) Beck depression inventory II. The psychological corporation. Harcourt Brace & Company, San Antonio

Carver CS (1997) You want to measure coping but your protocol's too long: consider the Brief COPE. Int J Behav Med 4(1):92–100

Carver CS, Scheier MF, Weintraub JK (1989) Assessing coping strategies: a theoretically based approach. J Pers Soc Psychol 56:267–283

Daly EJ, Donn PA, Galliher MJ, Zimmerman JS (1983) Biofeedback applications to migraine and tension headache: a double-blinded outcome study. Biofeedback Self Regul 8:135–152

De Fidio D, Sciruicchio V, Pastore B, Prudenzano MP, Di Pietro E, Tramontano A, Lorizio A, Granella F, Bussone G, Grazzi L, Sarchielli P (2000) Chronic daily headache: personality study by means of computerized MMPI-2. J Headache Pain 1(1):S67–S70

Duckro PN, Richardson WD, Marshall JE, Cassabaum S, Marshall G (1999) Taking control of your headaches: how to get the treatment you need. Guilford, New York

Eisenbud J (1937) The psychology of headache: a case studied experimentally. Psychiatr Quart 11(4):592–619

Franchini L, Bongiorno F, Dotoli D, Rainero I, Pinessi L, Smeraldi E (2004) Migraine headache and mood disorders: a descriptive study in an outpatient psychiatric population. J Affect Disord 81(2):157–160

Fulbright RK, Troche CJ, Skudlarski P, Gore JC, Wexler BE (2001) Functional MR imaging of regional brain activation associated with the affective experience of pain. Am J Roentgenol 177:1205–1210

Goldberg D (1981) The general health questionnaire. NFER-Nelson Publishing Company Ltd, Windsor

Harvey PG, Hay KM (1984) Mood and migraine – a preliminary prospective study. Headache 24(2):225–228

Holroyd KA, Drew JB (2006) Behavioral approaches to the treatment of migraine. Semin Neurol 26:199–207

Holroyd KA, O'Donnell FJ, Stensland M, Lipchick GL, Cordingley GE, Carlson BW (2001) Management of chronic tension-type headache with tricyclic antidepressant medication, stress management therapy, and their combination: a randomized controlled trial. J Am Med Assoc 285:2208–2215

Holroyd KA, Martin PR, Nash JM (2005) Psychological treatments of tension-type headache. In: Olesen J, Goadsby PJ, Ramadan N, Tfelt-Hansen P, Welch KM (eds) The headaches. Lippincott Williams & Wilkins, Philadelphia, pp 711–719

Jenkinson C (1990) Health status and mood state in a migraine sample. Int J Soc Psychiatry 36(1):42–48

Kaji Y, Hirata K (2009) Characteristics of mood disorders in Japanese patients with medication-overuse headache. Intern Med (Japan) 48(12):981–986

Kang EH, Park JE, Chung CS, Yu BH (2009) Effect of biofeedback-assisted autogenic training on headache activity and mood states in Korean female migraine patients. J Korean Med Sci 24(5):936–940

Kaushik R, Kaushik RM, Mahajan SK, Rajesh V (2005) Biofeedback assisted diaphragmatic breathing and systematic relaxation versus propanolol in long term prophylaxis of migraine. Complement Ther Med 13:165–174

Kuchemann C, Sanders D (2007) Understanding health anxiety: a self-help guide for sufferers and their families. Oxford University Press, Oxford

Lucas C, Lanteri-Minet M, Massiou H, Nachit-Ouinekh F, Pradalier A, Mercier F, El Hasnaoui A, Radat F (2007) The GRIM2005 study of migraine consultation in France II. Psychological factors associated with treatment response to acute headache therapy and satisfaction in migraine. Cephalalgia 27(12):1398–1407

MacGregor A, Jensen R (2008) Migraine and other primary headaches. Oxford University Press, Oxford

Marino E, Fanny B, Lorenzi C, Pirovano A, Franchini L, Colombo C, Bramanti P, Smeraldi E (2009) Genetic bases of comorbidity between mood disorders and migraine: possible role of serotonin transporter gene. Neurol Sci (Italia) 1:1590–1874

Mérelle SYM, Sorbi MJ, van Doornen LJP, Passchier J (2008a) Migraine patients as trainers of their fellow patients in non-pharmacological preventative attack management: short-term effects of a randomized controlled trial. Cephalalgia 28:127–138

Mérelle SYM, Sorbi MJ, van Doornen LJP, Passchier J (2008b) Lay trainers with migraine for a home-based behavioural training: a 6-month follow-up study. Headache 48:1311–1325

Merskey H (1992) Migraine and mood. Cephalalgia 12(2):68

Nideffer RM (1979) ACT attention control training: how to get control of your mind through total concentration. Wideview Books, New York

Prohaska TR, Leventhal EA, Leventhal H, Keller ML (1985) Health practices and illness cognition in young, middle aged, and elderly adults. J Gerontol 40:569–578

Pryse-Phillips WEM, Dodick DW, Edmeads JG, Gawel MJ, Nelson RF, Purdy RA, Robinson G, Stirling D, Worthington I (1998) Guidelines for the nonpharmacologic management of migraine in clinical practice. Can Med Assoc J 159(1):47–54

Richards JS, Nepomuceno C, Riles M, Suer Z (1982) Assessing pain behavior: the UAB Pain Behavior Scale. Pain 14(4):393–398

Sargent JD, Green EE, Walters ED (1972) The use of autogenic feedback training in a pilot study of migraine and tension headaches. Headache 12:120–124

Sargent JD, Walters ED, Green EE (1973) Psychosomatic self-regulation of migraine headaches. Semin Psychiatry 5:415–427

Schnider P, Maly J, Mraz M, Brantner Inthaler S, Zeiler K, Wessely P (1995) MMPI and critical flicker frequency (CFF) analysis in headache patients with and without drug abuse. Headache 35(1):17–20

Sorbi MJ, van der Vaart R (2010) User acceptance of an Internet training aid for migraine self-management. J Telemed Telecare 16(1):20–24

Usai S, Grazzi L, D'Amico D, Andrasik F, Bussone G (2009) Psychological variables in chronic migraine with medication overuse before and after inpatient withdrawal: results at 1-year follow-up. Neurol Sci (Italia) 30(Suppl 1):S125–S127, 1590–1874

Vilming ST, Ellertsen B, Troland K, Schrader H, Monstad I (1997) MMPI profiles in post-lumbar puncture headache. Acta Neurol Scand 95(3):184–188

Voils CI, Steffens DC, Flint EP, Bosworth HB (2005) Social support and locus of control as predictors of adherence to antidepressant medication in an elderly population. Am J Geriatr Psychiatry 13(2):157–165

Wall P (1999) Pain: the science of suffering. Weidenfeld & Nicolson, London

Wallston KA, Wallston BS, DeVellis R (1978) Development of the Multidimensional Health Locus of Control (MHLC) scales. Health Educ Monogr 6:160–170

Warner G, Lance JW (1975) Relaxation therapy in migraine and chronic tension headache. Med J Aust 1:298–301

Young JE (1999) Cognitive therapy for personality disorders: a schema-focused approach. Professional Resource Press, Florida

Zigmond AS, Snaith RP (1983) The hospital anxiety and depression scale. Acta Psychiatr Scand 67:361–370

Zsombok T, Juhasz G, Budavari A, Vitrai J, Bagdy G (2003) Effects of autogenic training on drug consumption in patients with primary headache: an 8-month follow-up study. Headache 43:251–257

34 Neurostimulation for Headache That Has Become Difficult to Treat

Thorsten Bartsch
University Hospital Schleswig-Holstein, University of Kiel, Kiel, Germany

Paolo Martelletti, Timothy J. Steiner (eds.), *Handbook of Headache*, DOI 10.1007/978-88-470-1700-9_34,
© Lifting The Burden 2011

Abstract: The acute and preventive medical treatment of patients with primary headache syndromes such as chronic migraine is challenging and side effects frequently complicate the course of medical treatment. Recently there has been considerable progress in neurostimulation techniques in medically intractable chronic headache syndromes. It is very well known that a non-painful stimulation of peripheral nerves can elicit analgesic effects. This phenomenon has been used in certain pain syndromes using non-invasive high- or low-frequency transcutaneous electrical nerve stimulation (TENS), percutaneous electrical nerve stimulation (PENS/acupuncture-like TENS or AL-TENS), and spinal cord stimulation (SCS). The analgesic effect is critically dependent on the intensity of the electrical stimulation. In recent years, minimally invasive neurostimulation techniques and neuromodulatory techniques, such as transcranial magnetic stimulation, have also been applied to patients with chronic headaches. This chapter summarizes the current concepts and outcome data of neurostimulation and neuromodulatory approaches. The studies suggest suboccipital neurostimulation can have an effect even decades after onset of headaches thus representing a possible therapeutic option in chronic patients with headaches difficult to treat and that do not respond to any medication. In a subset of patients with chronic cluster headaches, hypothalamic deep brain stimulation may be a treatment option.

Established Knowledge

The medical treatment of patients with chronic primary headache syndromes such as chronic migraine, chronic cluster headache, and hemicrania continua is challenging as adverse side effects frequently complicate the course of medical treatment. Traditionally, the effect of peripheral neurostimulation (PNS) has been attributed to the activation of non-noxious afferent nerve fibers (Aβ-fibers) which is thought to modulate Aδ- and C-fiber-mediated nociceptive transmission in the spinal cord, compatible with the "Gate Control Theory of Pain." The understanding of pain–modulatory mechanisms in the spinal cord as well as in the supraspinal structures has been greatly advanced by the Gate Control Theory by Ronald Melzack and Patrick D. Wall (Melzack and Wall 1965). Although considerably extended and modified since then, this framework in essence proposed that the transmission of pain in the spinal cord is modulated by excitatory and inhibitory influences (Dickenson 2002). These influences may arise from intrinsic factors within the spinal cord or from supraspinal projections onto the spinal cord, or both. This short- and long-lasting relay function of the spinal cord may play an important role in pathophysiological pain states, such as in persistent pain, central sensitization, hyperalgesia, and allodynia (Sandkuhler 2009). The concept of modulation also implies a changeable, plastic transmission. Besides the concept of modulation - mediated via decreasing excitation or increasing inhibition - a prerequisite of this arrangement is the convergence of different types of afferent activity. Another prerequisite of an adequate effect of PNS is an intact descending modulatory network. In accordance with the Gate Control Theory outlined above, a similar interplay of multiple mechanisms of segmental spinal inhibiting effects and descending pain inhibitory pathways may mediate the analgesic effects of PNS.

Occipital Nerve Stimulation in Primary Headache Disorders

In the past decade, a number of case reports, case series and some prospective studies have emerged on the application of ONS in the treatment of primary headache disorders as well as secondary headache disorders, including post-traumatic headache and cervicogenic headache, and cranial neuralgias, including occipital neuralgia (Weiner and Reed 1999). A careful work-up, including brain imaging, and an indomethacin test, seem mandatory baselines in classifying these phenotypes before procedures are considered. A clear IHS diagnosis (Headache Classification Committee of The International Headache Society 2004) IHS seems desirable before consideration of any device-based therapy.

Results on ONS in intractable chronic migraine, frequently in the context of medication overuse, have been encouraging (Matharu et al. 2004; Oh et al. 2004; Schwedt et al. 2007a) with the majority of patients (84%) experiencing at least a 50% improvement. A real effect of ONS is supported by recent data from a multicenter, prospective, randomized, single blind, controlled feasibility study (ONSTIM trial), awaiting full publication (Goadsby et al. 2009). The responder rate was defined as 50% drop in headache days/month or $\geq$3-point drop (on a 0–10 scale) in overall pain intensity from baseline at 3-month follow-up. As such, the responder rate was 39% in intractable chronic migraine patients treated with ONS, compared to 8% in a control stimulation group and 0% responder rate in the medical management group.

Trigeminal autonomic cephalalgias (TAC), including cluster headache, paroxysmal hemicrania and short-lasting unilateral neuralgiform headache attacks with conjunctival injection and tearing (SUNCT) can be devastating medically intractable conditions (Goadsby et al. 2008a). Clinical outcome data are in the literature for 26 patients with drug-resistant chronic cluster headache. In the two largest case series, one retrospective (Burns et al. 2009) and one prospective (Magis et al. 2007), at least a 50% improvement was noted in one-third to two-thirds of patients, respectively. Some cluster headache patients have been implanted bilaterally, even if they were suffering from strictly unilateral attacks (Burns et al. 2009). Indeed, contra-lateral development of cluster headache attacks has been described after trigeminal nerve section (Jarrar et al. 2003) and unilateral ONS (Magis et al. 2007).

Hemicrania continua is an indomethacin-responsive primary headache. Although it is a relatively rare condition, ONS data are available for nine patients at present. Hemicrania continua may experience the most robust response to ONS, as so far 7/9 (77%) patients reported at least 50% improvement after a mean follow-up of little over a year (Burns et al. 2008). Some patients with paroxysmal hemicrania, SUNCT and new daily persistent headache have been implanted, but their data have not yet been published in detail (Goadsby 2007; Paemeleire et al. 2008).

In general, procedural safety data are good, but surgical revisions are frequent. To date, not a single persistent iatrogenic neurological deficit has been reported. In experienced hands, the postoperative infection risk is low. Both traumatic and spontaneous electrode migration are frequently reported, often within the first year. Further, battery replacement and electrode fracture/malfunction may lead to repeated surgery. Some patients experience pain at the pulse generator site and a few had the stimulator explanted as they found ONS intolerable. Some turn their stimulator off at night to avoid paresthesia. Local discomfort, muscle recruitment and a shock-like sensation at the electrode site may occur, as well as slight neck stiffness persisting for some months after surgery. The stimulator may be accidentally switched off by strong magnetic fields. Despite these adverse events and frequent revisions, most patients state they would undergo the procedure again and recommend it to others (Burns et al. 2009).

Future prospects include careful clinical phenotyping which may include an indomethacin test is key to allow scientific evaluation of ONS and thus to identify headache disorders with higher likelihood of responding to ONS. It should further be tried to identify predictors of success with ONS, as response to an occipital nerve block is not (Schwedt et al. 2007b;

Paemeleire et al. 2008; Goadsby et al. 2009). Concomitant medication overuse may negatively affect outcome in chronic migraine patients, and patients should be withdrawn prior to ONS as withdrawal itself may account for improvement by itself (Paemeleire et al. 2008).

Several variants on the original Weiner and Reed implantation technique (Weiner and Reed 1999) have been described. In principle, the procedure can be performed under local or general anesthesia, with a subcutaneous lead (either a cylindrical or paddle style electrode) inserted to cross the greater, lesser, and least occipital nerves via an incision on the midline or a lateral incision close to the mastoid process (Trentman and Zimmerman 2008). Alternatively, a recent introduced miniaturized Bion device can be implanted in the suboccipital region (Lipton 2009). The stimulation parameters, including frequency, pulse width and voltage, are classically adjusted to make patients experience mild paresthesia in the stimulated area.

Occipital Nerve Stimulation: Current Research

Most likely, multiple mechanisms involving pain processing circuits in the central nervous system are participating in the analgesic effects of peripheral neurostimulation (Goadsby 2007; Goadsby et al. 2008a). Direct effects of electrical stimulation on peripheral nerve excitability such as transient slowing in conduction velocity, increase in electrical threshold, and decrease in response probability have been suggested (Ignelzi and Nyquist 1979). Interestingly though, ONS did not significantly alter pain thresholds in cluster headache patients (Magis et al. 2007). Secondly, as projection fibers within the spinal ascending tracts represent only a minority whereas propriospinal neurons and interneurons of the spinal dorsal horn outnumber these projection neurons it has been suggested that the segmental neural network might represent the site of the neuromodulatory effect (Chung et al. 1984; Doubell et al. 1999; Meyerson and Linderoth 2006). Indeed, it has been suggested that the somatosensory peripheral neurosti-mulation of afferent A-b fibers modulates the nociceptive transmission on a segmental level, thus revisiting the Gate Control Theory by Melzack and Wall (Kolmodin and Skoglund 1960; Woolf 1979; Chung et al. 1984; Garrison and Foreman 1996). Further, experimental data indicated that supraspinal structures, such as the periaquaeductal gray (PAG), are at least partly involved in mediating the anti-nociceptive effects of neurostimulation (Lindblom et al. 1977; Garrison and Foreman 1994). Using a neuropharmacological approach, the pharmaco-logical mechanisms of opioidergic and GABAergic receptor systems involved in ONS have just begun to be studied (Burns et al. 2009). Thirdly, there is recent experimental evidence indicating that supraspinal structures, such as the periaqueductal gray (PAG), are also involved in mediating the anti-nociceptive effects of neurostimulation (Lindblom et al. 1977; Garrison and Foreman 1994). A microdialysis study on transmitter release in the PAG of rats receiving spinal cord stimulation demonstrated that neurostimulation caused a decrease of gamma-aminobutyric acid (GABA) levels but not of serotonin or substance P. As GABA-neurons in the PAG exert a tonic inhibitory effect on the activity in descending pain inhibitory pathways, including trigeminovascular inputs (Knight et al. 2003), it is suggested that a decreased GABA level in this region following repeated spinal cord stimulation may lead to activation of descending anti-nociceptive projections with subsequent pain reduction (Duggan and Foong 1985; Stiller et al. 1995, 1996). Further effects were also observed at the thalamic level (Gildenberg and Murthy 1980; Olausson et al. 1994). Similar mechanisms, i.e., gate control at the segmental level as well as activation of descending pain inhibitory pathways, may be operative in ONS. However, the existence of a trigeminocervical complex adds an additional

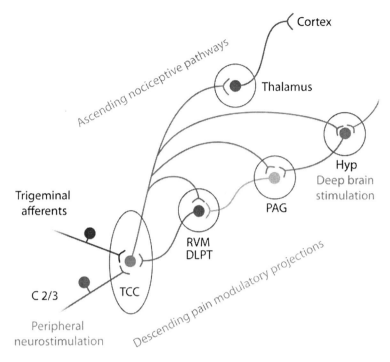

□ Fig. 34.1

Schematic drawing illustrating the functional anatomy of pain-modulatory pathways in the spinal cord and supraspinal structures. Nociceptive trigeminal fibers and C2-C3 afferents synapse and converge in the trigeminal nucleus caudalis (*TNC*) and dorsal horns of C2 and C3. The dorsal horns C1–3 and the TNC form a functional continuum, the trigeminocervical complex (*TCC*), from which information is relayed to higher centers of the brain, e.g., thalamus and cortex. Nociceptive and non-nociceptive information is relayed in the spinal dorsal horn where it is subject to segmental modulatory mechanisms either intrinsic or extrinsic from descending projections. The nociceptive input is transmitted to supraspinal relay sites, and is subject to inhibitory anti-nociceptive projections by pain-modulatory circuits in the brainstem (*RVM* rostral ventromedial medulla, *DLPT* dorsolateral pontomesencephalic tegmentum) and midbrain (*PAG* periaqueductal gray, *Hyp*, hypothalamus). Pain processing on different levels may be modulated by neurostimulation of occipital nerves and deep brain stimulation

level of complexity (❷ *Fig. 34.1*). It has been shown that nociceptive input from afferents in the trigeminal nerve and cervical afferents (C2–C3) converge on to the same nociceptive second-order neuron in the trigeminocervical complex that extends as a functional unit from the level of the trigeminal nucleus caudalis to at least the C2 segment. The resulting loss of spatial specificity helps to explains why ONS may have an anti-nociceptive effect in the territory of the trigeminal as well as occipital nerves (Goadsby 2007). Since the early studies on peripheral nerve stimulation (PNS), opioidergic mechanisms have been suggested to be involved in the effects of PNS and, at least partly, to contribute to the analgesic effect of PNS. In humans, experimental data show an increased concentration of β-endorphins and methionine–enkephalin in the cerebrospinal fluid after application of high frequency TENS. As discussed earlier, the involvement of pain modulating structures in the midbrain such as PAG and RVM also suggests an involvement of its opioidergic projections. Indeed, TENS elicits its analgesic effects by activation of μ- and δ-opioid receptors in the RVM and the spinal cord. With regard to TENS, low-frequency TENS elicits an anti-hyperalgesic effect through μ-opioid receptor activation whereas high-frequency TENS leads to anti-hyperalgesia through δ-opioid receptors in the spinal cord. Blockade of μ- and δ-opioid receptors in the spinal cord and RVM prevents the analgesic effect produced by TENS in arthritic rats.

Complementary neuroimaging studies investigating the role of supraspinal structures in mediating an anti-nociceptive effect in ONS suggest similar central mechanisms (Matharu et al. 2004). Eight patients with chronic migraine, who responded to a non-painful high-frequency stimulation (50–120 Hz) of afferents in the greater occipital nerve (GON) using bilaterally implanted neurostimulators, were PET scanned in different states: During stimulation when the patient was pain-free, during non-stimulation with pain and typical clinical features, and during partial activation of the stimulator with different levels of paresthesia (Matharu et al. 2004). Cerebral blood flow changes during the pain state were observed in the dorsal rostral pons, anterior cingulate cortex (ACC) and cuneus, sites that are known to be active in migraine (Weiller et al. 1995; Bahra et al. 2001). The activation in the dorsal rostral pons is highly suggestive of a role for this structure in the pathophysiology of chronic migraine. In the paresthesia state during neurostimulation, ACC and left pulvinar activation were observed indicating that ONS can modulate activity in the thalamus. Indeed, the pulvinar has been suggested to be involved in pain modulation as neurosurgical pulvinotomy has been performed in relieving intractable pain (Mayanagi and Bouchard 1976; Choi and Umbach 1977).

Deep Brain Stimulation in Chronic Cluster Headache

Cluster headache (CH) is a rare form of primary neurovascular headache, characterized by the sudden onset of excruciating unilateral periorbital pain. The pain is often accompanied by local signs of facial autonomic dysfunction such as lacrimation, rhinorrhea, sweating and flushing. Attacks last up to 3 h and occur in clusters of a few months with multiple attacks per day, often followed by periods of remission. In its chronic form, significant remission intervals are lacking as attacks appear on a daily base.

Neuroimaging studies have revealed structural and functional abnormalities in the posterior hypothalamic area in cluster headache patients suggesting dysfunctional hypothalamic activity being the pathophysiological correlate of CH attacks (Cohen and Goadsby 2006).

Thus, the posterior hypothalamic area has been chosen first by Leone et al. as a target for stereotactic neurostimulation leading to an effect on the severity and frequency of attacks in chronic cluster patients. Although this has been an effective strategy, it is not without risks and side effects (Schoenen et al. 2005).

Long-Term Outcome of Hypothalamic Deep Brain Stimulation (DBS)

To date, the outcome data from over 50 patients from 12 centers have been published (Bartsch et al. 2009).

These patients were selected after the published criteria for DBS surgery in cluster patients and were operated on the basis of the published stereotactic coordinates (Franzini et al. 2003; Leone et al. 2004). Patients showed multiple daily attacks that did not respond to drug treatment or where the side effects of the medication were unacceptable. The synopsis shows that from a total of 55 patients, 36 showed a beneficial effect of the hypothalamic deep brain stimulation. The follow-up range was between 1 and 6 years. The range of the effect, however, was quite different interindividually (Fontaine et al. 2010b; Starr et al. 2007).

Starr et al. (2007) reported an improvement after 1 year in two out of four patients after DBS, thus confirming the response rate in the literature of about 50%.

However, there are possible complications with this procedure as Schoenen et al. reported one fatal intracerebral hemorrhage among a series of six patients due to a hemorrhage along the electrode pathway. In another patient the intraoperative procedure had to be aborted due to a panic attack with autonomic disturbances (Schoenen et al. 2005). Another patient had an intraoperative TIA with a hemiplegia for 5 min (Starr et al. 2007). As all deep brain implantation procedures show a minor risk of intracerebral hemorrhage this procedure should be performed only in experienced DBS centers. Furthermore, due to anatomical considerations, the exact location of the effective target point of the deep brain stimulation in the posterior hypothalamic region either belonging to the hypothalamus or the periventricular gray matter region is a matter of discussion (Starr et al. 2007; Starr 2008). Usually, hypothalamic stimulation is well tolerated and side effects are rare. The most frequent side effects are vertigo and double vision. The effect of hypothalamic deep brain stimulation on cardiovascular parameters was studied in patients before and after surgery. It could be shown that baselines values were similar in both conditions. During the tilt test operated patients did show signs of an increased sympathoexcitatory tone (Cortelli et al. 2007). In two patients also the effects of hypothalamic DBS on sleep was evaluated showing an improved sleep structure and quality. More importantly, it was shown that the circadian rhythm was not altered during hypothalamic DBS (Vetrugno et al. 2007).

Hypothalamic DBS using the same coordinates has also been shown to be effective in another type of trigeminal autonomic cephalalgia classified as drug-resistant SUNCT (short-lasting unilateral neuralgiform headache attacks with conjunctival injection and tearing), since in this disorder an activation of the posterior inferior hypothalamus was also observed (Matharu et al. 2002; Leone et al. 2005; Lyons et al. 2008).

Deep Brain Stimulation: Current Research

It is well established that the nociceptive input from peripheral structures to the central nervous system is subject to a modulation from various levels of the central nervous system. Most importantly, inhibitory projections from brainstem structures, such as the periaqueductal gray (PAG), nucleus raphe magnus (NRM) and the rostroventral medulla (RVM), have a profound anti-nociceptive effect (Behbehani 1995), but other structures such as the hypothalamus including the posterior hypothalamus, thalamus and cortical regions seem also to be involved (Fontaine et al. 2010a).

The effect of hypothalamic neurostimulation is probably relayed via descending anti-nociceptive projections from the posterior hypothalamic area onto second-order neurons in the caudal trigeminal nucleus (Bartsch et al. 2004b; Bartsch et al. 2005). However, this stimulation-induced hypothalamic inhibition of nociceptive trigeminal neurons might involve further relay centers including the PAG (Veazey et al. 1982; Holstege 1987; Bartsch et al. 2004a). Additionally, investigations of cluster DBS patients studied with PET as well as the clinical observation that acute stimulation is not effective in aborting attacks suggest that the effect of DBS involves further neuroplastic mechanisms modulating hypothalamic and midbrain neuronal circuits (Fontaine et al. 2010a; Leone et al. 2006; May et al. 2006).

References

Bahra A, Matharu MS et al (2001) Brainstem activation specific to migraine headache. Lancet 357(9261): 1016–1017

Bartsch T, Knight YE et al (2004a) Activation of 5-HT1B/1D receptors in the periaqueductal grey inhibits meningeal nociception. Ann Neurol 56(3):371–381

Bartsch T, Levy MJ et al (2004b) Differential modulation of dural nociception to Orexin A and B receptor activation in the posterior hypothalamic area. Pain 109:367–378

Bartsch T, Levy MJ et al (2005) Inhibition of nociceptive dural input in the trigeminal nucleus caudalis by somatostatin receptor blockade in the posterior hypothalamus. Pain 117(1–2):30–39

Bartsch T, Paemeleire K et al (2009) Neurostimulation approaches to primary headache disorders. Curr Opin Neurol 22(3):262–268

Behbehani MM (1995) Functional characteristics of the midbrain periaqueductal gray. Prog Neurobiol 46(6):575–605

Burns B, Watkins L et al (2008) Treatment of hemicrania continua by occipital nerve stimulation with a bion device: long-term follow-up of a crossover study. Lancet Neurol 7(11):1001–1012

Burns B, Watkins L et al (2009) Treatment of intractable chronic cluster headache by occipital nerve stimulation in 14 patients. Neurology 72(4):341–345

Choi CR, Umbach W (1977) Combined stereotaxic surgery for relief of intractable pain. Neurochirurgia (Stuttg) 20(3):84–87

Chung JM, Lee KH et al (1984) Factors influencing peripheral nerve stimulation produced inhibition of primate spinothalamic tract cells. Pain 19(3):277–293

Cohen AS, Goadsby PJ (2006) Functional neuroimaging of primary headache disorders. Expert Rev Neurother 6(8):1159–1171

Cortelli P, Guaraldi P et al (2007) Effect of deep brain stimulation of the posterior hypothalamic area on the cardiovascular system in chronic cluster headache patients. Eur J Neurol 14(9):1008–1015

Doubell T, Mannion RJ, Woolf CJ (1999) The doral horn: state dependent sensory processing, plasticity and the generation of pain. In: Melzack PDWR (ed) Textbook of pain, vol 59, 4th edn. Churchill Livingstone, Edinburgh, pp 165–180

Duggan AW, Foong FW (1985) Bicuculline and spinal inhibition produced by dorsal column stimulation in the cat. Pain 22(3):249–259

Fontaine D, Lanteri-Minet M et al (2010a) Anatomical location of effective deep brain stimulation electrodes in chronic cluster headache. Brain 133(4):1214–1223

Fontaine D, Lazorthes Y et al (2010b) Safety and efficacy of deep brain stimulation in refractory cluster headache: a randomized placebo-controlled double-blind trial followed by a 1-year open extension. J Headache Pain 11(1):23–31

Franzini A, Ferroli P et al (2003) Stimulation of the posterior hypothalamus for treatment of chronic intractable cluster headaches: first reported series. Neurosurgery 52(5):1095–1099, discussion 1099–1101

Garrison D, Foreman R (1994) Decreased activity of spontaneous and noxiously evoked dorsal horn cells during transcutaneous electrical nerve stimulation (TENS). Pain 58(3):309–315

Garrison DW, Foreman RD (1996) Effects of transcutaneous electrical nerve stimulation (TENS) on spontaneous and noxiously evoked dorsal horn cell activity in cats with transected spinal cords. Neurosci Lett 216(2):125–128

Gildenberg PL, Murthy KS (1980) Influence of dorsal column stimulation upon human thalamic somatosensory-evoked potentials. Appl Neurophysiol 43(1–2):8–17

Goadsby PJ (2007) Neurostimulation in primary headache syndromes. Expert Rev Neurother 7(12):1785–1789

Goadsby PJ, Schoenen J et al (2006) Towards a definition of intractable headache for use in clinical practice and trials. Cephalalgia 26(9):1168–1170

Goadsby PJ, Bartsch T et al (2008a) Occipital nerve stimulation for headache: mechanisms and efficacy. Headache 48(2):313–318

Goadsby PJ, Cittadini E et al (2008b) Trigeminal autonomic cephalalgias: diagnostic and therapeutic developments. Curr Opin Neurol 21(3):323–330

Goadsby PJ, Dodick DW, Saper JR, Silberstein SD (2009) Occipital nerve stimulation (ONS) for the treatment of intractable chronic migraine (ONSTIM). Cephalalgia 29:133

Headache Classification Committee of The International Headache Society (2004) The International Classification of Headache Disorders (second edition). Cephalalgia 24(Suppl 1):1–160

Holstege G (1987) Some anatomical observations on the projections from the hypothalamus to brainstem and spinal cord: an HRP and autoradiographic tracing study in the cat. J Comp Neurol 260(1):98–126

Ignelzi RJ, Nyquist JK (1979) Excitability changes in peripheral nerve fibers after repetitive electrical stimulation. Implications in pain modulation. J Neurosurg 51(6):824–833

Jarrar RG, Black DF et al (2003) Outcome of trigeminal nerve section in the treatment of chronic cluster headache. Neurology 60(8):1360–1362

Knight YE, Bartsch T et al (2003) Trigeminal antinociception induced by bicuculline in the periaqueductal gray (PAG) is not affected by PAG

P/Q-type calcium channel blockade in rat. Neurosci Lett 336(2):113–116

Kolmodin GM, Skoglund CR (1960) Analysis of spinal interneurons activated by tactile and nociceptive stimulation. Acta Physiol Scand 50:337–355

Leone M, May A et al (2004) Deep brain stimulation for intractable chronic cluster headache: proposals for patient selection. Cephalalgia 24(11):934–937

Leone M, Franzini A et al (2005) Deep brain stimulation to relieve drug-resistant SUNCT. Ann Neurol 57(6):924–927

Leone M, Franzini A et al (2006) Acute hypothalamic stimulation and ongoing cluster headache attacks. Neurology 67(10):1844–1845

Lindblom U, Tapper DN et al (1977) The effect of dorsal column stimulation on the nociceptive response of dorsal horn cells and its relevance for pain suppression. Pain 4(2):133–144

Linderoth B, Foreman RD (1999) Physiology of spinal cord stimulation: review and update. Neuromodulation 2(3):150–164

Linderoth B, Foreman RD (2006) Mechanisms of spinal cord stimulation in painful syndromes: role of animal models. Pain Med 7(S1):S14–S26

Lyons MK, Dodick DW et al (2008) Responsiveness of short-lasting unilateral neuralgiform headache with conjunctival injection and tearing to hypothalamic deep brain stimulation. J Neurosurg 110:279–281

Magis D, Allena M et al (2007) Occipital nerve stimulation for drug-resistant chronic cluster headache: a prospective pilot study. Lancet Neurol 6(4):314–321

Matharu MS, Boes CJ et al (2002) SUNCT syndrome: prolonged attacks, refractoriness and response to topiramate. Neurology 58(8):1307

Matharu M, Bartsch T et al (2004) Central neuromodulation in chronic migraine patients with suboccipital stimulators: A PET study. Brain 127(1):220–230

May A, Leone M et al (2006) Hypothalamic deep brain stimulation in positron emission tomography. J Neurosci 26(13):3589–3593

Mayanagi Y, Bouchard G (1976) Evaluation of stereotactic thalamotomies for pain relief with reference to pulvinar intervention. Appl Neurophysiol 39(3–4): 154–157

Oh MY, Ortega J, Bradley Bellotte J, Whiting DM, Aló K (2004) Peripheral nerve stimulation for the treatment of occipital neuralgia and transformed migraine using a C1-2-3 subcutaneous paddle style electrode: a technical report. Neuromodulation 7(2):103–112

Olausson B, Xu ZQ et al (1994) Dorsal column inhibition of nociceptive thalamic cells mediated by gamma-aminobutyric acid mechanisms in the cat. Acta Physiol Scand 152(3):239–247

Paemeleire K, Van Buyten JP, Van Buynder M, Alicino D, Van Maele G, Smet I, Goadsby PJ (2008) Phenotype of patients responsive to sub-occipital neurostimulation for refractory head pain. Eur J Neurol 15(suppl 3):10

Schoenen J, Di Clemente L et al (2005) Hypothalamic stimulation in chronic cluster headache: a pilot study of efficacy and mode of action. Brain 128(Pt 4): 940–947

Schwedt TJ, Dodick DW et al (2007a) Occipital nerve stimulation for chronic headache–long-term safety and efficacy. Cephalalgia 27(2):153–157

Schwedt TJ, Dodick DW et al (2007b) Response to occipital nerve block is not useful in predicting efficacy of occipital nerve stimulation. Cephalalgia 27(3):271–274

Starr PA (2008) Commentary on Leone M et al., Lessons from 8 years' experience of hypothalamic stimulation in cluster headache. Cephalalgia 28(7):798

Starr PA, Barbaro NM et al (2007) Chronic stimulation of the posterior hypothalamic region for cluster headache: technique and 1-year results in four patients. J Neurosurg 106(6):999–1005

Stiller CO, Linderoth B et al (1995) Repeated spinal cord stimulation decreases the extracellular level of gamma-aminobutyric acid in the periaqueductal gray matter of freely moving rats. Brain Res 699(2):231–241

Stiller CO, Cui JG et al (1996) Release of gamma-aminobutyric acid in the dorsal horn and suppression of tactile allodynia by spinal cord stimulation in mononeuropathic rats. Neurosurgery 39(2):367–374, discussion 374–375

Trentman TL, Zimmerman RS (2008) Occipital nerve stimulation: technical and surgical aspects of implantation. Headache 48(2):319–327

Veazey RB, Amaral DG et al (1982) The morphology and connections of the posterior hypothalamus in the cynomolgus monkey (Macaca fascicularis). II. Efferent connections. J Comp Neurol 207(2):135–156

Vetrugno R, Pierangeli G et al (2007) Effect on sleep of posterior hypothalamus stimulation in cluster headache. Headache 47(7):1085–1090

Wall PD (1978) The gate control theory of pain mechanisms. A re-examination and re-statement. Brain 101(1):1–18

Weiller C, May A et al (1995) Brain stem activation in spontaneous human migraine attacks. Nat Med 1(7):658–660

Weiner R, Reed K (1999) Peripheral neurostimulation for control of intractable occipital neuralgia. Neuromodulation 2:217–221

Woolf CJ (1979) Transcutaneous electrical nerve stimulation and the reaction to experimental pain in human subjects. Pain 7(2):115–127

Woolf C, Thompson J (1994) Stimulation-induced analgesia: Transcutaneous electrical nerve stimulation (TENS) and vibration. In: Wall P, Melzack R (eds) Textbook of pain. Churchill Livingstone, New York, pp 1191–2008

35 What to Tell Patients About Headache Occurring on More Days Than Not

Timothy J. Steiner[1,2] · *Paolo Martelletti*[3]

[1]Norwegian University of Science and Technology, Trondheim, Norway
[2]Faculty of Medicine, Imperial College London, London, UK
[3]School of Health Sciences, Sapienza University of Rome, Rome, Italy

Parts of this contribution have also been published as part of a Springer Open Choice article which is freely available at springerlink.com – DOI 10.1007/s10194-007-0428-1

Paolo Martelletti, Timothy J. Steiner (eds.), *Handbook of Headache*, DOI 10.1007/978-88-470-1700-9_35,
© Lifting The Burden 2011

Abstract: Headache disorders are real – they are not just in the mind.

This chapter summarizes information suitable for communication to patients with headache occurring on more days than not – often referred to for convenience as "chronic daily headache". It describes types, symptoms, and treatment strategies. The information is aimed at helping patients to understand their headache, their diagnosis, and their treatment, and to work with their health-care provider in a way that will get best results for them.

Introduction

Chronic daily headache is not a diagnosis. It is a convenient description given to headache that happens on 15 or more days every month (that is, on more days than not) for more than 3 months.

What Are the Different Types of Chronic Daily Headache?

There are several different types of chronic daily headache, and they are generally defined by their causes. *Chronic tension-type headache* and *medication-overuse headache* are the most common. Medication-overuse headache (see below) can develop from migraine or tension-type headache.

Who Gets Chronic Daily Headache?

It is surprisingly common. About one in 20 people develops this problem at some time in their lives. It is more common in women than men, and it also happens in children.

What Are the Symptoms of Chronic Daily Headache?

The main feature is very frequent headache. This varies, but is often a dull pain. Other common symptoms, alongside headache, are feeling tired, feeling sick, being irritable, and difficulty sleeping. Sometimes headache seems relentless, although it may change as you go through the day. Medication-overuse headache is often at its worst on waking in the morning.

Will My Chronic Daily Headache Get Better?

How chronic daily headache is treated depends on the diagnosis and the cause. Getting the right treatment is very important, so medical care is usually necessary.

All types of chronic daily headache may be temporarily relieved by painkillers or anti-migraine treatments, but in many cases this relief is only partial and the effect diminishes over time. These treatments are not appropriate because they will make the condition worse.

If your headache is already being caused by overusing medication of this sort, then it is likely to improve once you stop taking the medication, and not otherwise.

Do I Need Any Tests?

Whatever the type of chronic daily headache, there are no tests to confirm the diagnosis. This is based on your description of your headaches and the lack of any abnormal findings when you are examined. Therefore, it is very important that you carefully describe your symptoms and how they developed. It is also very important that you say how many painkillers or other medications you are taking for your headaches, and how often you are taking them.

Your doctor should be able to tell quite easily whether you have an illness more serious than chronic daily headache. If he or she is not sure about the diagnosis or there is any sudden change in your headache, tests including a brain scan may be carried out to rule out other causes of your headache. However, these are not often needed. If your doctor does not ask for a brain scan, it means that it will not help to give you the best treatment.

What Is Medication-Overuse Headache?

Any medication you use to treat the symptoms of headache, when taken too often for too long, can cause medication-overuse headache. Aspirin, paracetamol, ibuprofen, and codeine – in fact, all painkillers, even those bought over the counter – are associated with this problem. And it is not just painkillers. Drugs that specifically treat migraine headache also lead to this problem when used too often. These include triptans and, most of all, ergotamine.

A similar headache (although not strictly medication-overuse headache) can result from taking too much caffeine. The usual source of this is coffee, tea, or cola drinks, but it can come from caffeine tablets or from caffeine included in many painkillers.

The exact way medication-overuse headache develops is not known, and may be different according to the nature of the medication. Triptans and ergotamine may cause a rebound effect, with headache returning after they wear off. Painkillers are believed to cause, over time, a change in pain-signaling systems in the brain. This means people become used to the effects of the medication so that they need more and more of it.

For most people with occasional headaches, painkillers are a safe and effective treatment. However, medication-overuse headache may develop in anyone taking headache treatments regularly on more than 3 days a week. Usually, the person with medication-overuse headache begins with occasional attacks of tension-type headache or (more commonly) migraine. For varying reasons, the headaches begin to happen more often. This may be through natural variation or because an extra headache has developed, perhaps due to stress or muscular pain. The increase in headache leads to use of more medication to try to control the symptoms, eventually until both happen every day.

Many people in this situation know that they are taking more medication than is wise, and try to reduce the amount. This leads them to have a withdrawal syndrome of worsening headache, for which they take more medication. It is easy to see how this results in a vicious circle, which can be difficult to break. It makes not so much difference how *much* you take – if you regularly use the full dose of painkillers on 1 or 2 days a week only, you are unlikely to develop medication-overuse headache. However, take just a couple of painkillers on most days and you may well be making your headaches worse. It is *frequent* use over a period of time that causes the problem.

What Can I Do to Help Myself?

The *only* way of treating this condition is to stop the overused medication (*withdrawal*). Clinical studies show that most people who withdraw from overused medication improve greatly. However, it can take up to 3 months before you see the full benefit. Even if headaches continue after that time, despite stopping the medication, their cause usually becomes clear and they will respond better to correctly prescribed specific treatment.

You can withdraw either by stopping in one go or by gradually reducing the amount taken over 2–3 weeks. Whichever way you choose, drink plenty of fluids while doing this (but avoid taking more caffeine). If you stop in one go, you will almost certainly have withdrawal symptoms – worsening headache, feeling sick, perhaps being sick, anxiety, and difficulty sleeping. These symptoms will appear within 48 h and may last, at worst, for up to 2 weeks. However, people who try to stop slowly seem more likely to fail, perhaps because it takes so much longer.

It makes sense to choose when to withdraw, and not begin shortly before an important event. Do warn your work colleagues that you may be unable to come into work for a few days.

What if I Just Carry on as I Am?

If medication overuse is causing your frequent headaches, carrying on as you are is not an option. You will continue to have ever-more frequent headaches, which will not respond to painkillers or to preventative medicine. Eventually you may do yourself other harm as well, such as damage to your liver and kidneys.

Are There Other Treatments I Can Take?

There are medications, which a doctor can prescribe, that you can take every day to help you withdraw. They work only if you stop all other headache medication, and even then it is uncertain how much they help. You will also have to stop these at some point, and, for most people, it is better to do without them.

How Can I Make Sure It Does Not Happen Again?

As it develops, medication-overuse headache largely replaces the original headache (migraine or tension-type headache) for which you took the medication in the first place. This means that, as your medication-overuse headache improves after withdrawal, you can expect your original type of headache to return.

If you need to, you can cautiously restart using medication for this headache once the pattern of headache has returned to normal. This is likely to be after at least several weeks.

Be careful, because there is a risk of following the same path as before. To prevent this, avoid treating headaches on more than 3 days in a row or on a regular basis on 3 or more days in a week. Always read the leaflet and packaging that come with any medicine.

If a headache does not get better or keeps returning, never continue taking medication without consulting your doctor or nurse.

Keep a Diary

You can use diary cards to record a lot of relevant information about your headaches – how often you get them, when they happen, how long they last, and what your symptoms are. They are valuable in helping with diagnosis and in assessing how well treatments work.

For people at risk of medication-overuse headache, diaries are especially important as they help keep track of just how much medication you are taking.

Acknowledgment

The text of this chapter is taken from a leaflet prepared by *Lifting The Burden: the Global Campaign Against Headache*. It was drafted by a small writing group, revised following review by an international panel whose principal responsibility was to ensure worldwide cross-cultural relevance and, finally, checked for ease of comprehension by the Campaign for Plain English. The leaflet is endorsed by the World Health Organization and has been published in *Journal of Headache and Pain* (2007).

Reference

Lifting The Burden. The Global Campaign to Reduce the Burden of Headache Worldwide (2007) Information for people affected by chronic daily headache. J Headache Pain 8(Suppl 1):S34–S36

Part 10

Common or Important Secondary Headaches and Facial Pains

36 Post-Traumatic Headache

Todd J. Schwedt[1] · *Maria Gabriella Buzzi*[2]
[1]Washington University in St. Louis School of Medicine, St. Louis, MO, USA
[2]IRCCS Fondazione Santa Lucia, Rome, Italy

Paolo Martelletti, Timothy J. Steiner (eds.), *Handbook of Headache*, DOI 10.1007/978-88-470-1700-9_36,
© Lifting The Burden 2011

Abstract: Post-traumatic headaches are those that are induced by trauma to the head and/or neck. Post-traumatic headaches are one of the most common secondary headache disorders. Diagnosis is based upon the temporal relationship of headache onset with trauma and exclusion of other potential headache causes. Post-traumatic headaches follow variable courses, with the majority resolving within the first 3 months (acute form) and some persisting beyond the initial 3 months (chronic form). Treatment often requires a multimodal approach, combining medications, cognitive-behavioral therapy, and physical therapies, all while ensuring avoidance of acute headache medication overuse.

Established Knowledge

Description

Post-traumatic headaches are headaches that are caused by injury of the head and/or neck. The current classification system (*International Classification of Headache Disorders II*, ICHD-II) includes post-traumatic headaches secondary to head injury and post-traumatic headaches due to whiplash (Headache Classification Subcommittee of the International Headache Society 2004). Headaches must begin within 7 days of head injury or whiplash or be present upon regaining consciousness after trauma. Post-traumatic headaches are considered "acute" if they resolve within 3 months of the injury and "chronic" if they persist after 3 months.

Post-traumatic headaches due to head injury are divided into those caused by mild head injury and those caused by moderate to severe head injury. Head injuries are classified as mild when there is no associated loss of consciousness or loss of consciousness lasting less than 30 min, a Glasgow Coma Scale (GCS) of at least 13 (see ❷ *Table 36.1*), and symptoms and/or signs of concussion. Head injuries are considered moderate or severe when there is loss of consciousness for greater than 30 min, GCS less than 13, post-traumatic amnesia lasting greater than 48 h, and/or imaging demonstration of traumatic brain injury. Imaging evidence for traumatic brain injury could include intracranial hemorrhage, brain contusion, and skull fracture.

Whiplash is an injury due to sudden acceleration and/or deceleration resulting in neck hyperextension followed by flexion. Whiplash most commonly occurs during a motor vehicle accident when the vehicle is hit from the front or from behind (Packard 1999;

❒ Table 36.1
Glasgow Coma Scale (range of total points is 3 [worst] to 15 [normal])

Points	Best eye opening	Best verbal	Best motor
6	NA	NA	Obeys
5	NA	Oriented	Localizes pain
4	Spontaneous	Confused	Withdraws to pain
3	To speech	Inappropriate	Flexion (decorticate)
2	To pain	Incomprehensible	Extensor (decerebrate)
1	None	None	None

Richter et al. 2000). There must be pain in the neck at the time of the trauma in order for headaches to be attributed to whiplash injury.

The pathogenesis of post-traumatic headaches is unclear, especially when there is no objective evidence for anatomic traumatic injuries. Post-traumatic headaches may be due to axonal injuries, alterations in cerebral metabolism and hemodynamics, psychopathology, and patient expectations of post-traumatic pain (Solomon 2009). Likely, post-traumatic headaches are explainable by a combination of these factors, perhaps superimposed upon an underlying genetic predisposition for headache.

Epidemiology

Head and neck injuries are common. According to the United States Center for Disease Control and Prevention, 1.4 million Americans suffer a traumatic brain injury each year [http://www.cdc.gov/ncipc/tbi/]. Leading causes of these injuries include falls (28%), motor vehicle–traffic crashes (20%), struck by/against events such as colliding with a moving or stationary object (19%), and assaults (11%) [http://www.cdc.gov/ncipc/tbi/Causes.htm]. Traumatic brain injury from falls are most common in the very young (aged 0–4 years) and elderly (75 years of age and older). Traumatic brain injury from motor vehicle accidents is most common in the 15–19-year-old age bracket. Men are about 1.5 times more likely than women to sustain a traumatic brain injury. Mild traumatic brain injuries are more common than moderate and severe traumatic brain injuries, accounting for greater than 75% of all brain injuries (Lee et al. 1992; Thornhill et al. 2000).

Whiplash has become more frequent in recent years due to the increased use of seatbelts and airbags (Richter et al. 2000). About one million cases of whiplash are thought to occur annually in the United States. (O'Neill et al. 1972). Approximately 30% of motor vehicle drivers wearing a seatbelt who have injuries from a motor vehicle accident have whiplash (Richter et al. 2000). Women are more likely than men to develop whiplash following a motor vehicle accident. Whiplash can result from multiple different types of motor vehicle accidents, although they most commonly occur after rear-end and front-end collisions (Richter et al. 2000). Whiplash injury may occur after minor accidents (low-speed at the time of impact) as well as after high-speed collisions (Richter et al. 2000).

Headaches secondary to head and/or neck trauma are amongst the most common types of secondary headaches and post-traumatic headache is the most common symptom after minor head injury (Packard 1999). The exact prevalence of these headaches is difficult to ascertain as a substantial proportion probably go unreported, especially those attributed to mild head injuries and/or whiplash injuries. A meta-analysis which included 12 studies and 1,670 traumatic brain injury patients found that 57.8% (95% confidence interval 55.5–60.2%) of patients suffered from chronic headaches after traumatic brain injury (Nampiaparampil 2008). This included patients with worsening of preexisting headache syndromes and those with new onset of headaches following traumatic brain injury. A Norwegian population study of chronic daily headache found the 1-year prevalence of secondary chronic headaches to be 2.14%, including a 1-year prevalence of 0.38% for post-traumatic headaches (Aaseth et al. 2008). This included a 1-year prevalence of chronic post-traumatic headache attributed to moderate or severe head injury of 0.04%, 0.17% prevalence of chronic post-traumatic headache attributed to mild head injury, and 0.17% 1-year prevalence of chronic headache attributed to whiplash injury (Aaseth et al. 2008).

Possible risk factors for development of post-traumatic headaches include presence of pre-injury headaches and less severe trauma (Obelieniene et al. 1999; Stovner et al. 2009). Some studies have found post-traumatic headaches to be more common after mild head injury than following severe head injury (Yamaguchi 1992). Yamaguchi found that severe post-traumatic headache occurred after mild head injury in 72% and in only 33% after severe injury (Yamaguchi 1992). Brain computed tomography abnormalities and mental impairment were negatively associated with presence of post-traumatic headache. However, some other studies have not found an inverse relationship between severity of traumatic brain injury and post-traumatic headache (Walker et al. 2005). Additional factors that may be associated with a higher likelihood of post-traumatic headache include female sex and presence of comorbid psychiatric disorders such as post-traumatic stress disorder, depression, and anxiety (Obelieniene et al. 1999).

Diagnosis

The diagnosis of post-traumatic headache is based upon operational diagnostic criteria and exclusion of other potential causes of the headache. It is essential to first exclude structural traumatic injuries that may need direct treatment in order to avoid further complications and to optimize headache treatment. Examples of such injuries include intracranial hemorrhage, hydrocephalus, skeletal fractures (skull, cervical spine), cervical artery dissection, and cerebrospinal fluid leaks. Thus, patients with post-traumatic headaches require brain and cervical spine imaging. Depending upon the specific clinical scenario, additional diagnostic tests may be indicated, including, but not limited to, evaluation of the cerebrovasculature. The vast majority of patients with post-traumatic headaches have no objective evidence for an anatomic abnormality relating to the pain. In addition to imaging, formal neurocognitive testing may be useful in the evaluation and monitoring of patients with complaints of post-traumatic cognitive dysfunction.

The ICHD-II diagnostic criteria for post-traumatic headaches are included in ❷ *Box 36.1*. Of note, there is ongoing debate about the utility of these current criteria and revisions are currently being conducted. Criticisms of these criteria include the necessity for headaches to begin within 7 days of injury, the arbitrary designation of 3 months as the tipping point differentiating "acute" from "chronic" post-traumatic headache, and the lack of specific headache characteristics required for the diagnosis. In addition, current criteria do not adequately differentiate worsening of preexisting headache patterns following trauma from onset of a new headache syndrome.

There are no specific headache characteristics that help differentiate a post-traumatic headache from other headache types. Most often, post-traumatic headaches resemble chronic or episodic tension-type headache, but may less frequently resemble chronic or episodic migraine, cervicogenic headache or occipital neuralgia. A systematic review of the literature found that 33.6% of patients with post-traumatic headache had headaches meeting criteria for tension-type headache, while 28.6% had headaches meeting diagnostic criteria for migraine (Lew et al. 2006). Infrequently, post-traumatic headaches resemble other headache disorders such as cluster headache and hemicrania continua.

Post-traumatic headaches may be part of a post-traumatic syndrome, a syndrome consisting of a constellation of symptoms and signs following traumatic brain injury. The most common symptoms of the post-traumatic syndrome include headache, dizziness, fatigue, reduced ability to concentrate, psychomotor slowing, mild memory problems, insomnia, anxiety, personality changes, and irritability (Evans 2004; Yang et al. 2009). Other symptoms include tinnitus, visual changes, photophobia, phonophobia, and decreased libido. Pscyhopathology, such as depression and anxiety, is common in patients with post-traumatic headaches and post-traumatic syndrome. Independent of pain severity, post-traumatic headache is associated with more psychopathology than migraine and tension-type headache (Ham et al. 1994). Furthermore, those with post-traumatic headaches are more likely to have depression and anxiety than patients with trauma without headaches (Tatrow et al. 2003a). The effects that post-traumatic symptoms have on occupational and social functioning may contribute to the development of or worsening of anxiety and depression (Packard 1999).

Box 36.1 International Classification of Headache Disorders Diagnostic Criteria for Post-Traumatic Headaches

Acute Post-Traumatic Headache Attributed to Moderate or Severe Head Injury

A. Headache, no typical characteristics known, fulfilling criteria C and D
B. Head trauma with ≥1 of the following:
    1. Loss of consciousness >30 min
    2. Glasgow Coma Scale (GCS) <13
    3. Post-traumatic amnesia for >48 h
    4. Imaging demonstration of a traumatic brain lesion
C. Headache develops within 7 days after head trauma or after regaining consciousness following head trauma
D. One or other of the following:
    1. Headache resolves within 3 months after head trauma
    2. Headache persists but 3 months have not yet passed since head trauma

Chronic Post-Traumatic Headache Attributed to Moderate or Severe Head Injury
Criteria A–C are the same as those above for "acute post-traumatic headache attributed to moderate or severe head injury"

Criterion D is different:

D. Headache persists for >3 months after head trauma

Acute Post-Traumatic Headache Attributed to Mild Head Injury

A. Headache, no typical characteristics known, fulfilling criteria C and D
B. Head trauma with all of the following:
    1. Either no loss of consciousness, or loss of consciousness of <30 min duration
    2. Glasgow Coma Scale (GCS) ≥13
    3. Symptoms and/or signs diagnostic of concussion
C. Headache develops within 7 days after head trauma
D. One or other of the following:
    1. Headache resolves within 3 months after head trauma
    2. Headache persists, but 3 months have not yet passed since head trauma

Chronic Post-Traumatic Headache Attributed to Mild Head Injury
Criteria A–C are the same as those above for "acute post-traumatic headache attributed to mild head injury"

· Criterion D is different:

D. Headache persists for >3 months after head trauma

Acute Headache Attributed to Whiplash Injury

A. Headache, no typical characteristics known, fulfilling criteria C and D
B. History of whiplash (sudden and significant acceleration/deceleration movement of the neck) associated at the time with neck pain
C. Headache develops within 7 days after whiplash injury
D. One or other of the following:
   1. Headache resolves within 3 months after whiplash injury
   2. Headache persists, but 3 months have not yet passed since whiplash injury

Chronic Headache Attributed to Whiplash Injury
Criteria A–C are the same as those above for "acute headache attributed to whiplash injury"

Criterion D is different:

D. Headache persists for >3 months after whiplash injury

Management

There is a lack of evidence-based guidelines from which to make decisions when treating post-traumatic headaches. Data from prospective, controlled trials are needed. However, benefits from divalproex sodium, propranolol, and amitriptyline have been suggested (Weiss et al. 1991; Packard 2000). In addition, uncontrolled studies have suggested benefit from relaxation therapy and biofeedback (Ham and Packard 1996; Tatrow et al. 2003b). Combination therapy with medication, relaxation therapy, and biofeedback may provide optimal benefits for the treatment of post-traumatic headache (Medina 1992).

At the current time, post-traumatic headaches are treated according to the primary headache disorder which they most resemble. In other words, the post-traumatic headache that resembles migraine would be treated like a migraine and the post-traumatic headache that most closely resembles tension-type headache is treated as such. However, it is essential to identify and treat comorbid disorders, such as myofascial pain and tightness, disorders of the skeleton (such as the temporomandibular joint dysfunction), psychiatric disorders (such as depression, anxiety, post-traumatic stress disorder), and sleep abnormalities. Outcomes will only be maximized when all potential aspects of the post-traumatic syndrome are treated appropriately, when present. In addition to prophylactic and abortive medications, treatments may include physical, occupational, and cognitive-behavioral therapies.

Overuse of medications used to abort the post-traumatic headache may lead to medication overuse headaches (often referred to as "rebound headaches"), and overuse must thus be avoided. Acute headache medication overuse is defined arbitrarily and according to the specific medication being overused. However, in general, if abortive medications are being used more often than 2–3 days per week, the patient is at risk for developing medication overuse headaches. Medication overuse can lead to an increased frequency of headaches and a reduced response to prophylactic and abortive medications.

Prognosis

The majority of patients with headache following trauma to the head and/or neck have resolution of symptoms within the first 3 months, while up to 25% develop symptoms that endure for years (Yang et al. 2009). Identified predictors of persistent symptoms include the presence of intracranial lesions at 1 and 2 weeks after trauma, dizziness at 2 weeks post-injury, report of fatigue or poor vision at 2 weeks post-injury, presence of headache, dizziness or nausea in the emergency room directly following mild head injury, presence of depression and anxiety, and the duration of post-traumatic amnesia (King 1996; King et al. 1999; De Kruijk et al. 2002; Borgaro et al. 2003; Yang et al. 2009).

Discussions about post-traumatic headaches typically include debate over the potential role of patient expectations for postaccident pain and litigation on the occurrence and persistence of post-traumatic headaches. Although malingering may be the driving force in a minority of patients who report post-traumatic headaches, the majority of evidence suggests a very limited effect of litigation on symptoms. Patients with litigation are similar to those without litigation in regard to headache characteristics, response to treatment, cognitive test results, and improvement in symptoms over time (Leininger et al. 1990; Weiss et al. 1991; Evans 2004). Furthermore, symptom resolution is generally not seen following legal settlements (Packard 1992). However, expectation of pain following a motor vehicle accident may play a role in the development and persistence of post-traumatic symptoms. Studies performed in Lithuania, a country in which there is very little expectation or awareness of developing chronic pain following a whiplash injury and a lack of insurance coverage for personal injury, suggest that chronic neck pain and headaches occur in equal proportions in the traumatized subjects and controls at 1 year postaccident (Obelieniene et al. 1999). Shortly after a rear-end motor vehicle accident, 47% of subjects reported pain. Neck pain alone was present in 10%, 18% had neck pain and headache, and 19% had headache alone. However, postaccident pain was relatively short-lived. The median duration of neck pain was 3 days and the median duration of headache was 4.5 h. At 1 year following the accident, there were no differences between the subjects involved in a motor vehicle accident and controls in regard to the proportion with frequent neck pain (>7 days per month; 4.0% of accident victims; 6.2% of controls) and frequent headaches (>7 days per month; 4.0% of accident victims; 6.7% of controls).

Current Research

The ICHD-II does not distinguish moderate traumatic brain injuries from severe/very severe traumatic brain injuries. The classification of brain injury as mild as opposed to moderate to severe is based upon a GCS score of >13. Future versions of diagnostic criteria may consider further distinguishing between severe and very severe traumatic brain injury based upon a GCS <8 and coma duration (Formisano et al. 2004, 2005). In addition, the current distinction of post-traumatic headaches as acute or chronic based upon the 3-month parameter appears inadequate (Formisano et al. 2009). In very severe traumatic brain injury, coma duration is longer than 15 days, often enduring for up to months, and post-traumatic amnesia may double the coma duration itself. Furthermore, the use of concomitant medication, such as anticonvulsants for seizures, propranol for neurovegetative disorders, or indomethacin for prevention of heterotopic ossification, may affect pain perception after regaining consciousness (Formisano et al. 2009). Post-traumatic stress disorder develops days or weeks after stress and tends to improve or disappear within 3 months after exposure; interestingly, this spontaneous timing is similar to post-traumatic headache and headache may well be part of post-traumatic stress disorder and post-concussion syndrome (Yehuda and LeDoux 2007). Therefore, an accurate psychological profiling is needed in post-traumatic headache patients. Patients with more improvement in cognitive functioning after severe traumatic brain injury are at higher risk of having headache, anxiety, and depression, probably due to a greater awareness of residual post-traumatic deficits (Buzzi et al. 2003).

After mild traumatic brain injury, advanced neuroimaging techniques such as fast sequence MRI, diffusion weighted imaging, and diffusion tensor imaging show structural changes in regions including frontal and temporal lobes, thalamus, and corpus callosum (McAllister et al. 1999). Functional imaging techniques may further identify brain damage (secondary injury) after mild traumatic brain injury (Metting et al. 2007). Identification of diffuse axonal injury in these patients may help to prognosticate after mild traumatic brain injury and support the hypothesis that organic lesions, although non-detectable with routine diagnostic procedures, may underlay the pain and associated symptoms (Bazarian et al. 2007; Metting et al. 2007). Finally, peripheral and central sensitization may contribute to perpetuation of pain in chronic post-traumatic headaches (Carlton et al. 2009).

References

Aaseth K, Grande RB et al (2008) Prevalence of secondary chronic headaches in a population-based sample of 30-44-year-old persons. The Akershus study of chronic headache. Cephalalgia 28(7):705–713

Bazarian JJ, Zhong J et al (2007) Diffusion tensor imaging detects clinically important axonal damage after mild traumatic brain injury: a pilot study. J Neurotrauma 24(9):1447–1459

Borgaro SR, Prigatano GP et al (2003) Cognitive and affective sequelae in complicated and uncomplicated mild traumatic brain injury. Brain Inj 17(3):189–198

Buzzi MG, Bivona U, Matteis M, Spanedda F, Formisano R (2003) Cognitive and psychological patterns in post-traumatic headache following severe traumatic brain injury. Cephalalgia 23:672, P4L22

Carlton SM, Du J et al (2009) Peripheral and central sensitization in remote spinal cord regions contribute to central neuropathic pain after spinal cord injury. Pain 147(1–3):265–276

De Kruijk JR, Leffers P et al (2002) Prediction of post-traumatic complaints after mild traumatic brain injury: early symptoms and biochemical markers. J Neurol Neurosurg Psychiatry 73(6): 727–732

Evans RW (2004) Post-traumatic headaches. Neurol Clin 22(1):237–249, viii

Formisano R, Carlesimo GA et al (2004) Clinical predictors and neuropsychological outcome in severe traumatic brain injury patients. Acta Neurochir (Wien) 146(5):457–462

Formisano R, Bivona U et al (2005) Early clinical predictive factors during coma recovery. Acta Neurochir Suppl 93:201–205

Formisano R, Bivona U et al (2009) Post-traumatic headache: facts and doubts. J Headache Pain 10(3): 145–152

Ham LP, Andrasik F et al (1994) Psychopathology in individuals with post-traumatic headaches and other pain types. Cephalalgia 14(2):118–126, discussion 78

Ham LP, Packard RC (1996) A retrospective, follow-up study of biofeedback-assisted relaxation therapy in patients with posttraumatic headache. Biofeedback Self Regul 21(2):93–104

Headache Classification Subcommittee of the International Headache Society (2004) International classification of headache disorders II. Cephalalgia 24(suppl 1):1–151.

King NS (1996) Emotional, neuropsychological, and organic factors: their use in the prediction of persisting postconcussion symptoms after moderate and mild head injuries. J Neurol Neurosurg Psychiatry 61(1):75–81

King NS, Crawford S et al (1999) Early prediction of persisting post-concussion symptoms following mild and moderate head injuries. Br J Clin Psychol 38(Pt 1):15–25

Lee LS, Shih YH et al (1992) Epidemiologic study of head injuries in Taipei City, Taiwan. Zhonghua Yi Xue Za Zhi (Taipei) 50(3):219–225

Leininger BE, Gramling SE et al (1990) Neuropsychological deficits in symptomatic minor head injury patients after concussion and mild concussion. J Neurol Neurosurg Psychiatry 53(4):293–296

Lew HL, Lin PH et al (2006) Characteristics and treatment of headache after traumatic brain injury: a focused review. Am J Phys Med Rehabil 85(7):619–627

McAllister TW, Saykin AJ et al (1999) Brain activation during working memory 1 month after mild traumatic brain injury: a functional MRI study. Neurology 53(6):1300–1308

Medina JL (1992) Efficacy of an individualized outpatient program in the treatment of chronic post-traumatic headache. Headache 32(4):180–183

Metting Z, Rodiger LA et al (2007) Structural and functional neuroimaging in mild-to-moderate head injury. Lancet Neurol 6(8):699–710

Nampiaparampil DE (2008) Prevalence of chronic pain after traumatic brain injury: a systematic review. JAMA 300(6):711–719

Obelieniene D, Schrader H et al (1999) Pain after whiplash: a prospective controlled inception cohort study. J Neurol Neurosurg Psychiatry 66(3):279–283

O'Neill B, Haddon W Jr et al (1972) Automobile head restraints–frequency of neck injury claims in relation to the presence of head restraints. Am J Public Health 62(3):399–406

Packard RC (1992) Posttraumatic headache: permanency and relationship to legal settlement. Headache 32(10):496–500

Packard RC (1999) Epidemiology and pathogenesis of posttraumatic headache. J Head Trauma Rehabil 14(1):9–21

Packard RC (2000) Treatment of chronic daily posttraumatic headache with divalproex sodium. Headache 40(9):736–739

Richter M, Otte D et al (2000) Whiplash-type neck distortion in restrained car drivers: frequency, causes and long-term results. Eur Spine J 9(2):109–117

Solomon S (2009) Post-traumatic headache: commentary: an overview. Headache 49(7):1112–1115

Stovner LJ, Schrader H et al (2009) Headache after concussion. Eur J Neurol 16(1):112–120

Tatrow K, Blanchard EB et al (2003a) Posttraumatic headache: biopsychosocial comparisons with multiple control groups. Headache 43(7):755–766

Tatrow K, Blanchard EB et al (2003b) Posttraumatic headache: an exploratory treatment study. Appl Psychophysiol Biofeedback 28(4):267–278

Thornhill S, Teasdale GM et al (2000) Disability in young people and adults one year after head injury: prospective cohort study. BMJ 320(7250):1631–1635

Walker WC, Seel RT et al (2005) Headache after moderate and severe traumatic brain injury: a longitudinal analysis. Arch Phys Med Rehabil 86(9):1793–1800

Weiss HD, Stern BJ et al (1991) Post-traumatic migraine: chronic migraine precipitated by minor head or neck trauma. Headache 31(7):451–456

Yamaguchi M (1992) Incidence of headache and severity of head injury. Headache 32(9):427–431

Yang CC, Hua MS et al (2009) Early clinical characteristics of patients with persistent post-concussion symptoms: a prospective study. Brain Inj 23(4):299–306

Yehuda R, LeDoux J (2007) Response variation following trauma: a translational neuroscience approach to understanding PTSD. Neuron 56(1):19–32

37 Cervicogenic Headache

Hans A. van Suijlekom[1] · *Fabio Antonaci*[2]
[1]Catharina Ziekenhuis, Eindhoven, The Netherlands
[2]University Consortium for Adaptive Disorders and Head Pain
(UCADH) and Headache Science Centre, Pavia, Italy

Paolo Martelletti, Timothy J. Steiner (eds.), *Handbook of Headache*, DOI 10.1007/978-88-470-1700-9_37,
© Lifting The Burden 2011

37

Abstract: Cervicogenic headache is pain referred to the head from nociceptive structures in the cervical spine. The prevalence of cervicogenic headache varies from 0.7% to 13.8%. The pathophysiology of the headache involves convergence between cervical and trigeminal afferents in the trigeminocervical nucleus. Cervicogenic headache is, in principle, a unilateral headache without side shift but it may also be bilateral. The pain starts in the neck and spreads to the ipsilateral oculofrontotemporal area. A diffuse, ipsilateral neck, shoulder, or arm pain may occur. A reliable diagnosis of cervicogenic headache can be made based on the criteria of Sjaastad and coworkers. The use of diagnostic blocks to diagnose cervicogenic headache is essential. Treatment of cervicogenic headache depends on the established pain source and varies from manual therapy, simple local injections, radiofrequency treatment to more invasive neurosurgical procedures.

Introduction

The concept that headache might stem from the neck is not new. Early publications based on the concept that headache could originate from structures in the neck were those by Barré and Bärtschi-Rochaix in the first half of the century (Barré 1926; Bärtschi-Rochaix 1948). According to this concept, the crucial feature delineating cervicogenic headache from the other headache syndromes is that the pain originates from nociceptive structures in the cervical spine.

In 1983, Sjaastad et al. introduced cervicogenic headache (CEH) as a clinically defined headache syndrome after a profound study over several years in 22 patients with a rather uniform headache profile (Sjaastad et al. 1983). Since the first cases of CEH were identified, considerable progress has been made. Particularly in the last two decades, there have been advances in therapeutic approaches and in defining the clinical picture and diagnostic criteria. In 1990, Sjaastad et al., on behalf of the Cervicogenic Headache International Study Group (CHISG), published the first criteria for CEH (Sjaastad et al. 1990). In 1998, refinements of the criteria for CEH were published (❷ *Table 37.1*) (Sjaastad et al. 1998).

CEH is a syndrome, not a disease or an entity *sui generis*. It constitutes a "final common pathway" for pain stemming from several neck disorders. These may involve such structures as nerves, nerve root ganglia, uncovertebral joints, intervertebral disks, facet joints, ligaments, muscles, and so on. CEH comprises all headaches stemming from the neck.

Epidemiology

The prevalence of CEH, according to Nilsson's questionnaire study, among the Danish population using the IHS criteria was 2.5% (Nilsson 1995). Monteiro, using the criteria from Sjaastad et al., showed in a population study a prevalence for CEH of 1% when six of a total of six criteria were employed (Monteiro 1995). Pfaffenrath and Kaube, using the criteria from Sjaastad et al., found in a hospital-based study a prevalence rate of 13.8% (Pfaffenrath and Kaube 1990). In another hospital-based study of D'Amico et al. the prevalence of CEH according the criteria from Sjaastad et al. was 0.7% among headache patients (D'Amico et al. 1994). In a recent population-based study (Vågå) from Sjaastad et al. the prevalence was 4.1% (Sjaastad and Bakketeig 2008). In conclusion: depending upon the population studied and which criteria have been used the prevalence has been reported between 0.7% and 13.8%.

◻ Table 37.1

Cervicogenic headache: summary of minimum requirements for diagnosis

Major criteria	Confirmatory combination	Provisional combination[a]
I. Neck involvement	Presence of a1 and/or a2	
(a) Precipitation of attacks (1) Subjectively (2) Iatrogenically		
(b) Reduced range of motion in neck		Present
(c) Ipsilateral shoulder/arm pain		Present
II. Anesthetic block effect	Positive	Positive
III. Unilaterality without sideshift	Present[b]	Present[b]
Pain characteristics		
IV. Non-throbbing pain, usually starting in the neck with episodes of varying duration, or a fluctuating continuous pain		
Other characteristics		
V. Only marginal effect of indomethacin		
Only marginal effect or lack of effect of ergotamine and sumatriptan		
A certain female preponderance		
Head or indirect neck trauma by history, usually of more than only medium severity		
Other descriptions of lesser importance		
VI. Various attack-related phenomena, only rarely present, and/or moderately expressed when present		
(a) Nausea		
(b) Phonophobia and photophobia		
(c) Dizziness		
(d) Ipsilateral "blurred vision"		
(e) Difficulties on swallowing		
(f) Ipsilateral edema, mostly in the periocular area		

[a]The provisional combination is tentative
[b]In nonscientific work "unilaterality without sideshift" does not need to be present

Pathophysiology

The role of the trigeminal nucleus in relation to pain in the face from the neck was established many years ago (Ray and Wolff 1940; Olszewski 1950). The trigeminal nucleus is divided in the main sensory nucleus and the spinal tract nucleus, which is located far caudally in the cervical cord. The nucleus caudalis is the most caudal subdivision of the spinal tract nucleus. The gray matter of the brain stem that constitutes the pars caudalis of the spinal tract nucleus of the trigeminal nerve is continuous with the gray matter of the dorsal horns of the spinal cord (Bogduk 1984). There is no intrinsic anatomical feature that demarcates where the spinal nucleus caudalis ends and the gray matter of the spinal cord begins. This functional continuum column of neural cells formed by the pars caudalis and the gray matter of the upper three cervical spinal cord segments could be regarded as the trigeminocervical nucleus (Bogduk 1992).

Connections between the trigeminocervical nucleus and the upper three cervical roots are the neuro-anatomical substrate for the spreading of pain from the cervical area to the head (Bogduk 1984). Convergence of primary afferents of the upper three cervical roots with those of the trigeminocervical nucleus has been established (Kerr 1972). This phenomenon of convergence of afferent input at the nucleus caudalis from the head and cervical region and from the main sensory trigeminal nucleus may serve as a pathway of referred pain impulses from the neck to the frontotemporal region of the head and vice versa (Bogduk 1984). This convergence forms the neuro-anatomical basis for the concept of CEH.

The nucleus caudalis contains two classes of neurons associated with sensory processing that are remarkably similar to those reported in the spinal cord. The first class is termed "nociceptive specific" (NS) and the second class is termed "wide dynamic" (WD) neurons. These "wide dynamic" neurons play a key role in sensitization and wind-up (Siddall and Cousins 1998). The concept in CEH is that nociception originates from anatomical structures in the occipital region of the head and the neck. Whether sensitization of "wide dynamic" neurons play a role in the pathogenesis of CEH needs to be established.

Clinical Picture

CEH has been defined, in principle, as a unilateral headache without sideshift, but is may also be bilateral. The pain typically starts in the neck or at the occipital-nuchal area and spreads to the ipsilateral oculofrontotemporal region where the maximal pain is frequently located.

Important diagnostic features are the symptoms and signs of neck involvement. Such signs are mechanical precipitation of attacks, reduced range of motion in the neck, diffuse ipsilateral neck/shoulder/arm pain of nonradicular nature or, occasionally, arm pain of radicular nature. Iatrogenically induced pain similar to the spontaneous one may be elicited by external pressure over tendon insertions in the occipital area. Intrinsic precipitation mechanisms may be activated by neck movements and/or sustained, awkward head positioning during sleep or during wakefulness. Ipsilateral shoulder/arm symptoms may be even more frequent than they seemed to be initially. One not infrequently encounters patients with marked, more or less constant arm pain of a nonradicular nature. However, these phenomena are not infrequently of low intensity, and may be more like a discomfort than a pain. The side-locked unilaterality of the headache combined with the ipsilaterality of the arm pain provides rather compelling evidence that headache on such occasions stems from neck structures, but not necessarily only from bony structures.

The duration of attacks/exacerbations varies widely with a strong tendency toward chronicity. The pain of attack starts in the neck, eventually spreading to the oculofrontotemporal area, where, during the acme, it may be as strong as or even stronger than in the occipital region. The duration of pain episodes is most frequently longer than in common migraine; the pain intensity is moderate, non-excruciating, and usually of a non-throbbing nature.

Autonomic symptoms and signs, like photo- and phonophobia, nausea, vomiting, and ipsilateral periocular edema, are infrequent – and mild if present – and some of them are clearly less marked than in common migraine.

X-Ray Investigations

The relationship between radiographic degenerative changes and pain is certainly not unequivocal (Heller et al. 1983; Schellhas et al. 1996). Fredriksen et al. did not find any abnormalities on standard X-rays of the cervical spine in patients with CEH (Fredriksen et al. 1989). This is in concordance with the results of Pfaffenrath et al. (1987).

Diagnosis

The diagnosis of CEH has been driven by two schools of practice, i.e., the clinical diagnosis school in Europe based on the application of diagnostic criteria (❯ Table 37.1) and the interventional school in Australia and North America only based on the use of diagnostic blocks to establish the diagnosis (Bogduk and Govind 2009). These differences are also reflected in the criteria of CEH according to Sjaastad et al. and the International Headache Society (IHS) criteria for CEH (Sjaastad et al. 1998; Headache Classification Committee of the International Headache Society 1988) (❯ Table 37.2).

Van Suijlekom et al. (1999) showed that the reliability in diagnosing CEH (kappa: 0.83 between the expert headache neurologists), when strictly applying the criteria from Sjaastad and coworkers, is similar to the reliability in diagnosing migraine and tension-type headache according the IHS criteria (Headache Classification Committee of the International Headache Society 1988).

An appropriate clinical history and accurate neurological examination, showing a reduced "range of movement" (ROM) (Antonaci et al. 2000) and precipitation mechanisms, are fundamental elements in distinguishing CEH from other ones. The combination of pain stemming from the neck and then spreading unilaterally to the frontal area on the same side fortifies the suspicion that one may be faced with a case of CEH. The site and radiation of pain, the temporal pattern, and the mechanical precipitation of attacks, both iatrogenically and subjectively, are important aspects of the clinical picture and may help in distinguishing between CEH on the one hand and migraine and tension-type headache on the other

◻ Table 37.2

Cervicogenic headache: IHS diagnostic criteria (Headache Classification Committee of the International Headache Society 1988)

Diagnostic criteria
A. Pain, referred from a source in the neck and perceived in one or more regions of the head and/or face, fulfilling criteria C and D
B. Clinical, laboratory and/or imaging evidence of a disorder or lesion within the cervical spine or soft tissues of the neck known to be, or generally accepted as, a valid cause of headache
C. Evidence that the pain can be attributed to the neck disorder or lesion based on at least one of the following: 1. Demonstration of clinical signs that implicate a source of pain in the neck   2. Abolition of headache following diagnostic blockade of a cervical structure or its nerve supply using placebo – or other adequate controls
D. Pain resolves within 3 months after successful treatment of the causative disorder or lesion

(Vincent and Luna 1999; Antonaci et al. 2001). In patients with bilateral pain, but still with a preponderance on the usual side, anesthetic blockades become mandatory even in clinical practice. In order to identify the correct level of affection, the blockades should be directed to the nerve or nerves, where most likely the pain originates/is elicited, on the side of prevailing pain (Bovim and Sand 1992).

In the IHS classification the criteria for headache associated with neck disorders has been largely revised (❯ *Table 37.2*) (Headache Classification Committee of the International Headache Society 1988) and the term "cervicogenic headache" and not "cervical headache" has been accepted for the first time. However, already under letter "A," it is stated that the pain can be in "... one or more regions of the head and/or face ..." a rather unspecific description meaning that there may be only facial pain and not a headache. Another shortcoming of the new classification is under letter "B," where it is stated: "Clinical, laboratory and/or imaging evidence...." According to what is written here, it can be interpreted as meaning: *imaging evidence* would suffice the diagnosis giving no importance to any headache (the examination better than the clinical evaluation !). Therefore, this criteria as it formulated provide a minimal importance of clinical evidence.

The IHS classification has deserved a minor importance to the property of CEH to be precipitated (i.e., both iatrogenically and subjectively induced); iatrogenically induced pain similar to the spontaneous one may be elicited by external pressure over tendon insertions in the occipital area. Pressure along the course of the major occipital nerve, over the groove immediately behind the mastoid process, and over the upper part of the sternocleido-mastoid muscle on the symptomatic side may also provoke similar pain. Intrinsic precipitation mechanisms may be activated by neck movements and/or sustained, awkward head positioning during sleep or during wakefulness (such as when washing the ceiling, speaking to one's neighbor at table during a party, and so forth). In addition, only in the IHS notes and not in the criteria is reported the important, ipsilateral shoulder/arm symptoms mentioned which aids in distinguishing CEH from a central affection. Unfortunately, these criteria, as the previous ones, may be somewhat unsuited for clinical headache work.

Differential Diagnosis

In the differential diagnosis of CEH, just as with other headaches, organic disorders such as a space-occupying lesion in the posterior fossa cerebellaris and other tumors, sinus thrombosis, arthritis of the cervical spinal column, etc., should be excluded.

Despite an apparent characteristic pattern of headache arising from the neck, there are still some difficulties in the differential diagnosis of CEH, which has symptoms that overlap with those of common primary headache syndromes. The differential diagnosis of CEH includes (a) migraine without aura; (b) tension-type headache; (c) cluster headache; (d) occipital neuralgia; (e) hemicrania continua.

The main diagnostic problem in patients with headache appears to be distinguishing CEH from migraine without aura and tension-type headache (Bovim and Sand 1992; Pöllmann et al. 1997).

Migraine Without Aura

Similarities between CEH and migraine without aura include: (1) unilaterality of the headache; (2) occurrence predominantly in women; (3) possible occurrence of nausea and vomiting.

However, there are also fundamental differences between migraine and CEH: (1) unilaterality without "side shift" in CEH, while in migraine without aura there can be a shift of the headache during the same headache attack as well as between the individual headache attacks. (2) CEH usually begins in the neck while migraine usually begins in the frontotemporal region. (3) CEH can be provoked by mechanical pressure in the upper lateral area of the cervical spinal column, on the symptomatic side, and/or with continuous backward tilting of the head; whereas, this usually does not occur with migraine. (4) In CEH, there is often a limitation of movement in the neck, which is not characteristic of migraine. (5) A nonradicular, ipsilateral diffuse shoulder/arm pain sometimes occurs in CEH but not in migraine.

Tension-Type Headache

CEH may present as a mild, non-throbbing, episodic pain that resembles tension-type headache. However, in tension-type headache there may be a "weight" or pressure-like sensation, and there is often the sensation of wearing a tight skullcap. In most cases, bilateral localization of the headache and the absence of mechanical trigger factors allow differentiation between tension-type headache and CEH.

Bilateral cases of CEH can complicate attempts to distinguish the condition from tension-type headache. In a study by Vincent and Luna that used the IHS criteria, only one patient with CEH was diagnosed as having tension-type headache (Vincent and Luna 1999).

Cluster Headache

CEH is easy to differentiate from cluster headache. Cluster headache is an excruciating unilateral headache that usually has a circadian rhythm. It can last from 20 min up to 3 h. During the attack, it is often difficult for the patient to stay still secondary to the severity of the pain. Also, cluster headache is characterized by associated autonomic symptoms.

Occipital Neuralgia

Paroxysmal lancinating pain is a key feature of neuralgia in general and is an essential diagnostic criterion for occipital neuralgia. Physical examination reveals a diminished sensation or dysesthesia in the affected area as well as tenderness to palpation in the distribution of the greater or lesser occipital nerves (Headache Classification Committee of the International Headache Society 1988).

Hemicrania Continua

Hemicrania continua is a rare, indomethacin-responsive headache disorder characterized by a continuous, moderately severe, unilateral headache that varies in intensity, waxing and waning without disappearing completely (Sjaastad and Spierings 1984). While hemicrania continua is not triggered by neck movements, tender points in the neck may be present.

A positive therapeutic response to indomethacin can distinguish hemicrania continua from CEH (Sjaastad et al. 1993).

Conservative Therapy

Generally, a conservative treatment should be the first option before interventional treatment is started. Conservative pain treatments include among others: medication, physiotherapy, manual therapy, and transcutaneous electrical nerve stimulation (TENS). Usually patients with CEH, seen in a Headache/pain management center, have already been extensively treated with conservative therapies.

Medication

Patients with CEH often take simple analgesics, such as paracetamol (acetaminophen) and NSAIDs. Clinical experience indicates that, in the majority of patients with mild CEH, these drugs provide only transient relief of the headache. Drugs such as morphine have only a marginal effect and are generally not indicated for CEH (Bovim and Sjaastad 1993).

Although ergotamine is a drug compound that is still widely used in the treatment of migraine, its use in CEH should not be recommended because it is completely ineffective in this condition (Martelletti 2000).

The triptans exert their agonist effects on the 5-HT1B/D receptors within the trigeminal system. The efficacy of these drugs has not been established in CEH.

Manual Therapy

Spinal manipulation is used in the treatment of neck pain and headache associated with symptomatic spinal segmental joint or dysfunction (Vernon 1991; Watson and Trott 1993). This manual examination, the so-called segmental spine examination, is performed to identify the precise localization of segmental dysfunction(s) and tenderness.

Only a small number of spinal manipulation trials have been conducted in patients with headache or patients with CEH (Whittingham et al. 1994; Schoensee et al. 1995; Nilsson 1995; Nilsson et al. 1997). Furthermore, the results were obtained 1–4 weeks after the final therapy session and a longer follow-up period will be required to establish the efficacy of spinal manipulation in CEH.

Although there are some risks with cervical spinal manipulation (e.g., traumatic myelopathy), their prevalence is extremely low (Van Zagten et al. 1993). Nevertheless, a very cautious approach when using this technique has been recommended (Martelletti et al. 1995).

TENS

Transcutaneous Electrical Nerve Stimulation (TENS) is an example of a noninvasive regularly used nerve stimulation technique. Farina et al. demonstrated in their nonrandomized study that TENS is an effective treatment method for CEH (Farina et al. 1986). A randomized study in patients with CEH patients, showed a significant improvement in headache symptoms after 3 months of TENS therapy compared with the placebo group (Sjaastad et al. 1997).

Interventional Therapy

Various interventional procedures for CEH have been published. A generally acceptable treatment method for CEH is not yet available. A number of invasive procedures for patients with CEH are described below. The selection of the type of invasive treatment is guided by the case history and physical examination.

Local Injections

Injections of the nervus occipitalis major with a local anesthetic with or without corticosteroids give a temporary positive effect for CEH (Anthony 1992; Gawell and Rothbart 1991; Vincent 1998). A randomized study by Naja et al. showed significant pain reduction after a follow-up of 2 weeks (Naja et al. 2006a). This study was continued as a prospective study whereby significant pain reduction was still achieved after a follow-up of 6 months. In this last study, 87% of the patients required an extra injection. In addition to an injection of the nervus occipitalis major, an injection of the nervus occipitalis minor was performed (Naja et al. 2006b).

Injection into the atlantoaxial joint with a local anesthetic and corticosteroid, in patients with CEH, was carried out when the clinical picture suggested atlantoaxial joint pain. There was no statistically significant difference after 6 months in this retrospective study (Narouze et al. 2007).

Martelletti et al. showed that cervical epidural injection with corticosteroids has no place in the therapeutic arsenal (Martelletti et al. 1998a, b).

Radiofrequency (RF) Treatment

In 1986, Hildebrandt et al. in an open study, reported a good result for 37%, an acceptable result for 28%, and no improvement for 35% of the patients with head and neck pain (Hildebrandt 1986). It is not known whether these patients had CEH. The average follow-up was 12 months (range 3–30).

In a prospective study in patients with CEH according to the criteria of Sjaastad, receiving RF treatment of the medial branch of the cervical facet joints C3–C6, the results were outstanding to good in 65%, average in 14%, and no improvement was seen in 21% of the patients, with an average follow-up of 16.8 months (range 12–22) (Van Suijlekom et al. 1998).

Stovner et al. included 12 patients with CEH according to the criteria of Sjaastad, and treated 6 patients with cervical facet denervation of C2 to C6 and 6 patients with a sham intervention (Stovner et al. 2004). Follow-up after 3, 12, and 24 months showed no difference between the two groups. Physical examination of the cervical facet joints was not carried out in this study.

Haspeslagh et al. included 30 patients with unilateral CEH according to the criteria of Sjaastad (Haspeslagh et al. 2006). Fifteen of these patients were treated with RF treatment of the cervical facet C3–C6 on the symptomatic side. The other 15 patients were treated with two injections of the nervus occipitalis major and ultimately followed with TENS therapy if necessary. Even though no significant difference between the two groups was found, there were patients in both groups with a significant visual analog scale (VAS) reduction and/or a positive effect on the global perceived effect scale. After a follow-up of 1 year there were 8 (53%) patients in the RF group and 7 (46%) in the injection/TENS group with a significant pain reduction. Physical examination for painful facet joints was an inclusion criterion of this study.

Govind and colleagues reported, in their retrospective study, 88% success rate (43/49 patients) with a median duration of headache relief of 297 days in patients with headache stemming from the C2–C3 joint (Lord et al. 1995; Govind et al. 2003). They performed a RF treatment of the nervus occipitalis tertius.

Surgical Treatments

Neurolysis of the nervus occipitalis major in patients with CEH, according to the criteria of Sjaastad, gave significant pain reduction after 1 week. Follow-up after a year showed that in 92% of the patients, the symptoms had completely returned (Bovim et al. 1992).

Microsurgical decompression of the dorsal root ganglion C2 (DRG) in 35 patients with CEH, according to the criteria of Sjaastad, showed that 37% of the patients were pain free, and in 51% a clear improvement was seen (Pikus and Phillips 1996). The average follow-up was 21 (3–70) months.

During microsurgical decompression of the DRG, ligament structures and veins around the ganglion were "removed" by means of electro-coagulation. Stechison claims that the results from Pikus et al. can also be attributed to the effects of electrocoagulation nearby the DRG, a kind of "radiofrequency lesion" (Stechison 1997).

References

Anthony M (1992) Headache and the greater occipital nerve. Clin Neurol Neurosurg 94:297–301

Antonaci F, Ghirmai S, Bono G, Nappi G (2000) Current methods for cervical spine movement evaluation: a review. Clin Exp Rheumatol 18(Suppl 19):45–52

Antonaci F, Ghirmai S, Bono G et al (2001) Cervicogenic headache: evaluation of the original diagnostic criteria. Cephalalgia 21:573–583

Barré M (1926) Sur un syndrome sympatique cervicale posterieur et sa cause fréquente: l'arthride cervicale. Rev Neurol 33:1246–1248

Bärtschi-Rochaix W (1948) Le diagnostic de l'encephalopathie posttraumatique d'orginal cervicale (« migraine cervicale »). Praxis 37:673–677

Bogduk N (1984) Headaches and the cervical spine. Cephalalgia 4(1):7–8

Bogduk N (1992) The anatomical basis for cervicogenic headache. J Manipul Physiol Ther 15(1):67–70

Bogduk N, Govind J (2009) Cervicogenic headache: an assessment of the evidence on clinical diagnosis, invasive tests and treatment. Lancet Neurol 8:959–968

Bovim G, Sand T (1992) Cervicogenic headache, migraine without aura and tension-type headache: diagnostic blockade of greater occipital and supraorbital nerves. Pain 51:43–48

Bovim G, Sjaastad O (1993) Cervicogenic headache: responses to nitroglycerin, oxygen, ergotamine and morphine. Headache 33:249–252

Bovim G, Fredriksen TA, Stolt-Nielsen A et al (1992) Neurolysis of the greater occipital nerve in cervicogenic headache. A follow up study. Headache 32:175–179

D'Amico D, Leone M, Bussone G (1994) Side-locked unilaterality and pain localization in long-lasting headaches: migraine, tension-type headache and cervicogenic headache. Headache 34:526–530

Farina S, Granella F, Malferrari G et al (1986) Headache and cervical spine disorders: classification and treatment with transcutaneous electrical nerve stimulation. Headache 26:431–433

Fredriksen T, Fougner R, Tangerud A, Sjaastad O (1989) Cic Headache. Radiological investigations concerning head/neck. Cephalalgia 9(2):139–146

Gawell M, Rothbart P (1991) Occipital nerve block in the management of headache and cervical pain. Cephalalgia 12:9–13

Govind J, King W, Bailey B et al (2003) Radiofrequency neurotomy for the treatment of third occipital headache. J Neurol Neurosurg Psychiatry 74:88–93

Haspeslagh SR, Van Suijlekom HA, Lame IE et al (2006) Randomised controlled trial of cervical radiofrequency lesions as a treatment for cervicogenic headache [isrctn07444684]. BMC Anesthesiol 16:1

Heller CA, Stanley P, Lewis-Jones B et al (1983) Value of x-ray examinations of the cervical spine. Br Med J (Clin Res Ed) 287:1276–1278

Hildebrandt J (1986) Percutaneaus nerve block of the cervical facets - a relatively new method in the treatment of chronic headache and neck pain. Man Med 2:48–52

Headache Classification Committee of the International Headache Society (1988) Classification and diagnostic criteria for headache disorders, cranial neuralgias and facial pain. Cephalalgia 8(S7):1–96

IHC IHSCS (2004) International classification of headache disorders, 2nd edn. Cephalalgia 24:1–160

Kerr F (1972) Central relationships of trigeminal and cervical primary afferents in the spinal cord and medulla. Brain Res 43(2):561–572

Lord SM, Barnsley L, Bogduk N (1995) Percutaneous radiofrequency neurotomy in the treatment of cervical zygapophysial joint pain: a caution. Neurosurgery 36:732–739

Martelletti P (2000) Proinflammatory pathways in cervicogenic headache. Clin Exp Rheumatol 18: S33–S39

Martelletti P, LaTour D, Giacovazzo M (1995) Spectrum of pathophysiological disorders in cervicogenic headache and its therapeutic indications. J Neuromusculoskelet Syst 3:182–187

Martelletti P, Di Sabato F, Granata M et al (1998a) Epidural corticosteroid blockade in cervicogenic headache. Eur Rev Med Pharmacol Sci 2:25–30

Martelletti P, Di Sabato F, Granata M et al (1998b) Failure of longterm epidural steroid injection in cervicogenic headache [letter]. Funct Neurol 13:148

Monteiro J (1995) Cefaleias: Estudo Epidemiologico e clinico de uma populacao urbana. Doctoral thesis, University Hospital Porto, Department of Neurology, Porto

Naja ZM, El-Rajab M, Al-Tannir MA et al (2006a) Occipital nerve blockade for cervicogenic headache: a double-blind randomized controlled clinical trial. Pain Pract 6:89–95

Naja ZM, El-Rajab M, Al-Tannir MA et al (2006b) Repetitive occipital nerve blockade for cervicogenic headache: expanded case report of 47 adults. Pain Pract 6:278–284

Narouze SN, Casanova J, Mekhail N (2007) The longitudinal effectiveness of lateral atlantoaxial intra-articular steroid injection in the treatment of cervicogenic headache. Pain Med 8:184–188

Nilsson N (1995a) The prevalence of cervicogenic headache in a random population sample of 20-59 year olds. Spine 20(17):1884–1888

Nilsson N (1995b) A randomised controlled trial of the effect of spinal manipulation in the treatment of cervicogenic headache. J Manip Physiol Ther 18:435–440

Nilsson N, Christensen HW, Hartvigsen J (1997) The effect of spinal manipulation in the treatment of cervicogenic headache. J Manip Physiol Ther 20:326–330

Olszewski J (1950) On the anatomical and functional organisation of the spinal trigeminal nucleus. J Comp Neurol 92:401–403

Pfaffenrath V, Kaube H (1990) Diagnostics of cervicogenic headache. Funct Neurol 5:159–164

Pfaffenrath V, Dandekar R, Pöllmann W (1987) Cervicogenic headache – the clinical picture, radiological findings and hypotheses on its pathophysiology. Headache 27(9):495–499

Pikus HJ, Phillips JM (1996) Outcome of surgical decompression of the second cervical root for cervicogenic headache. Neurosurgery 39:63–70

Pöllmann W, Keidel M, Pfaffenrath V (1997) Headache and the cervical spine: a critical review. Cephalalgia 17:801–816

Ray B, Wolff H (1940) Experimental study of headache. Arch Surg 41:813–856

Schellhas KP, Smith MD, Gundry CR et al (1996) Cervical discogenic pain. Prospective correlation of magnetic resonance imaging and discography in asymptomatic subjects and pain sufferers. Spine 21:300–311

Schoensee SK, Jensen G, Nicholson G et al (1995) The effect of mobilization on cervical headaches. J Orthop Sports Phys Ther 21:184–196

Siddall P, Cousins M (1998) Introduction to pain mechanisms. In: Cousins M, Bridenbaugh P (eds) Neural blockade: in clinical anaesthesia and management of pain, 3rd edn. Lippincott – Raven, New York, pp 675–714

Sjaastad O, Bakketeig LS (2008) Prevalence of cervicogenic headache: Vågå study of headache epidemiology. Acta Neurol Scand 117:173–180

Sjaastad O, Spierings EL (1984) "Hemicrania continua": another headache absolutely responsive to indomethacin. Cephalalgia 4:65–70

Sjaastad O, Saunte C, Hovdahl H, Breivik H, Gronbaek E (1983) Cervicogenic headache: an hypothesis. Cephalalgia 3:249–256

Sjaastad O, Fredriksen T, Pfaffenrath V (1990) Cervicogenic headache: diagnostic criteria. Headache 30:725–726

Sjaastad O, Joubert J, Vincent M et al (1993) Hemicrania continua and cervicogenic headache: separate headaches or two faces of the same headache? Funct Neurol 8:79–83

Sjaastad O, Fredriksen TA, Stolt-Nielsen A et al (1997) Cervicogenic headache: A clinical review with special emphasis on therapy. Funct Neurol 12: 305–317

Sjaastad O, Fredriksen T, Pfaffenrath V (1998) Cervicogenic headache: diagnostic criteria. The Cervicogenic Headache International Study Group. Headache 38:442–445

Stechison MT (1997) Outcome of surgical decompression of the second cervical root for cervicogenic headache. Neurosurgery 40:1105–1106

Stovner LJ, Kolstad F, Helde G (2004) Radiofrequency denervation of facet joints C2–C6 in cervicogenic headache: a randomized, double-blind, sham- controlled study. Cephalalgia 24:821–830

Van Suijlekom JA, van Kleef M, Barendse G et al (1998) Radiofrequency cervical zygapophyeal joint neurotomy for cervicogenic headache. A prospective study in 15 patients. Funct Neurol 13: 297–303

Van Suijlekom JA, De Vet HCW, Van den Berg SGM, Weber WEJ (1999) Interobserver reliability of diagnostic criteria for cervicogenic headache. Cephalalgia 19:817–823

Van Zagten MS, Troost J, Heeres JG (1993) Cervical myelopathy as complication of manual therapy in a patient with a narrow cervical canal. Ned Tijdschr Geneeskd 137:1617–1618

Vernon H (1991) Spinal manipulation and headaches of cervical origin: a review of literature and presentation of cases. J Manag Med 6:73–79

Vincent M (1998) Greater occipital nerve blockades in cervicogenic headache. Funct Neurol 13:78–79

Vincent M, Luna R (1999) Cervicogenic headache: a comparison with migraine and tension-type headache. Cephalalgia 19(Suppl 25):11–16

Watson D, Trott P (1993) Cervical headache: an investigation of natural head posture and upper cervical flexor muscle performance. Cephalalgia 13: 272–284

Whittingham W, Ellis WB, Molyneux TP (1994) The effect of manipulation (toggle recoil technique) for headaches with upper cervical joint dysfunction: a pilot study. J Manip Physiol Ther 17:369–375

38 Headache Attributed to Giant Cell (Temporal) Arteritis

Anne Ducros
Assistance Publique des Hôpitaux de Paris, Head and Neck Clinic,
Lariboisière Hospital, Paris, France

Paolo Martelletti, Timothy J. Steiner (eds.), *Handbook of Headache*, DOI 10.1007/978-88-470-1700-9_38,
© Lifting The Burden 2011

Abstract: Any new-onset headache in a subject >50 years raises the suspicion of giant cell arteritis (GCA). GCA may cause any type of headache, associated or not with other suggestive clinical features such as fatigue, fever, jaw claudication, temporal arteries abnormalities, shoulder and pelvic girdle pain, or visual alterations. The main risk is visual loss by anterior ischemic optic neuropathy. Diagnosis relies on clinical history (headache in a >50 years old), elevated ESR and CRP, and results of temporal artery biopsy. High-dose glucocorticosteroid therapy should be initiated immediately when clinical suspicion of GCA is raised, before the result of temporal artery biopsy if the clinical suspicion is high, in order to prevent complications. Efficacy of steroids is such dramatic that the persistence of headache after 4 days of treatment should prompt to consider an alternative diagnosis.

Established Knowledge

"Need to Know"

1. Early recognition and diagnosis of GCA is crucial in order to prevent visual loss due to anterior ischemic optic neuropathy (AION) and other ischemic end-organ damages.
2. Any new-onset headache in a patient aged >50 with an elevated erythrocyte sedimentation rate should raise the suspicion of GCA.
3. Urgent referral for specialist evaluation is suggested for all patients. Temporal artery biopsy (TAB) should be considered whenever the diagnosis is suspected, but should never delay the prompt institution of therapy.
4. Although modern imaging techniques show diagnostic promise, TAB remains the gold standard for investigation.
5. High-dose glucocorticosteroid therapy should be initiated immediately when clinical suspicion of GCA is raised.
6. Glucocorticosteroid reduction should be considered only in the absence of clinical symptoms, signs, and laboratory abnormalities suggestive of active disease.
7. Additional treatment should include bone protection, proton-pump inhibitors, and low-dose aspirin if no contraindications exist.

Definition and Background

Giant cell arteritis (GCA), the commonest of all the vasculitides, is a chronic vasculitis of large- and medium-sized blood vessels (Smeeth et al. 2006). The granulomatous inflammation process primarily affects the internal elastic membrane, with presence of characteristic multinucleated giant cells. GCA mainly affects the cranial branches of arteries arising from the aortic arch and respects the intracranial arteries, which lack internal elastic lamina. Superficial temporal arteries are involved in almost all patients, explaining that "temporal arteritis" is a synonym for GCA.

Any new-onset headache in a patient aged >50 with an elevated erythrocyte sedimentation rate (ESR) has to be considered as a GCA until the contrary is proven (Dasgupta et al. 2010). GCA is a medical emergency and is among the common causes of acute blindness. Visual loss occurs in up to one-fifth of patients and may be preventable by early diagnosis and treatment (Gonzalez-Gay et al. 2000; Salvarani et al. 2005; Loddenkemper et al. 2007) (❷ *Table 38.1*).

◻ **Table 38.1**

Clinical features that should raise the suspicion of GCA in a patient >50 years of age (Adapted from Dasgupta et al. 2010)

Clinical signs
• Abrupt-onset headache (unilateral or bilateral in the temporal area)
• Scalp tenderness
• Jaw and tongue claudication
• Visual symptoms (amaurosis fugax, visual blurring or loss, diplopia)
• Constitutional symptoms (fatigue, malaise, fever, weight loss, depression)
• Polymyalgic symptoms (neck, torso, shoulder, and pelvic girdle pain)
• Limb claudication (arms > legs)
Examination may show
• Abnormal superficial temporal artery: tender, thickened, reduced, or absent pulsation
• Scalp tenderness
• Transient or permanent visual loss
• Visual field defect
• Relative afferent papillary defect on the swinging flashlight test
• Pale, swollen optic disk with hemorrhages on fundoscopy (AION)
• Unilateral or bilateral central retinal artery occlusion
• Upper cranial nerve palsies
• Vascular bruits and asymmetry of pulses or blood pressure (large-vessel GCA)

The American College of Rheumatology (ACR) classification criteria for GCA (Hunder et al. 1990) are:

1. Age at disease onset >50 years: development of symptoms or findings beginning at the age of 50 years
2. New headache: new onset of or new type of localized pain in the head
3. Temporal artery abnormality: temporal artery tenderness to palpation or decreased pulsation, unrelated to arteriosclerosis of cervical arteries
4. Elevated ESR >50 mm/h by the Westergren method
5. Abnormal artery biopsy: biopsy specimen with artery showing vasculitis characterized by a predominance of mononuclear cell infiltration or granulomatous inflammation, usually with multinucleated giant cells

These criteria were designed to differentiate GCA from other vasculitides, and are not useful for diagnosing GCA at the level of individual patients (Salvarani et al. 2008). A patient shall be said to have GCA if at least three of these five criteria are present. The presence of any three or more criteria yields a sensitivity of 93.5% and a specificity of 91.2%.

The exact pathogenesis of GCA is unknown. GCA and polymyalgia rheumatica (PMR) often occur together, suggesting common mechanisms. PMR is characterized by aching and morning stiffness in the shoulder and pelvic girdles and neck (Salvarani et al. 2008).

The Incidence of GCA varies from 1.47 to 20 and more per 100,000 population older than 50 years. The lowest rate was found in Japan and the highest in Scandinavian countries and in Minnesota (USA), which has a population of similar ethnic background (Gonzalez-Gay et al. 2009).

The mean age at onset is 70 years and GCA is rare before age 50 years. The female-to-male ratio is about 3:1 (Dasgupta and Hassan 2007; Borg et al. 2008).

Headache and Craniofacial Pain

Headache is the most common presenting symptom (33%) and is a prominent symptom in 70% of the patients (Salvarani et al. 1987; Solomon and Cappa 1987; Gonzalez-Gay et al. 2005). The headache of GCA has no specific features. In a patient >50 years of age, the crucial point is to consider any new headache in a patient without history of headache, and any new type of headache in a patient with a history of chronic headaches, as possibly secondary to GCA. Pain mainly starts abruptly (and may rarely be of the thunderclap type) or rapidly progress over a few days. The pain is usually throbbing, generalized or unilateral, and continuous through the day, with eventual exacerbation during sleep. Focal temporal pain is usually present and patients report scalp tenderness when hair combing or lying head down on a cushion. Many patients have swollen, red, nodular, thickened, and/or painful superficial temporal arteries on direct palpation with decreased or absent pulsation.

Less often, the headache may predominate in the occipital or occipitonucchal areas. This posterior headache may either be the result of occipital arteries vasculitis, or be part of a more generalized pain syndrome in the setting of PMR, which occurs in about 58% of GCA patients (Caselli et al. 1988b; Salvarani et al. 2008).

Jaw claudication, i.e., pain when speaking or chewing, is almost pathognomonic of GCA and is due to ischemia of the maxillary arteries. It is rarely the initial symptom (4%) but occurs in about 40% of patients during the course of GCA (Caselli et al. 1988b). Other less frequent complaints include tongue claudication, and facial pain due to facial artery vasculitis. Finally, about 15% of the patients reported a unilateral or bilateral cervical pain, coined as "carotidynia" (Caselli et al. 1988b).

Systemic Symptoms

One or more systemic manifestations, including fever, malaise, fatigue, anorexia, and weight loss, are present in most patients (Salvarani et al. 1987; Solomon and Cappa 1987; Gonzalez-Gay et al. 2005). Fever is usually low grade, but it reaches 39–40°C in about 15% of patients and might be the presenting symptom or the only manifestation of GCA (Zenone 2007).

Neuro-Ophthalmic Symptoms

Irreversible partial or complete visual loss in one or in both eyes occurs in less than 20% of patients, is often an early feature, and may be the sole manifestation of an otherwise clinically silent GCA. Anterior ischemic optic neuropathy (AION) is the main cause (Gonzalez-Gay et al. 2000; Salvarani et al. 2005; Borg et al. 2008). Following monocular onset, the second eye is affected within a few days. Amaurosis fugax, found in 10–15% of patients, may precede permanent visual loss. A few patients may present with scintillating scotoma (Caselli et al. 1988b) which should also raise suspicion of AION and not be regarded as benign visual auras. Features predictive of permanent visual loss include jaw claudication and temporal artery abnormalities on physical examination. AION is mostly caused by narrowing or occlusion of the posterior ciliary arteries. Examination shows a partial or complete reduction in visual acuity and a relative afferent pupillary defect on the swinging flashlight test. Early fundoscopy shows slight pallor and edema of the optic disk, with scattered cotton-wool patches and small hemorrhages. Optic atrophy occurs 2–4 weeks later (Salvarani et al. 2008). Residual visual defects are usually altitudinal.

Less commonly, visual loss is caused by retinal artery occlusion or by retrobulbar ischemic optic neuropathy. In the latter case, funduscopy may show pallor and edema of the entire retina and optic disk together with a macular cherry red spot, and in the former case, initial normal fundus is followed by optic atrophy.

Diplopia may occur in GCA (6%). Any level of the oculomotor apparatus can be involved, including the extraocular muscles, the three oculomotor nerves, and the brain stem, but the muscles are most commonly involved. Diplopia may fluctuate daily similar to myasthenia gravis or may be static in the rare cases of ischemic oculomotor palsy. Ptosis and myosis may occur as part of Horner's syndrome, with or without other oculomotor disturbances.

Transient Ischemic Attacks (TIAs) and Ischemic Strokes

About 4% of patients have TIA or stroke at some point during the course of GCA (Caselli et al. 1988b). Atherosclerosis, hypertension, and cardiac disease are the most frequent causes of cerebral infarction in elderly patients with or without GCA. But the vasculitis may involve the extracranial portions of carotid and vertebral arteries, thus directly leading to TIAs and infarction. Infarcts may involve anterior and posterior circulations (either alone or in combination) and may lead to multi-infarct dementia (Solans-Laque et al. 2008).

Large-Vessel Involvement

Aortic arch syndrome occurs in about 10–15% of patients with GCA, presenting with claudication of the arms and rarely the legs; bruits over the carotid, subclavian, axillary, and brachial arteries; and absent or decreased pulses in the neck or arms; often in association with prominent systemic symptoms such as fever or cachexia (Salvarani et al. 2008; Borg and Dasgupta 2009). Ischemic complications may occur. Thoracic aortic aneurysms and dissection of the aorta are late complications of GCA (Nuenninghoff et al. 2003a, b).

Rare Manifestations

About 14% of all patients have neuropathies, including mononeuropathies and peripheral polyneuropathies of the upper or lower extremities (Caselli et al. 1988a).

Encephalopathy is rare in GCA and can be related to cerebral infarction (thalamic, mesial, temporal, or mesencephalic), to corticosteroid therapy (steroid psychosis, metabolic disorders, or infectious complications), or to causes unrelated to GCA, but related to older age (degenerative or vascular dementia, chronic subdural hematoma, sedating medications) (Salvarani et al. 2008).

Myelopathy occurs in less than 1% of GCA patient, presumably due to the extension of vasculitis to the anterior spinal artery.

Laboratory Investigations and Imaging

Blood tests should be performed as soon as the diagnosis is suspected and have to include full blood count, urea and electrolytes, liver function tests, CRP, and ESR (Dasgupta et al. 2010). An acute-phase response is the characteristic of GCA: raised ESR, CRP, anemia, thrombocytosis, abnormal liver function tests, particularly raised alkaline phosphatase, raised 1 and 2 globulins on serum electrophoresis. The American College of Rheumatology classification criteria for GCA include an ESR of 50 mm/h or more. However, GCA can occur in the face of lower levels of ESR and CRP (ESR <40 mm/h in 5.4% of patients) (Wong and Korn 1986).

Temporal artery biopsy (TAB) remains the gold standard for investigation (Robb-Nicholson et al. 1988; Mukhtyar et al. 2009). TAB should not delay the institution of steroid therapy and should be scheduled within 1 week of starting glucocorticosteroids (Achkar et al. 1994). Reports suggest that TAB may remain positive for 2–6 weeks following initiation of corticosteroids (Achkar et al. 1994; Ray-Chaudhuri et al. 2002). Patients should be referred to a surgical unit experienced in regular TAB. Biopsy samples should be long enough, ideally >2 cm (Mahr et al. 2006). Contralateral biopsy is usually not required (Hall et al. 2003) unless the size of the original biopsy specimen was suboptimal. The need to examine the specimen at multiple levels is controversial (Chakrabarty and Franks 2000).

TAB may be negative, due to the presence of skip lesions in some cases and suboptimal biopsy in others. Patients with negative biopsies should be managed as having GCA if there is a typical clinical and laboratory picture and response to glucocorticosteroids, or typical findings on ultrasound, or ischemic complications typical of GCA such as AION (Dasgupta et al. 2010).

Ultrasonography and 3T MRI have shown diagnostic promise to assess cranial arterial involvement in GCA. However, they do not replace TAB because they do not have the prognostic value of histology and are highly user or observer dependent. Ultrasonography can show a typical hypoechoic "halo" around affected temporal arteries, representing vessel wall edema, as well as arterial stenosis and occlusion (Karassa et al. 2005; Schmidt 2007). The possible role for ultrasound in cranial GCA may be in the selection of which patients should have a TAB (Dasgupta et al. 2010). High-resolution multi-slice 3T MRI using intravenous contrast may show increased vessel wall thickness and edema, with increased mural enhancement post contrast and luminal stenosis (Bley et al. 2005).

When large-vessel GCA is suspected, various arterial imaging modalities are used, including conventional angiography, CT, CT angiography, MRI, MR angiography, and ultrasonography (Blockmans et al. 2009; Dasgupta et al. 2010). Both catheter and noninvasive angiograms can show bilateral, smooth, tapering stenoses, or occlusions of the subclavian, axillary, and proximal brachial arteries. Leg arteries are less frequently involved. In addition, ultasonography and MRI can directly show inflammatory edema of the vessel wall (Blockmans et al. 2009). In addition, fluorodeoxyglucose PET seems to be a promising method in the detection of occult involvement of the aorta and large vessels in patients with suspected GCA, especially those presenting with fever of unknown origin (Blockmans et al. 2006).

Treatment

The mainstay of therapy remains high-dose corticosteroids, which should be initiated immediately when clinical suspicion of GCA is raised (Mukhtyar et al. 2009; Dasgupta et al. 2010). Recommended starting dosages are:

- Uncomplicated GCA (no jaw claudication or visual disturbance): 40–60 mg prednisolone daily (Kyle 1991)
- Evolving visual loss or amaurosis fugax (complicated GCA): 500 mg to 1 g of IV methyl-prednisolone for 3 days before oral corticosteroids (Chevalet et al. 2000; Mazlumzadeh et al. 2006)
- Established visual loss: 60 mg prednisolone daily to protect the contralateral eye (Chan et al. 2001; Foroozan et al. 2003)

Symptoms of GCA typically respond rapidly to this treatment, followed by resolution of the inflammatory response. Failure to do so, and especially persistence of headache after 4 days of treatment, should raise the question of an alternative diagnosis. If visual loss has occurred before start of treatment, it is usually not reversed.

Prescription of corticosteroids is accompanied by bone protection (calcium, vitamin D, and weekly bisphosphonates), proton-pump inhibitors for gastrointestinal protection, and low-dose aspirin (if no contraindications exist) to reduce cranial ischemic complications (Nesher et al. 2004; Dasgupta et al. 2010).

The initial dose of 40–60 mg prednisolone has to be continued until symptoms and laboratory abnormalities resolve (at least 3–4 weeks). Then a slow and gradual decrease is considered with a reduction by 10 mg every 2 weeks to 20 mg; then by 2.5 mg every 2–4 weeks to 10 mg; and then by 1 mg every 1–2 months provided there is no relapse. Although corticosteroids can be discontinued within 1–2 years in most cases, some patients will require long-term low-dose therapy.

Experience using conventional disease-modifying drugs such as methotrexate is mixed, and biological therapies require further evaluation for their steroid-sparing potential (Borg and Dasgupta 2009).

Patients should be closely monitored for evidence of relapse, disease-related complications, and glucocorticosteroid-related complications. Disease relapse should be suspected in patients with a return of symptoms of GCA, ischemic complications, unexplained fever, or polymyalgic symptoms. A rise in ESR/CRP is usually seen with relapse, but relapse can be seen with normal inflammatory markers. All patients in whom relapse is suspected should be treated with increased doses of glucocorticosteroids and referred for specialist assessment.

Recurrent relapse or failure to wean glucocorticosteroid dose requires the consideration of adjuvant therapy, such as methotrexate or other immunosuppressants. Biological therapies still require further study, and are not yet recommended.

Current Research

Prospective studies are needed to better evaluate predictors of earlier recognition and referral, different glucocorticosteroid doses, administration routes and tapering, TAB, and role of specific histological features, e.g., intimal hyperplasia. The role of glucocorticosteroid-sparing agents, such as methotrexate and biological therapies, needs to be established with well-designed randomized controlled trials (Salvarani et al. 2008). More studies are also required for early diagnosis and the identification and management of large-vessel GCA. Imaging techniques (ultrasound, MRI, and PET) show promise for the diagnosis and monitoring of GCA, but do not replace TAB for cranial GCA. Their role in early diagnosis of cranial GCA is an important area of future research (Dasgupta et al. 2010).

References

Achkar AA, Lie JT, Hunder GG, O'Fallon WM, Gabriel SE (1994) How does previous corticosteroid treatment affect the biopsy findings in giant cell (temporal) arteritis? Ann Intern Med 120:987–992

Bley TA, Weiben O, Uhl M, Vaith P, Schmidt D, Warnatz K, Langer M (2005) Assessment of the cranial involvement pattern of giant cell arteritis with 3T magnetic resonance imaging. Arthritis Rheum 52:2470–2477

Blockmans D, de Ceuninck L, Vanderschueren S, Knockaert D, Mortelmans L, Bobbaers H (2006) Repetitive 18F-fluorodeoxyglucose positron emission tomography in giant cell arteritis: a prospective study of 35 patients. Arthritis Rheum 55:131–137

Blockmans D, Bley T, Schmidt W (2009) Imaging for large-vessel vasculitis. Curr Opin Rheumatol 21:19–28

Borg FA, Dasgupta B (2009) Treatment and outcomes of large vessel arteritis. Best Pract Res Clin Rheumatol 23:325–337

Borg FA, Salter VL, Dasgupta B (2008) Neuro-ophthalmic complications in giant cell arteritis. Curr Allergy Asthma Rep 8:323–330

Caselli RJ, Daube JR, Hunder GG, Whisnant JP (1988a) Peripheral neuropathic syndromes in giant cell (temporal) arteritis. Neurology 38:685–689

Caselli RJ, Hunder GG, Whisnant JP (1988b) Neurologic disease in biopsy-proven giant cell (temporal) arteritis. Neurology 38:352–359

Chakrabarty A, Franks AJ (2000) Temporal artery biopsy: is there any value in examining biopsies at multiple levels? J Clin Pathol 53:131–136

Chan CC, Paine M, O'Day J (2001) Steroid management in giant cell arteritis. Br J Ophthalmol 85:1061–1064

Chevalet P, Barrier JH, Pottier P, Magadur-Joly G, Pottier MA, Hamidou M, Planchon B, El Kouri D, Connan L, Dupond JL, De Wazieres B, Dien G, Duhamel E, Grosbois B, Jego P, Le Strat A, Capdeville J, Letellier P, Agron L (2000) A randomized, multicenter, controlled trial using intravenous pulses of methylprednisolone in the initial treatment of simple forms of giant cell arteritis: a one year followup study of 164 patients. J Rheumatol 27:1484–1491

Dasgupta B, Borg FA, Hassan N, Alexander L, Barraclough K, Bourke B, Fulcher J, Hollywood J,

Hutchings A, James P, Kyle V, Nott J, Power M, Samanta A (2010) BSR and BHPR guidelines for the management of giant cell arteritis. Rheumatol 49(8):1594–1597

Foroozan R, Deramo VA, Buono LM, Jayamanne DG, Sergott RC, Danesh-Meyer H, Savino PJ (2003) Recovery of visual function in patients with biopsy-proven giant cell arteritis. Ophthalmology 110:539–542

Gonzalez-Gay MA, Garcia-Porrua C, Llorca J, Hajeer AH, Branas F, Dababneh A, Gonzalez-Louzao C, Rodriguez-Gil E, Rodriguez-Ledo P, Ollier WE (2000) Visual manifestations of giant cell arteritis. Trends and clinical spectrum in 161 patients. Medicine (Baltimore) 79:283–292

Gonzalez-Gay MA, Vazquez-Rodriguez TR, Lopez-Diaz MJ, Miranda-Filloy JA, Gonzalez-Juanatey C, Martin J, Llorca J (2009) Epidemiology of giant cell arteritis and polymyalgia rheumatica. Arthritis Rheum 61:1454–1461

Hall JK, Volpe NJ, Galetta SL, Liu GT, Syed NA, Balcer LJ (2003) The role of unilateral temporal artery biopsy. Ophthalmology 110:543–548, discussion 548

Hunder GG, Bloch DA, Michel BA, Stevens MB, Arend WP, Calabrese LH, Edworthy SM, Fauci AS, Leavitt RY, Lie JT et al (1990) The American College of Rheumatology 1990 criteria for the classification of giant cell arteritis. Arthritis Rheum 33:1122–1128

Karassa FB, Matsagas MI, Schmidt WA, Ioannidis JP (2005) Meta-analysis: test performance of ultrasonography for giant-cell arteritis. Ann Intern Med 142:359–369

Kyle V (1991) Treatment of polymyalgia rheumatica/giant cell arteritis. Baillières Clin Rheumatol 5:485–491

Loddenkemper T, Sharma P, Katzan I, Plant GT (2007) Risk factors for early visual deterioration in temporal arteritis. J Neurol Neurosurg Psychiatry 78:1255–1259

Mahr A, Saba M, Kambouchner M, Polivka M, Baudrimont M, Brocheriou I, Coste J, Guillevin L (2006) Temporal artery biopsy for diagnosing giant cell arteritis: the longer, the better? Ann Rheum Dis 65:826–828

Mazlumzadeh M, Hunder GG, Easley KA, Calamia KT, Matteson EL, Griffing WL, Younge BR, Weyand CM,

Goronzy JJ (2006) Treatment of giant cell arteritis using induction therapy with high-dose glucocorticoids: a double-blind, placebo-controlled, randomized prospective clinical trial. Arthritis Rheum 54: 3310–3318

Mukhtyar C, Guillevin L, Cid MC, Dasgupta B, de Groot K, Gross W, Hauser T, Hellmich B, Jayne D, Kallenberg CG, Merkel PA, Raspe H, Salvarani C, Scott DG, Stegeman C, Watts R, Westman K, Witter J, Yazici H, Luqmani R (2009) EULAR recommendations for the management of large vessel vasculitis. Ann Rheum Dis 68:318–323

Nesher G, Berkun Y, Mates M, Baras M, Rubinow A, Sonnenblick M (2004) Low-dose aspirin and prevention of cranial ischemic complications in giant cell arteritis. Arthritis Rheum 50:1332–1337

Nuenninghoff DM, Hunder GG, Christianson TJ, McClelland RL, Matteson EL (2003a) Incidence and predictors of large-artery complication (aortic aneurysm, aortic dissection, and/or large-artery stenosis) in patients with giant cell arteritis: a population-based study over 50 years. Arthritis Rheum 48:3522–3531

Nuenninghoff DM, Hunder GG, Christianson TJ, McClelland RL, Matteson EL (2003b) Mortality of large-artery complication (aortic aneurysm, aortic dissection, and/or large-artery stenosis) in patients with giant cell arteritis: a population-based study over 50 years. Arthritis Rheum 48:3532–3537

Ray-Chaudhuri N, Kine DA, Tijani SO, Parums DV, Cartlidge N, Strong NP, Dayan MR (2002) Effect of prior steroid treatment on temporal artery biopsy findings in giant cell arteritis. Br J Ophthalmol 86: 530–532

Robb-Nicholson C, Chang RW, Anderson S, Roberts WN, Longtine J, Corson J, Larson M, George D, Green J, Bryant G et al (1988) Diagnostic value of the history and examination in giant cell arteritis: a clinical pathological study of 81 temporal artery biopsies. J Rheumatol 15:1793–1796

Salvarani C, Cantini F, Hunder GG (2008) Polymyalgia rheumatica and giant-cell arteritis. Lancet 372: 234–245

Salvarani C, Cimino L, Macchioni P, Consonni D, Cantini F, Bajocchi G, Pipitone N, Catanoso MG, Boiardi L (2005) Risk factors for visual loss in an Italian population-based cohort of patients with giant cell arteritis. Arthritis Rheum 53:293–297

Salvarani C, Macchioni PL, Tartoni PL, Rossi F, Baricchi R, Castri C, Chiaravalloti F, Portioli I (1987) Polymyalgia rheumatica and giant cell arteritis: a 5-year epidemiologic and clinical study in Reggio Emilia, Italy. Clin Exp Rheumatol 5:205–215

Schmidt WA (2007) Technology insight: the role of color and power Doppler ultrasonography in rheumatology. Nat Clin Pract Rheumatol 3:35–42, quiz 59

Smeeth L, Cook C, Hall AJ (2006) Incidence of diagnosed polymyalgia rheumatica and temporal arteritis in the United Kingdom, 1990–2001. Ann Rheum Dis 65:1093–1098

Solans-Laque R, Bosch-Gil JA, Molina-Catenario CA, Ortega-Aznar A, Alvarez-Sabin J, Vilardell-Tarres M (2008) Stroke and multi-infarct dementia as presenting symptoms of giant cell arteritis: report of 7 cases and review of the literature. Medicine 87:335–344

Solomon S, Cappa KG (1987) The headache of temporal arteritis. J Am Geriatr Soc 35:163–165

Wong RL, Korn JH (1986) Temporal arteritis without an elevated erythrocyte sedimentation rate. Case report and review of the literature. Am J Med 80:959–964

Zenone T (2007) Fever of unknown origin in rheumatic diseases. Infect Dis Clin North Am 21:1115–1135, x–xi

39 Trigeminal Neuralgia

Giorgio Cruccu[1] · *Andrea Truini*[1] · *Joanna M. Zakrzewska*[2]
[1]Sapienza University of Rome, Rome, Italy
[2]Eastman Dental Hospital, UCLH NHS Foundation Trust, London, UK

Paolo Martelletti, Timothy J. Steiner (eds.), *Handbook of Headache*, DOI 10.1007/978-88-470-1700-9_39,
© Lifting The Burden 2011

Abstract: This chapter addresses the diagnostic and therapeutic problems of trigeminal neuralgia (TN). While classical TN has no apparent cause other than vascular compressions, symptomatic TN is caused by a demonstrable structural lesion such as cerebellopontine angle tumors or multiple sclerosis. Categorization of TN into typical and atypical forms is based on symptom constellation, and not etiology. Some clinical criteria that were used to distinguish between classic and symptomatic TN, such as age at onset, involvement of the ophthalmic division, and unresponsiveness to treatment, are no longer considered reliable. Bilateral pain and clinically manifest sensory deficits are rare occurrences even in symptomatic TN. Hence, MRI or trigeminal reflex testing is recommended in all patients. Carbamazepine (CBZ) and oxcarbazepine (OXC) are the first-choice medical treatment. Patients that reach adequate dosage of CBZ/OXC without getting sufficient pain relief should be made aware of the available surgical interventions. Some surgical procedures, that is, Gasserian ganglion percutaneous techniques, gamma knife, and microvascular decompression, are extremely efficacious with relatively few complications.

Established Knowledge

Definitions and Epidemiology

The International Association for the Study of Pain (IASP) defines TN as sudden, usually unilateral, severe, brief, stabbing, recurrent episodes of pain in the distribution of one or more branches of the trigeminal nerve. Trigeminal neuralgia (TN) can be distinguished in classic TN (with no apparent cause other than vascular compressions) and symptomatic TN (pain indistinguishable from that of classic TN but caused by a demonstrable structural lesion other than vascular compressions) (Headache Classification Subcommittee of IHS 2004; Cruccu et al. 2008; Gronseth et al. 2008). It should be noted that categorization of TN into typical and atypical forms is based on symptom constellation, and not etiology.

Recent epidemiological studies of general practice research databases reported a TN incidence ranging from 12.6 to 26.8 per 100,000/year, with the incidence increasing with age (16.3 in the fourth decade, 30.6 in patients older than 80 years) (Hall et al. 2006; Koopman et al. 2009). Classic TN is more common in women than in men (female-to-male ratio 3:2) and on the right side of the face (right-to-left ratio 3:2) (Cruccu et al. 2006; Koopman et al. 2009). Symptomatic TN occurs in about 15% of patients (Cruccu et al. 2008; Gronseth et al. 2008).

Clinical Features

Pain distribution is unilateral (bilateral TN may sometimes occur in multiple sclerosis). The maxillary division is the most frequently affected both in classic and symptomatic TN. The involvement of the ophthalmic division on its own is less common and was traditionally considered indicative of symptomatic TN, now it is more likely to be a case of a trigeminal autonomic cephalalgia. Strongly indicative of a symptomatic form, often a focal neuropathy, is pain in the tongue, which is usually spared in classic TN. The pain is very rarely felt directly in the teeth (Bowsher 2000). Pain, usually referred to as stabbing or electric-shock-like, is brief and paroxysmal, lasting a few seconds. Some patients will describe a prolonged burning, aching pain of decreased severity after these attacks and these patients have been termed to have atypical TN (see future research for more details). The condition may after weeks or months go into complete remission for many months. However, over time, the relapse rates gradually become more frequent and the pain-free periods fewer. Paroxysms may be provoked by stimulating cutaneous or mucous trigeminal territories (trigger zones), regardless of the distribution of the perceived pain. Gently touching the face, washing or shaving, talking, brushing the teeth, chewing, swallowing, or even a slight breeze, but not thermal or painful stimuli, can trigger the paroxysms. Pain provokes brief muscle spasms of the facial muscles, thus producing the tic. Lacrimation, rhinorrhea, or redness of the face is very rare. If these autonomic features are noted then the diagnosis of an autonomic cephalalgia must be considered.

Differential Diagnosis Between Classic and Symptomatic Forms

Several clinical features such as affected division, age at onset, and sensory deficits were traditionally considered useful for distinguishing symptomatic from classic TN. However, recent studies and systematic reviews of the evidence-based literature (Cruccu et al. 2006; Cruccu et al. 2008; Gronseth et al. 2008) came to different conclusions (❷ Fig. 39.1). The involvement of the ophthalmic division is equally rare (21% and 23%) in the two forms. The mean onset age is significantly lower in symptomatic (48 years) than in classic TN (57 years), but there is too much overlap in patients with classic TN and symptomatic TN for this predictor to be considered clinically useful. Although the presence of trigeminal sensory deficits or bilateral involvement of the trigeminal nerves increases the risk of symptomatic

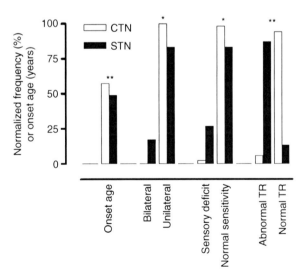

◘ Fig. 39.1
Differential diagnosis between classical (CTN) and symptomatic trigeminal neuralgia (STN). Onset age is lower in CTN than STN (**$P < 0.0001$). Bilateral neuralgia and sensory deficits only occur in STN (*$P < 0.001$). Trigeminal reflexes (TR) are abnormal in STN (87%) and normal in CTN (94%) (**$P < 0.0001$). (Modified from Cruccu et al. 2008, with permission)

TN, the absence of these features does by no means rule out symptomatic TN. Neuroimaging and neurophysiological studies are considered the best tools to distinguish symptomatic from classic TN (see paragraph on diagnostic test).

Pain Mechanisms

According to most investigators, classic TN is due to a vascular compression of the trigeminal root by tortuous or aberrant vessels (❷ *Fig. 39.2*). Microsurgical interventions in the posterior fossa have shown that the compressing vessel is most often the superior cerebellar artery (about 75% of cases) (Sindou et al. 2008). Support for this view comes from MRI studies reporting a frequent contact between vessels and the trigeminal root (Meaney et al. 1995). Nevertheless, other investigators do not support the view that a vascular compression is the main factor, because bilateral neurovascular contacts are frequent in patients with unilateral TN (71% according to Anderson et al. 2006), as well as unilateral or bilateral contacts in subjects who do not have TN (75% according to Kress et al. 2006). Possibly, several factors may contribute to the development of TN. Indeed, it is a fairly consistent finding that 25–30% of patients do not experience complete and persistent pain relief after microvascular decompression (Cruccu et al. 2008).

Symptomatic TN can be related to cerebellopontine angle tumors, which compress the trigeminal nerve root. Multiple sclerosis (MS) is the most commonly related disorder with TN

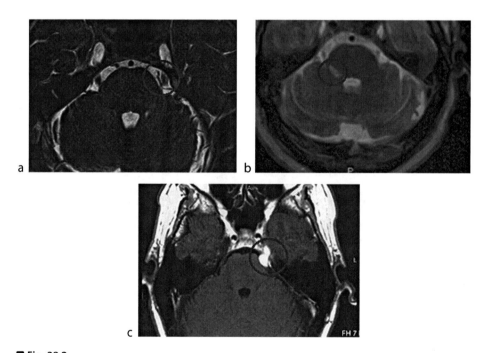

◘ Fig. 39.2

MRI findings in patients with trigeminal neuralgia. Neurovascular conflict between trigeminal root and a cerebellar artery in a patient with classical trigeminal neuralgia (a). Demyelinating plaque affecting the intra-axial course of the trigeminal afferents (b). Benign tumor compressing the trigeminal root (c) (courtesy of Dr. E. Tinelli)

with up to 2–4% of patients with TN having MS (Jensen 1982). Neurophysiological, neuroimaging, and pathological studies indicate that the demyelinating plaque that provokes TN affects the intrapontine presynaptic primary afferents near the root entry zone (Cruccu et al. 2009; Gass et al. 1997). Both in classic and symptomatic TN, the primary site of damage is thought to be peripheral near the root entry zone. Demyelination of the primary afferents is necessary (Love and Coakham 2001). Whether produced by multiple sclerosis or chronic compression exerted by a blood vessel or a benign tumor, demyelination increases the susceptibility of the nerve fibers to ectopic excitation, ephaptic transmission, and high-frequency discharges (Burchiel 1980). Although the primary cause of TN must necessarily affect the primary afferents, the pathophysiological mechanism may or may not secondarily involve the central neurons. Particularly for atypical TN, the sensitization of the second- or third-order neurons has been proposed as potential mechanisms (Obermann et al. 2007; Leonard et al. 2009).

Neurophysiological Testing

According to the EFNS guidelines on neuropathic pain assessment and the AAN-EFNS guidelines on trigeminal neuralgia management (Cruccu et al. 2008, 2010), the neurophysiological recording of trigeminal reflexes represents the most useful and reliable test in the neurophysiological diagnosis of trigeminal pains. The trigeminal reflexes consist of a series of reflex responses that assess function of trigeminal afferents from all trigeminal territories as well as trigeminal central circuits in the midbrain, pons, and medulla.

An objective demonstration of dysfunction is provided in all patients with pain secondary to a documented disease, such as symptomatic trigeminal neuralgia. As a tool for disclosing symptomatic TN, neurophysiological testing of trigeminal reflexes provides a diagnostic accuracy similar to that of MRI (Cruccu et al. 2006). In a meta-analysis of 10 trials in 628 patients, trigeminal reflexes were abnormal in STN (87%) and normal in CTN (94%) (Cruccu et al. 2008).

Trigeminal evoked potentials, regardless of the type of stimulation (laser or electrical), appear to be more sensitive than trigeminal reflexes in patients with facial pains secondary to structural lesions, such as trigeminal sensory neuropathy, postherpetic neuralgia, Wallenberg syndrome, multiple sclerosis, or cerbellopontine angle tumors (Leandri et al. 1987; Cruccu et al. 2001; Truini et al. 2003, 2008). Unfortunately, in typical TN their specificity is too low: in a meta-analysis of 209 patients the specificity was 64% (Cruccu et al. 2008; Gronseth et al. 2008).

Neuroimaging and Diagnostic Process

All patients with a facial pain of unclear origin or suspected of a symptomatic neurological lesion should undergo imaging studies. Currently, there are many facial pains of unknown origin which make it difficult to determine which patients need imaging. Furthermore, CT scans are not sufficiently accurate in conditions such as multiple sclerosis, small tumors, and vascular anomalies.

A diagnostic protocol for patients with trigeminal pain should rely primarily on trigeminal reflexes: the technique is easier and less invasive than that for evoked potentials and the finding of any abnormality implies an underlying structural lesion.

In all patients with TN we recommend to perform, at least once, MRI and/or trigeminal reflex testing, according to local availability.

Various MRI techniques are used prior to performance of a microvascular decompression to demonstrate neurovascular contacts. Unfortunately, no technique is currently considered reliable, both because neurosurgeons may find neurocompression at operation even if the MRI is negative and because of the high frequency of asymptomatic contacts (Cruccu et al. 2008; Gronseth et al. 2008). Hopefully in the future the problem may be solved by the MRI demonstration not only of a contact but also of nerve damage, as suggested by recent findings (Herweh et al. 2007).

Medical Treatment

Systematic reviews (Wiffen et al. 2010; Yang et al. 2011; Zakrzewska and Linskey 2009) and international guidelines (Cruccu et al. 2008; Gronseth et al. 2008) have all shown that the most effective drugs for this condition are the sodium-channel blocker antiepileptic drugs. One of the oldest drugs, carbamazepine (CBZ), still has the highest level of evidence. The other drug of choice recommended by international guidelines is oxcarbazepine (OXC) which is a derivative of CBZ. In a comparison between these two drugs, efficacy was shown to be very similar but tolerability is better with OXC. Unlike CBZ, OXC does not activate liver enzymes, which means that OXC has fewer drug interactions. Other drugs shown to be of limited efficacy in randomized controlled trials have included baclofen and lamotrigine (Cruccu et al. 2008; Gronseth et al. 2008). There is no data on the use of polytherapy as is common practice in epilepsy (❷ *Table 39.1*).

Practical Guidelines on Medical Therapies

The following need to be kept in mind when using these drugs

- Patients of Chinese and Thai origin need to be tested for their HLA status as they have a higher propensity to develop severe adverse events such as Stevens–Johnson syndrome when given carbamazepine.
- When using these drugs, it is essential to start with low doses and escalate the dose very slowly in order to decrease the likelihood of adverse events.
- Blood monitoring should take place on a regular basis when the drugs are first introduced and then repeated potentially on a yearly basis but more frequently if higher doses are used and significant side effects reported.
- Drug interactions are very common with carbamazepine including homeopathic medications and certain foods, for example, grapefruit.
- Patients with MS are often more resistant to drug therapy and these drugs may worsen their MS symptoms.

Surgical Treatment

With time, many patients will develop more intense pain and the drugs need to be raised to such a level that severe side effects begin to affect the quality of life. Clinical studies

◘ Table 39.1

Drugs used in management of trigeminal neuralgia

Drug	Average doses	Efficacy	Side effects	Comments
Baclofen	50–80 mg	NNT 1.4 (1–2.6) may be effective	Ataxia, lethargy, fatigue, nausea, vomiting	Evaluated in RCT useful as add-on therapy, beware rapid withdraw
Carbamazepine	300–1,000 mg	NNT 2.6 (2–4), effective	Drowsiness, ataxia, headaches, nausea, vomiting constipation, blurred vision, rash, reduced white cell count, hyponatremia higher doses	Introduce slowly, drug interactions retard form useful in controlled patients
Clonazepam	4–8 mg	Low	Severe drowsiness – 60%, addictive	Case series only
Gabapentin+ topical ropivacaine	1,800–3,600 mg, in RCT also trigger injection weekly	Good	Ataxia, dizziness, drowsiness, nausea, headache	One RCT with ropivacaine, other reports are case series
Lamotrigine	200–400 mg	NNT 2.1 (1.3–6.1) as add-on medication	Dizziness, drowsiness, constipation, ataxia, diplopia, irritability, rapid dose escalation leads to rashes	Slow escalation important
Oxcarbazepine	300–1,200 mg	Effective	Vertigo, fatigue, dizziness, nausea, hyponatremia in high doses	RCTs and case series. No major drug interactions, better tolerated than carbamazepine
Phenytoin	200–300 mg	Good	Ataxia, lethargy, nausea, headache, behavioral changes, folate deficiency in prolonged use, gingival hypertrophy	Case series only. Small margin for dose escalation, used intravenously for immediate effect
Pregabalin	150–600 mg	Good	Ataxia, dizziness, drowsiness, nausea, headache	Case series and cohort data. Rapid escalation possible
Valproic acid	600–1,200 mg	Poor	Irritability, restlessness, tremor, confusion, nausea, rash, weight gain	Case series only

RCT randomized controlled trials, *NNT* number needed to treat, check dosages in National Formularies

(Taylor et al. 1981; Zakrzewska and Patsalos 2002) in a long-term cohort study showed how the efficacy of carbamazepine and oxcarbazepine reduced over time. With the large range of antiepileptics now available, it is tempting to continue trying antiepileptics both as monotherapy and as polytherapy before considering a more surgical approach.

There is very little high-quality evidence to provide guidance as to when patients should be offered surgical procedures. Surveys among patients who have undergone surgery have suggested that on balance they would have preferred to have their surgical procedures early (Zakrzewska et al. 2005). However, hypothetical decision analysis about treatments among 156 patients showed that surgical treatments were only marginally more likely to be chosen than medical management (Spatz et al. 2007).

Surgical management can be carried out at three different levels (peripheral procedures, Gasserian ganglion procedures, and posterior fossa surgery) and each treatment has its pros and cons. Review of all surgical treatments was done when preparing international guidelines and Cochrane review on surgical management (in progress). The following data are based on these systematic reviews.

Peripheral Procedures

These treatments aim at the destruction of the trigger points and include neurectomy, laser therapy, streptomycin injections, and pulsed radiofrequency thermocoagulation. Those studies that include Kaplan–Meier survival graphs show that the mean time before 50% of patients have a recurrence of pain is 10 months (Zakrzewska and Thomas 1993). In many of these studies, patients have also had to continue some low dose levels of their antiepileptic drugs. There are relatively few side effects. These treatments have been largely abandoned.

Gasserian Ganglion Procedures

The Gasserian ganglion is the location for many of the ablative/destructive procedures, which aim to reduce pain transmission without compromising other sensory functions. These procedures are done under a short general anesthetic or heavy sedation. X-ray control is essential in order to locate the Gasserian ganglion lying above the foramen ovale. Patients tend to stay in overnight. These procedures can generally be carried out on all patients, even those who are medically unfit.

At this level the nerve can be:

- Coagulated by temperatures ranging between 60°C and 80°C – peripheral radiofrequency thermocoagulation (rhizotomy).
- Bathed in glycerol – percutaneous glycerol rhizotomy.
- Compressed by a Foley catheter balloon – balloon compression.

The average time to recurrence, a point at which 50% of patients will get a recurrence, is around 4 years (Cruccu et al. 2008; Gronseth et al. 2008). As these procedures are ablative, they inevitably result in sensory loss. This can be very varied both in extent and in severity. A very small percentage of patients can develop the condition of anesthesia dolorosa which is virtually untreatable. Up to 60% of patients can find these sensory changes to affect their quality of life (Zakrzewska et al. 1999). Most of the other side effects noted diminish with time. These procedures can be repeated.

Posterior Fossa Surgery

Microvascular decompression and partial sensory rhizotomy are major neurosurgical procedures which need to be done by neurosurgeons skilled in posterior fossa surgery. A postauricular incision is made in order to gain access to the posterior fossa where the vascular compression of the trigeminal nerve is identified. Compressing arterial vessels are carefully dissected off the nerve and then separated from the nerve by insertion of Teflon or use of a vascular sling. If venous compressions are found, the vessels can often be coagulated. After ensuring that the trigeminal nerve is free of any compressions, the area is meticulously closed in layers to prevent CSF leaks and encroachment on the mastoid air cells. Some neurosurgeons if they do not find a compression of the nerve will do a small partial sensory rhizotomy, which means that the patients are at risk of getting sensory changes.

This procedure offers the best long-term prognosis as at 10 years 70% of patients are still likely to be pain free (Cruccu et al. 2008; Gronseth et al. 2008). A recent study showed that patients with typical TN more likely are pain free immediately after surgery and less likely have a recurrence of pain within 2 years than patients with atypical TN (Miller et al. 2009a). However, as for any major neurosurgical procedure, posterior fossa surgery carries a small mortality risk of 0.2–0.4% (Cruccu et al. 2008; Gronseth et al. 2008). The other major complications are those of a stroke and postoperative CSF leak, which may require readmission. Aseptic meningitis and headaches are other more minor immediate operative complications. The most common long-term complication is that of ipsilateral hearing loss which can be as high as 4% (Cruccu et al. 2008; Gronseth et al. 2008).

Irradiation of Trigeminal Nerve

The final procedure that has been introduced most recently is that of gamma knife or other forms of radiation. Having located the trigeminal nerve in its path between the Gasserian ganglion and the brain, entry doses of radiotherapy between 60G and 90G are applied. This procedure is the least invasive of all and does not require inpatient admission. On average, pain relief is gained within a week but improvement may be noticed for up to 6 months. With increasing long-term reports it seems that the results are similar to other ablative procedures and 40–50% of patients can expect to be pain free at 5 years. Although initially these procedures were thought to have no risks attached to them, it is now found that up to 3% of patients may develop sensory loss which often occurs some 6 months after the procedure. Sensory loss may be mild but it can range up to the full-blown anesthesia dolorosa.

Psychological Support

Quality of life data and measures of depression and anxiety have shown that TN may affect the psychological well-being (Zakrzewska 2006). One way of helping the patients is to direct them to support groups who will enable contact with other patients, offer the opportunity to exchange views, and meet health-care professionals outside the conventional consulting room (Zakrzewska et al. 2009).

Current Research

Some studies on the basis of symptom constellation distinguish classic TN into two forms: typical and atypical (Obermann et al. 2007; Leonard et al. 2009; Miller et al. 2009a). Whereas in typical TN the patient is usually pain free between paroxysms, in patients with atypical TN a dull, burning, continuous background pain persist in between. A recent clinical study (Miller et al. 2009a) showed that the two groups of patients differ in several clinical features. Patients with typical are younger and have a more frequent right-sided pain than those with atypical TN. A neurovascular contact and a longer remission period after surgery are more frequent in patients with typical than in those with atypical TN (Miller et al. 2009b; Zacest et al. 2010). Although some patients progress from typical to atypical TN, usually the two forms represent distinct clinical entities. Although studies by Miller and Zacest proposed clear-cut differences between the two forms of TN, and identified the typical as a type 1 and the atypical as a type 2 TN, further studies are needed to elucidate whether the two forms are distinct entities and the clinicians have to differently approach them.

Although TN is universally considered the best-known facial pain in clinical practice, further research is needed in several areas: epidemiological studies to investigate risk factors, and the role of heredity and genetics, neurophysiological and neuroimaging studies to clarify the underlying mechanisms of atypical forms of TN (Obermann et al. 2007), and neuroimaging studies to propose widely agreed imaging techniques able to assess not only the mere neurovascular contact but also the actual nerve damage (Herweh et al. 2007). Larger, higher-quality RCTs are needed to assess emerging drugs, the use of polypharmacy, and the management of patients with TN associated to multiple sclerosis. Studies directly addressing the appropriateness of referral to surgery are needed and it is essential that there are more high-quality RCTs and long-term prospective trials of surgical procedures and that these are compared in head-to-head studies.

References

Anderson VC, Berryhill PC, Sandquist MA, Ciaverella DP, Nesbit GM, Burchiel KJ (2006) High-resolution three-dimensional magnetic resonance angiography and three-dimensional spoiled gradient-recalled imaging in the evaluation of neurovascular compression in patients with trigeminal neuralgia: a double-blind pilot study. Neurosurgery 58: 666–673

Bowsher D (2000) Trigeminal neuralgia: a symptomatic study of 126 successive patients with and without previous interventions. Pain Clin 12:93–101

Burchiel KJ (1980) Ectopic impulse generation in focally demyelinated trigeminal nerve. Exp Neurol 69: 423–429

Cruccu G, Leandri M, Iannetti GD, Mascia A, Romaniello A, Truini A, Galeotti F, Manfredi M (2001) Small-fiber dysfunction in trigeminal neuralgia: carbamazepine effect on laser-evoked potentials. Neurology 56:1722–1726

Cruccu G, Biasiotta A, Galeotti F, Iannetti GD, Truini A, Gronseth G (2006) Diagnostic accuracy of trigeminal reflex testing in trigeminal neuralgia. Neurology 66:139–141

Cruccu G, Gronseth G, Alksne J, Argoff C, Brainin M, Burchiel K, Nurmikko T, Zakrzewska JM (2008) AAN-EFNS guidelines on trigeminal neuralgia management. Eur J Neurol 15:1013–1028

Cruccu G, Biasiotta A, Di Rezze S, Fiorelli M, Galeotti F, Innocenti P, Mameli S, Millefiorini E, Truini A (2009) Trigeminal neuralgia and pain related to multiple sclerosis. Pain 143:186–191

Cruccu G, Sommer C, Anand P, Attal N, Baron R, Garcia-Larrea L, Haanpaa M, Jensen TS, Serra J, Treede RD (2010) EFNS guidelines on neuropathic pain assessment: revised 2009. Eur J Neurol 17(8):1010–1018. [8 Mar Epub ahead of print]

Gass A, Kitchen N, MacManus DG, Moseley IF, Hennerici MG, Miller DH (1997) Trigeminal neuralgia in patients with multiple sclerosis: lesion localization with magnetic resonance imaging. Neurology 49:1142–1144

Gronseth G, Cruccu G, Alksne J, Argoff C, Brainin M, Burchiel K, Nurmikko T, Zakrzewska JM (2008) Practice parameter: the diagnostic evaluation and treatment of trigeminal neuralgia (an evidence-based review): report of the quality standards subcommittee of the American Academy of Neurology and the European Federation of Neurological Societies. Neurology 71:1183–1190

Hall GC, Carroll D, Parry D, McQuay HJ (2006) Epidemiology and treatment of neuropathic pain: the UK primary care perspective. Pain 122:156–162

Headache Classification Subcommittee of IHS (2004) The international classification of headache disorders. Cephalalgia 24(Suppl 1):1–160

Herweh C, Kress B, Rasche D, Tronnier V, Tröger J, Sartor K, Stippich C (2007) Loss of anisotropy in trigeminal neuralgia revealed by diffusion tensor imaging. Neurology 68:776–778

Jensen TS, Rasmussen P, Reske-Nielsen E (1982) Association of trigeminal neuralgia with multiple sclerosis: clinical and pathological features. Acta Neurol Scand 65(3):182–189

Koopman JS, Dieleman JP, Huygen FJ, de Mos M, Martin CG, Sturkenboom MC (2009) Incidence of facial pain in the general population. Pain 147(1–3):122–127

Kress B, Schindler M, Rasche D, Hähnel S, Tronnier V, Sartor K (2006) Trigeminal neuralgia: how often are trigeminal nerve-vessel contacts found by MRI in normal volunteers. Rofo 178:313–315

Leandri M, Parodi CI, Zattoni J, Favale E (1987) Subcortical and cortical responses following infraorbital nerve stimulation in man. Electroencephalogr Clin Neurophysiol 66:253–262

Leonard G, Goffaux P, Mathieu D, Blanchard J, Kenny B, Marchand S (2009) Evidence of descending inhibition deficits in atypical but not classical trigeminal neuralgia. Pain 147:217–223

Love S, Coakham HB (2001) Trigeminal neuralgia: pathology and pathogenesis. Brain 124:2347–2360

Meaney JF, Eldridge PR, Dunn LT, Nixon TE, Whitehouse GH, Miles JB (1995) Demonstration of neurovascular compression in trigeminal neuralgia with magnetic resonance imaging. Comparison with surgical findings in 52 consecutive operative cases. J Neurosurg 83:799–805

Miller JP, Acar F, Burchiel KJ (2009a) Classification of trigeminal neuralgia: clinical, therapeutic, and prognostic implications in a series of 144 patients undergoing microvascular decompression. J Neurosurg 111:1231–1234

Miller JP, Magill ST, Acar F, Burchiel KJ (2009b) Predictors of long-term success after microvascular decompression for trigeminal neuralgia. J Neurosurg 110:620–626

Obermann M, Yoon MS, Ese D, Maschke M, Kaube H, Diener HC, Katsarava Z (2007) Impaired trigeminal nociceptive processing in patients with trigeminal neuralgia. Neurology 69:835–841

Sindou M, Leston JM, Decullier E, Chapuis F (2008) Microvascular decompression for trigeminal neuralgia: the importance of a noncompressive technique – Kaplan-Meier analysis in a consecutive series of 330 patients. Neurosurgery 63:341–350

Spatz AL, Zakrzewska JM, Kay EJ (2007) Decision analysis of medical and surgical treatments for trigeminal neuralgia: how patient evaluations of benefits and risks affect the utility of treatment decisions. Pain 131:302–310

Taylor JC, Brauer S, Espir MLE (1981) Long-term treatment of trigeminal neuralgia. Postgrad Med J 57: 16–18

Truini A, Haanpää M, Zucchi R, Galeotti F, Iannetti GD, Romaniello A, Cruccu G (2003) Laser-evoked potentials in post-herpetic neuralgia. Clin Neurophysiol 114:702–709

Truini A, Galeotti F, Haanpaa M, Zucchi R, Albanesi A, Biasiotta A, Gatti A, Cruccu G (2008) Pathophysiology of pain in postherpetic neuralgia: a clinical and neurophysiological study. Pain 140:405–410

Wiffen PJ, Collins S, McQuay HJ, Carroll D, Jadad A, Moore RA (2010) Anticonvulsant drugs for acute and chronic pain. Cochrane Database Syst Rev 20 Jan 2010(1):CD001133

Yang M, Zhou M, He L, Chen N, Zakrzewska JM (2011) Non-antiepileptic drugs for trigeminal neuralgia. Cochrane Database Syst Rev 1:CD004029

Zacest AC, Magill ST, Miller J, Burchiel KJ (2010) Preoperative magnetic resonance imaging in type 2 trigeminal neuralgia. J Neurosurg 113(3):511–515. [29 Jan Epub ahead of print]

Zakrzewska JM (2006) Insights: facts and stories behind trigeminal neuralgia. Trigeminal Neuralgia Association, Gainesville

Zakrzewska JM, Linskey ME (2009) Trigeminal neuralgia. Clin Evid pii:1207

Zakrzewska JM, Patsalos PN (2002) Long-term cohort study comparing medical (oxcarbazepine) and surgical management of intractable trigeminal neuralgia. Pain 95(3):259–266

Zakrzewska JM, Thomas DG (1993) Patient's assessment of outcome after three surgical procedures for the management of trigeminal neuralgia. Acta Neurochir Wien 122:225–230

Zakrzewska JM, Sawsan J, Bulman JS (1999) A prospective, longitudinal study on patients with trigeminal neuralgia who underwent radiofrequency thermocoagulation of the Gasserian ganglion. Pain 79:51–58

Zakrzewska JM, Lopez BC, Kim SE, Coakham HB (2005) Patient reports of satisfaction after microvascular decompression and partial sensory rhizotomy for trigeminal neuralgia. Neurosurgery 56:1304–1311

Zakrzewska JM, Jorns TP, Spatz A (2009) Patient led conferences – who attends, are their expectations met and do they vary in three different countries? Eur J Pain 13:486–491

40 Persistent Idiopathic Facial Pain

Rigmor Jensen[1] · *Dimos D. Mitsikostas*[2] · *Christian Wöber*[3]
[1]Glostrup Hospital, University of Copenhagen, Glostrup, Copenhagen, Denmark
[2]Athens Naval Hospital, Athens, Greece
[3]Medical University of Vienna, Vienna, Austria

Paolo Martelletti, Timothy J. Steiner (eds.), *Handbook of Headache*, DOI 10.1007/978-88-470-1700-9_40,
© Lifting The Burden 2011

Abstract: Persistent Idiopathic Facial Pain (PIFP) is a moderate or severe continuous pain disorder in the facial region. The pain is usually deep and poorly localized, and the quality is of burning, cramping, or dull quality. The incidence is estimated to 2–4 per 100,000 but exact epidemiological data are lacking. Persistent idiopathic facial pain is a difficult diagnostic group compared to other pain categories and symptomatic causes must always be sought. The underlying pathophysiology is yet unknown and therapy is widely unspecific and ineffective. The existing literature is reviewed and summarized, the possible differential diagnoses are listed, and the existing treatment strategies are presented. The optimal outcome is achieved by a multidisciplinary approach focusing on a combination of symptomatic medication, patient education, cognitive therapy, and coping strategies. In conclusion, patients with PIFP remain a complicated group to diagnose and to treat. The scientific evidence for a specific entity, a clear pathophysiological mechanism and effective treatment strategies are still lacking. Further field testing and clinical characterizations of these severely affected patients are highly needed and the noncommittal title *Persistent Idiopathic Facial Pain* is preferable until further evidence is available.

Clinical Features

By definition, the persistent idiopathic facial pain (PIFP) is localized in the specific anatomical region, where the boundaries of the face are defined by the hairline, the frontal area to the caudal limitation of the lower jaw. The pain is persistent, that is, present for more than 3 months and present on a daily basis, underlining the continuous and chronic pain in contrast to the paroxysmal but otherwise chronic pain disorders with pain-free intervals during the day, as cluster headaches and trigeminal neuralgia (TN). The pain is deep and poorly localized, and fairly intense in most cases (Zebenholzer et al. 2005; Headache Classification Committee of the International Headache Society 2004). The quality of pain may vary and words such as burning, cramping, tearing, or dull quality are most often reported. Patients present with unilateral location around the cheek and/or lower jaw although bilateral affliction may develop over time (Headache Classification Committee of the International Headache Society 2004; Zebenholzer et al. 2005; Graff-Radford 2009). Like TN, there is no specific nocturnal pain and the sleep is rarely severely affected.

The exact prevalence is still unknown as large-scale epidemiological studies and a clear consensus among specialties about the diagnostic criteria are lacking (Brenoliel et al. 2008; Graff-Radford 2009; Cornelissen et al. 2009). Like in most other pain disorders, a majority of females, representing around 75% of patients, is reported whereas the relation to age is actually unknown. In our hands, the typical patient is a middle-aged woman, with a clinical presentation as a complicated, doubtful patient with a fairly typical pain history, numerous investigations, and prior contacts to dentists and pain specialists. In an earlier study from a pain clinic, one third of the patients also reported the pain to be preceded by an operation or a trauma, challenging the applied term *idiopathic.*

Diagnostic Criteria

PIFP does not have the characteristics of the cranial neuralgias and is not attributed to another disorder. The ICHD-II diagnostic criteria are presented in ❷ *Table 40.1.* The criteria have been studied in several papers and several suggestions for revisions have been introduced

◘ Table 40.1

Diagnostic criteria group 13.18.4 persistent idiopathic facial pain (Headache Classification Committee of the International Headache Society 2004)

A. Pain in the face, present daily and persisting for all or most of the day, fulfilling criteria B and C
B. Pain is confined at onset to a limited area on one side of the face, and is deep and poorly localized
C. Pain is not associated with sensory loss or other physical signs
D. Investigations including x-ray of face and jaws do not demonstrate any relevant abnormality

(Zebenholzer et al. 2005; Zebenholzer et al. 2006; Brenoliel et al. 2008; Cornelissen et al. 2009). Especially, dental and oromaxillar pain specialists have challenged the present ICHD-II criteria but so far no consensus has been reached and the ICHD-II criteria are very widely used and accepted.

The term "persistent and idiopathic" is also well accepted and clearly better than the former term "atypical facial pain."

In a detailed study from an Austrian pain clinic, it was found that the pain is quite intense and not as mild to moderate as previously believed (Zebenholzer et al. 2005). The patients may also report bilateral pain but in most cases they present as unilateral cases and then progress over time.

In the ICHD-II classification, it is commented that PIFP may be initiated by surgery or injury to the face, teeth, or gums but persists without any demonstrable local cause, thereby challenging the term idiopathic. In the prior study mentioned above, a large group of patients could not be classified according to ICHD-II as their symptoms were precipitated by external stimuli, various procedures (especially dental procedures) and they presented with sensory disturbances or with facial pain spreading to the head. In future field testing studies, it may therefore be of importance to include and classify all these types of facial pain irrespective of the various diagnostic criteria system as the field is difficult and complex and all patients do not fit into these systems irrespective their similarities. A minor revision of the criteria addressing these concerns has thus been proposed (Zebenholzer et al. 2005; Zebenholzer et al. 2006).

Laboratory Examinations and Imaging

Only limited evidence for investigations exists but there is a general consensus that these patients should be extensively evaluated by an oral/maxillofacial and ear–nose–throat specialist as well as by a neurologist. Unfortunately, there is no specification as to which additional test or imaging should be applied. The increasing frequency of posterior fossa exploration and magnetic resonance imaging in TN has demonstrated that many, possibly most, patients with this condition have compression of the trigeminal root by tortuous or aberrant vessels but so far no such consistent abnormalities have been noted in PIFP. In our hands, a minimum of laboratory examinations containing inflammatory and rheumatological biomarkers and an MR-scan including an MRA of the brain, the face, and the trigeminal nerves are recommended.

Differential Diagnosis

The term idiopathic indicates that the pain disorder rather is a diagnosis of exclusion than a specific diagnostic entity. In a comparative study of the diagnostic criteria, ICHD-I and II,

97 cases with facial pain were analyzed and of these 20 patients were diagnosed with PIFP (Zebenholzer et al. 2005). Hereof, the pain was preceded by traumas, operations, dental or other procedures in 7 patients leaving this group as a very difficult diagnostic group compared to other pain categories (Zebenholzer et al. 2005). The possible differential diagnoses are numerous and symptomatic causes are and must always be sought (Graff-Radford 2009). In all consultations, a clear and detailed history and clinical examination intra- and extraorally including a sensory examination are required before any treatment attempts are initiated. The most frequent causes in the differential diagnosis are listed and commented in ❷ *Table 40.2*. The distinction between TN and PIFP rarely represents any problem as the TN patient presents with a completely different pain quality, very intense paroxysms, and is asymptomatic between paroxysms of TN although a dull background pain may also persist in some long-standing TN cases. A clear history of a trauma or dental treatment preceding the pain may alert the physician to search for a nerve lesion although causal relations are very difficult to prove in these severely affected patients with very long-lasting pain disorders. Recently, the use of specific local analgesics in 4% solutions for mandibular blocks is suspected to cause permanent nerve lesions resulting in persistent pain and sensory disturbances within the affected facial area (Hillerup and Jensen 2006; Hillerup et al. 2011). Although rare, the neurotoxic lesions are permanent, and these individuals should be identified and the use of these high concentrations of analgesics should be avoided (Hillerup et al. 2011). Likewise molar extractions in the lower jaw may also leave the patient with a permanent painful lesion within the mandibular division

◘ Table 40.2

The most frequent differential diagnosis to persistent idiopathic facial pain

Diagnosis	Clinical features
Trigeminal neuralgia	Repeated attacks of severe neuralgiform pain lasting seconds without accompanying symptoms, usually pain free between attacks
SUNCT	Short seconds lasting neuralgiform pain attacks with associated conjunctival injection and tearing
Migraine, lower facial location	Hours-days lasting typical attacks with associated symptoms with pain dominance in the face
Cluster headache	30 min to 3 h, repeated attacks located around the eye and with accompanying autonomous symptoms. Rarely a constant facial pain
Lesions of the trigeminal nerve	Constant and/or paroxysmal pain with or without sensory disturbances in the affected area, also intraorally. Usually a related history of dental procedures, local analgesic, or surgery
Other trauma	Related history of trauma and eventual objective signs with sensory disturbances
Malignant disorders	Progression of pain, referred pain around the ear and associated symptoms
Dental or temporomandibular disorders	Functional pain related to eating, yawning, talking, or chewing
Atypical odontalgia	Continuous pain in the teeth or in a tooth socket after extraction

of the trigeminal nerve. Facial pain around the ear or temple may precede the detection of an ipsilateral lung carcinoma causing referred pain by invasion of the vagus nerve. The term *atypical odontalgia* has been applied to a continuous pain in the teeth or in a tooth socket after extraction in the absence of any identifiable dental cause (List et al. 2008; Baad-Hansen 2008).

Patient Education

Patients with PIFP frequently relate their pain to dental or jaw problems, surgery, or trauma. They undergo numerous examinations and often are dissatisfied because "the cause" of their pain could not be found. In a first step, physicians dealing with PIFP must emphasize that they believe in the patient's pain. Patients in whom other conditions have been ruled out by an appropriate multidisciplinary approach should be advised that further search for "the cause" of the pain will not be helpful. Patients with chronic pain are often desirous of a concrete cause and treatment, and will therefore request surgery (Madland and Feinmann 2001). In this case, patients should be advised that surgical procedures, for example, of the sinuses and jaws as well as dental or other surgery are only indicated, if a causative disorder has been demonstrated. It will be necessary to direct the patient's focus from diagnostic procedures unsuccessfully trying to find "the cause" of pain to treatment of pain following a multidisciplinary approach and focusing on symptomatic medication, cognitive behavioral therapy, and coping strategies specifically aimed at reducing interference with life. It is crucial that physicians and patients reach an agreement about how to manage the pain and it is crucial to define realistic goals of treatment.

Treatment of PIFP

There is no evidence-based treatment for PIFP. Additionally, treatment is difficult and often requires a multidisciplinary approach including behavioral, pharmacological, and physical interventions. If treatment fails, additional diagnostic tests are required to reestablish the diagnosis. The gold standard is the combination of behavioral treatment with pharmacotherapy while surgery has little importance.

Pharmacotherapy

Potential effective drugs involve the tricyclic antidepressants (TCAs), the antiepileptics (AEDs) used in treating neuropathic facial pain, and some selective serotonin reuptake inhibitors (SSRIs) or selective noradrenalin and serotonin inhibitors (SNRIs) (Benoliel and Eliav 2008). Since the etiology of PIFP is poorly understood, these drugs are used empirically. Like in other chronic pain states, amitriptyline could be the drug of first choice at doses 25–100 mg per day (Evans and Agostoni 2006; Benoliel and Eliav 2008; Sardella et al. 2009; Cornelissen et al. 2009). Fluoxetine at dose 20–40 mg per day may be considered too (Cornelissen et al. 2009). However, venlafaxine is the only antidepressant tested in a randomized, placebo-controlled trial for atypical facial pain, a term previously used for PIFP. Thirty patients were treated with 75 mg venlafaxine daily for 4 weeks and then crossed over to placebo for another 4-week period. Eight patients discontinued due to adverse events, and two patients were excluded because of noncompliance. Venlafaxine was superior to placebo in pain relief and escape medication use but not in pain intensity indicating that the drug was only modestly effective (Forssell et al. 2004). However, the dose used in this study might have been too low and treatment for 4 weeks too short.

Among AEDs those that block sodium channels may be preferable, because they display high efficacy in facial neuropathic pain. Carbamazepine and lamotrigine are the most common drugs of this category. Although the efficacy of carbamazepine may be used as a diagnostic marker for trigeminal neuralgia, atypical facial pain may also respond to this medication (Sato et al. 2004). In another report, lamotrigine was of little utility in facial pain (Delvaux and Schoene 2001). However, combinations of two agents may be more useful. Since PIFP often is comorbid with affective disorders, the combination of AEDs with antidepressants is highly rational. There is one report favoring the use of topiramate 100 mg hs, combined with imipramine 50 mg (Volcy et al. 2006). Combination of lamotrigine (200–400 mg per day) with venlafaxine (150–225 mg) could be an alternative pharmacological choice for those that do not respond to monotherapy or who co-suffer from anxiety or depression-like disorders. Considering evidence and experience in other pain disorders, gabapentin and pregabaline may also be used.

Behavioral Treatment

For a long time, the usefulness of psychotherapy has been recognized in atypical facial pain sufferers, who may co-suffer from psychiatric disturbances (Baile and Myers 1986). Most often, PIFP patients have experiences with various unsuccessful and painful dental or orofacial surgical procedures. Illustrating the underlying psychodynamic mechanisms associated with pain in these patients may help in pain management, but most importantly helps in understanding the role of learning, the family system, and other factors in producing chronic pain syndromes. Hypnosis seems to offer clinically relevant pain relief in PIFP, particularly in highly susceptible patients. Importantly, hypnosis activates specific cerebral areas in PIFP patients (Derbyshire et al. 2004). However, stress-coping skills and unresolved psychological problems need to be included in a comprehensive management plan in order also to address psychological symptoms and quality of life (Abrahamsen et al. 2008).

Other Therapies

When the pharmacological and behavioral treatment fails, pulsed radiofrequency treatment of the ganglion pterygopalatinum (sphenopalatinum) can be considered (Cornelissen et al. 2009), although often pain relapses (Balamucki et al. 2006). In the longest and largest case report, 20 patients with PIFP were treated with gamma knife surgery (80–90 Gy) and followed up for 19.1 ± 11.2 months. Pain relief was reported by 60% of patients whereas in 33.3% the pain recurred. Excellent outcome (complete pain relief without additional medication use) was reported by 15% of treated patients (Balamucki et al. 2006). Other interventions include percutaneous radiofrequency rhizotomy (Teixeira et al. 2006) and deep brain stimulation of the posterior hypothalamus (Broggi et al. 2007), again with poor results. Most experts suggest avoidance of invasive treatments like surgery and endodontics (Baad-Hansen 2008; Broggi et al. 2005, 2007).

Current Research and Established Knowledge

In a study based on primary care medical records (Koopman et al. 2009), the incidence rates of atypical facial pain (AFP), trigeminal neuralgia (TN), and cluster headache (CH) were 4.4, 12.6, and 12.5 per 100,000 person years, respectively, suggesting a AFP:TN/CH ratio of 1:2.8. Scientific evidence regarding our understanding of persistent idiopathic facial pain (PIFP)/ (AFP) is limited. Given that the incidence ratio of AFP to TN or Cluster is roughly 1:2.8 as mentioned above, the paucity of literature on AFP or PIFP is disheartening. Searching Medline for "persistent idiopathic facial pain," "atypical facial pain," "trigeminal neuralgia," and "cluster headache" results in 21, 245, 5635, and 2330 references, respectively. Taking PIFP and AFP together, the ratio of the published literature is 1:21 compared to TN and 1:8.8 compared to CH. Comparing incidence rates and number of scientific papers gives an impression of the scientific neglect of PIFP.

In 2000, Woda and Pionchon reviewed the pathophysiology of idiopathic orofacial pain. They discussed the role of female hormones, osteoporosis, neuralgia-inducing cavitational osteonecrosis, similarities with complex regional pain syndrome, local inflammatory, infectious, or mechanical irritation as well as minor nerve trauma and psychosocial factors. The authors stressed that none of these factors can currently be considered as the sole etiologic factor, and hypothesized that the idiopathic pain entities depend on one or several neuropathic mechanisms such as nociceptor sensitization, phenotypic changes, and ectopic activity from the nociceptors as well as central sensitization possibly maintained by ongoing activity from initially damaged peripheral tissues, sympathetic abnormal activity, alteration of segmental inhibitory control, and hyper- or hypoactivity of descending controls. However, in the decade since the article by Woda and Pionchon was published, only a few original papers have been added (Woda and Pionchon 2000).

Lang et al. (2005) examined the trigeminal root entry zone in patients with PIFP by means of MRI 3D visualization in 12 patients with unilateral pain. The frequency of contact between an artery or vein on the symptomatic and asymptomatic sides did not differ significantly. Sensitivity was 58% and specificity 33%. The authors conclude that PIFP cannot be attributed to a contact between a vessel and trigeminal root entry zone, and therefore, pain relief after microvascular decompression cannot be expected.

Forssell and coworkers used blink reflex recordings and quantitative sensory testing in patients with AFP and trigeminal neuropathic pain and found abnormalities less frequently in AFP than in trigeminal neuropathic pain, but when present, type and pattern of findings were similar in both conditions (Forssell et al. 2004). List et al. demonstrated somatosensory abnormalities in atypical odontalgia. These findings suggest a continuum in the level and extent of neuropathic involvement.

In another small study from the same group (Hagelberg et al. 2003), positron emission tomography (PET) was applied to assess striatal presynaptic dopaminergic function and dopamine D1 and D2 receptor availabilities. There was a tendency of increased D2 receptor availability in the left putamen ($P = 0.056$), and the D1/D2 ratio in the putamen was decreased bilaterally by 7.7% ($P = 0.002$) in patients when compared to controls. In a voxel-based analysis, the uptake of $[^{11}C]$raclopride was increased in the left putamen ($P = 0.025$). The increase in D2 receptor availability in the left putamen and the decrease in D1/D2 ratio imply that alterations in the striatal dopaminergic system as evaluated by PET may be involved in chronic orofacial pain conditions. In 2010, Schmidt-Wilcke and coworkers confirmed for PIFP what was demonstrated earlier in other chronic pain conditions, that is, altered brain morphology in brain regions known to be part of the pain system (Schmidt-Wilcke et al. 2010). Using voxel-based morphometry, they found a decrease in gray matter volume in the left anterior cingulate gyrus and left temporo-insular region, as well as in the left and right sensory-motor area, projecting to the representational area of the face.

In conclusion, patients with PIFP remain a complicated group to diagnose and to treat. The scientific evidence for a specific entity, a clear pathophysiological mechanism and effective treatment strategies are still lacking. Further field testing and clinical characterizations of these severely affected patients are highly needed and the noncommittal title *Persistent Idiopathic Facial Pain* is preferable until further evidence is available.

References

Abrahamsen R, Baad-Hansen L, Svensson P (2008) Hypnosis in the management of persistent idiopathic orofacial pain – clinical and psychosocial findings. Pain 136(1–2):44–52. Epub 6 Aug 2007

Baad-Hansen L (2008) Atypical odontalgia – pathophysiology and clinical management. J Oral Rehabil 35(1):1–11

Baile WF Jr, Myers D (1986) Psychological and behavioral dynamics in chronic atypical facial pain. Anesth Prog 33(5):252–257

Balamucki CJ, Stieber VW, Ellis TL, Tatter SB, Deguzman AF, McMullen KP, Lovato J, Shaw EG, Ekstrand KE, Bourland JD, Munley MT, Robbins M, Branch C (2006) Does dose rate affect efficacy? The outcomes of 256 gamma knife surgery procedures for trigeminal neuralgia and other types of facial pain as they relate to the half-life of cobalt. J Neurosurg 105(5):730–735

Benoliel R, Eliav E (2008) Neuropathic orofacial pain. Oral Maxillofac Surg Clin North Am 20(2):237–254, vii

Brenoliel R, Birman N, Eliav E, Shrav Y (2008) The international classification of headache disorders accurate diagnosis of orofacial pain. Cephalalgia 28:752–762

Broggi G, Ferroli P, Franzini A, Galosi L (2005) The role of surgery in the treatment of typical and atypical facial pain. Neurol Sci 26(Suppl 2):s95–s100

Broggi G, Franzini A, Leone M, Bussone G (2007) Update on neurosurgical treatment of chronic trigeminal autonomic cephalalgias and atypical facial pain with deep brain stimulation of posterior hypothalamus: results and comments. Neurol Sci 28(Suppl 2):S138–S145

Cornelissen P, van Kleef M, Mekhail N, Day M, van Zundert J (2009) Evidence-based interventional pain medicine according to clinical diagnoses. 3. Persistent idiopathic facial pain. Pain Pract 9(6):443–448

Delvaux V, Schoenen J (2001) New generation antiepileptics for facial pain and headache. Acta Neurol Belg 101(1):42–46

Derbyshire SW, Whalley MG, Stenger VA, Oakley DA (2004) Cerebral activation during hypnotically induced and imagined pain. Neuroimage 23(1):392–401

Evans RW, Agostoni E (2006) Persistent idiopathic facial pain. Headache 46(8):1298–1300

Forssell H, Tasmuth T, Tenovuo O, Hampf G, Kalso E (2004) Venlafaxine in the treatment of atypical facial pain: a randomized controlled trial. J Orofac Pain 18(2):131–137

Forssell H, Tenovuo O, Silvoniemi P, Jääskeläinen SK (2007) Differences and similarities between atypical facial pain and trigeminal neuropathic pain. Neurology 69(14):1451–1459

Graff-Radford SB (2009) Facial pain. Neurologist 15:171–177

Hagelberg N, Forssell H, Aalto S, Rinne JO, Scheinin H, Taiminen T, Någren K, Eskola O, Jääskeläinen SK (2003) Altered dopamine D2 receptor binding in atypical facial pain. Pain 106(1–2):43–48

Headache Classification Committee of the International Headache Society (2004) Classification and diagnostic criteria for headache disorders, cranial neuralgia and facial pain, 2nd Edition. Cephalalgia 24(Suppl 1):1–164

Hillerup S, Jensen R (2006) Nerve injury caused by mandibular block analgesia. Int J Oral Maxillofac Surg 35:437–443

Hillerup S, Jensen R, Ersbøll B (2011) Trigeminal nerve injury associated with injection of local anaesthetics. Needle lesion or neurotoxicity? [Epub ahead of print]

Koopman JS, Dieleman JP, Huygen FJ, de Mos M, Martin CG, Sturkenboom MC (2009) Incidence of facial pain in the general population. Pain 147(1–3):122–127

Lang E, Naraghi R, Tanrikulu L, Hastreiter P, Fahlbusch R, Neundörfer B, Tröscher-Weber R (2005) Neurovascular relationship at the trigeminal root entry zone in persistent idiopathic facial pain: findings from MRI 3D visualisation. J Neurol Neurosurg Psychiatry 76(11):1506–1509

List T, Leijon G, Svensson P (2008) Somatosensory abnormalities in atypical odontalgia: a case-control study. Pain 139(2):333–341

Madland G, Feinmann C (2001) Chronic facial pain: a multidisciplinary problem. J Neurol Neurosurg Psychiatry 71(6):716–719

Sardella A, Demarosi F, Barbieri C, Lodi G (2009) An up-to-date view on persistent idiopathic facial pain. Minerva Stomatol 58(6):289–299

Sato J, Saitoh T, Notani K, Fukuda H, Kaneyama K, Segami N (2004) Diagnostic significance of carbamazepine and trigger zones in trigeminal neuralgia. Oral Surg Oral Med Oral Pathol Oral Radiol Endod 97(1):18–22

Schmidt-Wilcke T, Hierlmeier S, Leinisch E (2010) Altered regional brain morphology in patients with chronic facial pain. Headache 50(8):1278–1285. [Epub ahead of print 5 Mar 2010]

Teixeira MJ, Siqueira SR, Almeida GM (2006) Percutaneous radiofrequency rhizotomy and neurovascular decompression of the trigeminal nerve for the treatment of facial pain. Arq Neuropsiquiatr 64(4):983–989

Volcy M, Rapoport AM, Tepper SJ, Sheftell FD, Bigal ME (2006) Persistent idiopathic facial pain responsive to topiramate. Cephalalgia 26(4):489–491

Woda A, Pionchon P (2000) A unified concept of idiopathic orofacial pain: pathophysiologic features. J Orofac Pain 14(3):196–212

Zebenholzer K, Wöber C, Vigl M, Wessely P, Wöber-Bingöl C (2005) Facial pain in a neurological tertiary care centre – evaluation of the international classification of headache disorders. Cephalalgia 25:689–699

Zebenholzer K, Wöber C, Vigl M, Wessely P, Wöber-Bingöl C (2006) Facial pain and the second edition of the international classification of headache disorders. Headache 46:259–263

41 Acute Headache in the Emergency Department

Dominique Valade[1] · *Anne Ducros*[2] · *Susan W. Broner*[3]
[1]Lariboisière Hospital, Assistance Publique des Hôpitaux de Paris, Paris, France
[2]Assistance Publique des Hôpitaux de Paris, Head and Neck Clinic, Hôpital Lariboisière, Paris, France
[3]St. Luke's-Roosevelt Hospital, New York, NY, USA

Paolo Martelletti, Timothy J. Steiner (eds.), *Handbook of Headache*, DOI 10.1007/978-88-470-1700-9_41,
© Lifting The Burden 2011

Abstract: In emergency departments, the top priority is to establish a precise etiologic diagnosis and to classify the headache as a primary headache, a benign secondary headache, such as from influenza, or a secondary headache due to a serious condition, requiring further exploration or emergency treatment (meningeal hemorrhage, meningitis, intracranial hypertension, amongst others). The crucial part of this diagnostic step is the interview. This step, supplemented by the clinical examination, will determine the differential diagnosis and, ultimately, will steer any tests that need to be done emergently and the course of treatment. Depending on the headache diagnosis, the patient may be treated and released for outpatient follow-up or may need to be admitted to the hospital for either further evaluation and/or treatment.

The physician must also identify headaches occurring in patients already hospitalized for another reason. It is important to rule out any iatrogenic causes such as drug induced headaches or headaches caused by hypotension of the cerebral spinal fluid (CSF) such as secondary to a persisting fistula after lumbar puncture or other procedure that enters into the CSF space.

Finally, some patients diagnosed with a primary headache may sometimes require hospitalization either because of an acute exacerbation of their primary headache in a particular psychological context, or, especially, for detoxification for chronic daily headache associated with medication overuse.

Introduction

Headache is an extremely common complaint in the emergency department, accounting for 1–16% of all visits according to the studies (Dhopesh et al. 1979; Dickman and Masten 1979; Leicht 1980; Fodden et al. 1989; Silberstein 1992; Luda et al. 1995; Ramirez-Lassepas et al. 1997; Morgenstern et al. 1998; Newman and Lipton 1998; Stevenson et al. 1998; Cortelli et al. 2004). Emergency department patients with headache are mostly young adults with a female preponderance. While primary headaches are the most frequently seen, serious and sometimes potentially life-threatening conditions are disclosed in 5–15% of the cases. The first priority, therefore, is to establish a precise etiologic diagnosis and to distinguish between primary headaches, benign secondary headaches – such as headache due to influenza – and serious secondary headaches requiring emergent investigations and treatment (subarachnoid hemorrhage, meningitis, intracranial hypertension). The crucial part of establishing a diagnosis is the patient interview, complemented by the physical examination. It is these that determine the management of the patient. Management may include administration of specific acute headache treatments (some of which may be conducted on an outpatient basis for primary headaches), investigations if needed followed by treatment on an outpatient basis for benign secondary headaches, and finally, emergent investigations and treatment in the hospital setting for possible secondary headaches with serious underlying causes. The treatment of secondary headaches requires the treatment of the underlying cause, for example, embolization or surgery of a ruptured intracranial aneurysm, antibiotics for infectious meningitis, or steroids for temporal arteritis. It is useful to administer a symptomatic treatment to patients suffering from acute unusual headaches; however, physicians should be aware that headaches might be alleviated even when they are symptomatic of a serious cause. A good response should not be a reason for postponing etiologic investigations.

Steps in the Initial Diagnosis of a Headache Seen in the Emergency Room

Obtaining a Detailed History of Present and Previous Headaches

The first step in establishing a diagnosis is to obtain a history from the patient by interview. This can be difficult for a patient suffering from an intense headache, but can be manageable in a quiet, dark room. Interviewing the patient's family or friends is often useful. When the patient and the physician do not speak the same language, and if there is no available translator, severe headaches should be considered and investigated as potential secondary headaches symptomatic of a serious cause: a cerebral CT scan and a CSF analysis, if deemed safe, are mandatory.

Mode of Onset and Time Course of the Actual Headache

Primary headaches account for the vast majority of emergency department visits for headache. The most important part of the interview is thus to ascertain if the patient is affected by a definite primary headache disorder – the most frequent being migraine, episodic, or chronic tension-type headache and cluster headache – or not. The first two questions to ask to the patients are the following:

(a) When did your actual headache start? (acute or chronic headache)
(b) Have you ever had this same type of headache before? (an unusual headache or an attack of their known headache pattern)

According to the responses to these two questions, there are three different situations. Firstly, the patient is able to say that he has already suffered from several similar headaches for months or years. In such cases, a primary headache disorder is the most likely cause and the description of headache characteristics – age of onset, duration of headache attacks, pain location, associated signs and symptoms, trigger factors – will help to make a precise diagnosis. Secondly, the patient denies a previous headache history and reports having headaches for the first time in his life for some hours, days, weeks, or months. In such cases, a secondary headache has to be excluded and investigations have to be performed. Finally, the patient reports a history of definite primary headaches but states that his acute headache is different from his usual headaches attacks. In such cases, a secondary headache has to be suspected and investigations are noteworthy. In both latter cases of acute unusual headaches, additional questions have to be asked:

(a) How did the headache begin? (sudden or progressive onset)
(b) How has the pain changed since its onset? (improvement, worsening, or stability)

Unusual headaches with a sudden onset may reveal a wide range of serious conditions including mainly vascular disorders such as subarachnoid hemorrhage. Unusual progressive headaches are the mode of presentation of multiple conditions including intracranial hypertension, meningitis or meningoencephalitis, local cranial disorders, tumors, and temporal arteritis.

Circumstances of Onset

The circumstances surrounding the onset of a headache can sometimes guide the physician to an immediate diagnosis: cranial trauma (hemorrhage or cerebral contusion), medication or drugs recently taken, recent lumbar puncture, peridural (epidural) or spinal anesthesia causing CSF hypotension, fever associated with general disease, etc. However, the circumstances surrounding onset can also be misleading: an exertional headache can be benign but also a symptom of a subarchnoid hemorrhage; a headache after lumbar puncture is generally caused by a low CSF pressure but can sometimes be caused by a cerebral venous thrombosis (Benzon et al. 2003), or an infection.

Characteristics of the Headache

The intensity of the pain does not help to distinguish between a primary and a secondary headache. Nevertheless, any sudden and severe headache (thunderclap headache) must be regarded as secondary and further explored in the emergency department. It is important to consider the concordance between the intensity of the pain described by the patient and the consequences of the pain on his affect and activities (e.g., does he require bed rest, or have difficulties in expressing himself). A wide range of pain types may be described (pulsatile, continuous, "electric shock," crushing, pressure, discomfort) but none is specific for a particular etiology. Topography may sometimes be an element in favor of a particular etiology, such as the temporal pain in temporal arteritis, however it is usually not specific for a particular disease.

Associated Symptoms

Any recent and unusual headache associated with a neurological symptom, such as consciousness impairment, epileptic seizures, or focal signs, should always be assumed to be due to an intracranial lesion until proven otherwise. A headache with deterioration of health or claudication of the jaw in a patient of more than 50 years of age should immediately point to a possible diagnosis of temporal arteritis. On the other hand, nausea, vomiting, photophobia, and phonophobia are nonspecific symptoms that may be part of a meningeal syndrome but are also associated with migraine, so do not readily help determine the diagnosis without other clues. Importantly, the absence of any associated symptom does not eliminate a secondary headache and should not postpone the initiation of investigations if the headache is recent, unusual, and persistent.

Medical History

The patient's medical history must be obtained in a systematic way because it may guide the diagnosis. Cardiovascular disease and hypertension (strokes), postpartum or previous history of venous thrombosis of the lower limbs (cerebral venous thrombosis), cancer (cranial metastases), known HIV seropositivity (cerebral toxoplasmosis), anxiety and depression (decompensation with tension-type headache or *migraine*), and consumption of psychotropic drugs can all affect headache diagnosis.

Physical Examination

The first step is to assess blood pressure, pulse rate, and body temperature. An elevated blood pressure is often the consequence and not the cause of a severe head pain, although if extremely elevated may indicate a hypertensive encephalopathy as the cause of the pain. Headache associated with fever immediately points to an infectious disorder. Skin has to be examined in all febrile headache patients suspected of bacterial meningitis in order to search for purpuric lesions. The rest of the clinical examination should include a focal head and neck exam as well as a neurological examination. Any abnormality in either the neurological or physical examination indicates the need for further evaluation. On the other hand, a strictly normal clinical examination does not eliminate the possibility of a serious cause and should not preclude investigations depending on the history.

Neurologic Examination

The first step is to assess the state of consciousness and to search for a meningeal syndrome. Then, the physician should check for a focal neurological deficit that the interview could have missed. Eyelids and pupils are crucial to examine. A painful Horner's sign points to a dissection of the homolateral internal carotid artery. Headaches associated with a unilateral mydriasis or a complete third cranial nerve paralysis points to an aneurysm of the posterior communicating artery or the termination of the internal carotid artery compressing the third nerve. Patients have to be checked for a static or kinetic cerebellar syndrome that may be overlooked in a patient lying down with severe headaches, vomiting, and reluctant to move. Moreover, the visual field has also to be carefully ascertained even in patients who do not complain of visual troubles. Indeed, a right-handed patient with a right occipital lesion may have a left-sided homonymous hemianopia and complain only about headaches because he is anosognosic of the visual deficit. Finally, a fundoscopic examination will search for papillary edema indicating intracranial hypertension or for hypertensive retinopathy possibly indicating hypertensive encephalopathy.

Local Physical Examination

The local cranial examination should include inspection for redness of the eyes, exophthalmy or swelling of the eyelids, palpation of the temporal arteries, of the eyeballs, and of the cranial sinuses to search for an unusual sensitivity to pressure, nuchal rigidity, and focal rashes or lesions and, finally, auscultation of the vessels for cervical or cranial murmurs. It is also important to palpate the cervical and chewing muscles, which are very often contracted and painful in the case of a tension-type headache.

Identifying Headache Emergencies and Urgencies

The golden rule is to consider all recent and unusual headaches as secondary to an organic cerebral cause and to perform adequate investigations. In all patients with an acute brutal headache (thunderclap headache) and in all patients with an acute progressive and persistent

◻ **Table 41.1**

Clinical features in favor of a secondary headache requiring investigations

Recent de novo headache (either sudden or progressive)
Unusual headache in a subject suffering from primary headaches
Thunderclap headache
Focal neurological deficit (except typical migrainous aura in a patient)
Consciousness impairment or confusion
Abnormal neurological examination
Papillary oedema
Neck stiffness
Fever
Serious medical disorder, including immunosuppression
Severe elevated blood pressure
Painful and inflammatory temporal arteries
Headache aggravated by Valsalva maneuver
Headache that awakens the patient from sleep

headache, investigations have to be started in the emergency room (❷ *Table 41.1*). Hospitalization is necessary when a serious underlying cause is rapidly found and has to be treated, but is also often necessary when the first investigations have not permitted a firm diagnosis and additional investigations are required. When a benign secondary headache is obvious after the clinical interview and examination (e.g., headache due to influenza), the patient can be managed as an outpatient. Finally, primary headaches or idiopathic facial neuralgias may show acute exacerbations with intractable pain or impossibility to eat or drink with a risk of dehydration. These are pain urgencies that may require a hospitalization over a few days to give a parenteral treatment.

Strategy of the Diagnostic Evaluations

The usual blood examinations are seldom conclusive, except for an increased erythrocyte sedimentation rate, which indicates temporal arteritis or an infectious state. An elevated C-reactive protein may also support the diagnosis of temporal arteritis. Any recent headache which is unusual and persistent, whether of sudden or progressive onset, requires two basic examinations to be carried out in a systematic way: a computed tomography (CT) scan without contrast injection and a lumbar puncture (Boulan et al. 2004).

CT Scan

A cerebral CT scan is the first investigation to perform. Images have to be carefully examined for the presence of abnormal hyperdensities indicating blood either in the subarachnoid spaces or in the cerebral or cerebellar parenchyma, for dilatation of the ventricules indicating hydrocephalus, for a localized hypodensity (ischemia) or a localized mass effect indicating an expansive lesion (tumor, abscess, infarct with oedema). Those abnormalitis will then have to be further investigated later by CT scan with injection or, better, with an MRI (Prager and Mikulis 1991). If there is a possibility of acute sinusitis, a scan of the sinuses is the procedure of choice. Importantly, a normal CT scan does not preclude an organic cause: 5–10% of meningeal hemorrhages, 30–50% of cerebral venous thrombosis, most cervical arterial dissections with isolated headaches and local signs, and the vast majority of meningitis present with a normal CT scan and require further investigations.

Lumbar Puncture (LP)

A LP should be performed in all patients with unusual or persistent headaches whether the onset was sudden or progressive. Analyzing the CSF is the only way to diagnose a meningitis. Moreover, the LP will catch a diagnosis of a subarchnoid hemorrhage in the 5% of patients who have an aneurysm with a normal CT scan. In headache patients, the LP has to be performed after brain imaging (CT scan or MRI) to rule out a contraindication, that is, a space-occupying lesion with mass effect and risk of brain herniation. Rarely, an LP may be performed without previous brain imaging when a bacterial meningitis is highly suspected and the patient has a normal consciousness and fundoscopic exam and has no other focal neurological signs. It is essential to measure the CSF opening pressure. Intracranial hypertension with normal CT scan requires checking for a cerebral venous thrombosis or a dural fistula.

Cervical and Transcranial Ultrasound Examination

This examination must be conducted when the clinical picture is in favor of a carotid or a vertebral artery dissection. Isolated headache may be seen with a cervical or vertebral arterial dissection (Arnold et al. 2006). Echography can visualize a hematoma in the arterial wall and cervical and transcranial duplex scanning evaluate the hemodynamic repercussion. However, both examinations can be strictly normal when the dissection affects an intracranial portion of the artery or when the hematoma does not produce a significant arterial stenosis. In such cases, investigations have to be continued with an MRI (cervical and cranial axial sequences with Fat Sat) and a cervical and cerebral MR angiography (MRA).

Magnetic Resonance Imaging (MRI)

MRI is much more sensitive than CT scan for a number of disorders that may be revealed by isolated headaches. A cerebral MRI has to be performed in all patients with an unusual severe and persistent headache even after a normal CT scan and a normal or near-normal LP. Indeed, several conditions revealed by an acute headache may present with a normal CT scan and a normal LP. A large number of sequences are necessary: diffusion-weighted sequences (acute ischemic lesions), FLAIR (small cortical subarchnoid hemorrhage, pituitary necrosis, posterior leukoencephalopathy), Fat Sat axial cervical and cerebral sequences (arterial dissection), T1 and $T2^*$ weighted sequences as well as MR veinography (cerebral venous thrombosis). T1 weighted sequences with gadolinium enhancement are needed to search for pachymeningeal enhancement when an idiopathic low CSF pressure syndrome is suspected. MRA may disclose an arterial aneurysm, a dissection, or segmental spasms consistent with cerebral vasoconstriction syndrome. If an MR apparatus is not available, CT veinography and angiography are helpful.

Conventional Cerebral Angiography

Conventional cerebral angiography is indicated in the event of acute headaches in only two cases. First, if CT or MR angiography is nondiagnostic, some patients with a subarachnoid hemorrhage must have a conventional angiogram in order to search for a ruptured aneurysm. Second, a conventional angiogram may be discussed in some patients with a sudden and severe headache, if all preceding investigations are normal and the headaches persists or worsens. Indeed, MR or CT angiography may sometimes be insufficient to formally exclude a cerebral venous thrombosis, an arterial dissection especially a vertebral dissection, or a cerebral vasoconstriction syndrome.

Diagnosis and Management of the Most Frequent Causes of Headaches

Epidemiological studies about headaches in the emergency room are rare (Bourrier et al. 2001). Patients are characterized by a female preponderance and a mean age close to 35–40 years old. Most patients are affected by primary headaches and benign, secondary headaches (upper tract respiratory infections, general viral syndromes). Among primary headaches, tension-type headaches and migraine are the two most frequently seen. However, 5–15% of the patients have a serious secondary cause. The following chapter deals with the most frequent serious and benign nontraumatic causes (❷ *Fig. 41.1*). Patients with a severe acute post-traumatic headache, with *or without* focal neurological signs and/or consciousness impairment, need an emergent CT scan. Patients with an epidural hematoma or a traumatic subdural hematoma require immediate neurosurgery.

Thunderclap Headaches

A thunderclap headache (TCH) is a severe and explosive headache that reaches its maximal intensity in less than 1 min (Schwedt et al. 2006). Every thunderclap headache has to be considered as symptomatic of an organic cause and immediately investigated. Indeed, 30–80% of the thunderclap headaches reveal an underlying disorder, the most frequent being vascular disorders. The location and the type of thunderclap headaches are not specific to a particular cause. Duration may range according to the various causes from some minutes to several days. A thunderclap headache may be unique or be recurrent over a few days. It may start spontaneously or be triggered by Valsalva maneuvers, physical effort, or sexual activity. The first cause to search for is a subarachnoid hemorrhage (SAH): 11–33% of thunderclap headaches are due to a SAH (Linn et al. 1994, 1998; Lledo et al. 1994; Landtblom et al. 2002) and 70% of SAH present with isolated headaches consistent with a thunderclap headache in 50% of the cases. A CT scan has to be performed immediately followed by a LP if the CT is normal. Patients have

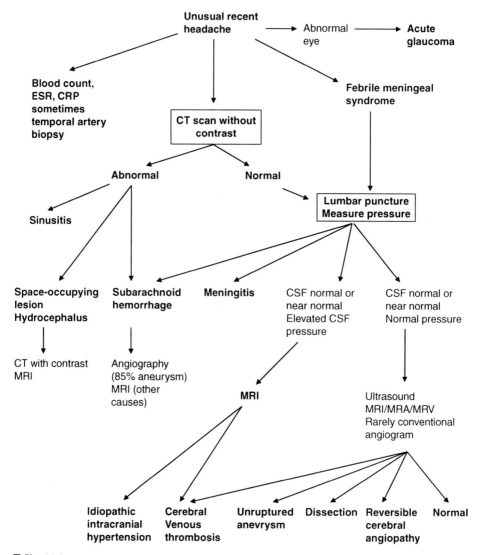

□ Fig. 41.1

Strategy of investigations in an acute headache patient with a suspicion of an organic cause

to be hospitalized to undergo a conventional angiogram. In 85% of cases of SAH, a ruptured aneurysm is the cause, and the definitive treatment requires a neurosurgical intervention or an intra-arterial embolization. Other intracranial hemorrhages account for 5–10% of the thunderclap headaches (Fodden et al. 1989; Lledo et al. 1994; Landtblom et al. 2002).

Isolated TCH that mimic SAH are frequently seen in patients with cerebellar or intraventricular hemorrhages. TCH are rarely seen in some patients with supratentorial parenchymal hematomas especially right frontal or temporal hematomas in right-handed persons. Finally, a thunderclap headache can rarely reveal a subdural hematoma. CT scan easily makes the diagnosis of these cerebral hemorrhages.

Ischemic infarcts with the same topography may also be revealed by isolated brutal headaches (Schwedt and Dodick 2006). The initial CT scan may be normal, but MRI with diffusion-weighted imaging is much more sensitive (Schwedt and Dodick 2006). Patients with cerebellar infarcts or hemorrhages have to be hospitalized in intensive care units close to a neurosurgery department because they may deteriorate acutely: compression of the fourth ventricle can provoke an acute hydrocephalus and result in brain herniation and death.

Numerous other vascular disorders may present with isolated thunderclap headaches including about 5% of cervical or intracranial artery dissections, 2–3% of cerebral venous thrombosis, some pituitary necrosis, rare cases of temporal arteritis, and the majority of reversible cerebral vasoconstriction syndromes (also known as reversible or benign cerebral angiopathy) (Dodick and Wijdicks 1998; Cumurciuc et al. 2005; Arnold et al. 2006; Chen et al. 2006). In all these causes, CT scan and LP may be normal; therefore, an MRI with MRA and MRV is mandatory. When these diagnoses are confirmed, patients have to be hospitalized in a stroke unit (if possible) to receive a specific treatment by a neurologist or vascular specialist. These treatments may include heparin for cerebral venous thrombosis, blood-pressure control and heparin for cervical arteries dissections, and nimodipine for cerebral vasoconstriction syndromes.

Finally, the existence of thunderclap headaches due to an unruptured aneurysm is still debated. The rule to perform a systematic MRI/MRA/MRV in all patients with one or several thunderclap headaches will allow visualization of aneurysms having a diameter of at least 2–3 mm. Any patient with an aneurysm needs to be evaluated by specialized neurovascular teams.

An isolated thunderclap headache may also reveal a nonvascular condition: acute blocked sinusitis, parenchymal or intraventricular tumors with hydrocephalus (colloid cyst of the 3rd ventricle), some meningitis, and some cases of low CSF pressure syndrome. Indeed, about 15% of cases of idiopathic low CSF pressure syndromes present with a thunderclap headache. Diagnosis is made on the postural character of the headache (alleviated by lying down) and the typical MRI features (meningeal enhancement, cranio-caudal displacement of the brain structures, subdural collections). If bed rest during a few days does not improve the headache, one or two autologous lumbar epidural blood patches may be performed (Berroir et al. 2004), followed, in case of failure, by a search for the source of leak with subsequent guided epidural blood patch or surgical intervention, depending on the location. Rarely TCH may be the presenting symptom of myocardial infarction or ischemia in patients with cardiac risk factors. An EKG may be appropriate in this subgroup of patients.

Unusual Headaches with a Progressive Onset

The list of etiologies is large, including all causes of thunderclap headaches that may also provoke progressive headaches, all causes of intracranial hypertension, all causes of meningitis and meningoencephalitis, temporal arteritis, and all extracerebral head and neck lesions (eyes, ears, teeth, oropharyngeal tract, skull. . .).

Intracranial Hypertension

Intracranial hypertension is suspected when a patient describes progressive worsening headaches worsened by cough, effort, or lying down. It may be associated with nausea or vomiting and sometimes with horizontal diplopia due to VIth nerve paralysis and visual eclipses. Bilateral papillary oedema is an important clinical finding, though not always present. However, headaches from intracranial hypertension may not have associated symptoms especially at the initial phase. CT scan may reveal hydrocephalus (stenosis of the sylvian aqueduct), effacement of the sulci and most of the space-occupying lesions sufficiently important to cause an intracranial hypertension. But CT may miss posterior fossa lesions and infectious causes of intracranial hypertension. Therefore, a contrast-enhanced CT scan or, better, a cerebral MRI with and without gadolinium is needed when there is a suspicion of a posterior fossa lesion. If these studies are normal, an LP including measurement of the CSF pressure is mandatory. A high opening CSF pressure (above 25 cm of water) is consistent with intracranial hypertension and other secondary causes need to be sought. These include cerebral venous thrombosis or dural fistula. The LP has the added benefit of removing CSF which in itself can alleviate the headache. If the CT scan, the CSF analysis, and the MRI/MRA/MRV are normal and the pressure is elevated it will be concluded that the patient has a "benign" intracranial hypertension, which may be due to drugs (steroids, vitamin A) or be idiopathic, seen more commonly in young obese women.

Meningitis and Meningoencephalitis

A febrile headache with neck stiffness, nausea/vomiting, and photophobia points to an infectious meningitis. An LP is the only way to confirm the diagnosis and guide the choice of the treatment. However, fever may be absent if the patient has used over-the-counter antipyretics and the meningeal syndrome may be absent. This favors the rule to systematically perform an LP in patients complaining of a new onset headache and having a normal CT scan. In some patients with meningoencephalitis, headache may be the presenting symptom before the onset of focal deficits, consciousness impairment, or seizures. Empiric treatment covering bacterial and viral etiologies when an infection is suspected, including coverage for herpes zoster, must be initiated immediately after the LP while awaiting the CSF results. PCR of CSF is the test of choice for herpes zoster.

Temporal Arteritis

Every patient aged above 50 years old complaining from a new onset, unusual headache should be evaluated for temporal arteritis. Diagnosis is made on an elevated ESR and C-reactive protein and a temporal artery biopsy. When the clinical suspicion is strong (fatigue, febricula, inflammatory signs on temporal arteries, jaw claudicating, girdle pain, loss of vision), steroids have to be initiated before the results of the temporal artery biopsy. The efficacy of steroids on the headache in case of temporal arteritis is so important that the persistence of headaches after 4 days should lead to consideration of an alternative diagnosis.

Local Cranial Lesions

In case of an unusual recent headache without any neurological signs or symptoms, two main causes have to be considered: acute sinusitis and acute glaucoma. Acute sinusitis often provokes severe acute headaches, increased by putting the head down or lying down. Pain may be isolated in case of a blocked sinusitis and especially in sphenoid sinusitis (Gordon-Bennett et al. 2006). Indeed, purulent rhinorrhea as well as fever are not constant. Diagnosis requires a cranial CT scan of the sinuses. Antibiotic and anticongestant therapy are required and, if appropriate, sinus drainage may be carried out. An acute angle-closure glaucoma has to be suspected in case of a severe periorbital pain with a red eye and unilateral visual loss. However, the clinical features are sometimes misleading (Gordon-Bennett et al. 2006) Examination may disclose an areactive semi-mydriasis pupil. Diagnosis requires measuring the intraocular pressure. Treatment is based on miotics such as systemic acetazolamide, pilocarpine, eye drops of betablockers, or surgery.

Carbon Monoxide Poisoning

Carbon monoxide (CO) is a colorless and odorless gas. Most intoxications are due to dysfunctions of heating or cooking apparatus, in which combustion systems produce CO. Headache is the most frequent symptom and the most frequent presenting symptom (90%) of chronic or acute CO intoxications. These headaches have no specific characteristics. They usually precede other symptoms including dizziness, syncope, visual troubles, and general weakness. Severe symptoms such as seizures, coma, dysrhythmias, and cardiac ischemia occur later on (Kao and Nanagas 2006). The intensity of symptoms is correlated with the level of blood carboxyhemoglobin (HbCO). From 10% to 20% of HbCO, the headache is generally isolated. With HbCO percentages above 20%, the headache is associated with nausea, vomiting, fatigue, and irritability. When the level is above 30%, the headaches become intractable, the patient becomes confused and then comatose. Blood has to be drawn as soon as possible, if possible in the place of intoxication, because the level of HbCO immediately decreases when the exposure to the CO stops and may even be normal if the blood is drawn too late. Some characteristics in favor of the diagnosis include headache during the night that improves in the morning and headaches that improve when the patient is outside. The diagnosis is more easily made when the intoxication involves a household, affecting multiple persons. Treatment consists of oxygen therapy, supportive care, and, in selected cases, hyperbaric oxygen therapy. Eradication of the source of contamination is crucial to prevent recurrences.

Primary Headaches in the Emergency Room

The most important step is to make an exact diagnosis: Is it a migraine attack? An exacerbation of tension-type headaches in the setting of stress, anxiety, or depression? Or a cluster headache? Patients have to be carefully interviewed because the diagnosis is based on the description of the characteristics of headache attacks and on a normal physical and neurological examination. By consequence, emergency physicians have to be familiar with the diagnostic criteria of these primary headache disorders.

Management of Migraine Attacks in the Emergency Room

Treatment of the attack adjusted to previous therapies, to contraindications, and to any excessive use of medicinal products, should be offered to the patient (Valade 2006).

In the aftermath of the attack, the patient should be managed by his or her family doctor, neurologist, or a headache specialist. The risk of medication overuse should be systematically explained to the patient. If medication overuse is present, withdrawal should be planned and the advice of a headache specialist for a preventive migraine treatment is crucial.

It frequently occurs that a patient comes to the emergency department without having taken any treatment, and then it may be sufficient to initiate therapy with a single 1-g oral dose of aspirin or even with an NSAID, either by oral route or, in case of nausea, in suppository form. Metoclopramide or metopimazine in suppositories or by IV administration are given in combination with the above-mentioned drugs if nausea or serious vomiting is present.

If the patient has already taken either aspirin, an NSAID, or paracetamol (acetaminophen) possibly combined with caffeine, codeine, or dextropropoxyphene, the use of a specific anti-migraine therapy is indicated, preferably by nasal or subcutaneous route (20 mg sumatriptan nasal spray or 6 mg/0.5 ml subcutaneous sumatriptan).

In case of a known allergy to triptans, it is possible to use dihydroergotamine (DHE) either by nasal route (spray) or injectable route (IM, SC, or IV), for example, DHE 1 mg/ml. DHE, like the triptans, should not be given to patients with uncontrolled risk factors for heart attack or stroke or with prolonged or complex neurological symptoms with their migraines. Either metoclopramide or metopimazine in suppository form or by injectable route must always been administered in combination with therapy as it can cause nausea.

When specific anti-migraine drugs are not effective or are contraindicated, preference should be given to the parenteral route of administration. Depending on individual habits and types of medication previously taken by the patient for treatment of the attack, the following can be administered:

- 1 g paracetamol (acetaminophen) over a short 20-min IV infusion in the absence of a previous excessive self-medication with paracetamol (acetaminophen).
- Ketoprofen (100 mg) infusion under the same conditions.
- Nefopam in infusion under the same conditions.
- 30 mg of intravenous or intramuscular ketorolac can also be very effective. If given IV, it can be given IV piggy back in 50 cc of normal saline over 20–30 min.
- Metoclopromide, given intravenously, has been shown to not only reduce the nausea and vomiting that can accompany migraine, but has also been shown to be effective in reducing pain. Studies have shown that doses ranging from 10 to 20 mg given as an intravenous infusion over 15–20 min can be as effective as sumatriptan and other migraine treatments. Akesthesia is a common side effect but is easily reversed with diphenhydramine.
- 25 to 50 mg of diphenydramine in 50 cc of normal saline infused over 20–30 min can be given in addition to an NSAID to help reduce the pain.
- A 20- or 50-mg ampoule of clorazepate can be added to the IV infusion depending on the patient's anxiety condition; in case of nausea or vomiting, a 10-mg ampoule of metoclopramide can also be added.

In the event of failure of the above-mentioned infusions, or in case of excessive use of medications not allowing the use of the above-mentioned drugs, 50 mg amitriptyline and 1 mg/ml clonazepam can be administered, especially if the acute attack is accompanied by tension-type headache. Amitriptyline and clonazepam are infused slowly over approximately 2 h, after informing the patient that, as a result of the sedative effect of these drugs, it will be necessary for him or her to be escorted home by another person. Intravenous infusions of valproate may also be effective in stopping an intractable migraine. Nonpharmacological treatments that may be beneficial include isotonic IV fluids, especially in the case of vomiting, ice packs, and deep relaxation.

In case of *status migrainosus*, or headaches that continue despite emergency department treatment, the patient should be hospitalized for a more prolonged course of treatment under the care of a neurologist or headache specialist. In case of medication overuse, withdrawal should be planned in a second phase.

For pregnant or nursing women: IV paracetamol may be used as first-line therapy in the absence of contraindication (previous excessive oral intake). Oxygen delivered via face mask at a rate of 10 l/min for 30 min may be administered. One thousand milligram of IV magnesium may also be of benefit.

For young children, the recommended first-line therapies are as follows:

– 20 mg/ml ibuprofen: 0.5 ml/kg, that is, 10 mg/kg of body weight, for children over 6 months of age
– Diclofenac 25 mg suppositories starting at 16 kg body weight, that is, children over 4 years of age
– 275 mg naproxen starting at 25 kg body weight, that is, children over 6 years of age
– Paracetamol (acetaminophen) alone or in combination with metoclopramide under the same conditions as described above
– Ergotamine tartrate one tablet in children over 10 years of age, never exceeding the dose of six tablets/week
– Sumatriptan 20 mg nasal spray starting at 35 kg body weight, that is, over 12 years of age

The rectal route or nasal spray should be given preference in the event of nausea/vomiting.

A child presenting with migraine disease should be referred for relaxation therapy as soon as possible.

Management of Cluster Headache in the Emergency Room

Even if the cluster headache attacks are short-lived, patients with cluster headache very often visit the emergency room for a lot of reasons. First, patients may have cluster headache and the diagnosis has not been made before. The delay between the first attacks of cluster headache and the diagnosis is often of several years. Secondly, these patients come because they have very severe pain and may not have received effective treatment as an outpatient. If they are seen during an attack, the two only efficient acute treatments are subcutaneous sumatriptan (6 mg/ml) and oxygenotherapy (10–12 l/min for 15 min via non-rebreather facial mask). Patients known to be affected by episodic or chronic cluster headache may also visit the emergency department for other reasons: the urgent need of a prescription because they have used their last subcutaneous sumatriptan during the previous night; an increase in the number of daily attacks since a few days; or a fear of adverse reactions because they have treated six or seven attacks with sumatriptan in the same day (which is absolutely not recommended – the maximum dose is 12 mg per 24 h). In case of an increase in the number of daily attacks, oxygen should always be tried because it may represent a good option in patients having more than two attacks a day. A preventive treatment with high doses of verapamil should be initiated and the patient should be referred for outpatient follow-up consultation. Several authors add a tapering oral steroids regime to verapamil, but others avoid it and use instead intranasal lidocaine 1 g intravenous of hydrocortisone or greater occipital nerve blocks.

Management of Tension-Type Headaches in the Emergency Room

Although patients with episodic tension-type headaches and chronic tension-type headaches are believed to rarely visit the emergency department because the pain in this disorder is typically mild to moderate, they do sometimes present in the setting of stress, anxiety, or sometimes depression or when they can no longer cope. They often have an intense fear of having a cerebral lesion such as a brain tumor or an aneurysm and ask for brain imaging. A careful interview and clinical examination is necessary to make the appropriate diagnosis. If there is no diagnostic doubt, investigations are not necessary and it is important to provide the patients with explanations about tension-type headaches. A treatment with tranquilizers such as lorazepam or muscle relaxants such as clonazepam may be initiated, as well as anti-inflammatories. In case of frequent episodic or chronic tension-type headache, a follow-up with a neurologist or a headache specialist must be scheduled.

References

Arnold M, Cumurciuc R, Stapf C, Favrole P, Berthet K, Bousser MG (2006) Pain as the only symptom of cervical artery dissection. J Neurol Neurosurg Psychiatry 77:1021–1024

Benzon HT, Iqbal M, Tallman MS, Boehlke L, Russell EJ (2003) Superior sagittal sinus thrombosis in a patient with postdural puncture headache. Reg Anesth Pain Med 28:64–67

Berroir S, Loisel B, Ducros A, Boukobza M, Tzourio C, Valade D, Bousser MG (2004) Early epidural blood patch in spontaneous intracranial hypotension. Neurology 63:1950–1951

Boulan P, Ducros A, Berroir S, and Bousser MG (2004) Les céphalées aiguës. In: Niclot P, Amarenco P (eds) Urgences neurologiques. Puteaux, Da Te Be, pp 13–26

Bourrier P, Perroux D, Lannehoa Y, Thomas O (2001) Epidémiologie des céphalées de l'adulte dans les services d'urgences. In: Bourrier P (ed) Céphalées en urgence. Paris, Masson, pp 3–10

Chen SP, Fuh JL, Lirng JF, Chang FC, Wang SJ (2006) Recurrent primary thunderclap headache and benign CNS angiopathy: spectra of the same disorder? Neurology 67:2164–2169

Colman I, Brown MD, Innes GD et al (2004) Parenteral metoclopramide for acute migraine: meta-analysis of randomized controlled trials. Br Med J 329:1369

Cortelli P, Cevoli S, Nonino F, Baronciani D, Magrini N, Re G, De Berti G, Manzoni GC, Querzani P, Vandelli A (2004) Evidence-based diagnosis of nontraumatic headache in the emergency department: a consensus statement on four clinical scenarios. Headache 44:587–595

Cumurciuc R, Crassard I, Sarov M, Valade D, Bousser MG (2005) Headache as the only neurological sign of cerebral venous thrombosis: a series of 17 cases. J Neurol Neurosurg Psychiatry 76:1084–1087

Dhopesh V, Anwar R, Herring C (1979) A retrospective assessment of emergency department patients with complaint of headache. Headache 19:37–42

Dickman RL, Masten T (1979) The management of non-traumatic headache in a university hospital emergency room. Headache 19:391–396

Dodick DW, Wijdicks EF (1998) Pituitary apoplexy presenting as a thunderclap headache. Neurology 50:1510–1511

Fodden DI, Peatfield RC, Milsom PL (1989) Beware the patient with a headache in the accident and emergency department. Arch Emerg Med 6:7–12

Friedman BW, Corbo J, Lipton RB et al (2005) A trial of metoclopramide vs. sumatritpan for the emergency department treatment of migraines. Neurology 64:463–468

Gordon-Bennett P, Ung T, Stephenson C, Hingorani M (2006) Misdiagnosis of angle closure glaucoma. Br Med J 333:1157–1158

Kao LW, Nanagas KA (2006) Toxicity associated with carbon monoxide. Clin Lab Med 26:99–125

Landtblom AM, Fridriksson S, Boivie J, Hillman J, Johansson G, Johansson I (2002) Sudden onset headache: a prospective study of features, incidence and causes. Cephalalgia 22:354–360

Leicht MJ (1980) Non-traumatic headache in the emergency department. Ann Emerg Med 9: 404–409

Linn FH, Wijdicks EF, van der Graaf Y, Weerdesteyn-van Vliet FA, Bartelds AI, van Gijn J (1994) Prospective study of sentinel headache in aneurysmal subarachnoid haemorrhage. Lancet 344:590–593

Linn FH, Rinkel GJ, Algra A, van Gijn J (1998) Headache characteristics in subarachnoid haemorrhage and benign thunderclap headache. J Neurol Neurosurg Psychiatry 65:791–793

Lledo A, Calandre L, Martinez-Menendez B, Perez-Sempere A, Portera-Sanchez A (1994) Acute headache of recent onset and subarachnoid hemorrhage: a prospective study. Headache 34:172–174

Luda E, Comitangelo R, Sicuro L (1995) The symptom of headache in emergency departments. The experience of a neurology emergency department. Ital J Neurol Sci 16:295–301

Morgenstern LB, Luna-Gonzales H, Huber JC Jr, Wong SS, Uthman MO, Gurian JH, Castillo PR, Shaw SG, Frankowski RF, Grotta JC (1998) Worst headache and subarachnoid hemorrhage: prospective, modern computed tomography and spinal fluid analysis. Ann Emerg Med 32:297–304

Newman LC, Lipton RB (1998) Emergency department evaluation of headache. Neurol Clin 16:285–303

Prager JM, Mikulis DJ (1991) The radiology of headache. Med Clin North Am 75:525–544

Ramirez-Lassepas M, Espinosa CE, Cicero JJ, Johnston KL, Cipolle RJ, Barber DL (1997) Predictors of intracranial pathologic findings in patients who seek emergency care because of headache. Arch Neurol 54:1506–1509

Schwedt TJ, Dodick DW (2006) Thunderclap stroke: embolic cerebellar infarcts presenting as thunderclap headache. Headache 46:520–522

Schwedt TJ, Matharu MS, Dodick DW (2006) Thunderclap headache. Lancet Neurol 5:621–631

Shahien R, Saleh SA, Bowirrat A (2010) Intravenous valproate sodium (Orfiril i.v.) aborts migraine headaches rapidly. Acta Neurol Scand

Shrestha M, Singh R, Moreden J et al (1996) Ketorolac vs chlorpromazine in the treatment of acute migraine without aura. A Prospective, randomized, double blind trial. Arch Intern Med 156(15): 1725–1728

Silberstein SD (1992) Evaluation and emergency treatment of headache. Headache 32:396–407

Stevenson RJ, Dutta D, MacWalter RS (1998) The management of acute headache in adults in an acute admissions unit. Scott Med J 43:173–176

Swidan SZ, Lake AE III, Saper R JR (2005) Efficacy of intravenous diphenhydramine versus intravenous Swidan SZ, Lake AE III, and R. Saper JR. Treatment of severe migraine headache. Curr Pain Headache Rep 5(1):65–70

Valade D (2006) Headache in the emergency room. In: Olesen J, Goadsby PJ, Ramadan NM, Tfelt-Hansen P, Welch KMA (eds) The headaches. Lippincott Williams & Wilkins, Philadelphia, pp 1133–1138

42 Headache in the Tropics: Sub-Saharan Africa

Redda Tekle Haimanot
Addis Ababa University, Addis Ababa, Ethiopia

Paolo Martelletti, Timothy J. Steiner (eds.), *Handbook of Headache*, DOI 10.1007/978-88-470-1700-9_42,
© Lifting The Burden 2011

Abstract: Relatively very limited studies have addressed the epidemiology of headache in tropical countries. The few that have been published are mainly on migraine. Headache in general and migraine in particular, are under-recognized and underdiagnosed in the tropics. Nevertheless, chronic headache appears to be less prevalent in the tropics than in North America and Europe. There are a number of clinical features that make headache in the tropics different from the rest of the world. Headaches due to organic causes, mainly infectious, are common occurrences in the tropics. Contrary to beliefs in the past, migraine is not a rare entity among Africans. Its clinical manifestations are similar to other countries but classical migraine appears to be rare. Food items seem to play a minor role as triggering factors of migraine. Hot climatic conditions tend to exacerbate all types of headache. Due to lack of awareness and limited access to health care facilities, only a small percentage of the headache sufferers in the tropics get modern treatment. Headache symptoms are either tolerated or the sufferer uses herbal medication or goes to the traditional healer for treatment. The disability impact of headache and its effect on quality of life have not been very well evaluated in tropical countries. Considering the paucity of evidence-based data, there is a need for future population-based epidemiological studies of headaches in different tropical countries using standardized protocols in conformity with the classification of the International Headache Society.

Introduction

When talking of tropical countries, one traditionally is reminded of sub-Saharan Africa and the Indian subcontinent. This chapter deals with headache in the tropics. One may ask if there are major differences in the prevalence and manifestation of headache in tropical countries compared to the rest of the world to deserve a separate chapter in a textbook on headache? There are a number of reasons to justify this approach if the tropical Africa is taken into consideration.

The literature on the prevalence and health burden of headache in Africa is scanty. In addition to the limited available published materials, one has to rely on the personal experience of prominent neurologists to get a broad picture of the magnitude of the problem in the continent. Countries south of the Sahara have more or less similar sociodemographic characteristics, which may provide possibilities to make comparisons and some guarded conclusions on the burden of headache in tropical Africa.

In as far as the global picture of headache is considered, there are similarities and differences between the situation in the North (i.e., Europe and North America) and the tropical South. Headache in Africa is commonly encountered, although less frequent that the North. A meta-analysis of prevalence studies indicated migraines are more common in North America, less prevalent in South America and Europe, and far less in Africa and Asia (Rasmussen 1995). Genetic risk factors are believed to contribute to this difference (Stewart et al. 1996).

Sub-Saharan Africa has its own characteristics and particularities in as far as disease patterns are concerned. Because of the low life expectancy in African countries, prevalence studies tend to deal with relatively young populations. Socioeconomically, low incomes, poor infrastructures, and inadequate healthcare coverage make the disease burden of headache different from the rich and developed North. Environmentally, there is the role of the tropical hot climate and the high prevalence of infectious diseases. According to the experience of clinicians that have worked in Africa, pain in the African culture is tolerated more than in the West. On top of this, diseases in rural Africa are perceived in the magico-religious context where traditional healers play a big role.

It is to be noted that headache due to organic pathologies is a common occurrence in Africa. There are the localized ENT and ophthalmic pathologies. Meningitis and encephalitis from different etiologies are commonly encountered. What are even more prevalent are the systemic diseases primarily of infectious origin such as malaria, tuberculosis, cysticercosis, relapsing fever, typhus, typhoid, pneumonia, and tuberculosis where headache may be the chief complaint. These etiologies are extremely uncommon in the West and are rarely brought into the differential diagnosis of severe headache. Undiagnosed hypertension is fairly common in Africa and contributes to the causation of chronic headaches. These particularities have their direct and indirect consequences on headache as a medical problem. In most African countries, there are often delays in seeking medical care as well as in the diagnosis of organic causes of headache. As a result, headache is often under-recognized and underdiagnosed.

Epidemiology of Headache in Tropical Countries

Population-based studies on headache in tropical countries are very scanty. The few that exist are mostly on migraine. A recent review of research on headache in Developing Countries over the past decade revealed that only 10.6% of publications came from low-income countries and most of them were on migraine (Mateen et al. 2008). In fact, until the early 1970s, there was hardly any publication on headache in Africa. Spillane's 1973 Textbook of Tropical Neurology brought together neurologists to share their rich experiences on the prevalence of neurological disorders including headache. Their reports were based on hospital population studies. Authors in the book did not mention migraine as a problem in Senegal (Collomb et al. 1973) and Uganda (Billinghurst 1973). It was reported to be very rare in Zimbabwe (Rachman 1973; Levy and Axton 1973) and South Africa (Cosnett 1973). The neurologists in both Zimbabwe and South Africa specifically remarked on the extreme rarity of the condition. They claimed to have seen only one or two cases of migraine a year. However, Osuntokun in Nigeria (Osuntokun 1973), Harris in Kenya (Harris 1973), and Haddock in Ghana (Haddock 1973) already recognized its existence with prevalences of 3%, 3.5%, and 6.3%, respectively, in hospital populations. Subsequent to this collected experiences published in Spillane's 1973 book hardly anything appeared in the literature on headache in Africa until the early 1980s.

Primary and Tension-Type Headache

There are only a few epidemiological studies from Africa that have addressed the prevalence of headaches and tension-type headache, in particular. Winkler et al. (2009) probably undertook the most extensive and well designed study on tension headache in Africa. They recorded a prevalence of 12.1% for headache and 7% for tension headache in a Tanzanian rural community. Similarly, Dent et al. (2004) also recorded a 23.1% prevalence of headache in another rural part of Tanzania. Tekle Haimanot et al. (1995) in a rural population-based study in Ethiopia found a much lower prevalence of 4.7% for chronic headache and 1.7% for tension headache. It is to be noted that the Ethiopian study did not include participants below the age of 20 years. In addition, the investigators searched specifically for repeated headache episodes rather than a lifetime occurrence. Compared to the Norwegian large population-based study (Hagen et al. 2000), the prevalence of headache is much lower in Africa (23.1% vs 38%).

Migraine Headache

Surveys among students, workers, and hospital-based studies in primary care and referral clinics produced significantly varying prevalence rates of migraine that ranged from 4.5% to 42.4% – ❷ *Table 42.1* (Amayo et al. 1996; Matuja 1991; Getahun et al. 2008; Ogunyemi 1984; Wahab and Ugheoke 2009; Lisk 1987; Adoukonou et al. 2009). It is evident that hospital-based studies and those that surveyed special groups like students do not generally reflect the prevalence of diseases in the general population. The different study populations and survey methodologies employed in these studies do not therefore lend to comparisons and conclusions on the true prevalence of migraine in Africa. However, all the studies confirm that migraine is not a very rare entity in the Africa as it was earlier assumed.

The population-based epidemiological surveys in Nigeria (Osuntokun et al. 1982; Osuntokun et al. 1992; Longe and Osuntokun 1988), Ethiopia (Tekle Haimanot et al. 1995), Tanzania (Winkler et al. 2009; Dent et al. 2004), Zimbabwe (Levy 1983), and Benin (Houinato et al. 2010) produced prevalence rates of 3–6.9% among adults. Two Nigerian studies put the prevalence of migraine among children at 5.7% and 6.8% (Okobo 1991; Oniji and Iloeje 1997). These prevalence rates are lower than in Europe as evidence in the Norwegian headhunt study which revealed a rate of 12%. The Norwegian prevalence estimate is similar to findings in population-based studies in other Western countries using the IHS criteria (Hagen et al. 2000). The clinical features of migraine in Africans as described in all the available studies are similar to those described among Caucasians. An obvious female preponderance of 1: 1.8–2.8 was documented in the studies. Analysis of the age distribution of migraine sufferers in the different African studies yielded different patterns. It was therefore difficult to draw general conclusions on peak prevalence. However, a decline of prevalence of migraine is seen after the age of 40 years.

Migraine with aura is relatively rare in the African (❷ *Table 42.1*). The population-based studies from Nigeria (Longe and Osuntokun 1988), Ethiopia (Tekle Haimanot et al. 1995), and Tanzania (Dent et al. 2004) recorded prevalence rates that ranged from 0.3% to 3.6%. Levy from Zimbabwe did not encounter migraine with aura in his survey of a large urban population of 5,028 (Levy 1983). The relative rarity of migraine with aura among Africans is commented upon by Lisk in Sierra Leone who found the condition to be comparatively more common among Lebanese residing in Sierra Leone than among indigenous Africans (Lisk 1987).

In as far as precipitating factors for migraine are concerned, most studies show that hot climate, particularly exposure to the sun, physical and emotional stress were the most important trigger factors. Alcohol and menstruation in women have their contributions. However, food items play a very minor role in triggering migraine attacks (Tekle Haimanot et al. 1995; Ogunyemi 1984).

Cluster headache is extremely rare in the African according to the available literature (Tekle Haimanot et al. 1995; Matuja 1991; Getahun et al. 2008; Wahab and Ugheoke 2009).

With regard to associated conditions, epilepsy was seen in 8% and 10.8% of migraine sufferers in two studies in Nigeria. In the same country, hemoglobinopathies (sickle cell SS, AS) were associated with migraine in 20–60% of cases. This association was relatively more frequent with migraine with aura (Osuntokun and Osuntokun 1972). Family history of

□ Table 42.1

Prevalences of headache and migraine in studies in Africa

Country, author, year	Age (Years)	Number respondents	Study method migraine def.	Time period prevalence	Headache	Migraine headache ± aura	Migraine headache + aura	Migraine headache − aura	Cluster headache
Nigeria, Osuntokun et al. (1982)	All ages	906 (Rural)	Questionnaire AHC	?		6.9			
Osuntokun et al. (1992)	All ages	2,925 (Rural)	Questionnaire	?		6.3	0.4	5.9	
Ogunyemi (1984)	Youngsters	1,756 Med. students	Questionnaire AHC	?	60	28.2	3.9	12.9	0.3
Longe and Osuntokun (1988)	All ages	18,954 (Urban)	Questionnaire AHC	Lifetime	51	5.3			
Ojini et al. (2009)	Youngsters	(Med. students)	Questionnaire	1 year	46	6.4			
Wahab and Ugheoke (2009)		1,513 (Students)	Questionnaire IHS	Lifetime		9.6			
Seirra Leone, Lisk (1987)	All ages	250 (Neurology referral)	Questionnaire	?	25	42.4	10.0	32.4	0.8
Tanzania, Matuja (1991)	All ages	675 (Clinic)	Questionnaire		20.6	30.8			
Dent et al. (2004)	All ages	3,351 (Rural)	Questionnaire IHS		23.1	5.0	3.6	1.4	
Winkler et al. (2009)	All ages	7,412 (Rural)	Questionnaire IHS	1 year		4.3			
Kenya, Amayo et al. (1996)	All ages	711 (Med. students)	Questionnaire	1 year	62	38			
Ethiopia, Tekle Haimanot et al. (1995)	≥20	15,000 (Rural)	Questionnaire IHS	1 year	16.4	3.0	0.3	2.7	0.03
Getahun et al. (2008)	All ages	1,105 (Semi-urban)	Questionnaire IHS			6.2			
Zimbabwe, Levy (1983)	≥5	5,028 (Urban)	Questionnaire AHC	1 year		4.2	0	4.2	0.45
Benin, Houinato et al. (2010)	All ages	1,113 (Rural)	Questionnaire IHS	Lifetime		3.3			
Adoukonou et al. (2009)	Youngsters	336 (Students)	Questionnaire IHS	Lifetime		11.3			

migraine was found in 30–68% of the migraineurs in the different countries where studies were undertaken (Tekle Haimanot et al. 1995; Matuja 1991; Lisk 1987; Longe and Osuntokun 1988; Levy 1983).

It is perhaps appropriate to expand on the reasons for the low prevalence of migraine in the African populations. First, there is the issue of underdiagnosis, which may arise from a number of reasons. From our surveys, we have observed that rural people have a big tolerance to pain. Headache, even if persistent and recurrent, is often perceived as a trivial problem. Nevertheless, all these situations considered the prevalence of migraine among African populations is still lower than Europeans. One possible explanation may be genetic. According to Stewart, the prevalence of migraine among female African Americans was found to be lower (16.2%) than in Caucasian females (20.4%) (Stewart et al. 1996). This racial difference seen in the United States may suggest that migraine through genetic determinants may be less prevalent among Africans.

Treatment of Headaches in the Tropics

The study of Amayo et al. (1996) provides a representative picture of the therapeutic approach to migraine in Africa. There were only very few migraineurs on specific medication and only 11.2% used analgesics. Wahab and Ugheoke in Nigeria (Lisk 1987) found that only 35.8% of university students with moderate to severe disability caused by migraine were on preventive treatment. Among the majority of the rural poor, other more basic and demanding problems take higher priority. Most rural headache sufferers come from low socioeconomical bracket and are less educated. They lack the awareness and are therefore less likely to seek proper medical attention. Many go for the traditional and herbal treatments. One should also not ignore the fact that medical practitioners in the African setting do not pay a great deal of attention to the problem of headache, which may appear trivial compared with infectious diseases and malnutrition that pose greater threats to public health.

Disability Impacts of Headaches

The impact of migraine on individual sufferers and the public has been acknowledged and measured in the West. Not so in communities in sub-Saharan Africa. The impact of migraine on absenteeism and productivity has not been measured accurately in Africa. However, there are a few studies that have addressed the issue. Onji and Iloeje reported on the high incidence of absenteeism among Nigeria schoolchildren with migraine (Ojini et al. 2009). In Kenya, Amayo et al. (Matuja 1991) found that 23.5% of medical students missed at least 1 day of work or school in 1 year as a direct result of headache. Among 1,540 urban workers and students of higher education in Dar es Salaam, Tanzania, Matuja et al. found that 175 cases had an average of 11.3 lost work days per year due to headache compared with controls with only 5.7 lost workdays per year for reasons other than headache (Matuja et al. 1995). Getahun et al. (2008) found that 34.8% of Ethiopian factory workers with primary headache had on the average lost 13.8 work days per year. The figure was even higher for migraine, 16 lost working days per year. A great deal needs to be investigated on disability impact of headache in Africa through well-designed measurements of the disability and health-related quality of life.

Conclusion

Migraine in Africans is not as rare as it was reported in earlier reports. It is however under-recognized and accorded very low priority. Its clinical manifestations in Africans are similar to that seen in other populations. It is an undertreated condition where a very low percentage of the sufferers receive specific treatment. The majority of migraineurs in rural areas resort to herbal and traditional healers. There are few studies that have addressed the issue of disability assessment. Hence, the impact on health facility utilization and sickness absence from work is not very well documented. The prevalence and impact of chronic tension-type headache has also been poorly investigated in African populations. Future headache epidemiological investigations will have to be comprehensive and use protocols that are closely related to the classification of the International Headache Society (Headache Classification Committee of the International Headache Society 1988). Migraine disability assessment will also be very essential because, as Lipton observed "disability is a powerful predictor of treatment needs, failure to include it in the evaluation of a patient with migraine is a major barrier to health care" (Lipton 2001).

References

Adoukonou T, Houinato D, Kankouan J, Makoutode M, Paraiso M, Tehindrazanarivelo A, Vlader F, Preux P-M (2009) Migraine among university students in Cotonou (Benin). J Headache Pain 49:887–893

Amayo EO, Jowi JO, Njeru EK (1996) Migraine headaches in a group of medical students at Kenyatta National Hospital, Nairobi. East Afr Med J 73: 594–597

Billinghurst JR (1973) Neurological disorders in Uganda. In: Spillane JD (ed) Tropical Neurology. Oxford University Press, London, pp 191–206

Collomb H, Dumas M, Girard PL (1973) Neurological disorders in Senegal. In: Spillane JD (ed) Tropical Neurology. Oxford University Press, London, pp 131–142

Cosnett JE (1973) Neurological disorders in Natal. In: Spillane JD (ed) Tropical Neurology. Oxford University Press, London, pp 259–272

Dent W, Spiss HK, Helbok R, Matuja WBP, Scheunemann S, Schmutzhard E (2004) Prevalence of migraine in a rural area in South Tanzania: a door-to-door survey. Cephalalgia 24:960–966

Getahun MT, Tekle Haimanot R, Martelletti P (2008) Prevalence and burden of primary headache in Akaki textile mill workers, Ethiopia. J Headache Pain 9:119–128

Haddock DRW (1973) Neurological disorders in Ghana. Uganda. In: Spillane JD (ed) Tropical Neurology. Oxford University Press, London, pp 143–160

Hagen K, Zwart J-A, Vatten L, Stovner LJ (2000) Bovini G Prevalence of migraine and non-migrainous headache-head-HUNT, a large population-based study. Cephalalgia 20:900–906

Harris JR (1973) Neurological disorders in Kenya. In: Spillane JD (ed) Tropical Neurology. Oxford University Press, London, pp 207–222

Headache Classification Committee of the International Headache Society (1988) Classification and diagnostic criteria for headache disorders, cranial neuralgias and facial pain. Cephalalgia 8(Suppl 7):1–96

Houinato D, Adoukonou T, Ntsiba F, Adjien C, Avode D-G, Preux P-M (2010) Prevalence of migraine in rural community in south Benin. Cephalalgia 30:62–87

Levy LM (1983) An epidemiological study of headache in an urban population in Zimbabwe. Headache 23:2–9

Levy LF, Axton J (1973) Neurosurgery in Rhodesia. In: Spillane JD (ed) Tropical Neurology. Oxford University Press, London, pp 223–236

Lipton RB (2001) Epidemiology and burden of headache. Adv Stud Med 1:442–445

Lisk Dr (1987) Severe headache in the African: report on 250 cases from Sierra Leone, West Africa. Headache 27:477–483

Longe AC, Osuntokun BO (1988) Prevalence of migraine in Udo, a rural community in southern Nigeria. East Afr Med J 65:621–624

Mateen FJ, Dua T, Steiner T, Saxena S (2008) Headache disorder in developing countries: research over the past decade. Cephalalgia 28:1107–1114

Matuja WBP (1991) Headache: pattern and features as experienced in a neurology clinic in Tanzania. East Afr Med J 68:359–362

Matuja WB, Mteza IB, Rwiza HT (1995) Headache in a nonclinical population in Dar es Salaam Tanzania. A community-based study. Headache 35:273–276

Ogunyemi AO (1984) Prevalence of headache among Nigerian university students. Headache 24:127–130

Ojini FI, Okubadejo NU, Danesi MA (2009) Prevalence and clinical characteristics of headache in medical students of the University of Lagos, Nigeria. Cephalalgia 29(4):472–477

Okobo ME (1991) Migraine in Nigerian children – a study of 51 patients. Headache 31:673–676

Oniji GI, Iloeje SO (1997) Childhood migraine in Nigeria: a community-based study. West Afr J Med 16:208–217

Osuntokun BO (1973) Neurological disorders in Nigeria. In: Spillane JD (ed) Tropical Neurology. Oxford University Press, London, pp 161–190

Osuntokun BO, Osuntokun O (1972) Complicated migraine and haemoglobin AS in Nigerians. Br Med J 1:621–622

Osuntokun BO, Schoenberg BS, Nottidge VA, Adeuja AOG, Kale O, Adeyefa A et al (1982) Migraine headache in a rural community in Nigeria: results of a pilot study. Neuroepidemiology 1:31–39

Osuntokun BO, Adeuja AD, Nottidge VA, Bademosi O, Olumide AO, Ige O et al (1992) Prevalence of headache and migrainous headache in Nigerian Africans: a community based study. East Afr Med J 69: 196–199

Rachman I (1973) Neurological disorders in Rhodesia. In: Spillane JD (ed) Tropical Neurology. Oxford University Press, London, pp 237–246

Rasmussen BK (1995) Epidemiology of headache. Cephalalgia 15:44–67

Stewart WF, Lipton RB, Liberman J (1996) Variation in migraine prevalence by race. Neurology 46:52–59

Tekle Haimanot R, Seraw B, Forsgren L, Ekbom K, Ekstedt J (1995) Migraine, chronic tension-type headache, and cluster headache in an Ethiopian rural community. Cephalalgia 15:482–488

Wahab KW, Ugheoke AJ (2009) Prevalence and associated disabilities among Nigerian undergraduates. Cephalalgia 36:216–221

Winkler AS, Stelzhammer B, Kerschaumsteiner K, Meindl M, Dent W, Kaaya J, Matuja W, Schmutzhard E (2009) The prevalence of headache with emphasis on tension-headache in rural Tanzania: a community-based study. Cephalalgia 29:1317–1315

43 Headache in the Tropics: India

K. Ravishankar
Jaslok Hospital and Research Centre, Lilavati Hospital and Research Centre, Mumbai, India

Paolo Martelletti, Timothy J. Steiner (eds.), *Handbook of Headache*, DOI 10.1007/978-88-470-1700-9_43,
© Lifting The Burden 2011

Abstract: Headache management in the Tropics is somewhat different from what prevails in the Temperate zones primarily because of the many regional factors that impact a primary headache disorder like migraine. There are different geographical factors, different environmental problems and different cultural attitudes. The aim of this chapter is to try and appraise a worldwide audience of these factors that influence headache prevalence and treatment in the Tropics.

India with a population of 1.2 billion is the second most populous country in the world and is located in the Tropics to the north of the equator. Some of the epidemiological studies on headache from this region have been detailed. Medication overuse headache is not so common in India as in the West. Barriers to care have been divided into those that are patient-related, physician-related and regional. Overpopulation, low literacy levels, low income, growing urbanization, different triggering factors and nonavailability of latest treatment options are some of the more important regional problems. Alongside are listed the efforts needed to overcome these barriers.

Special measures are therefore required to tackle the burden of headache in India. Addressing these issues will also go a long way to providing headache relief in other Tropical regions where similar conditions prevail and where more than 40% of the world population lives.

Introduction

The Tropics refers to the region by the Equator limited in the north by the Tropic of Cancer and in the south by the Tropic of Capricorn and largely includes sub-Saharan Africa, the Indian subcontinent, rest of Asia, Central and South America, and parts of Australia. Approximately 40% of the world's population lives in the tropical zone. Being close to the Equator, the climate is hot and humid for most parts of the year and there are also many socioeconomic factors that are different in this region. Therefore when we talk of headache in the Tropics, what we actually mean is factors that impact on headache because of situations existing in tropical regions and different from temperate zones. With a view to appraising a worldwide audience of the important role of regional differences, the author reviews here factors that impact on "Headache" in India and discusses the different "Barriers to Care" and "Efforts" needed to improve the headache situation in this setting. Some of the more important contributions to headache literature from India have also been listed.

Primary headaches are more common in practice than secondary headaches. Though there may not be too many variations in the clinical presentations of primary headaches across different regions of the world, treatment outcomes may vary depending on differences in genes, geography, and environment. Attitudes, awareness, and health-care policies all have an influence on the way headaches are perceived and managed. Migraine is the main cause of headache burden worldwide. When you look at the factors that can impact on "Migraine," there are many differences between the Tropics and the Temperates. Some secondary headaches that are more commonly seen in the Tropics are those due to intracranial granulomas, neurocysticercosis, meningeal infections, and cerebral venous thrombosis.

Headache in India

India is located to the north of the equator and besides the heat and humidity there are other migraine-triggering factors that contribute to the burden of headache. Against the backdrop of other health concerns, headache management in India is not given the priority it deserves in the health-care system. Like elsewhere in the world, there is limited teaching on "headache" in medical schools and headache diagnosis and treatment are often suboptimal. Headache medicine is still not a recognized subspeciality in India. Myths and misunderstandings abound and headache patients end up being seen by many different specialists, each of whom looks at the problem through the window of their own speciality. For all these reasons, headache patients in India do not receive adequate sympathy, care, and attention. There are many additional barriers to headache care in India.

With a population of more than one billion, India has 16% of the world population and therefore health priorities keep changing. Low literacy levels make it more difficult for patients to understand the treatment plan and expectations are always high. The health-care system in the country is also not geared to supporting effective headache treatment. Less than 5% in India seek private care or managed care. With a significant part of the population being in the lower income group, financial constraints and fixed notions lead to poor compliance. Twenty-five percent of the Indian population lives in the cities and 75% in villages. Growing urbanization leads to infrastructural breakdown and increase in stress levels. Most of the rural population tries alternative treatment methods such as homeopathy, ayurveda, and unani. Physicians do not understand the true misery of headaches and time constraints and overcrowded clinics add to the problems of patients with headache. Headache diaries are not maintained, disability levels are not evaluated, and the true burden cannot be assessed.

Regional Epidemiological Data

There have been no standardized population-based epidemiological studies that can be quoted as indicative of the true prevalence. Gourie-Devi et al. (2004) did an epidemiological study of neurological disorders in Southern India that included evaluation of patients with headache. Ravishankar (1997) analyzed the pattern of headaches seen at a tertiary referral center in India. Out of 1,000 patients who presented with headache, 86% had primary headaches that were classifiable, 11% were unclassifiable, and 3% had secondary headaches. Of the primary headaches, 55% had migraine, 28.3% had tension-type headache, 22.2% had cluster headache and 0.5% had miscellaneous primary headaches. There is also a paucity of headache literature from India. Shah and Nafee (1999) studied 2,982 patients from the Kashmir Valley and analyzed the various headache patterns and cranial neuralgias. They found Ramadan fasting to be a significant factor for precipitating migraines. Shukla et al. (2001a, b) investigated blood nitrite levels and showed that platelet aggregation response and blood nitrite levels were not significantly altered after an attack in patients with migraine. They also evaluated platelet ketanserin binding in migraine patients. Garg et al. (2004) have reported on patients with solitary cysticercus granuloma and seizures who also complained of disabling headache. Sixteen patients with new onset disabling headache and solitary cysticercus granuloma with seizures were treated with a short course of prednisolone and obtained long-lasting relief. Chakravarty (2003) and Chakravarty et al. (2004) analyzed chronic daily headache (CDH) in adults and children and also studied the prevalence of trigeminal autonomic cephalalgias (TACs) seen at their center in the eastern part of India. They found that CDH remains relatively unexplored in the Indian setting and analgesic overuse is often not recognized. The average dose of analgesics implicated in CDH seems much less than what is reported in the West. They found that TACs are relatively uncommon in their center.

Medication overuse headache (MOH) is not as big a problem in India as in the West. There is however a need for more evidence on this. There have been only two clinic-based references. Ravishankar (2008a) from a headache clinic analysis noted that there were only 184 patients with MOH fulfilling I H S criteria out of a total of 6,000 patients who presented to the Headache Clinic between 2000 and 2007. Chakravarty (2003) analyzed his patients with chronic daily headache and found a comparatively low incidence of MOH as well. The commonest drug causing MOH in India is ergotamine. Triptans are costly for the average Indian migraine patient, combination analgesics and opioids are limited in number, and short-acting barbiturates are not used for headache treatment in India.

Panda and Tripathi (2005) have reported an observational study on the clinical characteristics of migraineurs from India. They reported a low frequency of patients with a positive family history of headache. Gupta and Bhatia (2006) found that 73.1% of their migraine patients had autonomic features. Ophthalmoplegic migraine (OM), is a unique disorder characterized by recurrent attacks of ophthalmoplegia, following severe migrainous headaches. Lal (2010) reported 62 adult patients with OM in a cohort of 7,000 patients with migraine seen in a tertiary care hospital in India. These patients developed acute ophthalmoplegia with severe attacks of migraine. Isolated abducens palsy was seen in 35 (56.5%) patients at presentation thus suggesting that abducens nerve palsy is not as rare as previously reported.

The advent of gadolinium magnetic resonance imaging (GdMRI) studies provided new insights into the pathogenesis of OM and triggered a sea change in the perception of the entity. The initial literature on MRI changes in OM was mostly confined to single case reports. In the first large series of OM in the post-MRI era in 1998, Mark et al. (1998) reported six patients with recurrent third nerve palsy associated with thickening and enhancement of the involved nerves on GdMRI. Besides cases with enhancement, lack of third nerve enhancement on GdMRI is also well documented in the literature. Lal reported 62 adult patients (age 15–68 years) of OM from India. None of the patients had any nerve enhancement. Ravishankar and Karthik (2007) and Ravishankar (2008b) also reported lack of enhancement in four patients of OM with involvement of third nerve. Thus, most of the patients who are diagnosed with OM in the Indian setting do not show enhancement as happens in the West.

Barriers to Care

Ravishankar (2004) reported on barriers to headache care in India and the efforts that are needed to improve the situation. The barriers were grouped as patient-related, physician-related and regional. Local problems that pertain to headache management, some unusual triggers seen in India and the inadequacies of the health-care system have been outlined below.

1. *Patient-related barriers:* Myths and misconceptions about headaches, patients' own presumptive diagnoses, and delays in seeking treatment are all barriers to care (❷ *Table 43.1*). Financial constraints commonly lead to failure to comply with follow-up consultation and long-term prophylactic treatment. Treatment of a primary headache is perceived as an unnecessary waste of money by many patients and their families for a recurrent disorder with no permanent cure. Cheap and easy access to CT scans can be detrimental. Walk-in CT scans are obtained and all further treatment is given up once they are told that the scan is normal. Low literacy levels lead to an inability to understand migraine and the reasons for

☐ Table 43.1

Barriers to care: Where do patients go wrong?

Their own myths and misconceptions
1. That headaches are caused by a defect in visual acuity
2. That headaches are caused by sinus infection
3. That headaches are caused by acidity or constipation
4. That headaches are caused by emotional upset
5. That there is no permanent cure, so you might as well live with it!
Delay in the seeking of treatment
1. Because of self-medication
2. Because of alternative treatment options
3. Because of the fear of side effects of allopathic drugs
Poor compliance due to:
1. Financial constraints
2. Frequent change of doctors
3. Poor control of triggers
4. Wrong expectation levels

☐ Table 43.2

Barriers to care: Where do physicians go wrong?

Wrong diagnosis
1. Low emphasis of headache in medical curriculum
Wrong treatment
2. Faulty drug choice
3. Suboptimal dosages
4. Inadequate duration of prophylaxis
Under-use of non-pharmacological strategies
Wrong referrals
Lack of efforts to educate patients

recurrent head pain. Many patients change doctors frequently, consult different specialists, do not recognize the importance of trigger-control measures, and lapse from care if they are not assured of a permanent cure.

2. *Physician-related barriers*: In India, as in most countries, all doctors treating headaches are not aware of the recent advances in migraine management and do not have the right attitude toward headache (❷ *Table 43.2*). Most physicians do not appreciate the true misery caused by headache, and the medical curriculum does not adequately train in the treatment of headache disorders. Overcrowded clinics with no regulated system of consultation by prior appointment make it more difficult for the general neurologist who also has to treat

◘ Table 43.3

Barriers to care: region-based issues

1. Over population
2. Growing urbanization
3. Cultural and social diversities
4. Triggers peculiar to India
5. Inadequacies of the health-care system
6. Availability of alternative treatment options
7. Low literacy levels
8. Low income levels

epilepsy and stroke, to devote much time to patients with headache. Assessment of burden with the migraine disability assessment (MIDAS) score is difficult in India because of the lack of records about days of work lost due to headache, and, therefore, care is not stratified. Patients and family practitioners do not readily accept in-patient management for chronic recurrent headaches, even for status migrainosus. Drug rebound headaches go unrecognized, alternative routes for drugs are unknown, and the latest treatment options are not used.

3. *Regional barriers:* These barriers (❷ *Table 43.3*) are beyond the control of both patient and physician, vary widely, and may have a direct bearing on the prevalence, the frequency, the severity, and the intractability of headaches. The barriers peculiar to each geographic setting must be understood if we are to make a joint effort to decrease the burden of headache worldwide. Eight major region-specific factors have an effect on the management of migraine in India.

    (a) *Over population:* With a population of more than 1 billion, India is the second most populous country in the world, second only to China. India has 16% of the world population and with an annual population growth rate of 19·5%, India's population is expected to reach 1·2 billion by the year 2011. This population growth also puts significant strain on the health-care system. Our health priorities also keep changing and so long as other major health problems such as tuberculosis, malaria, HIV, etc., are not brought under control, we cannot expect focus on an invisible misery like headache.

    (b) *Low literacy:* Low literacy has a direct bearing on the way patients perceive primary headaches and the way they set their expectations and understand treatment plans. Our national literacy level is 59·5% (men 70·2% and women 48·3%). Because migraine is more prevalent in women than in men, and owing to the high level of illiteracy in women, quality-of-life on the basis of work-related functional disability is not easily assessed, hence the estimation of the true burden of migraine is difficult.

    (c) *Low income:* Despite the fact that India has an emerging middle class of more than 250 million, there are still 350–400 million people living in lower-middle class conditions. So, with basic wants not being fulfilled, it is difficult for patients to seek treatment for their headaches.

    (d) *Growing urbanization:* Unlike many other countries with a high degree of urbanization, 25% of India's population live in cities and 75% live in rural villages, where proper infrastructural facilities are lacking. Rural areas also have no access to specialized care of headache. As India has become more urban, more doctors have moved into cities, and now 70% of physicians paradoxically are based in urban areas.

(e) *Cultural and social diversity*: India has to deal with major cultural and social differences. There are 24 major languages, with many different traditions, customs, habits, beliefs, all of which have a bearing on the attitude to the seeking of care for headaches. This also makes it difficult for migraine to be perceived and treated in the same way all over the country.

(f) *Unusual triggers*: India is located to the north of the equator in the eastern hemisphere and the heat and humidity are conducive to increased frequency and severity of migraine. Some parts of the country can have temperatures of up to 38°C for more than 8 months of the year. The hot and humid weather for most of the year, the increased light and noise levels, the different food triggers, the fasting habits in different communities, the application of henna, stressful school education, and the stress of travel in crowded conditions can all contribute to more frequent headaches that may not respond to medical treatment. Besides the established triggers that are better known, Ravishankar (2006) has described hair-wash or head-bath as an unusual trigger that is not seen in the West.

(g) *Inadequacies of the health-care system*: In India, the health-care system is represented by three sectors. The public-health sector is the state-managed free service in which doctors have no scope for ideal headache management particularly in the face of so many other pressing medical problems. The private sector or self-paid care is where patients can expect to get proper treatment for their headaches; however, because of the costs, less than 5% of people in India seek private care. As a result, only the higher strata of society can get their headaches treated correctly. In insurance-funded or managed health care, insurance agencies do not perceive primary headaches as a biological problem needing specific treatment (and sometimes hospitalization). This view not only prevents effective treatment but also wrongly indicates to the community that headache is not a disorder that needs to be taken seriously.

(h) *Easy availability of alternative therapies*: Most of the rural population try alternative methods of treatment, such as homeopathy, ayurveda, and unani. There are also unqualified practitioners and local chemists who treat patients unsuccessfully. Failed attempts at treatment only serve to reaffirm the idea that headache is difficult to treat.

Conclusion

To alleviate the burden of headache worldwide, in addition to the application of standard guidelines, we need to (a) focus regionally, (b) change the attitude to headache of both patients and physicians, (c) educate doctors about recent advances, and (d) influence insurance agencies, and improve health-care systems.

Special efforts are therefore needed to tackle the headache problem in India. Awareness and education on headache needs to improve and insurance agencies must recognize headache as a valid biological disorder. We need more tertiary care clinics and lay support groups. The health-care system should be modified to include headache care for all.

In India, there are many other important health problems and so headache is still low on the priority list. But if we address these additional barriers to care, headache burden can be reduced substantially and headache relief can get the priority it deserves.

References

Chakravarty A (2003 Jun) Chronic daily headaches: clinical profile in Indian patients. Cephalalgia 23(5):348–353

Chakravarty A, Mukherjee A, Roy D (2004 Oct) Trigeminal autonomic cephalagias and variants: clinical profile in Indian patients. Cephalalgia 24(10):859–866

Garg RK, Kar AM, Singh MK (2004 Apr) Prednisolone-responsive headache in patients with solitary cysticercus granuloma and seizures. Headache 44(4):365–369

Gourie-Devi M, Gururajb G, Satishchandraa P, Subbakrishnac DK (2004) Prevalence of neurological disorders in Bangalore, India: A community-based study with comparison between urban and rural areas. Neuroepidemiology 23: 261–268

Gupta R, Bhatia MS (2006) A report of cranial autonomic symptoms in migraineurs. Cephalalgia 27:22–28

Lal V (2010 Jan-Feb) Ophthalmoplegic migraine: Past, present and future. Neurol India 58(1):15–19

Mark AS, Casselman J, Brown D et al (1998) Ophthalmoplegic migraine: reversible enhancement and thickening of the cisternal segment of the oculomotor nerve on contrast enhanced MRI images. Am J Neuroradiol 19:1887–1891

Panda S, Tripathi M (2005 Feb) Clinical profile of migraineurs in a referral centre in India. J Assoc Physicians India 53:111–115

Ravishankar K (1997) Headache pattern in India: A headache clinic analysis of 1000 patients. Cephalalgia 17:316–317, 1

Ravishankar K (2004 Sep) Barriers to headache care in India and efforts to improve the situation. Lancet Neurol 3(9):564–567

Ravishankar K (2006 Nov) 'Hair wash' or 'head bath' triggering migraine: observations in 94 Indian patients. Cephalalgia 26(11):1330–1334

Ravishankar K (2008a) Medication overuse headache in India. Cephalalgia 28(11):1223–1226

Ravishankar K (2008b) Ophthalmoplegic migraine: still a diagnostic dilemma? Curr Pain Headache Rep 12(4):285–291

Ravishankar K, Karthik G (2007) Ophthalmoplegic migraine-suggestions for revision of nosology based on normal imaging in four patients [abstract]. Cephalalgia 27:1182

Shah PA, Nafee A (1999 Nov) Clinical profile of headache and cranial neuralgias. J Assoc Physicians India 47(11):1072–1075

Shukla R, Barthwal MK, Srivastava N, Nag D, Seth PK, Srimal RC, Dikshit M (2001a) Blood nitrite levels in patients with migraine during headache-free period. Headache 41(5):475–481

Shukla R, Khanna VK, Pradeep S, Husain M, Tandon R, Nag D, Dikshit M, Srimal RC, Seth PK, Platelet H (2001b) Ketanserin binding in migraine. Cephalalgia 21(5):567–572

Part 11

Childhood and Adolescent Headache

44 Diagnosing Headache in Young People

Çiçek Wöber-Bingöl[1] · *Andrew D. Hershey*[2] · *Marielle A. Kabbouche*[2]
[1]Medical University of Vienna, Vienna, Austria
[2]Cincinnati Children's Hospital Medical Center, University of Cincinnati College of Medicine, Cincinnati, OH, USA

Paolo Martelletti, Timothy J. Steiner (eds.), *Handbook of Headache*, DOI 10.1007/978-88-470-1700-9_44,
© Lifting The Burden 2011

Abstract: Headache is the most common somatic complaint in children and adolescents. Diagnosis is based on thorough history with the patient and the caregiver. History is the prerequisite for differentiating primary from secondary headaches and for recognizing potentially life-threatening disorders. Red flags include the first or worst headache ever in the life, recent headache onset, increasing severity or frequency, occipital location, awakening from sleep because of headache, headache occurring exclusively in the morning associated with severe vomiting, and headache associated with straining. History must cover all features required for headache diagnosis according to the International Classification of Headache Disorders (ICHD) as well as general medical problems, especially possible comorbid disorders, family history, social background, life events, lifestyle, as well as factors precipitating and alleviating headache. History has to be completed by detailed general and neurological examinations. The question whether imaging, laboratory tests, or other investigations are required is based on the clinical findings, i.e., history and clinical examination. In patients with recurrent or chronic headache, a headache diary is recommended particularly for differentiating migraine from tension-type headache and for assessing use and efficacy of abortive medication. A thorough evaluation of recurrent headache in children and adolescents is necessary to make a specific diagnosis and initiate treatment, bearing in mind that children with headache are more likely to experience psychosocial adversity and to grow up with an excess of both headache and other physical and psychiatric symptoms, thus creating an important healthcare problem for their future life.

Established Knowledge

Epidemiology

Headache disorders in children and adolescents show a high incidence and prevalence, and are associated with considerable individual burden and societal cost (Bille 1962; Hämäläinen et al. 1996). The vast majority of headaches are primary and classified as migraine or TTH (Lipton et al. 2001; Wöber-Bingöl et al. 1995).

Prevalence of headache increases throughout childhood reaching a peak at about 11–13 years of age in both sexes. By age 3, headache occurs in 3–8% of children. At age 5, 19.5% have headache, and by age 7, 37–51.5% have headache. In 7–15-year-olds, headache prevalence ranges from 26% to 82% (Sillanpää et al. 1991; Bugdayci et al. 2005).

Most of the epidemiological studies found that TTH was the most frequent headache in children aged 8–12 years. The prevalence of TTH in schoolchildren has been reported as 0.9–72.8% relating to study design and psychosocial events. The prevalence of TTH increases with age (Anttila 2006).

Migraine is the second most common cause of chronic recurrent headache in schoolchildren. The prevalence ranges from 3.2% to 14.5%. Positive family history for headache is commonly reported with a frequency of 60–77.5% (Lipton et al. 2001; Özge et al. 2002).

Principles of Clinical Diagnosis

A thorough evaluation of headache in children and adolescents is necessary to make the correct diagnosis and initiate treatment. The evaluation is based on a detailed history including observations by parents, teachers, and other child-carers. One has to keep in mind that some symptoms may be referred from the child's behavior only (e.g., stopping to watch a favorite movie, interrupting a computer game, or the child's wish to go to bed in a quiet, darkened room during daytime). Children may also be asked to draw a picture of their headache, since children, especially younger ones, communicate better through pictures than verbally (Stafstrom et al. 2005). History is completed by detailed general and neurological examinations.

History

Taking the history requires sufficient time and patience and should be done with age-appropriate terminology. Questions need to be directed to both the child and parents. Questions important to be included in the history are summarized in ❷ *Table 44.1*. Headache severity of children and adolescents should be quantified using a pain-rating scale, visual-analogue scale, or other equivalents according to age and cognitive levels of subjects. Combined scales may be more useful than one-way scales. Biological parameters of pain and observations of other family members should be noted also. History should also include pregnancy period of mother, birth and developmental history, injuries, operations and dietary habits of early

❑ Table 44.1

Questions for taking the history in young patients presenting with headache

– Do you have one or more types of headache?
– How did the headaches begin?
– When did the headaches begin?
– Are the headaches progressive, staying the same, or improving?
– How often does each headache type occur every month (or every day)?
– How long do the headaches last?
– Do the headaches occur at any special time or under any special circumstances?
– Are the headaches related to specific foods, situations, medications, or activities?
– Are there warning symptoms before headache onset?
– Where is the pain located?
– What is the quality of the pain?
– Are there associated symptoms during the headaches?
– What do you do during your headaches?
– What makes the headaches better?
– Does anything make the headaches worse?
– Do symptoms continue between headaches?
– Are you being treated for or do you have any other medical problems?
– Do you take medication for any other problem on a regular on intermittent basis?
– Does anyone else in the family have headaches?
– What do you think is causing your headaches?
– How is your daily routine?

childhood, history of substance use, psychological and psychiatric disorders, as well as family relationships, school, peer group, and psychosocial status both of the child and parents. Patients with recurrent or chronic headache should be asked to keep a headache diary (assisted by the parents) depicting the main headache characteristics and associated symptoms over a period of some weeks to document the headache frequency and duration, the degree of disability, and the occurrence of associated symptoms as well as the use of medication.

Physical Examination

The examiners should keep in mind the tentative diagnosis and substantiate their clinical impression while performing general examination.

Neurological Examination

A complete neurological examination should be performed focusing particularly on level of consciousness; meningeal signs; visual disturbances; focal neurological deficits; disorders of coordination, gait, and speech; auditory disorders; and localized tenderness of scalp or any body areas. In addition, a psychiatric interview of children and parents should be performed when needed. In the majority of patients with primary headache disorders, the general physical and neurological examinations are normal (Özge et al. 2002).

Psychological Examination

Repeated pain experience has some negative effects on daily living activities (i.e., sleep, appetite, play, attention, etc.). During the prepuberty and puberty period, changes of emotional status and personality stand in the forefront. It should be differentiated whether the emotional problem or change is a comorbidity or the main problem. Symptoms of depression, which include sadness, tearfulness, withdrawal from activities, and hopelessness, need to be checked (Karwautz et al. 1999). The evaluation process should be completed with scales (including depression, anxiety, self-esteem, CBCL, etc.) and family interview.

Principles of Diagnostic Testing

Primary headache and migraine diagnosis is usually based on the clinical history as well as physical examination (Bille 1962). Additional testing is needed if the history does not fit diagnostic criteria or physical examination shows some neurological abnormality (Lewis and Winner 2001).

Testing in these cases will be necessary not directly for primary headache diagnostic as much as to rule out any secondary headaches.

Reviews on when to refer to diagnostic testing in headache in general as well as pediatric headache have been reported in the literature (Silberstein and Rosenberg 2000; Lewis et al. 2002; Kabbouche et al. 2009). The American Academy of Neurology has also published its own guidelines in the adult and pediatric population (Silberstein and Rosenberg 2000).

These guidelines mostly focus on the role of neuroimaging in the diagnosis of headache. There is a lack of consensus regarding the role of EEG, lumbar puncture, and other laboratory testing.

Neuroimaging

Evans published an interesting manuscript detailing guidelines in when to consider imaging when a child presents with headaches (Evans and Lewis 2001). He states that clinical interviewing would give clues to the provider on the necessity of imaging, and these clues include the following:

(a) Subacute headache with rapidly progressive increase in severity
(b) New onset of headache in immunosuppressed patient
(c) Headache of new onset in patient younger than 5 years old
(d) Associated systemic symptoms, such as fever, nuchal rigidity, high blood pressure
(e) Headache with focal neurological abnormalities on physical examination

It is important to understand that other factors during the general visit should be considered in the younger population that increases the suspicion of a secondary headache. These factors were described by Medina as major in classifying a child with headache as high risk for a space occupying lesion and include (Medina et al. 1997):

(a) Headache of less than 1 month duration.
(b) Absence of family history of migraine/primary headache.
(c) Abnormal neurological examination.
(d) Gait abnormality.
(e) Seizure.
(f) Sleep-related headaches, vomiting, and confusion.
(g) Lewis did add in his comment, and this was included in the American Academy of neurology guidelines in the evaluation of headaches in children that any occipital headache in children should be evaluated for a space occupying lesion (Lewis et al. 2002).

In 2002, Lewis et al. did publish a literature review evaluating the necessity of neuroimaging when a child presents with headaches (Lewis et al. 2002). The studies reviewed included altogether 117 CT scans, 483 MRI scans, with 75 using both techniques.

Abnormalities revealed by these imaging were as follow:

(a) Sixteen percent had incidental, nonsurgical findings, including Chiari Malformation, arachnoid cysts without mass effect, paranasal sinus disease, occult vascular abnormalities, and others (cavum septi pellucidi, pineal cyst, ventricular asymmetry).
(b) Three percent had a surgically treatable lesion or lesion needing medical intervention such as a pituitary gland abnormality.
(c) Only ten patients had a tumor such as medulloblastoma, cerebellar astrocytoma, arachnopid plexus papilloma, sarcoma, primitive neuroectoderma tumor, glioblastoma.

Lewis had the same results from his review compared to Medina's publication as far as predictive value for increased risk of a space occupying lesion.

The recommendation for children was then reported by the Quality standards subcommittee of the American Academy of Neurology and the Practice Committee of the Child Neurology Society (Lewis et al. 2002) as follows:

(a) Obtaining a neuroimaging on a routine basis is not indicated in children with recurrent headache and a normal neurological examination.

(b) Neuroimaging should be considered in children with an abnormal neurological examination and/or in whom there are historical features suggesting recent onset of headache, change in type of headache, neurological dysfunction, as well as occipital location of the headache.

The 12 rule of thumb in considering getting a brain imaging in children evaluated for headache are summarized in ❷ *Table 44.2.*

EEG

EEG was previously part of the routine evaluation of children with headache due to the increase risk of post-ictal headache (Chen et al. 1994; Kramer et al. 1997). Rarely this testing is of value in headache these days. The only prominent response was a prominent response during photic stimulation (the H response). This response was of no clinical value for diagnosis and treatment of children with headache, and was neither sensitive nor specific to children with primary headache (Whitehouse et al. 1967). An EEG would be warranted if the headache is associated with suspicious symptoms for seizures. Children, especially younger kids, have a wide variety of atypical symptoms, including the periodic syndrome of childhood as well as migraine variants. These clinical syndromes share a similar symptomatology with seizure disorders in this age group, and in these cases, an EEG would be warranted to rule out an underlying seizure or epilepsy syndrome.

Lumbar Puncture

The indication for a lumbar puncture in children are as follows (Quality Standard Subcommittee of the American Academy of Neurology: Practice Parameters: Lumbar Puncture. 1993):

❏ Table 44.2

The 12 rule of thumb in considering a brain imaging in children evaluated for headache

– Abnormal neurological examination
– Atypical presentation of the headache: vertigo, intractable vomiting, headache waking the child from sleep
– Recent headache of less than 6 months
– Child of less than 6 years of age
– No family history of migraine or primary headache
– Occipital headache
– Change in type of headache
– Subacute progressive headache severity
– New onset headache in an immunosuppressed child
– First and/or worst headache
– Systemic symptoms and signs
– Headache associated with confusion, focal neurological complaints, seizures

(a) First and/or worst headache to rule out a subarachnoid hemorrhage, especially if suspicion is high and the CT brain is normal
(b) Headache with fever in an immunosuppressed patient
(c) Headache with fever/nuchal rigidity or other signs of meningitis and or encephalitis
(d) Evaluation for an increased/decreased intracranial pressure

Clinical Laboratory Testing

Clinical laboratory testing is not of routine recommendation for primary headache. When requested, these tests usually are targeting to rule out suspected secondary headache from anemia, thyroid diseases, or other underlying systemic disorders.

Routine testing is usually recommended prior or during preventive therapies with specific medications such as antiepileptic medication used for headache treatment (Sargent and Solbach 1983). Some headache centers do have on their protocol to evaluate the Vitamin B2, Coenzyme Q10, as well as Vitamin D levels in children who necessitate preventive therapies due to the frequency of their headache since headache frequency can be associated with low level of the above-mentioned vitamins.

Migraine

A child or adolescent suffering from an acute migraine attack usually stops playing or studying, looks "sick," wants to lie down, and may wish to sleep. Onset of headache is acute or gradual. The headache is often severe, localized on one or both sides, typically on the forehead (in contrast to adults, hemicrania is infrequent in children), and may get worse by physical activity (Wöber-Bingöl et al. 2004). Associated symptoms may consist of nausea, vomiting, photophobia, phonophobia, or osmophobia. Headache usually lasts a few hours (sometimes less than 1 h; migraine with aura is less common in children than in adolescents), whereas the neurological symptoms should subside within an hour.

Over the last five decades, several definitions of pediatric migraine have been proposed. Definitions by Vahlquist (1955), followed by Bille (1962) (Prensky and Sommer 1979) have been followed by IHS proposing a new set of criteria (1988). Revising the IHS headache duration criterion, i.e., decreasing minimum headache duration from 2 h to 1 h, the utility of the IHS criteria for migraine performed 47–86.6% sensitivity and 92.4–98.6% specificity (Wöber-Bingöl et al. 1995; Winner et al. 1995). In 2004, the International Classification of Headache Disorders (ICHD-II) was published (2004). ICHD-II inlcudes the following criteria or comments specific to pediatric migraine without aura:

1. Attacks may last 1–72 h.
2. Migraine headache is commonly bilateral.
3. Photophobia and phonophobia may be inferred from behavior.

These specific features have improved the sensitivity of the criteria (Hershey et al. 2005; Kienbacher et al. 2006).

A bidirectional relationship between migraine and depression suggests a neurobiological link. Adverse experiences, particularly childhood maltreatment, may alter neurobiological systems, and predispose to a multiplicity of adult chronic disorders. The majority of the studies with clinical populations show slightly higher scores on at least one of the anxiety or depression scales in the migraine group as compared to the control group. However, in all 11 studies, the average score on the anxiety and depression scales obtained by children with migraine did not reach a pathological level, according to the norms established by the validated scales. Findings point to above average levels of anxiety or depression, rather than diagnosed psychopathologies. Therefore, certain authors use the term "subclinical." None of the three studies carried out in the general population revealed differences between the anxiety and depression scores in children with migraine as opposed to children in the control group. The difference in results from studies in the general population and clinical populations can most likely be explained by a recruitment bias. The association of childhood sexual abuse with migraine and depression is amplified if abuse also occurs at a later age (Guidetti and Galli 2002; Tietjen et al. 2007; Amouroux and Rousseau-Salvador 2008).

Migraine Variants

Familial hemiplegic migraine (FHM) is an uncommon and genetically heterogeneous autosomal dominant subtype of migraine with aura in which the aura consists of hemiparesis. Three subtypes of FHM have been described: FHM1, FHM2, and FHM3 (Thomsen et al. 2007).

Basilar-type migraine is a migraine variant that is classified as part of the spectrum of migraine with aura in the ICHD-II classification. The diagnostic criteria comprise vertigo, visual disturbances in both hemifields, bilateral sensory symptoms, and ataxia. The sudden appearance of diplopia, vertigo, and vomiting must prompt consideration of disorders within the posterior fossa such as arteriovenous malformations, cavernous angiomas, tumors, or congenital malformations (Kirchmann et al. 2006).

"Alice in Wonderland" Syndrome originates from Lewis Carol's novel and characterized by bizarre visual illusions and spatial distortions which precede headaches. The children may describe bizarre or vivid visual illusions such as micropsia, macropsia, metamorphopsia, and teleopsia (Lewis and Winner 2001).

Acute confusional migraine (ACM) is a rare type of migraine described as acute confusional states, lasting 4–24 h, associated with agitation and aphasia commonly seen in juvenile migraineurs. ACM may be a presenting feature and important clue, enabling CADASIL to be recognized. Therefore, a brain MRI and/or testing for Notch3 mutations should be considered in adult patients with ACM (Ehyai and Fenichel 1978; Sathe et al. 2009).

Migraine Equivalents

Migraine equivalents of infancy, childhood, and adolescence are recognized periodic, paroxysmal syndromes without associated headache that are thought to be migrainous in etiology. The following equivalents are presently recognized.

1. Cyclical vomiting (ICHD-II 1.3.1)
2. Abdominal migraine (ICHD-II 1.3.2)
3. Benign paroxysmal vertigo (ICHD-II 1.3.3)
4. Benign paroxysmal torticollis (ICHD-II A1.3.5)

Tension-Type Headache

Although TTH and migraine are the two most common types of headache in children and adolescents, most articles address migraine headache. The smaller genetic effect on TTH than on migraine suggests that the two disorders are distinct. However, many believe that TTH and migraine represent the same pathophysiological spectrum.

TTH may be hard to differentiate from migraine in children as some of the symptoms overlap. A headache diary is a useful method for the differentiation of headache types. Regarding the frequency of TTH, ICHD-II differentiates infrequent episodic TTH occurring less than once a month, frequent episodic TTH present on up to 14 days per month, and chronic TTH occurring at least on 15 days per month or 180 days per year. TTH is characterized by a pressing tightness occurring bilaterally anywhere on cranium or suboccipital region. The pain is mild to moderate in intensity and usually not aggravated by physical activity. Associated symptoms are absent or limited to one out of photophobia and phonophobia in episodic TTH and one out of mild nausea, photophobia, and phonophobia in chronic TTH. The clinical features of TTH show only minor differences between children, adolescents, and adults (Wöber-Bingöl et al. 1996). ICHD-II does not provide specific criteria for pediatric TTH.

In children, a connection seems possible between TTH and psychosocial stress, psychiatric disorders, muscular stress, or oromandibular dysfunction. Children and adolescents with chronic diseases and stressful family events have an increased risk for chronic TTH. Of children with chronic TTH, over 50% have had predisposing physical or emotional stress factors. Compared to migraine group, children with TTH had greater psychological and temperamental difficulties (Kaynak et al. 2004; Anttila 2006).

Cluster Headache and Other Trigeminal Autonomic Cephalalgias

Cluster headache (CH) is the most painful of the primary headaches. The condition usually begins in the second decade of life; the prevalence of childhood onset is approximately 0.1% and the sex ratio is approximately the same as in adults (M:F ~3.2:1). Onset may be as soon as 3 years, but there is a relatively low number of cases with onset <10 years old (Ekbom et al. 2002).

Paroxysmal hemicrania and short-lasting unilateral neuralgiform headache attacks with conjunctival injection and tearing (SUNCT) have been reported very rarely in young patients (Seidel and Wöber 2009).

Differential Diagnosis of Chronic Headache

In children and adolescents, chronic headache is an exceptionally challenging type of headache to treat. The most important subtypes are chronic migraine (CM), chronic tension-type headache (CTTH), and new daily persistent headache (NDPH). Chronic headache has different expressions in children and adults; the different expressions may reflect several different etiologies or a developmental continuum. Although a positive family history predisposes children to develop headache, many environmental, biological, and psychological processes may share a role in the etiology (McGrath 2001; Seshia et al. 2008; Kung et al 2009).

Comorbid chronic migraine and CTTH was the most frequent subtype of chronic headache. Childhood adversities may contribute to greater risk of the development of chronic headache in young adolescents (Galli et al. 2004). NDPH is the least studied form of CDH. Most adolescents with NDPH do not overuse acute medication, and most have prominent migraine features (Kung et al. 2009).

Current Research

There remain many gaps in our current understanding of pediatric headache, although recent work has begun to fill in some of these areas. As noted elsewhere in this text, headaches can be divided into primary and secondary headaches. In the study of primary headaches in pediatrics, most of the research has focused on pediatric migraine and chronic migraine (CM) (reviewed (Hershey)), while the research studies into TTH has been much less studied (reviewed Seshia et al. 2009). For trigeminal autonomic cephalalgias (TACs), there have been a few reports on cluster headaches and only case reports for the remainder. For secondary headaches, there have been few dedicated studies examining secondary headaches with a great need to further exam the role of head trauma, allergies, and sinus disease.

Recent areas of research focus for pediatric specific headaches have included epidemiology and disease characterization, acute treatment, preventative treatment, psychological interventions and influences, and comorbid conditions, with limited advances into the unique pathophysiological components of childhood headaches. There are needs to fill in all of these areas, some of which have been described elsewhere.

Disease Characterization

The scientific diagnosis of headaches is based on ICHD-II (Headache Classification Subcommittee of the International Headache Society 2004). These criteria have pediatric specific footnotes added for migraine without aura, while the remainder of the criteria are not pediatric specific. The specificity and sensitivity of these criteria have been addressed by several studies (Hershey et al. 2005; Kienbacher et al. 2006). The common findings within these studies are that shorter duration migraine without aura occurs frequently in children and that the criteria could have an increase in the sensitivity by lowering the minimum duration of headache. This is included as one of the footnotes in ICHD-II, but further detailed characterization of this time association across different developmental ages and the corresponding sensitivity and specificity of shorter duration migraine.

Another disease characterization that was noted in the ICHD-II was the allowance for parental observation, especially of photophobia and phonophobia, to be utilized in defining the associated symptoms. Although this does allow for increased ability to meet criteria, the correlation between the parental observation and the actual occurrence of these symptoms needs to be further defined. In addition, there may be additional associated symptoms that may assist with improving the sensitivity and specificity of the ICHD-II, including osmophobia (as noted in the appendix to the ICHD-II (2004) and Corletto (Corletto et al. 2008)), as well as lightheadedness and difficulty thinking (Hershey et al. 2005). Additional headache characteristics including cutaneous allodynia due to central sensitization may also improve disease characterization and their sensitivity and specificity should be determined.

Frequency of the headaches separates migraine without aura into episodic migraine (less than 15 headaches per month) from chronic migraine (15 or more headaches per month with at least meeting IHCD-II for migraine without aura). This division is somewhat arbitrary with other divisions including infrequent, frequent but not chronic, chronic but not daily, daily intermittent and daily continuous, as well as others. It appears in adults that there may be a frequency which when exceeded promotes the worsening of headache frequency – sometimes referred to as "chronification." This has lead to the pathophysiological study of migraine progression. Further study is needed in pediatrics and adolescents to characterize if there is a similar risk point of progression, as well as the reversibility with treatment.

For TTH, the disease characteristics and criteria have not been studied in enough detail to differentiate specific pediatric-related characteristics. The lower severity level of TTH results in TTH to be less likely brought to the child's family or healthcare providers and thus has not been as well studied, and further work is needed to determine if there are pediatric modifications needed for the diagnosis of TTH.

For TACs and secondary headaches, pediatric specific disease characterization studies are also largely lacking. For the TACs, this is due to the low frequency of these disorders in pediatrics, while for many of the secondary headaches, the symptoms are confused between the true secondary headaches and the triggering of migraine by the presumed secondary etiology. One of the most common occurrences of this in adults is the misdiagnosis of migraine as a "sinus headache." It has not been well delineated the frequency with which pediatric migraine is being misdiagnosed as sinus headaches, but it can be assumed that it may be comparable to adults.

Another secondary headache that warrants further disease characterization is post-traumatic headaches. Head trauma from mild to severe is common in pediatrics and adolescents, especially in those children involved in contact sports. Although it is clear that when significant head trauma occurs, there can be corresponding brain injury, the majority of the sports-related head injuries are mild to moderate, associated with spontaneous recovery, yet may have long-term effects on headaches and cognitive functioning. Not only is there a need for better characterization of the headaches that occur in children with a head trauma, but there is also a need for research into the pathophysiology, treatment, and outcome.

Epidemiology

The epidemiology of migraine continues to add to our understanding of frequency and contributing/confounding factors (reviewed (Hershey 2010)). This has included epidemiological studies in specific regions (Turkey (Unalp et al. 2007), Germany (Kroner-Herwig et al. 2007; Gassmann et al. 2008; Kroner-Herwig et al. 2009), Thailand (Visudtibhan et al. 2007), USA (Bigal et al. 2007)). Some of the recent observations that have resulted from these studies include the rather consistent frequency of migraine from 5% to 20% and the frequency of CM at ~1%, the influence of socioeconomic factors, and the role of parents and environment. One aspect that is missing is identical epidemiological studies across geographical and cultural regions to identify if there are true differences in prevalence and incidence, or if the differences are due to sample and protocol variations.

Comorbid Conditions

A variety of comorbid conditions have recently been demonstrated to be associated with pediatric headache. These include asthma and allergic disorders (Gurkan et al. 2000; Ku et al. 2006), obesity (Pinhas-Hamiel et al. 2008; Hershey et al. 2009), epilepsy (Pellock 2004; Yamane et al. 2004; Piccinelli et al. 2006; Stevenson 2006), sleep disorders (Bruni et al. 1997; Miller et al. 2003; Luc et al. 2006; Gilman et al. 2007; Isik et al. 2007; Pakalnis et al. 2009), and psychological/emotional disorders (Pakalnis et al. 2007; Kroner-Herwig et al. 2008; Vannatta et al. 2008). Understanding how these comorbid conditions influence the expression of primary headaches and the effectiveness of interventions is needed to be further studied.

One comorbid condition that is of increasing concern is the role of obesity. As obesity is become epidemic in proportion in many areas of the world, there appears to be not only an association of increased frequency and disability, but there may also be a treatment effect when the children normalize their weight. It is not clear if this is due to the combined effect of both conditions, or if it is directly due to pathophysiological interactions.

Pathophysiology

The pathophysiology of primary and secondary headaches in pediatrics and adolescents should be expected to be similar to adults. Two factors may have a greater influence in the pathophysiolgcal expression of headaches – genetics and hormonal effects of puberty.

Several older genetic studies have demonstrated that for children and adolescents, the influence of inheritance for migraine with aura is approximately 60–70%, with environmental influences accounting for the rest of the expression (Ulrich et al. 1999). For migraine that starts or worsens in adults, this genetic influence also exists but does not appear to be strong. This suggests that the study of the genetics of migraine may be more appropriately studied in children as having a "more pure" disease expression.

During adolescents, the effects of pubertal hormones can have a significant effect on a child's life that is influenced by both the direct effects of the hormones on the developing brain, as well as the psychodynamic and sociological effects of puberty itself. In addition, it is at this time that the expression of menstrual migraine becomes evident. As this is a time period that the epidemiology studies demonstrate the most rapid rise in the presentation of migraine, this biological influence of pubertal hormones needs further investigation.

References

Amouroux R, Rousseau-Salvador C (2008) Anxiety and depression in children and adolescents with migraine: a review of the literature. Encephale 34 (5):504–510

Anttila P (2006) Tension-type headache in childhood and adolescence. Lancet Neurol 5(3):268–274

Bigal ME, Lipton RB et al (2007) Migraine in adolescents: association with socioeconomic status and family history. Neurology 69(1):16–25

Bille BS (1962) Migraine in school children. A study of the incidence and short-term prognosis, and a clinical, psychological and electroencephalographic comparison between children with migraine and matched controls. Acta Paediatr 51 (Supp 136): S1–S151

Bruni O, Febrizi P et al (1997) Prevalence of sleep disorders in childhood and adolescence with headache: a case-control study. Cephalalgia 17: 492–498

Bugdayci R, Özge A, Sasmaz T, Kurt AO, Kaleagasi H, Karakelle A, Tezcan H, Siva A (2005) Prevalence and factors affecting headache in Turkish schoolchildren. Pediatr Int 47(3):316–322

Chen JH, Wang PJ et al (1994) Etiological classification of chronic headache in children and their electroencephalographic features. Zhonghua Min Guo Xiao Er Ke Yi Xue Hui Za Zhi 35(5):397–406

Corletto E, Dal Zotto L et al (2008) Osmophobia in juvenile primary headaches. Cephalalgia 28(8): 825–831

Ehyai A, Fenichel GM (1978) The natural history of acute confusional migraine. Arch Neurol 35(6):368–369

Ekbom K, Svensson DA, Traff H, Waldenlind E (2002) Age at onset and sex ratio in cluster headache: observations over three decades. Cephalalgia 22:94–100

Evans RW, Lewis DW (2001) Is an MRI scan indicated in a child with new-onset daily headache? Headache 41(9):905–906

Galli F, Patron L, Russo PM, Bruni O, Ferini-Strambi L, Guidetti V (2004) Chronic daily headache in childhood and adolescence: clinical aspects and a 4-year follow-up. Cephalalgia 24(10):850–858

Gassmann J, Morris L et al (2008) One-year course of paediatric headache in children and adolescents aged 8–15 years. Cephalalgia 28(11):1154–1162

Gilman DK, Palermo TM et al (2007) Primary headache and sleep disturbances in adolescents. Headache 47(8):1189–1194

Guidetti V, Galli F (2002) Psychiatric comorbidity in chronic daily headache: pathophysiology, etiology, and diagnosis. Curr Pain Headache Rep 6(6): 492–497

Gurkan F, Ece A et al (2000) Parental history of migraine and bronchial asthma in children. Allergol Immunopathol (Madr) 28(1):15–17

Hämäläinen ML, Hoppu K, Santavuori PR (1996) Pain and disability in migraine or other recurrent headache as reported by children. Eur J Neurol 3:528–532

Headache Classification Committee of the International Headache Society (1988) Classification and diagnostic criteria for headache disorders, cranial neuralgia and facial pain. Cephalalgia 8(Suppl 7):S1–S96

Headache Classification Subcommittee of the International Headache Society (2004) The international classification of headache disorders: 2nd edition. Cephalalgia 24(Suppl 1):1–160

Hershey AD (2010) Current approaches to the diagnosis and management of paediatric migraine. Lancet Neurol 9(2):190–204

Hershey AD, Winner P, Kabbouche MA, Gladstein J, Yonker M, Lewis D et al (2005) Use of the ICHD-II criteria in the diagnosis of pediatric migraine. Headache 45(10):1288–1297

Hershey AD, Powers SW et al (2009) Obesity in the pediatric headache population: a multicenter study. Headache 49(2):170–177

Isik U, Ersu RH et al (2007) Prevalence of headache and its association with sleep disorders in children. Pediatr Neurol 36(3):146–151

Kabbouche MA, Powers SW et al (2009) Inpatient treatment of status migraine with dihydroergotamine in children and adolescents. Headache 49(1):106–109

Karwautz A, Wöber C, Lang T, Böck A, Wagner-Ennsgraber C, Vesely C et al (1999) Psychosocial factors in children and adolescents with migraine and tension-type headache: a controlled study and review of the literature. Cephalalgia 19:32–43

Kaynak Key FN, Donmez S, Tuzun U (2004) Epidemiological and clinical characteristics with psychosocial aspects of tension-type headache in Turkish college students. Cephalalgia 24:669–674

Kienbacher C, Wöber C, Zesch HE, Hafferl-Gattermayer A, Posch M, Karwautz A et al (2006) Clinical features, classification and prognosis of migraine and tension-type headache in children and adolescents: a long-term follow-up study. Cephalalgia 26(7):820–830

Kirchmann M, Thomsen LL, Olesen J (2006) Basilar-type migraine: clinical, epidemiologic, and genetic features. Neurology 66(6):880–886

Kramer U, Nevo Y et al (1997) Electroencephalography in the evaluation of headache patients: a review. Isr J Med Sci 33(12):816–820

Kroner-Herwig B, Heinrich M et al (2007) Headache in German children and adolescents: a population-based epidemiological study. Cephalalgia 27(6): 519–527

Kroner-Herwig B, Morris L et al (2008) Biopsychosocial correlates of headache: what predicts pediatric headache occurrence? Headache 48(4):529–544

Kroner-Herwig B, Morris L et al (2009) Agreement of parents and children on characteristics of pediatric headache, other pains, somatic symptoms, and depressive symptoms in an epidemiologic study. Clin J Pain 25(1):58–64

Ku M, Silverman B et al (2006) Prevalence of migraine headaches in patients with allergic rhinitis. Ann Allergy Asthma Immunol 97(2):226–230

Kung E, Tepper SJ, Rapoport AM, Sheftell FD, Bigal ME (2009) New daily persistent headache in the paediatric population. Cephalalgia 29:17–22

Lewis DW, Winner P (2001) Migraine, migraine variants, and other primary headache syndromes. In: Winner P, Rothner AD (eds) Headache in children and adolescents. BC Decker, London, pp 60–86

Lewis DW, Ashwal S et al (2002) Practice parameter: evaluation of children and adolescents with recurrent headaches: report of the Quality Standards Subcommittee of the American Academy of Neurology and the Practice Committee of the Child Neurology Society. Neurology 59(4):490–498

Lipton RB, Maytal J, Winner P (2001) Epidemiology and classification of headache. In: Winner P, Rothner AD (eds) Headache in children and adolescents. BC Decker, Hamilton, pp 87–115

Luc ME, Gupta A et al (2006) Characterization of symptoms of sleep disorders in children with headache. Pediatr Neurol 34(1):7–12

McGrath PA (2001) Chronic daily headache in children and adolescents. Curr Pain Headache Rep 5(6): 557–566

Medina LS, Pinter JD et al (1997) Children with headache: Clinical predictors of surgical space-occupying lesions and the role of neuroimaging. Pediatr Radiol 202:819–824

Miller VA, Palermo TM et al (2003) Migraine headaches and sleep disturbances in children. Headache 43(4):362–368

Özge A, Bugdayci R, Sasmaz T, Kaleagasi H, Kurt O, Karakelle A et al (2002) The sensitivity and specificity of the case definition criteria in diagnosis of headache: a school-based epidemiological study of 5562 children in Mersin. Cephalalgia 22:791–798

Pakalnis A, Butz C et al (2007) Emotional problems and prevalence of medication overuse in pediatric chronic daily headache. J Child Neurol 22(12):1356–1359

Pakalnis A, Splaingard M et al (2009) Serotonin effects on sleep and emotional disorders in adolescent migraine. Headache 49(10):1486–1492

Pellock JM (2004) Understanding co-morbidities affecting children with epilepsy. Neurology 62(5 Suppl 2): S17–S23

Piccinelli P, Borgatti R et al (2006) Relationship between migraine and epilepsy in pediatric age. Headache 46(3):413–421

Pinhas-Hamiel O, Frumin K et al (2008) Headaches in overweight children and adolescents referred to a tertiary-care center in Israel. Obesity (Silver Spring) 16(3):659–663

Prensky AL, Sommer D (1979) Diagnosis and treatment of migraine in children. Neurology 29:506–510

Quality Standard Subcommittee of the American Academy of Neurology (1993) Practice parameters: lumbar puncture. Neurology 43:625–627

Sargent JD, Solbach P (1983) Medical evaluation of migraineurs: review of the value of laboratory and radiologic tests. Headache 23(2):62–65

Sathe S, DePeralta E, Pastores G, Kolodny EH (2009) Acute confusional migraine may be a presenting feature of CADASIL. Headache 49(4):590–596

Seidel S, Wöber C (2009) Paroxysmal hemicrania with visual aura in a 17-year-old boy. Headache 49:607–609

Seshia SS, Phillips DF, von Baeyer CL (2008) Childhood chronic daily headache: a biopsychosocial perspective. Dev Med Child Neurol 50(7):541–545

Seshia SS, Abu-Arafeh I et al (2009) Tension-type headache in children: the Cinderella of headache disorders! Can J Neurol Sci 36(6):687–695

Silberstein SD, Rosenberg J (2000) Multispecialty consensus on diagnosis and treatment of headache. Neurology 54:1553

Sillanpää M, Piekkala P, Kero P (1991) Prevalence of headache at preschool age in an unselected child population. Cephalalgia 11(5):239–242

Stafstrom CE, Goldenholz SR, Dulli DA (2005) Serial headache drawings by children with migraine: correlation with clinical headache status. J Child Neurol 20(10):809–813

Stevenson SB (2006) Epilepsy and migraine headache: is there a connection? J Pediatr Health Care 20(3): 167–171

Thomsen LL, Kirchmann M, Bjornsson A, Stefansson H, Jensen RM, Fasquel AC et al (2007) The genetic spectrum of a population-based sample of familial hemiplegic migraine. Brain 130(Pt 2):346–356

Tietjen GE, Brandes JL, Digre KB, Baggaley S, Martin VT, Recober A et al (2007) History of childhood maltreatment is associated with comorbid depression in women with migraine. Neurology 69(10):959–968

Ulrich V, Gervil M et al (1999) The inheritance of migraine with aura estimated by means of structural equation modelling. J Med Genet 36(3):225–227

Unalp A, Dirik E et al (2007) Prevalence and clinical findings of migraine and tension-type headache in adolescents. Pediatr Int 49(6):943–949

Vahlquist B (1955) Migraine in children. Int Arch Allergy Appl Immunol 7(4–6):348–355

Vannatta K, Getzoff EA et al (2008) Multiple perspectives on the psychological functioning of children with and without migraine. Headache 48(7):994–1004

Visudtibhan A, Siripornpanich V et al (2007) Migraine in Thai children: prevalence in junior high school students. J Child Neurol 22(9):1117–1120

Whitehouse D, Pappas JA et al (1967) Electroencephalographic changes in children with migraine. N Engl J Med 276(1):23–27

Winner P, Martinez W, Mante L, Bello L (1995) Classification of pediatric migraine: proposed revisions to the IHS criteria. Headache 35:407–410

Wöber-Bingöl C, Wöber C, Karwautz A, Vesely C, Wagner-Ennsgraber C, Amminger GP et al (1995) Diagnosis of headache in childhood and adolescence: a study in 437 patients. Cephalalgia 15:13–21

Wöber-Bingöl Ç, Wöber Ch, Karwautz A, Schnider P, Vesely Ch, Wagner-Ennsgraber Ch, Zebenholzer K, Wessely P (1996) Tension-type headache in different age groups at two headache centers. Pain 67: 53–58

Wöber-Bingöl Ç, Wöber Ch, Karwautz A, Auterith A, Serim M, Zebenholzer K, Aydinkoc K, Kienbacher Ch, Wanner Ch, Wessely P (2004) Clinical features of migraine: a cross-sectional study in patients aged three to sixtynine. Cephalalgia 24:12–17

Yamane LE, Montenegro MA et al (2004) Comorbidity headache and epilepsy in childhood. Neuropediatrics 35(2):99–102

45 Managing Headache in Young People

Çiçek Wöber-Bingöl[1] · *Isabel Pavão Martins*[2]
[1]Medical University of Vienna, Vienna, Austria
[2]Lisbon Faculty of Medicine, Portugal Hospital de Sta Maria,
Lisbon, Portugal

Paolo Martelletti, Timothy J. Steiner (eds.), *Handbook of Headache*, DOI 10.1007/978-88-470-1700-9_45,
© Lifting The Burden 2011

Abstract: Headache is a frequent complaint in childhood and adolescence, and its prevalence increases with age. Although the most common causes of chronic or recurrent headaches in this group are benign primary headaches, migraine, and TTH, they may have a significant impact in children's lives, disrupting school and social activities.

Appropriate management requires an individually tailored strategy giving due consideration to both nonpharmacologic and pharmacologic treatments. Reassurance, education, and information of patients and family are important intervention measures. Longitudinal studies have demonstrated that childhood migraine tends to improve with age and early diagnosis and intervention may be important to avoid persistence of symptoms.

In migraine, acetaminophen and ibuprofen are effective in the acute treatment of the attacks, but oral therapy can fail due to vomiting. Nasal sumatriptan, nasal zolmitriptan, and oral almotriptan have been approved for use in patients above 11 years of age. Supplementary measures such as rest in a quiet, darkened room are recommended. In chronic TTH, patients should be advised to take acute therapy only when the pain is severe, in order to avoid analgesic overuse.

Prophylactic management of migraine and TTH should include strategies relating to daily habits, family, school, and leisure-time activities. Nonpharmacologic treatments include relaxation training, biofeedback, cognitive-behavioral therapy, other psychotherapeutic approaches, or combinations of these treatments. Pharmaco-prophylaxis is indicated if headache are frequent and severe despite lifestyle modifications. Although many prophylactic medications have been tried in pediatric migraine, there are only a few medications that have been studied in controlled trials (particularly flunarizine and topiramate).

Multidisciplinary treatment is an effective strategy for children and adolescents with improvement of multiple outcome variants including frequency and severity of headache and school days missed because of headache.

Established Knowledge

Headache can have a significant impact in children's lives, a fact that is not quite recognized in primary care. On a study of children between the ages of 12 and 15 years, 20% of whom suffering from headache one or more times a week, it was found that those with headache were more likely to miss school and had a worse quality of life compared to children with asthma or diabetes (Kernick et al. 2009).

In this chapter, we will describe migraine and tension-type headache (TTH) in young people focusing on its therapeutic approaches and management and we will briefly address the treatment of cluster headache.

The general principles of management of headache in children and adolescents can be summarized as follows:

- Establish the diagnosis.
- Look for possible somatic and psychiatric comorbidities.
- Ask for triggers and assess degree of disability.
- Educate the child and family about the condition.
- Use a headache calendar to establish the characteristics of headache and associated symptoms.
- Establish realistic expectations and set appropriate goals.
- Reduce the emotional mechanisms (on a personal level, within the family and at school) that provoke stress and may favor headache attacks.

- Advise to maintain a sound rhythm in daily life, which includes regular meals, sufficient fluid intake, physical exercise, and sleep.
- Advise how to cope with trigger factors.
- Prescribe acute medication, if needed, and advise how to use it.
- Recommend specific nonpharmacological treatment, if needed.
- Assess the need of prophylactic medication and advise how to use it.
- Discuss the expected benefits of therapy and the time course to achieve them.

In comparison to adults, headache management in young patients requires an age related approach. The history is taken with the child as well as with the parents, and worries of the parents are taken seriously, e.g., regarding the referral for neuroimaging. Clinical and diagnostic issues are presented in ❱ Chap. 44.

Migraine

Migraine is a chronic recurrent disorder, and like any other chronic disorder requires "good doctoring," an empathic and trusting relationship, where patients and parents have an active role in therapy and can manifest their preferences and disagreements (Wöber-Bingöl 2002). Therapeutic intervention should be made at different levels and includes: (a) reassurance about the benign nature of migraine, though keeping a clear awareness of its impact in child's life; education of the patient and family about this disorder and instructions about the record of the attacks in the form of a paper or an electronic diary (preferred by adolescents); (b) attempts to the identification of the precipitant factors and implementation of lifestyle changes that can reduce the frequency of the attacks, namely, sufficient intake of fluid, avoiding long periods of fasting, and regular sleep; (c) acute attack therapy to reduce its duration and severity; and (d) prophylactic interventions to improve attack frequency. The latter is required when there are three or more attacks per month or if the attacks are unusually severe, long, or unresponsive to therapy.

There is ongoing research trying to identify precipitants of attacks in children, and headache diaries are recommended to facilitate their identification. In many cases, it is possible to identify at least one trigger factor (Chakravarty et al. 2009). The most common reported are school-related stress, weather changes or environmental factors (hot humid weather, smoke, and noise), prolonged fasting, lack of sleep or prolonged sleep, fever, minor head trauma (during football, rugby, or other sports), and menstrual period in adolescent girls (Kröner-Herwig and Vath 2009; Hershey 2010). Alcohol is a common precipitant and should be sought in older adolescents. Although some children relate the attacks to specific foods like chocolate, cheese, orange juice, or food additives, on large studies this relation is not clear since most of those studies are retrospective and can be biased by selective memory.

Pharmacological Treatment

The pharmacological treatment of migraine consists of symptomatic and prophylactic therapy. The former is aimed at headache resolution and return to normal function within 1–2 h, whereas prophylactic therapy, which requires the daily intake of medication for a certain period of time, is aimed at reduction of headache frequency to, e.g., 1–2 headaches per month for 4–6 months and reduction of headache related disability.

Recent practice guidelines, systematic reviews, and meta-analyses about the pharmacological treatment have repeatedly stressed that there is insufficient evidence about drug treatment of childhood migraine. There is a marked lack of controlled studies and an "urgent need for new, evidence-based approaches" (Lewis et al. 2004a, b; Damen et al. 2005a, b, c; Lewis and Winner 2006; Víctor and Ryan 2006; Hershey 2010; Papetti et al. 2010). It is also remarked that in most studies, there is a lack of planning of sample size, small samples, and that the evidence of lack of effect for some drugs is inconclusive due to these methodological constraints. It has also been recognized that the placebo effect in childhood migraine is quite marked and may conceal the results of active drugs, thus requiring specific trial designs to control this effect, namely, crossover trials or the exclusion of placebo responders (Fernandes et al. 2008; Evers et al. 2009). On the other hand, the placebo effect is a psychobiological phenomenon that can be attributed to different mechanisms (Benedetti et al. 2005), and it should be properly used by the physician, simply bearing in mind that any medical treatment is surrounded by a psychosocial context that affects the therapeutic outcome.

Symptomatic Medication

The goal of treatment should be a quick response with return to normal activity and without relapse. Yet symptomatic medication may not be required if the attack is short lasting and ease spontaneously after vomiting or with sleep. Regarding the use of medication, several key concepts should be emphasized to patients and parents. It is generally recommended that medication should be taken shortly after onset of migraine headache to optimize the effect, but clear scientific evidence supporting this recommendation in children is lacking. Indeed, in adults, the occurrence of allodynia, a phenomenon that indicates the development of central sensitization and is manifested by scalp tenderness, is associated with poor response to triptans, and this finding supports the need for early recognition of headache and early intervention. Prominent scalp symptoms include sensitivity to touch and difficulty brushing hair (Burstein and Collin 2000; Eidlitz-Markus et al. 2007; Hung and MacGregor 2008). Allodynia is often not routinely evaluated during a headache history even though there may be potential therapeutic implications. In fact, it has been shown to be present in 37% of children during their migraine. This suggests that medication should be available to the patients also at school to allow an early intervention, and school should be informed about its administration.

Furthermore, it is important to use medication in an appropriate dose, but also to give clear limitations to avoid medication overuse. Since attacks are often short lasting and young children tend to vomit early in the attack, alternatives to oral administration have been tried. Rectal administration of acetomiphen is often recommended but is not practical for children who are in school. Drugs with a rapid onset of action delivered intranasally or sublingually could be of great help.

Details of studies on symptomatic drugs are given in ❯ *Tables 45.1* and ❯ *45.2.* In summary, ibuprofen (7.5 mg/kg/dose), acetaminophen (15 mg/kg), nasal sumatriptan, oral zolmitriptan, and rizatriptan have shown superiority over placebo in at least one double-blind, randomized, placebo-controlled trial (Termine et al. 2011).

Although there are several published trials demonstrating the effectiveness of triptans in the treatment of acute attacks in children and adolescents, so far only nasal sumatriptan and nasal zolmitriptan have been approved by the European Medicines Agency (EMEA) and oral

◘ Table 45.1

Symptomatic drugs for migraine management evaluated in placebo-controlled and open clinical trials

First author	Drug	Dose	Age (years)	Number of patients	Responders (%) Active drug	Placebo	p-value
Hämäläinen et al. (1997a)	Ibuprofen	10 mg/kg	4–16	88	68	37	<0.05
Lewis et al. (2002)	Ibuprofen	7.5 mg/kg	6–12	84	76	53	0.006
Evers et al. (2006)	Ibuprofen	200–400 mg	6–18	32	69	28	<0.05
Hämäläinen et al. (1997a)	Acetaminophen	15 mg/kg	4–16	88	54	37	<0.05
Hämäläinen et al. (1997b)	Dihydroergotamine	20 µg/kg, 40 µg/kg	5–15	12	58	16	NS
Uebarall (1999)	Sumatriptan nasal	20 mg	6–10	14	86	43	0.03
Winner et al. (2000)	Sumatriptan nasal	5–10–20 mg	12–17	510	66[a]	53	<0.05
Ahonen et al. (2004)	Sumatriptan nasal	10–20 mg	8–17	83	64	39	0.003
Winner et al. (2006)	Sumatriptan nasal	20 mg	12–17	738	61	52	NS
Hämäläinen et al. (1997c)	Sumatriptan oral	50–100 mg	8–16	23	30	22	NS
Mac Donald 1994	Sumatriptan sc.	3–6 mg	6–16	17	64	–	–
Linder 1996	Sumatriptan sc.	0.06 mg/kg	6–18	50	78	–	–
Winner et al. (2002)	Rizatriptan	5 mg	12–17	196	66	56	NS
Visser et al. (2004)	Rizatriptan	5 mg	12–17	234	68	69	NS
Visser et al. (2004)	Rizatriptan	5 mg	12–17	686	77	–	–
Ahonen (2006)	Rizatriptan	5–10 mg	6–17	96	73–74	35	<0.001
Linder and Dowson (2000)	Zolmitriptan oral	2.5–5 mg	12–17	38	70–88	–	–
Evers et al. (2006)	Zolmitriptan oral	2.5 mg	6–18	32	62	28	<0.05
Rothner (2006)	Zolmitriptan oral	2.5–10 mg	12–17	850	53–57	58	NS
Charles 2006	Almotriptan oral	6.25–12.5 mg	11–17	15	86	–	–

NS no statistically significant difference between active drug and placebo
[a]5 mg

◻ Table 45.2
Summary of the efficacy of medication used to treat acute migraine attacks in children and adolescents (45)

	Outcome			
	Pain relief	Pain-free	Recurrence	Need for rescue medications
Oral medication				
Acetaminophen (n = 1)	+	−	−	−
DHE (n = 1)	−	−	−	−
Ibuprofen (n = 3)	+	+/−	−	+/−
Rizatriptan (n = 4)	+/−	−	−	+/−
Sumatriptan (n = 1)	−	+/−	−	−
Zolmitriptan (n = 3)	+/−	+/−	−	+
Intranasal medication				
Sumatriptan (n = 4)	+/−	+/−	−	+/−
Intravenous medication				
Prochlorperazine (n = 1)	+	?	−	?
Ketorolac (n = 1)[a]	?	?	?	? +/−

+ studies showing consistent positive results or a study showing positive result, − studies showing consistent negative results or a study showing negative result, +/− studies showing inconsistent results, ? not evaluated
[a]Used as a comparative agent against prochlorperazine

almotriptan by the Food and Drug Administration (FDA) for use in adolescents between 12 and 17 years of age (see Hershey 2010 for a detailed review).

Intravenous therapy might be necessary in rare occasions. A systematic review (Damen et al. 2005a) concluded that there is moderate evidence that IV prochlorperazine is more effective than IV ketorolac in the reduction of symptoms 1 h after intake.

Prophylactic Medication

Pharmaco-prophylaxis is recommended when migraines are occurring with sufficient frequency (usually 3–4 per month) and severity to impact a patient's daily function or quality of life (e.g., missing school), and whenever lifestyle modification and nonpharmacological prophylaxis alone are not effective. Although many prophylactic medications have been tried in pediatric migraine, there are only a few medications that have been studied in controlled trials. To minimize adverse effects, prophylactic medications are started at the lowest dose and titrated upward as needed. They have to be given over a period of at least 4–6 months usually. Both comorbidities and side effects of the drug have to be taken into consideration (Wöber-Bingöl and Hershey, in press; Hung and MacGregor 2008).

■ Table 45.3
Prophylactic drugs for migraine management evaluated in placebo-controlled and open clinical trials

First author	Drug	Daily dose	Age (years)	Patients (n)	Study design	% responders or p-values (*)
Antihypertensive drugs						
Ludvigsson (1974)	Propranolol	60–120 mg	7–16	28	RCT	82% vs. 14%
Forsythe et al. (1984)	Propranolol	80 mg	9–15	39	RCT	NS
Olness et al. (1987)	Propranolol	3 mg/kg	6–12	28	RCT	NS
Sillanpaa (1977)	Clonidine	25–50 µg	≤15	57	RCT	NS
Sills et al. (1982)	Clonidine	0.07–0.1 mg	7–14	43	RCT	NS
Calcium channel blockers						
Guidetti et al. (1987)	Flunarizine	5 mg	10–13	12	OT	66%
Sorge et al. (1988)	Flunarizine	5 mg	5–11	63	RCT	$p < 0.001$ (HA frequency)
						$p < 0.01$ (HA duration)
Visudtibhan et al. (2004)	Flunarizine	5–10 mg	7–15	21	OT	66%
Battistella et al. (1990)	Nimodipine	10–20 mg	7–18	37	RCT	NS
Serotonergic drugs						
Gillies et al. (1986)	Pizotifen	1–1.5 mg	7–14	47	RCT	NS
Lewis et al. (2004b)	Cyproheptadine	2–8 mg	3–12	30	OT	83%
Antidepressants						
Battistella et al. (1993)	Trazodone	1 mg/kg	7–18	35	RCT	NS
Hershey et al. (2000)	Amitriptyline	1 mg/kg	9–15	192	OT	80%
Lewis et al. (2004a)	Amitriptyline	10 mg	3–12	73	OT	89%
Anticonvulsants						
Caruso et al. (2000)	Divalproex sodium	15–45 mg/kg	7–16	42	OT	76%
Serdaroglu et al. (2002)	Divalproex sodium	500–1,000 mg	9–17	10	OT	$p = 0.000$ (HA severity)
						$p = 0.002$ (HA frequency)
						$p = 0.001$ (HAduration)
Apostol et al. (2008)	Divalproex sodium	250–1,000 mg	12–17	300	RCT	NS

◘ Table 45.3 (Continued)

First author	Drug	Daily dose	Age (years)	Patients (n)	Study design	% responders or p-values (*)
Hershey et al. (2002)	Topiramate	1.4±0.7 mg/kg	8–15	75	OT	p < 0.001 (HA frequency)
Winner et al. (2005)	Topiramate	2–3 mg/kg	6–15	162	RCT	NS
Lewis et al. (2009)	Topiramate	100 mg	12–17	103	RCT	72%
Miller (2004)	Levetiracetam	250–1,500 mg	3–17	19	OT	p < 0.0001 (HA frequency)
Pakalnis et al. (2007)	Levetiracetam	250–1,500 mg	6–17	20	OT	p < 0.0001 (HA frequency)
Belman et al. (2001)	Gabapentin	15 mg/kg	6–17	18	OT	80%
Pakalnis and Kring (2006)	Zonisamide	5.8 mg/kg	10–17	12	OT	66%

NS no statistically significant difference between active drug and placebo, HA headache, RCT randomized controlled trial, OT open trial (*) % expressed as overall % of responders (OT) or active drug vs. placebo % of responders (RCT), p-values refer to active drug vs. placebo comparisons (RCT) or pretreatment vs. post-treatment comparison of headache characteristics (OT)

Prophylactic drugs evaluated in placebo-controlled and open label trials for migraine have been summarized in ❯ Table 45.3. Following findings should be stressed (Termine et al. 2011):

- Flunarizine 5 mg is an effective drug. Its use is limited by daytime sedation found in 10% of the patients and weight gain in more than 20%. Because of probable D2 receptor interaction, intake should be limited to 3 months (given in the evening can avoid daytime sleepiness).
- Propranolol was superior to placebo in one randomized controlled trial and not effective in two others. It was found to activate asthma in subjects with atopic disorders or a positive history of atopic disorders.
- Topiramate is an effective drug for the reduction of headache frequency, severity, and duration. The most common side effects reported were cognitive (12.5%), weight loss (5.6%), and sensory (2.8%).
- There are limited data from open trials on cyproheptadine, amitriptyline, divalproex sodium, levetiracetam, gabapentin, and zonisamide reporting response rates of 66–89%.
- Clonidine, nimodipine, pizotifen, trazodone, and divalproex sodium were not superior to placebo in one randomized controlled trial each.

Nonpharmacological Treatment

Behavioral therapy is aimed at lifelong headache control through maintenance of healthy habits. Behavioral interventions, particularly biofeedback and relaxation therapy, have demonstrated their effectiveness in the treatment of children with migraine in controlled trials. The physiological basis for their effectiveness is unclear, but data from one trial suggest that levels of plasma beta-endorphin can be altered by relaxation and biofeedback therapies. The data supporting the effectiveness of behavioral therapies are less clear-cut in children than in adults, but that is also true for the data supporting medical treatment. This is due in part to methodological issues, especially the lack of specific tests for migraine, which has hampered research and helped leading to an inappropriate de-emphasis on care for childhood headache. In addition, migraine headaches in children are often briefer and have a higher rate of spontaneous remission than those experienced by adults, making it difficult to separate effective from ineffective treatments (Baumann 2002; Andrasik et al. 2003; Damen et al. 2005b).

Relaxation and cognitive-behavioral techniques have been found to reduce the intensity and frequency of headache in children and adolescents (Kazdin 2002; Eccleston et al. 2003).

The specialists involved in the assessment and care of headache patients should strive to increase their knowledge of alternative therapies, so as to be better equipped to guide patients toward safe, economical, and potentially effective treatments, rather than useless, costly, or dangerous ones.

Outcome

The long-term follow-up of migraine in childhood has produced encouraging results (Bille 1997; Kienbacher et al. 2006; Kröner-Herwig and Vath 2009). Most children tend to improve with age. Early diagnosis and intervention may reduce the chance to chronicity.

Tension-Type Headache

Most TTH is best managed by primary care. Episodic TTH is self-limiting, but children and their parents generally consult doctors when headaches become frequent and are no longer responsive to analgesics. Medication overuse can be a common problem in patients with frequent headache. The treatment of migraine and TTH overlaps. Both require acute treatment, either behavioral or pharmaceutical. Behavioral treatment is needed for all types of TTH. Preventive pharmaceutical treatment is needed for frequent TTH if lifestyle modification and nonpharmacological treatment alone are not effective. Although childhood TTH is often treated with medication, few studies have been published on the efficacy of medication in pediatric TTH (Wöber-Bingöl and Hershey 2006). More studies in children need to be done regarding the treatment of this common disorder. The lack of availability and cost of nonpharmacological interventions might diminish the use of some treatment modalities (Anttila 2006).

For acute treatment of episodic TTH, paracetamol, aspirin, and combination analgesics are effective and inexpensive drugs. In children younger than 15 years, aspirin is not recommended because of the concern of Reye's syndrome. Paracetamol seems to be safe even in young children (Anttila 2006; Pini et al. 2008; Dooley 2009).

Prophylactic pharmacological treatment should be considered in chronic TTH if nonpharmacological management is inadequate. For children with frequent headache, amitriptyline might be beneficial, but no placebo-controlled studies have been performed (Hershey et al. 2000).

Cluster Headache

Cluster headache is a rare condition in children. Several treatment alternatives have been tried in cases reported in the literature. According to these data, the most effective symptomatic treatments are oxygen, sumatriptan, and acetylsalicylic acid (Termine et al. 2011). Prophylactic treatments tried in literature are prednisone/prednisolone, indomethacin, pizotifen, verapamil, methysergide, loratadine, astemizole, and flunarizine (Termine et al. 2011). No controlled study has been reported.

Considering the unbearable pain intensity, off-label use of sumatriptan nasal spray or subcutaneous sumatriptan may be necessary. Lidocaine applied with a spray bottle or by dropping in the nostril ipsilateral to pain achieves moderate pain relief, and it may be useful as an adjunctive therapy. Although the reason for steroid efficacy is unknown, the use of cortisone in the acute period can stop the attacks and may help to prevent further attacks. In adolescents, a marked relief of cluster headache in 77% of 77 episodic cluster headache patients, and a partial relief in another 12% of patients treated with prednisone was reported (D'Cruz 1994). For prophylactic treatment, the efficacy of verapamil has been attributed to a possible stabilization of vascular tone. It can be used in combination with corticosteroids and sumatriptan (Dodick and Campbell 2000; Majumdar et al. 2008).

Current Research

The impact of migraine in children has been the focus of study only in recent years (Kernick et al. 2009). An adaptation of the adult scale MIDAS has been developed for children (PedMIDAS) and can now be used as a measure of disability, criteria for prophylaxis, or outcome for clinical trials, for instance (Hershey et al. 2001).

Health-related quality of life (QOL) is an emerging area of headache research with a direct impact on patient adherence, patient satisfaction, and treatment effectiveness. On the other hand, the assessment of QOL in children is difficult, since measures must consider children's changing cognitive and social development (Powers et al. 2004; Akyol et al. 2007). Data-based analyses revealed that children with frequent or severe headaches (FSH) were significantly more likely than those without FSH to exhibit high levels of emotional, conduct, inattention-hyperactivity, and peer problems, and were significantly more likely than children without FSH to be upset or distressed by their difficulties and to have their difficulties interfere with home life, friendships, classroom learning, and leisure activities (Strine et al. 2006). Subjects familiar with headache experienced more stress, fatigue, depression, and somatic symptoms; they felt less strong, had a less cheerful mood, and reported lower satisfaction with health and with life in general than the subjects who never had headaches (Karwautz et al. 1999). The impact of headaches on QOL is similar to that found for other chronic illness conditions, with impairments in school and emotional functioning being the most prominent (Powers et al. 2003). Headache is the third most common cause among illness-related causes of school absenteeism, resulting in substantial impairment among pediatric patients (Newacheck and Taylor 1992).

Migraine comorbidities have also been systematically investigated in the last decade. It may shed light on the pathogenesis of this disorder and help to tailor therapy according to the special needs of each patient (Wöber-Bingöl and Hershey, in press).

It has been found that children with migraine are more likely to suffer from sleep-disordered breathing, disrupted sleep architecture with reduced rapid eye movement, and slow-wave sleep, especially in severe and chronic migraine (Vendrame et al. 2008; Pakalnis et al. 2009). This stresses the need of screening for sleep disturbances in this group and its possible participation in the aggravation of migraine (Heng and Wirrell 2006).

The association between migraine and epilepsy has also been of particular interest more recently. Both are transient neurological disorders, may share some genetic predisposition, quite evident in cases of familial hemiplegic migraine (de Vries et al. 2009), and are associated with increased cortical excitability and respond to antiepileptic drugs. All this communalities have raised the possibility of an association between the two disorders. Clinical studies have shown that children with migraine, particularly those with aura, have an increased risk of epilepsy (Toldo et al. 2010). In addition, there are some primary types of benign epilepsies of childhood associated and confounded with migraine. One of them, the primary epilepsy with occipital spikes (Caraballo et al. 2008), begins with visual disturbances, followed by a motor or generalized seizure, and is followed by an intense headache. Other primary epileptic syndrome of childhood with autonomic manifestations (vomiting, pallor, syncope) can be confused with migraine equivalents of abdominal pain or repeated vomiting (Covanis 2006).

As already stated, there is much need of therapeutic trials in migraine both for acute and prophylactic treatment. It is possible that response may vary with the child's age and stratified analysis by age can be useful. Placebo response is also much more marked in younger children, and this can require specific trial designs.

References

Ahonen K, Hämäläinen ML, Rantala H, Hoppu K (2004) Nasal sumatriptan is effective in the treatment of migraine attacks in children. Neurology 62:883–887

Ahonen K, Hämäläinen ML, Eerola M, Hoppu K (2006) A randomized trial of rizatriptan in migraine attacks in children. Neurology 67:1135–1140.

Akyol A, Kiylioglu N, Aydin I, Erturk A, Kaya E, Telli E et al (2007) Epidemiology and clinical characteristics of migraine among school children in the Menderes region. Cephalalgia 27(7):781–787

Andrasik F, Grazzi L, Usai S, D'Amico D, Leone M, Bussone G (2003) Brief neurologist-administered behavioral treatment of pediatric episodic tension-type headache. Neurology 60:1215–1216

Anttila P (2006) Tension-type headache in childhood and adolescence. Lancet Neurol 5:268–274

Apostol G, Cady RK, Laforet GA, Robieson WZ, Olson E, Abi-Saab WM, Saltarelli M (2008) Divalproex extended-release in adolescent migraine prophylaxis: results of a randomized, double-blind, placebo-controlled study. Headache 48:1012–1025

Battistella PA, Ruffilli R, Moro R, Fabiani M, Bertoli S, Antolini A et al (1990) A placebo-controlled crossover trial of nimodipine in pediatric migraine. Headache 30:264–268

Battistella PA, Ruffilli R, Cernetti R, Pettenazzo A, Baldin L, Bertoli S et al (1993) A placebo-controlled crossover trial using trazodone in pediatric migraine. Headache 33(1):36–39

Baumann RJ (2002) Behavioral treatment of migraine in children and adolescents. Paediatr Drugs 4(9): 555–561

Belman AL, Milazo M, Savatic M (2001) Gabapentin for migraine prophylaxis in children. Ann Neurol 50(Suppl 1):S109

Benedetti F, Mayberg HS, Wager TD, Stohler CS, Zubieta JK (2005) Neurobiological mechanisms of the placebo effect. J Neurosci 25:10390–10402

Bille B (1997) A 40-year follow-up of school children with migraine. Cephalalgia 17:488–491

Burstein R, Collin B (2000) An association between migraine and cutaneous allodynia. Ann Neurol 47:614–624

Caraballo R, Koutroumanidis M, Panayiotopoulos CP, Fejerman N (2008) Idiopathic childhood occipital epilepsy of Gastaut: a review and differentiation from migraine and other epilepsies. J Child Neurol 24:1536–1542

Caruso JM, Brown WD, Exil G, Gascon GG (2000) The efficacy of divalproex sodium in the prophylactic treatment of children with migraine. Headache 40:672–676

Chakravarty A, Mukherjee A, Roy D (2009) Trigger factors in childhood migraine: a clinic-based study from eastern India. J Headache Pain 10:375–380

Charles JA (2006) Almotriptan in the acute treatment of migraine in patients 11–17 years old: an open-label pilot study of efficacy and safety. J Headache Pain 7:95–97

Covanis A (2006) Panayiotopoulos syndrome: a benign childhood autonomic epilepsy frequently imitating encephalitis, syncope, migraine, sleep disorder, or gastroenteritis. Pediatrics 118:1237–1243

D'Cruz OF (1994) Cluster headaches in childhood. Clin Pediatr 33:241–242

Damen L, Bruijn JK, Verhagen AP, Berger MY, Passchier J, Koes BW (2005a) Symptomatic treatment of migraine in children: a systematic review of medication trials. Pediatrics 116:295–302

Damen L, Bruijn JK, Verhagen AP, Berger MY, Passchier J, Koes BW (2005b) Prophylactic treatment of migraine in children. Part 1. A systematic review of non-pharmacological trials. Cephalalgia 26:373–383

Damen L, Bruijn JK, Verhagen AP, Berger MY, Passchier J, Koes BW (2005c) Prophylactic treatment of migraine in children. Part 2. A systematic review of pharmacological trials. Cephalalgia 26:497–505

de Vries B, Stam AH, Kirkpatrick M, Vanmolkot KR, Koenderink JB, van den Heuvel JJ, Stunnenberg B, Goudie D, Shetty J, Jain V, van Vark J, Terwindt GM, Frants RR, Haan J, van den Maagdenberg AM, Ferrari MD (2009) Familial hemiplegic migraine is associated with febrile seizures in an FHM2 family with a novel de novo ATP1A2 mutation. Epilepsia 50:2503–2504

Dodick D, Campbell JK (2000) Cluster headache. Diagnosis, management, and treatment. In: Silberstein SD, Lipton RB, Dalessio DJ (eds) Wolff's headache and other head pain, 7th edn. Oxford University Press, New York, pp 283–309

Dooley J (2009) The evaluation and management of paediatric headaches. Paediatr Child Health 14:24–30

Eccleston C, Yorke L, Morley S, Williams AC, Mastroyannopoulou K (2003) Psychological therapies for the management of chronic and recurrent pain in children and adolescents. Cochrane Database Syst Rev (1):CD003968

Eidlitz-Markus T, Shuper A, Gorali O, Zeharia A (2007) Migraine and cephalic cutaneous allodynia in pediatric patients. Headache 47:1219–1223

Evers S, Rahmann A, Kraemer C, Kurlemann G, Debus O, Husstedt IW et al (2006) Treatment of childhood migraine attacks with oral zolmitriptan and ibuprofen. Neurology 67:497–499

Evers S, Marziniak M, Frese A, Gralow I (2009) Placebo efficacy in childhood and adolescence migraine: an analysis of double-blind and placebo-controlled studies. Cephalalgia 29:436–444

Fernandes R, Ferreira JJ, Sampaio C (2008) The placebo response in studies of acute migraine. J Pediatr 152:527–533

Forsythe WI, Gillies D, Sills MA (1984) Propranolol (Inderal) in the treatment of childhood migraine. Dev Med Child Neurol 26:737–741

Gillies D, Sills M, Forsythe I (1986) Pizotifen (Sandomigran) in childhood migraine. A double-blind placebo controlled trial. Eur Neurol 25:32–35

Guidetti V, Moscato D, Ottaviano S, Fiorentino D, Fornara R (1987) Flunarizine and migraine in childhood: an evaluation of endocrine function. Cephalalgia 7:263–266

Hämäläinen ML, Hoppu K, Valkeila E, Santavuori P (1997a) Ibuprofen or acetaminophen for the acute treatment of migraine in children: a double-blind, randomized, placebo-controlled, crossover study. Neurology 48:102–107

Hämäläinen ML, Hoppu K, Santavuori PR (1997b) Oral dihydroergotamine for therapy-resistant migraine attacks in children. Pediatr Neurol 16:114–117

Hämäläinen M, Hoppu K, Santavuori P (1997c) Sumatriptan for migraine attacks in children: a randomized placebo-controlled study. Do children with migraine respond to oral sumatriptan differently than adults? Neurology 48:1100–1103

Heng K, Wirrell E (2006) Sleep disturbance in children with migraine. J Child Neurol 21:761–766

Hershey AD (2010) Current approaches to the diagnosis and management of paediatric migraine. Lancet Neurol 9:190–204

Hershey AD, Powers SW, Bentti AL, Degrauw TJ (2000) Effectiveness of amitriptyline in the prophylactic management of childhood headaches. Headache 40:539–549

Hershey AD, Powers SW, Vockell AL, LeCates S, Kabbouche MA, Maynard MK (2001) PedMIDAS: development of a questionnaire to assess disability of migraines in children. Neurology 57(11):2034–2039

Hershey AD, Powers SW, Vockell AL, LeCates S, Kabbouche M (2002) Effectiveness of topiramate in the prevention of childhood headache. Headache 42:810–818

Hung RM, MacGregor DL (2008) Management of pediatric migraine: current concepts and controversies. Indian J Pediatr 75:1139–1148

Karwautz A, Wöber C, Lang T, Böck A, Wagner-Ennsgraber C, Vesely C et al (1999) Psychosocial factors in children and adolescents with migraine and tension-type headache: a controlled study and review of the literature. Cephalalgia 19:32–43

Kazdin AE (2002) The state of child and adolescent psychotherapy research. Child Adolesc Ment Health 2:53–59

Kernick D, Reinhold D, Campbell JL (2009) Impact of headache on young people in a school population. Br J Gen Pract 59:678–681

Kienbacher CH, Wöber CH, Zesch H, Hafferl-Gattermayer A, Posch M, Karwautz A, Zormann A, Berger G, Zebenholzer K, Konrad A, Wöber-Bingöl Ç (2006) Clinical features, classification and prognosis of migraine and tension-type headache in children and adolescents: a long-term follow-up study. Cephalalgia 26:820–830

Kröner-Herwig B, Vath N (2009) Menarche in girls and headache-a longitudinal analysis. Headache 49:860–867

Lewis DW, Winner P (2006) The pharmacological treatment options for paediatric migraine: an evidence-based appraisal. NeuroRx 3:181–191

Lewis DW, Kellstein D, Dahl G, Burke B, Frank LM, Toor S et al (2002) Children's ibuprofen suspension for the acute treatment of pediatric migraine headache. Headache 42:780–786

Lewis D, Ashwal S, Hershey A, Hirtz D, Yonker M, Silberstein S, American Academy of Neurology Quality Standards Subcommittee; Practice Committee of the Child Neurology Society (2004a) Practice parameter: pharmacological treatment of migraine headache in children and adolescents: report of the American Academy of Neurology Quality Standards Subcommittee and the Practice Committee of the Child Neurology Society. Neurology 63:2215–2224

Lewis DW, Diamond S, Scott D, Jones V (2004b) Prophylactic treatment of pediatric migraine. Headache 44:230–237

Lewis D, Winner P, Saper J, Ness S, Polverejan E, Wang S, Kurland CL, Nye J, Yuen E, Eerdekens M, Ford L (2009) Randomized, double-blind, placebo-controlled study to evaluate the efficacy and safety of topiramate for migraine prevention in pediatric subjects 12 to 17 years of age. Pediatrics 123(3):924–934

Linder SL (1996) Subcutaneous sumatriptan in the clinical setting: the first 50 consecutive patients with acute migraine in the pediatric neurology office practice. Headache 36:419–422

Linder SL, Dowson AJ (2000) Zolmitriptan provides effective migraine relief in adolescents. Int J Clin Pract 54:466–469

Ludvigsson J (1974) Propranolol used in prophylaxis of migraine in children. Acta Neurol 50:109–115

Mac Donald JT (1994) Treatment of juvenile migraine with subcutaneous sumatriptan. Headache 34:581–582

Majumdar A, Ahmed MA, Benton S (2008) Cluster headache in children-experience from a specialist headache clinic. Eur J Paediatr Neurol 13(6):524–529

Miller GS (2004) Efficacy and safety of levetiracetam in pediatric migraine. Headache 44:238–243

Newacheck PW, Taylor WR (1992) Childhood chronic illness: prevalence, severity, and impact. Am J Public Health 82:364–371

Olness K, Macdonald JT, Uden DL (1987) Comparison of self-hypnosis and propranolol in the treatment of juvenile classic migraine. Pediatrics 79:593–597

Pakalnis A, Kring D (2006) Zonisamide prophylaxis in refractory pediatric headache. Headache 46(5):804–807

Pakalnis A, Kring D, Meier L (2007) Levetiracetam prophylaxis in pediatric migraine – an open-label study. Headache 47(3):427–430

Pakalnis A, Splaingard M, Splaingard D, Kring D, Colvin A (2009) Serotonin effects on sleep and emotional disorders in adolescent migraine. Headache 49:1486–1492

Papetti L, Spalice A, Nicita F, Paolino MC, Castaldo R, Iannetti P, Villa MP, Parisi P (2010) Migraine treatment in developmental age: guidelines update. J Headache Pain 11(3):267–276 [Epub ahead of print]

Pini LA, Del Bene E, Zanchin G, Sarchielli P, Di Trapani G, Prudenzano MP et al (2008) Tolerability and efficacy of a combination of paracetamol and caffeine in the treatment of tension-type headache: a randomised, double-blind, double-dummy, crossover study versus placebo and naproxen sodium. J Headache Pain 9(6):367–373

Powers SW, Patton SR, Hommel KA, Hershey AD (2003) Quality of life in childhood migraines: clinical impact and comparison to other chronic illnesses. Pediatrics 112(1 Pt 1):e1–e5

Powers SW, Patton SR, Hommel KA, Hershey AD (2004) Quality of life in paediatric migraine: characterization of age-related effects using PedsQL 4.0. Cephalalgia 24:120–127

Rothner AD, Wasiewski W, Winner P, Lewis D, Stankowski J (2006) Zolmitriptan oral tablet in migraine treatment: high placebo responses in adolescents. Headache 46:101–109.

Serdaroglu G, Erhan E, Tekgul H, Oksel F, Erermis S, Uyar M et al (2002) Sodium valproate prophylaxis in childhood migraine. Headache 42:819–822

Sillanpaa M (1977) Clonidine prophylaxis of childhood migraine and other vascular headache. A double blind study of 57 children. Headache 17:28–31

Sills M, Congdon P, Forsythe I (1982) Clonidine and childhood migraine. Dev Med Child Neurol 24:837–841

Sorge F, De Simone R, Marano E, Nolano M, Orefice G, Carrieri P (1988) Flunarizine in prophylaxis of childhood migraine. A double-blind, placebo-controlled crossover study. Cephalalgia 8:1–6

Strine TW, Okoro CA, McGuire LC, Balluz LS (2006) The associations among childhood headaches, emotional and behavioral difficulties, and health care use. Pediatrics 117(5):1728–1735

Termine C, Özge A, Antonaci F, Natriashvili S, Guidetti V, Wöber-Bingöl Ç (2010) Overview of diagnosis and management of paediatric headache. Part II: therapeutic management. J Headache Pain. Epub ahead of print

Toldo I, Perissinotto E, Menegazzo F, Boniver C, Sartori S, Salviati L, Clementi M, Montagna P, Battistella PA (2010) Comorbidity between headache and epilepsy in a pediatric headache center. J Headache Pain 11(3):235–240 [Epub ahead of print]

Uebarall MA (1999) Intranasal sumatriptan for the acute treatment of migraine in children. Neurology 52:1507–1510

Vendrame M, Kaleyias J, Valencia I, Legido A, Kothare SV (2008) Polysomnographic findings in children with headaches. Pediatr Neurol 39:6–11

Víctor S, Ryan SW (2006) Drugs for preventing migraine headaches in children. Cochrane Database Syst Rev CD002761

Visser WH, Winner P, Strohmaier K, Klipfel M, Peng Y et al; Rizatriptan Protocol 059 and 061 Study Groups (2004) Rizatriptan 5 mg for the acute treatment of migraine in adolescents: results from a double-blind, single-attack study and two open-label, multiple-attack studies. Headache 44:891–899

Visudtibhan A, Lusawat A, Chiemchanya S, Visudhiphan P (2004) Flunarizine for prophylactic treatment of childhood migraine. J Med Assoc Thai 87(12): 1466–1470

Winner P, Rothner AD, Saper J, Nett R, Asgharnejad M, Laurenza A et al (2000) A randomized, double-blind, placebo-controlled study of sumatriptan nasal spray in the treatment of acute migraine in adolescents. Pediatrics 106:989–997

Winner P, Lewis D, Visser WH, Jiang K, Ahrens S, Evans JK, Rizatriptan Adolescent Study Group (2002) Rizatriptan 5 mg for the acute treatment of migraine in adolescents: a randomized, double-blind placebo-controlled study. Headache 42:49–55

Winner P, Pearlman EM, Linder SL, Jordan DM, Fisher AC, Hulihan J, Topiramate Pediatric Migraine Study Investigators (2005) Topiramate for migraine prevention in children: a randomized, double-blind, placebo-controlled trial. Headache 45(10):1304–1312

Winner P, Rothner AD, Wooten JD, Webster C, Ames M (2006) Sumatriptan nasal spray in adolescent migraineurs: a randomized, double-blind, placebo-controlled, acute study. Headache 46: 212–222

Wöber-Bingöl Ç (2002) What does it mean to treat headache in children and adolescents? Dealing with patients, dealing with parents, dealing with teachers. In: Guidetti V, Russell G, Sillanpää M, Winner P (eds) Headache and migraine in childhood and adolescence. Martin Dunitz, London, pp 459–466

Wöber-Bingöl Ç, Hershey (2011) A, Migraine co-morbidities in children. In: Schoenen J, Sandor P, Dodick D (eds) Co-morbidity in migraine – clinical aspects, prevalence, mechanisms and management. Blackwell, Oxford, pp 122–132

Wöber-Bingöl Ç, Hershey AD (2006) Tension-type headaches and other primary headaches in the pediatric population. In: Olesen J, Goadsby P, Ramadan N, Tfelt-Hansen P, Welch KMA (eds) The headaches, 3rd edn. Lippincott, Williams and Wilkins, Philadelphia, pp 1079–1081

Part 12

Headache in the Elderly

46 Diagnosing Headache in Older People

Andreas Straube
University of Munich, Munich, Germany

Paolo Martelletti, Timothy J. Steiner (eds.), *Handbook of Headache*, DOI 10.1007/978-88-470-1700-9_46,
© Lifting The Burden 2011

Abstract: Headaches become relatively less prevalent in older patients but still more than 50% of people older than 65 years complain about regularly occurring headaches. Most of these headaches are primary headaches, with tension-type headache much more prevalent than migraine headache. The proportion of secondary headaches increases in older patients and remains about 2.2%. Subjects who complain about headaches for the first time after the age of 64 have a clearly elevated risk of having a symptomatic headache (about 15.3%) compared to the general population with 7–8%. There are some changes in the symptoms of primary headache syndromes. In particular, migraine attacks may have other symptoms in older patients with nausea and vomiting less often and a dull and holozephalic pain and isolated auras more often. There are also some headache syndromes that occur almost exclusively in older patients, namely, hypnic headache, giant cell arteritis, and sleep apnea–associated headache. Diagnostic interventions in older patients generally do not differ from those in younger patients.

Introduction

Demographic developments in industrial nations in the coming years will result in an increasing number of people over the age of 65. In 2037, it is expected that about 45% of the population in Germany will be older than 65. Despite this background, for a number of disorders it is not clear how they are influenced by higher age. There are several reasons for this: (1) In order to speak about diagnostic constraints in older people, we have to define who is an older patient. This is not as clear as it might first appear. In the literature, there is no generally accepted definition of "older." When most authors speak about older patients, they mean those above 60 years and patients above 75 years are considered to be elderly. (2) In headache in particular, only a very limited number of studies deal with older people. Thus, most of the therapy trials even excluded patients above 65 years.

We have to be aware that there is only limited data on the epidemiology and clinical characteristics of headache in older people. Below we will first discuss the epidemiology of headaches and then the clinical characteristics of primary headaches in older patients. At the end of each paragraph, we will also discuss the value of specific diagnostic measurements.

General Epidemiology

In the older population, 50% of females and males report headaches with a tendency to less frequent headache with increasing age (Prencipe et al. 2001). In a population-based investigation in Italy, 44.5% of the older population complained about tension-type headache, 11% about migraine (12-month prevalence), and 2.2% about symptomatic headache; females were affected twice as often as males (Prencipe et al. 2001). In an epidemiological study by the German Headache Society, the 6-month prevalences in the 65–75-year-old group were about 3.5% for migraine and about 12.5% for tension-type headache, with females affected 1.5–2 times more often (Pfaffenrath et al. 2009). Subjects who complain about headaches for the first time after the age of 64 have a clearly elevated risk of having symptomatic headache (about 15.3%) compared to the general population with 7–8% (Prencipe et al. 2001). In summary, headaches are still an often reported symptom in the elderly and, while primary headaches are most often the reason for this, secondary headaches are diagnosed relatively more often than in younger patients.

Migraine: Epidemiology and Clinical Characteristics

In another population-based study, the prevalence of migraine after the 75th year was 2.7% for males and 7.6% for females (Schwaiger et al. 2009). The available data suggest that older patients with migraine on average have headache on more days (41% on 10–14 days/month) (Bigal et al. 2006; Martins et al. 2006) than the general population, where only 15.5% of migraine patients have headache on more than 6 days (Straube et al. 2009). About two-thirds of the patients report a reduction in the attack frequency, but the remaining third may have even more attacks. In a population-based study in Northern Italy, about 20% of the female migraine patients lose their migraine with every 10 years of lifetime after the menopause (Schwaiger et al. 2009). Clinically, there is a shift in the symptomatology with nausea and vomiting and a pulsating character of the headaches less often; otherwise, the headache is more often located in the neck (Wöber-Bingöl et al. 2004). Amplification of the headache due to physical activity is also reported less often (Wöber et al. 2007). Acute medication seems to influence the attacks better than in younger patients (Kelman 2006). Aura symptoms with headache but also without accompanying headache seem to occur more often in the elderly; in the group of 18–29-year-olds about 15.2% have auras compared to 41% of the patients aged 70 years and older (Bigal et al. 2006; Kelman 2006; Wöber et al. 2007).

Diagnostic problems can be that aura-like phenomena can also be triggered by cortical ischemia and therefore diagnostic tests may be necessary in each patient with aura for the first time or with changes in the symptoms of the aura compared to previous one. MRI imaging including diffusion-weighted images is the best way to clarify this.

Tension-Type Headache: Epidemiology and Clinical Characteristics

The prevalences of episodic and chronic tension-type headache in the general population are 42% and about 3% (Stovner et al. 2007). Based on the available data, the decrease in the prevalence is less in tension-type headache than in migraine (Kaniecki 2006, 2007). In a study in Southern Tyrol, the 12-month prevalence of episodic tension-type headache in older people was about 36% and 2.1% of the patients had chronic tension-type headache (Schwaiger et al. 2009). Clinical characteristics of tension-type headache older patients do not differ from those in younger patients. It can be problematic that migraine attacks are more difficult to distinguish from tension-type headache attacks in the elderly and that most secondary headaches can also be confused with tension-type headache. A consequence of this is that the diagnosis of primary tension-type headache in the elderly can only be established after exclusion of secondary headaches, especially, medication-overuse headache, idiopathic intracranial hypertension, and sleep apnea–associated headache.

Trigeminal Autonomic Headaches: Epidemiology and Clinical Characteristics

No epidemiological studies have been published on cluster headache and hypnic headache in older people. There are reports on first manifestation of cluster headache above 65 years of age (Fischera et al. 2005). There are no reports on the clinical symptoms or age-related changes in symptoms in older patients. Since there are several case reports of symptomatic cluster headache (Straube et al. 2007; Rigamonti et al. 2007), especially in older patients with the first manifestation of an otherwise typical cluster headache, MRI imaging of the head, including an imaging of the cervical vessels, is mandatory. In some patients with cluster headache, a persisting miosis on the affected side may be observed, but these can also be seen in symptomatic cases due to carotidal artery dissection.

In general, hypnic headache is a primary headache form that manifests in patients older than 50–55 years; on average the patients are 61 years old at the time at which the diagnosis is established (Donnet and Lanteri-Minet 2009; Evers and Goadsby 2003). No changes in clinical characteristics with increasing age are known. An imaging study at the point of diagnosis is strongly recommended.

Secondary Headaches: Epidemiology and Clinical Characteristics

It is generally accepted that the cumulative prevalence of secondary headaches increases with age, although primary headaches are still more prevalent than secondary (Prencipe et al. 2001). Important causes of secondary headaches in older patients are cerebrovascular diseases, brain tumors, giant cell arteritis, zoster neuritis and, for facial pain, trigeminal neuralgia.

Ischemic brain infarcts as well as intracerebral bleeding increase with increasing age. Thus the annual incidence increases from 9–14/100,000 people for the 25–34-year-old group to 837–996/100,000 people for the 75–84-year-old group (Truelsen et al. 2006). Headache is reported in about 32% of the ischemic lesions and 64.5% of the bleedings, with a correlation of the extent of the lesion and the cortical involvement and the probability of developing headache (Arboix et al. 1994, 2005; Ferro et al. 1998). Headache is also reported more often after ischemic lesions in the posterior circulation than after lesions in the carotid area. A possible explanation for this is that lesions of the visual cortex in particular may be able to trigger a cortical spreading depression, which may then activate trigeminal afferences. In all older patients with unexplained sudden headaches or first manifestation of aura symptoms MRI imaging, including diffusion-weighted images, should be discussed, such imaging is mandatory if focal neurological symptoms or reduced consciousness are present. In the case of intracerebral bleeding, a CT scan is as sensitive and specific as MRI scans with flair-weighted sequences.

The main symptoms of giant cell arteritis are pain and general sickness. This special form of a vasculitis occurs almost exclusively in patients older than 50 years with a prevalence of 70–133/100,000 (Boesen and Sorensen 1987). Females are more often affected than males. The clinical hallmarks are persistent holocephalic dull headaches (in 60%), fatigue, increased sweating, weight loss, acute monocular visual loss, and anemia (Ward and Levin 2005). A special case is polymyalgia rheumatica where the pain is located in the upper limb girdle. The diagnosis can be suggested if, in addition to the typical clinical symptoms, C-reactive protein is elevated and the IL-2 level and the alpha2 fraction of the serum electrophoresis are increased. Doppler investigation of the temporal artery may show up a so-called halo sign of the vessel wall. In 80% of the patients, FDG-PET also shows an involvement of the aortic arc. The diagnosis is confirmed by the typical histological finding with segmental affection of the temporal artery wall by inflammatory cells.

In older patients, the prevalence of any type of carcinoma as well as of the most prevalent brain tumors increases. Brain gliomas and meningeomas reach maximum incidence between 45 and 70 years (Lipton et al. 1993). About 60% of patients with brain tumor complain about headaches and most of them describe a tension-type like headache. In the case of a known primary headache in these patients, 82.5% of the patients describe a change in the symptoms of the headache during the tumor disease; headache was the exclusive symptom of the tumor in only 2% of the patients (Schankin et al. 2007). The symptoms in pituitary tumors, where 30% of the patients described migraine-like headaches and cluster-like headaches are also reported (Levy et al. 2005), are a special case. In general, there is no clear relationship between headache prevalence and intensity and tumor dimension. As mentioned above, only rarely are headaches the only symptom of a brain tumor and focal neurological signs in combination with headaches call for cranial imaging.

Like most other disorders, pulmonary disorders are also more prevalent in older people. Obstructive sleep apnea in particular can cause mild to moderate holocephalic dull headaches in the morning, which have some similarities with tension-type headache. The average manifestation age of sleep apnea is between 50 and 70 years and about 2% of all females and 4% of all males may be affected (Provini et al. 2006). Eleven to forty percent of these patients report such a headache; females are affected relatively more often than males and there may be a correlation to the amount of the hypercapnia and hypoxia in the night (Goksan et al. 2009). Typically, the patients are obese and report about snoring and often also sleepiness in the daytime. The diagnostic gold standard is the sleep polysomnographic registration of the sleep apnea, associated hypoxia, and arousal in the EEG. The improvement of the headache with nasal continuous positive airway pressure treatment of the sleep apnea proves the diagnosis.

Arterial hypertension can be found in about 50% of the over fifties (Wittchen et al. 2003). The relationship between headaches and arterial hypertension is not completely understood. Headaches are without doubt one of the main symptoms of an acute arterial hypertensive crisis (Cortelli et al. 2004). Conflicting data have been published concerning headaches in only mild to moderate increased arterial hypertension. In one study the probability of suffering from headache was increased by a factor of 2 (Bulpitt et al. 1976), in other studies there was no significant increase (Rasmussen and Olesen 1992; Muiesan et al. 2006), and in another study a protective effect of arterial hypertension was described (Tronvik et al. 2008). Otherwise, it can be considered as proven that migraine is a risk factor for arterial hypertension regardless of the age of the patient (Rasmussen and Olesen 1992; Bigal et al. 2010). In order to establish such a relationship between headache and arterial hypertension, a long-term blood pressure recording in combination with the documentation of the headache phases may be necessary.

Headaches due to substance use or withdrawal from substances are not an isolated problem of the older patient, but, due to the fact that the number of drugs taken daily increases with increasing age, it is clear that in older patients with headaches such a cause has to be ruled out before other diagnoses are discussed. Drugs that quite regularly induce headache are phosphodiesterase inhibitors, NO donors, calcium antagonists, calcineurin inhibitors, immunoglobulins, some biologics, and others. Furthermore, the mean age of patients with medication-overuse headache is roughly 7 years higher than that of patients with chronic daily headache and no overuse (Colás et al. 2004). The mean percentage of patients with medication overuse is 1–1.5% in the general population (Straube et al. 2010; Jensen and Bendtsen 2008) and 1.9% in patients older than 65 years (Prencipe et al. 2001). Thus, there is evidence that medication-overuse headache is more prevalent in the older population than in the general population. The clinical complaints in older patients do not differ from those in younger patients. As is generally required in secondary headaches, the symptoms should improve after cessation of intake of the substances.

There is the general opinion that headaches attributed to disorder of the neck become more prevalent with older age since degenerative cervical joint diseases and degeneration of the cervical disks are more often in older people. In contrast to this generally accepted opinion, there is only a sparse published literature on that topic. There are no epidemiological data published about the prevalence of headaches attributed to disorder of the neck. For the cervicogenic headache, a subgroup, Sjaastad and colleagues (2008) found in Norway a prevalence of 4.1% in the age group of 18–65 years, older subjects were not investigated and they used the "Sjaastad criteria," which are different to the IHS criteria. The age at onset of the cervicogenic headache was 32,7 years in this study. In another study from Australia, which was not population based, the age of onset was 49,5 years compared to 34,7 years in a migrainous group (Anthony 2000). A further problem in the diagnosis of neck-related headaches is that musculoskeletal dysfunction can be also found in patients with headaches classifiable as migraine or tension-type headache. But more of these symptoms (impaired range of motion, muscle tenderness of the neck muscles, cervical joint dysfunction, muscle strength, etc.) can be found in patients with more classical cervicogenic headache (Uthaikhup et al. 2009). There are also no specific MRI findings that can be attributed to neck pain (Nordin et al. 2009). No differences in the symptoms of the headache was seen between a group of patients with proven cervical spondylosis compared to a group without spondylosis and the overall incidence of headache in the patients with spondylosis was low (Iansek et al. 1987). Therefore, it is also not surprising that blockades of the occipital nerve were effective in patients diagnosed as cervicogenic headache as well as migraine of cluster headache (Anthony 2000).

In conclusion, the attribution of headache to the neck is still difficult due to the lack of specific symptoms, specific clinical findings, specific radiological findings, and the unspecific effect of therapeutic interventions. The combination of stretching the cervical muscles in combination with an endurance and strength training may be the best therapy recommendation (Ylinen et al. 2010).

Cranial Neuralgias: Epidemiology and Clinical Characteristics

Cranial neuralgias are much more common in older patients than in younger patients. This is true for classic trigeminal neuralgia as well as for zoster neuritis of the trigeminal or facial nerve. Furthermore, the higher incidence of diabetic cranial neuropathy is due to the fact that diabetes is more often a disorder of older people.

Classic trigeminal neuralgia has an incidence of 4/100,000 people in the 20–30-year-old group and 20/100,000 in the 60–70-year-old group (Straube 2009). Females are affected 1.5 times more often than males. Clinically there is no difference in the symptoms between younger and older patients. Generally the paroxysmal pain is described as electrifying and stabbing, lasts for seconds to a maximum of 1 min, and is located in the second or third branch of the trigeminal nerve (Bennetto et al. 2007). At the beginning of the neuralgia spontaneous remission may occur, but with longer disease duration the neuralgia becomes chronic. Especially in younger patients with an involvement of the first branch, secondary trigeminal neuralgia should be considered. Clinical examination does not show a deficit, although after some years a slight persisting sensory deficit can occur. MRI scans sometimes show a compression of the trigeminal nerve root in the area of the exit at the pontine brainstem by a vessel, generally the superior cerebellar artery. Electrophysiological as well as radiological structural damage of the nerve can be shown statistically in group comparisons but this does not help to establish the diagnosis in the individual patient.

In contrast to classic trigeminal neuralgia, zoster neuritis typically involves the first branch of the trigeminal nerve (ophthalmic nerve) or the sensory part of the facial nerve. The reason for zoster neuritis is the reactivation of the varicella virus, a herpes virus, which is incorporated into the genome of the dorsal spinal ganglion neurons after primary infection with chicken pox during childhood. The prevalence increases with increasing age and is 45–100/100,000 for patients aged 80 years (Straube 2009). The lifetime prevalence is 25% and roughly a quarter of all zoster cases are located cranially. Clinically the first symptoms are burning and stabbing pain in the area of the first trigeminal nerve and facial nerve. Some days later, the typical skin lesions can be detected and this establishes the diagnosis. Serological or radiological tests are only necessary in cases with different clinical courses or symptoms. Only very rarely is there no skin lesion in patients with a severely suppressed immune system; in these patients the serological test can also be negative and a PCR is necessary to detect virus DNA. Besides the intense pain, motor paresis can also develop: In the case of trigeminal neuritis, the eye muscle and also the optical nerve can be affected; in the case of the facial nerve, a paresis of the mimic muscles can be seen. Rarely vasculitis of the carotid artery occurs. Patients with chronic diseases such as HIV, carcinomas, diabetes, or immunosuppression have a higher risk of suffering from zoster neuritis. Older patients, females, involvement of the cranial nerves and, pronounced skin lesions indicate an increased risk for the development of so-called postherpetic pain. In such a case, the pain persists for longer than 6 weeks after healing of the skin lesions. Such patients typically complain about paroxysmal pain in the innervation area and/or an allodynia in this area.

The third cranial neuropathy that occurs more often in older people is diabetic cranial nerve neuralgia. In a case series of 105 patients with eye muscle paresis, 9% were classified as diabetic and the mean age was 63 years (Batochi AP et al. 1997). The oculomotor nerve was involved significantly more often than the abducens nerve (Batochi et al. 1997). About half of the patients describe a mild to moderate pain. The course of the disorder is monophasic and the paresis generally has a good prognosis. Diagnostically, a diabetic cranial neuropathy can only be considered if other causes have been ruled out by proper imaging techniques. The diagnosis is supported by a slightly elevated protein count in the cerebral spinal fluid without signs of an inflammation.

Headaches and Psychiatric Comorbidities in Older People

There is a significant relationship between headaches and depression, which has been shown in several epidemiological studies (Breslau et al. 2003; Lake et al. 2005). This relationship is shown for migraine as well as tension-type headache and in both headaches depression is about three times more frequent than in the controls. Furthermore, there is also a relationship between anxiety disorder and migraine, with these disorders being 4–8 times more common in migraine patients than in controls (Juang et al. 2000; Wang et al. 1999). There are no studies available that focus on the relationship between headaches and psychiatric comorbidities in the elderly in particular but it seems to be the case that depression occurs more often in older patients with migraine than in the control population without headache. The prevalence of major depression in the population above 65 years of age is estimated to be 1–5%, with females affected more often than males (Fiske et al. 2009), and the prevalence of depressive syndromes increases with age (Snowdon 2001). Depression in older headache patients is not only influenced by the current headache situation but also by the previous headache history (Wang et al. 1999).

No differences are reported in the pain-related psychopathology. Generally, older patients tend to report somatic complaints more often and emotional symptoms less often than younger patients (Allaz 2006). As with younger patients, older patients with headaches also have lower scores in quality of life ratings compared to subjects of the same age without headaches (Jelicic et al. 1998).

Summary

1. Primary headaches are still the most common cause of headaches in older people but secondary causes are roughly twice as common as in younger people.
2. Hypnic headache and giant cell arteritis are two headache syndromes that occur almost solely in the elderly. Zoster neuritis, brain tumor–associated headaches, stroke-related headaches, and sleep apnea–related headaches are also more prevalent in the elderly.
3. Diagnostic interventions in older patients do not differ from those in younger headache patients. For most questions, MR imaging including diffusion-weighted imaging and MR angiography is the procedure of choice.

Acknowledgment

The author would like to thank Miss K. Ogston for her help in editing the manuscript.

References

Allaz AF (2006) Psychological components of chronic pain in the elderly. Psychol Neuropsychiatr Vieil 4:103–108

Anthony M (2000) Cervicogenic headache: prevalence and response to local steroid therapy. Clin Exp Rheumatol 18(2 Suppl 19):S59–S64

Arboix A, Massons J, Oliveres M, Arribas MP, Titus F (1994) Headache in acute cerebrovascular disease: a prospective clinical study in 240 patients. Cephalagia 14:37–40

Arboix A, Gracia-Trallero O, Gracia-Eroles L, Massons J, Comes E, Targa C (2005) Stroke-related headache: a clinical study in lacunar infarction. Headache 45:1345–1352

Batochi AP, Evoli A, Majolini L, Lo Monaco M, Padua L, Ricci E, Dickman A, Tonali P (1997) Ocular palsies in the absence of other neurological or ocular symptoms: analysis of 105 cases. J Neurol 244:639–645

Bennetto L, Patel NK, Fuller G (2007) Trigeminal neuralgia and its management. Brit Med J 27:201–205

Bigal ME, Libermann JN, Lipton RB (2006) Age-dependent prevalence and clinical features of migraine. Neurology 67(2):246–251

Bigal ME, Kurth T, Santanello N, Buse D, Golden W, Robbins M, Lipton RB (2010) Migraine and cardiovascular disease: a population-based study. Neurology 74(8):628–635

Boesen P, Sorensen SF (1987) Giant cell arteritis, temporal arteritis, and polymyalgia rheumatica in a Danish county. A prospective investigation, 1982-1985. Arthritis Rheum 30:294–299

Breslau N, Lipton RB, Stewart WF, Schultz LR, Welch KM (2003) Comorbidity of migraine and depression: investigating potential etiology and prognosis. Neurology 60(8):1308–1312

Bulpitt CJ, Dollery CT, Carne S (1976) Change in symptoms of hypertensive patients after referral to hospital clinic. Br Heart J 38:121–128

Colás R, Muñoz P, Temprano R, Gómez C, Pascual J (2004) Chronic daily headache with analgesic overuse: epidemiology and impact on quality of life. Neurology 62(8):1338–1342

Cortelli P, Grimaldi D, Guaraldi P, Pierangeli G (2004) Headache and hypertension. Neurol Sci 25(Suppl 3): S132–S134

Donnet A, Lantéri-Minet M (2009) A consecutive series of 22 cases of hypnic headache in France. Cephalalgia 29(9):928–934

Evers S, Goadsby PJ (2003) Hypnic headache: clinical features, pathophysiology, and treatment. Neurology 60(6):905–909

Ferro JM, Melo TP, Guerreiro M (1998) Headache in intracerebral hemorrhage survivors. Neurology 50:203–207

Fischera M, Anneken K, Evers S (2005) Old age of onset in cluster-headache patients. Headache 45 (5):615

Fiske A, Wetherell JL, Gatz M (2009) Depression in older adults. Annu Rev Clin Psychol 5:363–389

Goksan B, Gunduz A, Karadeniz D, Ağan K, Tascilar FN, Tan F, Purisa S, Kaynak H (2009) Morning headache in sleep apnoea: clinical and polysomnographic evaluation and response to nasal continuous positive airway pressure. Cephalalgia 29(6):635–641

Iansek R, Heywood J, Karnaghan J, Balla JI (1987) Cervical spondylosis and headaches. Clin Exp Neurol 23:175–178

Jelicic M, Kepmen G, Passchier J (1998) Psychological well-being in older adults suffering from chronic headache. Headache 38:292–294

Jensen R, Bendtsen L (2008) Medication overuse headache in Scandinavia. Cephalalgia 28(11):1237–1239

Juang KD, Wang SJ, Fuh JL, Lu SR, Su TP (2000) Comorbidity of depressive and anxiety disorders in chronic daily headache and its subtypes. Headache 40:818–823

Kaniecki RG (2006) Tension-type headache in the elderly. Curr Pain Headache Rep 10:448–453

Kaniecki RG (2007) Tension-type headache in the elderly. Curr Treat Options Neurol 9:31–37

Kelman L (2006) Migraine changes with age: impact on migraine classification. Headache 46:1161–1171

Lake AE, Rains JC, Penzien DB, Lipchik GL (2005) Headache and psychiatric comorbidity: historical context, clinical implications, and research relevance. Headache 45:493–506

Levy MJ, Matharu MS, Meeran K, Powell M, Goadsby PJ (2005) The clinical characteristics of headache in patients with pituitary tumours. Brain 128:1921–1930

Lipton RB, Pfeffer D, Newman LC, Solomon S (1993) Headaches in the elderly. J Pain Symptom Manage 8:87–97

Martins KM, Bordini CA, Bigal ME, Speciali JG (2006) Migraine in the elderly: a comparision with migraine in young adults. Headache 46:312–316

Muiesan ML, Padovani A, Salvetti M, Monteduro C, Poisa P, Bonzi B, Paini A, Cottini E, Agosti C, Castellano M, Rizzoni D, Vignolo A, Agabiti-Rosei E (2006) Headache: prevalence and relationship with office or ambulatory blood pressure in a general population sample (the Vobarno study). Blood Press 15(1):14–19

Nordin M, Carragee EJ, Hogg-Johnson S, Weiner SS, Hurwitz EL, Peloso PM, Guzman J, van der Velde G, Carroll LJ, Holm LW, Côté P, Cassidy JD, Haldeman S (2009) Assessment of neck pain and its associated disorders: results of the bone and joint decade 2000-2010 task force on neck pain and its associated disorders. J Manipulative Physiol Ther 32(2 Suppl):S117–S140

Pfaffenrath V, Fendrich K, Vennemann M, Meisinger C, Ladwig KH, Evers S, Straube A, Hoffmann W, Berger K (2009) Regional variations in the prevalence of migraine and tension-type headache applying the new IHS criteria: the German DMKG Headache Study. Cephalalgia 29(1):48–57

Prencipe M, Casini AR, Ferretti C, Santini M, Pezzella F, Scaldaferri N, Culasso F (2001) Prevalence of headache in an elderly population: attack frequency, disability, and use of medication. J Neurol Neurosurg Psychiatry 70:377–381

Provini F, Vetrugno R, Lugaresi E, Montagna P (2006) Sleep-related breathing disorders and headache. Neurol Sci 27(Suppl 2):S149–S152

Rasmussen BK, Olesen J (1992) Symptomatic and nonsymptomatic headaches in a general population. Neurology 42:1225–1231

Rigamonti A, Iurlaro S, Zelioli A, Agostoni E (2007) Two symptomatic cases of cluster headache associated with internal carotid artery dissection. Neurol Sci 28(Suppl 2):S229–S231

Schankin CJ, Ferrari U, Reinisch VM, Birnbaum T, Goldbrunner R, Straube A (2007) Characteristics of brain tumour-associated headache. Cephalalgia 27(8):904–911

Schwaiger J, Kiechl S, Seppi K, Sawires M, Stockner H, Erlacher T, Mairhofer ML, Niederkofler H, Rungger G, Gasperi A, Poewe W, Willeit J (2009) Prevalence of primary headaches and cranial neuralgias in men and women aged 55-94 years (Bruneck study). Cephalalgia 29(2):179–187

Sjaastad O, Bakketeig LS (2008) Prevalence of cervicogenic headache: Vågå study of headache epidemiology. Acta Neurol Scand 117(3):173–180

Snowdon J (2001) Is depression more prevalent in old age? Aust N Z J Psychiatry 35:782–787

Stovner LJ, Hagen K, Jensen R, Katsarava Z, Lipton R (2007) The global burden of headache: a documentation of headache prevalence and disability worldwide. Cephalagia 27:193–210

Straube A (2009) Diagnostik und Therapie von Gesichtsschmerzen. Angew Schmerzther Palliativmedizin 4:40–46

Straube A, Freilinger T, Rüther T, Padovan C (2007) Two cases of symptomatic cluster-like headache suggest the importance of sympathetic/parasympathetic balance. Cephalalgia 27(9):1069–1073

Straube A, Pfaffenrath V, Ladwig KH, Meisinger C, Hoffmann W, Fendrich K, Vennemann M, Berger K (2010) Prevalence of chronic migraine and medication overuse headache in Germany-the German DMKG headache study. Cephalalgia 30(2):207–213

Tronvik E, Stovner LJ, Hagen K, Holmen J, Zwart JA (2008) High pulse pressure protects against headache: prospective and cross-sectional data (HUNT study). Neurology 70(16):1329–1336

Truelsen T, Piechowski-Józwiak B, Bonita R, Mathers C, Bogousslavsky J, Boysen G (2006) Stroke incidence and prevalence in Europe: a review of available data. Eur J Neurol 13(6):581–598

Uthaikhup S, Sterling M, Jull G (2009) Cervical musculoskeletal impairment is common in elders with headache. Man Ther 14(6):636–641

Wang SJ, Liu HC, Fuh JL, Liu CJ, Wang PN, Lu SR (1999) Comorbidity of headaches and depression in the elderly. Pain 82:239–243

Ward TN, Levin M (2005) Headache in giant cell arteritis and other arteritides. Neurol Sci 26:134–137

Wittchen HU, Krause P, Hofler M, Pfister H, Ritz E, Goke B, Lehnert H, Tschope D, Kirch W, Pittrow D, Sharma AM, Bramlage P, Kupper B, Unger T (2003) Hypertension, diabetes mellitus and comorbidity in primary care. Fortschr Med Orig 27:19–27

Wöber C, Brannath W, Schmidt K, Kapitan M, Rudel E, Wessely P, Wober-Bingol C (2007) Prospective analysis of factors related to migraine attacks: the PAMINA study. Cephalagia 27:304–314

Wöber-Bingöl C, Wöber C, Karwautz A, Auterith A, Serim M, Zebenholzer K, Aydinkoc K, Kienbacher C, Wanner C, Wessely P (2004) Clinical features of migraine: a cross-sectional study in patients aged three to sixty-nine. Cephalalgia 24(1):12–17

Ylinen J, Nikander R, Nykänen M, Kautiainen H, Häkkinen A (2010) Effect of neck exercises on cervicogenic headache: a randomized controlled trial. J Rehabil Med 42(4):344–349

47 Managing Headache in Older People

Simona Sacco · Antonio Carolei
University of L'Aquila, L'Aquila, Italy

Paolo Martelletti, Timothy J. Steiner (eds.), *Handbook of Headache*, DOI 10.1007/978-88-470-1700-9_47,
© Lifting The Burden 2011

Abstract: Adults aged 20–50 years are the most likely headache sufferers but elderly individuals are affected too. In the elderly, as the prevalence of primary headache disorders decreases, the prevalence of secondary headaches increases, but primary headaches remain the main forms also in this age group. Scientific evidence referring to non-pharmacological and pharmacological treatment of headaches in the elderly is poor. So far, most of the available clinical trials excluded old subjects. When treating headache in the elderly, particular caution should be adopted in deciding for acute attack treatment or prevention since the elderly often present comorbid diseases, take polytherapy, and are at increased risk of adverse effects. For this reason, selection of available medications should be made at the individual level considering the above reported factors. Simplification of the drug regimens and downward of dosing are often the most adequate measures.

Headache is a symptom of a range of neurobiological disorders, including some of the most common and ubiquitous. Adults aged 20–50 years are the most likely sufferers but elderly individuals are affected too. In the elderly, as the prevalence of primary disorders such as tension-type headache, migraine, and cluster headache decreases, the prevalence of secondary headaches due to an underlying condition increases. However, primary headaches remain the most frequent headaches reported by older people and even if secondary headache disorders more often occur in the elderly, they account for no more than 10–20% of the headaches diagnosed over the age of 65 years (Edmeads 2000; Lipton et al. 1993). The substantial number of high-quality studies in young and middle-aged individuals contrasts with the considerable paucity of data on headache in the elderly.

Primary Headaches in the Elderly

To diagnose a primary headache disorder, a history must be taken, and the patient needs a thorough physical (including neurologic) examination. There are no diagnostic tests for any of the primary headache disorders. The medical history is all-important. Potential secondary causes of headache need to be considered and ruled out. Details referring to clinical characteristics of migraine, tension-type headache, cluster headache and other trigeminal autonomic cephalalgias, and other primary headache disorders can be found in ❷ Chaps. 15, ❷ 19, ❷ 23, and ❷ 28, respectively.

Migraine

Onset of migraine is from childhood onward but most commonly in the 20s and 30s and relatively infrequent after the age of 40 years. Just around 2% of the migraineurs report the onset of migraine after the age of 50 years (Lipton et al. 2001; Bigal et al. 2006). In migraineurs, with age progression, usually the attacks remit or their frequency and intensity reduce (Lyngberg et al. 2005; Mattson et al. 2000). Around 40% of migraineurs stop having attacks (Cologno et al. 1998; Eriksen et al. 2004; Lyngberg et al. 2005; Nachit-Ouinekh et al. 2005). The decrease begins in the fifth or sixth decade of life (Rasmussen and Lipton 2006) and occurs not only in women, but also in men. Also gender ratio varies with age; while female to men ratio is around 3:1 in young and middle-aged patients, it is around 2:1 at the age of 70 years (Lisotto et al. 2004; Stewart et al. 1992). Prevalence of migraine over 65 years of age is 7–14% for females and 4–7% for males (Lipton and Stewart 1994; Prencipe et al. 2001; Stewart et al. 1992). In the elderly, a low proportion of migraineurs present with the hallmarks of the disease such as unilateral pain, pain aggravated by exercise, and photo- and/or phonophobia. Aura shows the opposite pattern and is more common with age. Transformed migraine seems to be more prevalent at middle and older ages than in younger subjects, suggesting that some individuals with migraine transform to chronic daily headache over time (Castillo et al. 1999; Scher et al. 2003).

Tension-Type Headache

Tension-type headache is the most widespread of headache disorders. Onset is often in the teenage years and prevalence peaks in the fourth decade and then declines. Overall, 1-year prevalence of tension-type headache ranges from 44 to 61% (Prencipe et al. 2001; Rasmussen at al. 1991). A large part of the population have mild and infrequent tension-type headache (once per month or less), with 20–30% experiencing headache episodes more often. Frequency, characteristics, and severity of tension-type headache do not change substantially with advancing age (Schwaiger et al. 2002).

Other Primary Headaches and Facial Neuralgias

They are considered rare disease entities in the elderly (Schwaiger et al. 2002). Hypnic headache has a prevalence of 0.5% in the elderly, thunderclap headache has a prevalence of 0.3%, whereas the frequency is 0.2–1.2% for primary stabbing, cough, and exertional headache, and <0.2% for cluster headache, hemicrania continua, new daily persistent headache, and sexually induced headaches (Schwaiger et al. 2002).

Secondary Headaches in the Elderly

As already reported, secondary headaches become more likely in the elderly. Headache is secondary to serious disorders in around 15% of elderly patients while the corresponding proportion in patients aged less than 65 years is around 2% (Pascual and Berciano 1994) and secondary headaches may represent 10–20% of headaches in the elderly that are seen by clinicians. Because the likelihood of secondary headaches increases with age, it seems prudent for the clinician to be particularly cautious in the evaluation of patients with headache and a lowered threshold for obtaining laboratory and neuroimaging testing is appropriate. While in the young only headaches associated with "red flags" deserve consideration for secondary headaches, in the elderly any headache of new onset or any change in headache pattern deserves caution since it may reflect an underlying disease. Warning features may be represented by headache that is new or unexpected in an individual patient, thunderclap headache (intense headache with abrupt or "explosive" onset), headache with atypical aura, progressive headache worsening over weeks or longer, headache associated with postural change, headache waking up the patient, headache precipitated by physical exertion or Valsalva manouvre (e.g., coughing, laughing, or straining), new onset headache in a patient with a history of cancer, and new onset headache in a patient with a history of HIV or another infection. Other features that may indicate a secondary headache include focal neurological symptoms, non-focal neurological symptoms (e.g., cognitive disturbances), abnormal neurological examination, jaw claudication or visual disturbances, neck stiffness, fever, and risk factors for cerebral venous sinus thrombosis.

Secondary headache in the elderly include head or neck trauma, stroke, unruptured vascular malformations, arteritis, carotid or vertebral artery pain, cerebral venous thrombosis, other intracranial vascular disorders, intracranial hypertension or hypotension, intracranial inflammatory or infectious diseases, intracranial tumors, substance abuse or withdrawal, disorders of hemostasis, arterial hypertension, diseases of the head, eyes, ears, nose, throat, and cervical spine, systemic illnesses, and neuralgias (trigeminal, glossopharyngeal, and postherpetic). Common and important causes of secondary headaches and facial pain are described elsewhere in this text (❯ Chaps. 36, ❯ 37, ❯ 38, ❯ 39 and ❯ 41). 14–18% of chronic headaches are cervicogenic in origin, i.e., result from a musculoskeletal dysfunction in the cervical spine (Zito et al. 2006). Cervicogenic headache may be a frequent complaint in the elderly. An extensive description of the condition is reported in ❯ Chap. 37. It consists of a unilateral or bilateral pain localized to the neck and occipital region which may project to regions on the head and/or face. Pain may be precipitated or aggravated by particular neck movements or sustained neck postures and is associated with alterations in neck posture, movements, muscle tone, and/or muscle tenderness. Manual examination identifying articular mobility, muscle extensibility and range of motion, in the form of flexion and extension may assist diagnosis. Neck examination should be carried out in all patients presenting with headache including assessment of neck posture, range of movement, muscle tone, and of muscle tenderness. A new headache in any patient over 50 years of age should raise the suspicion of giant cell arteritis. An extensive description of the condition is reported in ❯ Chap. 38. Headache is the best known but not an inevitable symptom of giant cell arteritis. It is variable, likely to be persistent when present, often worse at night, and it can be very severe indeed. In only a minority of cases it is localized to the temple. Jaw claudication is so suggestive that, in its presence, the diagnosis is that of giant cell arteritis until proved otherwise. Furthermore, the patient with giant cell arteritis is systemically unwell. Marked scalp tenderness is common on examination, and may be a presenting complaint, and the temporal artery may be inflamed, and tender, tortuous, and thickened to palpation. Most patients have an erythrocyte sedimentation rate >50 mm/h, but this can be lower or it may be raised in the elderly for other reasons so temporal artery biopsy is usually necessary to secure the diagnosis. Treatment is represented by steroids in high dosage that however may be toxic in the long-term and particularly in the elderly. Nonspecific headache, particularly in the elderly, may be a symptom of primary angle-closure glaucoma. This is rare before middle age, when its prevalence is close to 1:1,000. Family history, female gender, and hypermetropia are recognized risk factors (Coleman 1999). Primary angle-closure glaucoma may present dramatically with acute ocular hypertension, a unilateral painful red eye with the pupil mid-dilated and fixed, associated nausea and vomiting, and, essentially, impaired vision. In other cases, headache or eye pain may be episodic and mild, with the diagnosis of primary angle-closure glaucoma suggested if the patient reports colored haloes around lights (Coleman 1999). The diagnosis of primary angle-closure glaucoma is confirmed by skilled slit-lamp examination and gonioscopy. A diagnosis of glaucoma should not be missed, and should prompt immediate referral. Rarely do intracranial tumors produce headache until quite large (although pituitary tumors are an exception to this rule). Usually they become evident for other reasons, but 3–4% present as headache. Raised intracranial pressure is apparent in the history. Epilepsy is a cardinal symptom of intracerebral space occupying lesions, and loss of consciousness should be viewed very seriously. In all likelihood, focal neurological signs will be present. Problems are more likely to occur with slowly growing tumors, especially those in neurologically "silent" areas of the frontal lobes. Subtle personality changes may result in treatment for depression, with headache attributed to it. Investigation may be prompted eventually by non-response to treatment, but otherwise some of these can be very difficult to pick up, whilst their infrequency does not justify routine brain scanning. Heightened suspicion is appropriate in patients who develop new headache and are known to have cancer elsewhere, or a suppressed immune system.

Established Knowledge

When treating headache in the elderly, particular caution should be adopted in deciding for acute attack treatment and prevention since the elderly often present comorbid diseases, take polytherapy, and are at increased risk of adverse events. For this reason, selection of available medications should be made at the individual level.

Treatment of Primary Headaches in the Elderly

A thorough initial assessment and appropriate diagnostic evaluation are always necessary and may reveal disease-modifying interventions that can potentially relieve the headache at source. Interdisciplinary assessment during the evaluation process may help identify all such treatable contributing factors. Several drugs, commonly used in the aged, can aggravate headache symptoms or cause headache de novo (Haan et al. 2006; Lipton et al. 1993). Examples of medications that exacerbate headache are nitrate-containing drugs, estrogen replacement therapies, and vasodilating antihypertensive drugs, such as nifedipine. As in younger age groups, before drug treatment of headache is tried, non-pharmacological measures, such as avoiding headache or migraine triggers, should be advised. Moreover, biofeedback, stress management, relaxation therapy, and cognitive-behavioral therapy have been shown to have some efficacy (Ward 2002). In selected cases, physical measures such as exercise and physical therapy may be appropriate. When general measures are not effective, treatment of the headache attacks, or a combination of attack treatment and preventive treatment, can be considered.

The approach to headache management in older persons differs from that for younger people. Aging is characterized by several physiological and pathological changes that together alter the effects of drug treatment. Physiological changes include gastric factors (decline of gastric acid secretion, slowing of gastric emptying, decreased peristalsis, and changes in gut wall metabolism), hepatic factors (40% reduction of blood flow to the liver, reduction of liver mass, and changes in liver metabolism), renal factors (decline in glomerular filtration rate and 25% reduction in kidney mass), and changes in body composition and in vascular control systems (McLean and Le Couteur 2004). Moreover, the elderly are more likely to have coexistent medical conditions, which present both therapeutic limitations and opportunities when selecting acute and preventive treatments for headache. Vascular diseases, such as hypertension and diabetes, lead not only to heart disease and stroke in the elderly, but also to decreased hepatic and renal function. The aging kidney, for example, is characterized by increased fibrosis, tubular atrophy, and arteriosclerosis. Advancing age changes the risk–benefit ratio of many drugs since age-related changes make older subjects more susceptible to the adverse effects of medication. The incidence of adverse drug reactions correlates with age (Chutka et al. 2004) since altered pharmacokinetics and pharmacodynamics in the older age groups may increase the likelihood of adverse effects and drug interactions. The increased incidence of adverse drug reactions is due not only to altered pharmacokinetics, but also to comorbidity and polytherapy. When adverse drug reactions occur in older people, they are more likely to be severe, and are even estimated to be the fourth to sixth greatest cause of death (McLean and Le Couteur 2004). Because the risk/benefit ratio of drug therapy can be less favorable in the elderly, it is important to use drugs with documented effectiveness and the lowest toxicity. Moreover, elderly people with multiple diseases often take multiple drugs simultaneously; with multiple medicines, there is an increased chance of adverse effects, interactions between different medicines and problems taking them correctly. Dose must often be reduced in the elderly, although dose requirements vary considerably (up to fivefold) from person to person. In addition, the physical effects of aging, such as arthritis and failing eyesight and memory, can also cause issues in taking medicines. Complexity of drug regimens (multiple drugs, frequent dosing, variable doses) increases the risk of noncompliance. If a patient has more than one disorder (e.g., hypertension and angina), it may be possible to treat both conditions with a single drug (e.g., a β-blocker or a calcium channel blocker), thus reducing the number of drugs prescribed. Drugs with once- or twice-daily dosing (long-acting or slow-release preparations) enable better compliance than do those with more frequent dosing. Downward dose adjustments and simplifying medication regimens are often appropriate. Moreover, cost of drugs can impose a major financial burden, particularly for elderly patients who rely on fixed incomes. Prescribers need to be aware of drug costs and to discuss cost. When cost is a factor, the least expensive comparable therapy should first be considered.

In the elderly, difficulties in treating migraine or tension-type headache depends on the exclusion from the majority of clinical trials of patients aged >60 or >65 years without further explanation (Landy and Lobo 2005). It is likely that this has been done to improve the efficacy outcome of the study treatment and to decrease possible adverse events. This has led to an unjustified, scientifically unproven concern about perceived adverse events and to undertreatment of older patients (Prencipe et al. 2001). Many physicians also feel uncertain with treating attacks or prescribing preventive drugs in elderly patients (Gladstone et al. 2004). Treatment options are considered to be restricted and this often leads to a failure of both elderly patients and their physicians to address specifically the topic of preventive treatment (Gloth 2001). Coincidental diseases and medication, however, rarely fully hinder the use of medications. When the various aspects are taken into account, treating headache in the elderly can be successful and satisfying. Persistent headache or its inadequate treatment is associated with a number of adverse outcomes in older people, including functional impairment, falls, mood changes (depression and anxiety), decreased socialization, sleep and appetite disturbance, and greater health-care use and costs (American Geriatrics Society Panel 2009). Although appropriate treatment can reduce these adverse events, the treatments themselves may incur their own risks and morbidities. Persistent pain can also be as distressing for the caregiver as for the patient. Caregiver strain and negative caregiver attitudes can substantially affect the patient's experience of pain and should be evaluated and discussed during the clinical encounter, if present. Although older patients are generally at higher risk of adverse drug reactions, analgesic and pain-modulating drugs can still be safe and effective when comorbidities and other risk factors are carefully considered. Recommendations for age-adjusted dosing are not available for most drugs. In reality, dosage for most patients requires initiation with low doses followed by careful upward titration, including frequent reassessment for dosage adjustments and optimum pain relief and for adverse events.

Acute Attack Treatment

The present part will deal about specific details of available medications for headaches referring to the elderly. Details referring to treatment and prevention of primary headaches are reported in ❯ Chaps. 17, ❯ 21, ❯ 25, ❯ 32 and ❯ 33. In terms of acute treatment, migraine can be managed with available substance groups such as analgesics, non-steroidal anti-inflammatory drugs (NSAIDs), ergotamine derivatives, and triptans, with their different modes of administration. Notably, triptans are also effective in the acute treatment of cluster headache, and perhaps other types of primary or even secondary headache (Brennum et al. 1992; Goadsby and Sprenger 2010; Limmroth et al. 2002; Rosenberg and Silberstein 2005). New strategies in acute treatment are very promising and the calcitonin gene-related peptide (CGRP) receptor antagonists and serotonin 5-HT$_{1F}$ agonists are in the late stages of development. To minimize adverse effects, all pain-modulating drugs must be carefully titrated and monitored frequently. Regular phone contact and follow-up visits should be scheduled to assess therapeutic effects and monitor for adverse events.

Acetaminophen or paracetamol can be used for the treatment of acute attacks of migraine and of tension-type headache. It should be considered as initial and ongoing pharmacotherapy in the treatment of elderly patients owing to its demonstrated effectiveness and good safety profile. Because hepatic metabolism is reduced in the elderly, it is advised to monitor liver function, especially when the drug is used regularly. It is contraindicated in the presence of liver failure while it should be used with caution in the presence of hepatic insufficiency, chronic alcohol abuse or dependence. The maximum dose is usually of 4 g daily. The dose should be reduced of around 50–75% in the presence of hepatic insufficiency or history of alcohol abuse. The addition of caffeine to acetaminophen does not lead to an increased risk of adverse events in the elderly.

NSAIDs can be used for the treatment of acute attacks of migraine and of tension-type headache but their prescription requires caution particularly in elderly patients and demands individualized consideration (Gloth 2001). Key issues in the selection of NSAID therapy are pain amelioration, frequency of use, cardiovascular risk, nephrotoxicity, drug interactions, and gastrointestinal toxicity. Frequency of attacks, comorbidities, concomitant medications, and associated risk factors all affect the decision to introduce such treatment. In some individuals, particularly in those with a previous positive experience with use of NSAIDs, decision-making must weigh the potential benefits of the improved function and health status that NSAIDs may provide against their risk profile. Most of the concerns raised with NSAIDs use refer to patients with bone and/or articular diseases or other conditions in which those drugs are used daily or nearly daily and they are difficult to be extrapolated to patients with headache. In older persons, NSAID-associated adverse events include relevant gastrointestinal toxicity (Ofman et al. 2002), which increases in frequency and severity with age (Boers et al. 2007). An estimated 15–35% of all the reported peptic ulcer complications are secondary to NSAID use (Chutka et al. 2004). At least in part, the gastrointestinal toxicity of NSAIDs is dose related and time dependent (Ofman et al. 2003; Richy et al. 2004). The concern for gastrointestinal bleeding in chronic NSAIDs users is heightened in the setting of co-administration with low-dose aspirin, often employed as an antithrombotic treatment in the elderly (de Abajo and Garcia Rodriguez 2001; McKellar et al. 2008). In individuals in whom NSAID therapy is considered and in whom gastrointestinal risk is low, it may be reasonable to recommend or prescribe ibuprofen or naproxen. Concomitant administration of misoprostol, H2-receptor antagonists, or proton pump inhibitors may reduce the risk for gastrointestinal ulceration in chronic NSAID users and should be prescribed if gastrointestinal risk is high (Hawkey et al. 2007; Rostom et al. 2002). Whether an NSAID prescribed along with a proton pump inhibitor provides superior protection from incident dyspepsia, bleeding, or other gastrointestinal tract complications remains unclear (Hur et al. 2006; Spiegel et al. 2006). NSAIDs may adversely affect blood pressure control (Aw et al. 2005; Izhar et al. 2004; Whelton et al. 2001), renal function (Juhlin et al. 2005; Niccoli et al. 2002), and heart-failure management (Juhlin et al. 2004). When NSAIDs are used, renal function, liver function, and gastrointestinal adverse events should be monitored (Burris 2004). NSAIDs interact with anticoagulants, hypoglycaemics, digoxin, antihypertensive agents, and diuretics (Lipton et al. 1993). Some traditional NSAIDs also have the in vitro capacity to interfere with the antiplatelet effect of aspirin therapy (Gladding et al. 2008). To this end, the Food and Drug Administration (FDA) issued a warning in 2006 concerning the co-administration of aspirin and ibuprofen (but the true clinical impact of this remains to be elucidated, as it remains unclear whether this is unique to ibuprofen or may hold true for other NSAIDs). Absolute contraindications to NSAIDs include current active peptic ulcer disease, chronic kidney disease, and heart failure while relative contraindications and cautions include arterial hypertension, Helicobacter pylori, history of peptic ulcer disease, and concomitant use of corticosteroids. Of the traditional NSAIDs, diclofenac has been identified as possessing potentially higher risk for adverse cardiovascular events (Kearney et al. 2006; McGettigan and Henry 2006). Naproxen sodium has been implicated as possessing less cardiovascular toxicity than other agents; ketorolac is not recommended for its high potential for gastrointestinal and renal toxicity (American Geriatrics Society Panel 2009). The addition of anti-emetics or prokinetics, such as domperidone (Dowson et al. 2000; Macgregor et al. 1993) or metoclopramide (Geraud et al. 2002), to NSAIDs might improve the efficacy of these drugs with an independent anti-nociceptive effect and help patients to deal with migraine-associated nausea. However, the evidence for their additional use is weak (Goldstein et al. 1999; Lipton et al. 1998; Tfelt-Hansen et al. 1980; Tfelt-Hansen et al. 1995). Besides, these drugs, particularly caffeine-containing analgesics (Scher et al. 2004), might carry an increased risk of medication overuse headache, although no prospective studies have been done. The use of antiemetic drugs, such as metoclopramide, favor the risk of extrapyramidal adverse events in the elderly (Lipton et al. 1993).

Cyclooxygenase-2 (COX-2) selective inhibitors were introduced in the hopes of mitigating traditional NSAIDs-related adverse effects (Christensen et al. 2007). For example, celecoxib appeared to have fewer significant gastrointestinal adverse events (Goldstein et al. 2001; Moore et al. 2005; Singh et al. 2006a). However, the protection afforded by COX-2 selective inhibition against gastrointestinal bleeding is not complete, and other NSAIDs-related toxicities are no different with COX-2 inhibitors (Moore et al. 2006). COX-2 inhibitors have also proven effective in migraine treatment with similar efficacy to NSAIDs (Silberstein et al. 2004). However, the COX-2 inhibitors rofecoxib, the best studied COX-2 inhibitor in migraine, and valdecoxib were withdrawn from the market because of the associated risk of adverse cardio-vascular events (Setakis et al. 2008). COX-2 inhibitors such as celecoxib can cause lower-limb edema (Burris 2004) and may also increase the risk of stroke. Moreover, there is no evidence to support the use of those agents in the treatment of headache despite they are sometimes prescribed in the clinical setting.

Opioids may represent a further possibility for the treatment of headache, especially in patients at risk for NSAIDs-related adverse effects (Singh et al. 2006b). However, no strong evidence exists regarding the efficacy of those drug in the treatment of primary headaches and also the potential adverse events associated with opioids can present a barrier to treatment. In the elderly the use of opioid analgesics is limited by sedation and cognitive side effects (Biondi and Saper 2000; Kalso et al. 2004; Noble et al. 2008). Adverse events such as constipation and urinary retention must be monitored (Burris 2004). Respiratory depression, which affects respiratory rate, minute volume, and oxygen saturation, is the most serious adverse event and therefore deserves special consideration and usually results from excessively rapid dosing increases, drug–drug interactions with other central nervous system depressants (most notably benzodiazepines, alcohol, and barbiturates), and drug accumulation or accidental overdose from opioids with variable pharmacokinetic profiles, such as methadone (Fishman et al. 2002; Santiago and Edelman 1985). Tramadol often causes nausea and vomiting, and in higher doses can cause seizures (Gloth 2001). Propoxyphene can cause ataxia and dizziness (Gloth 2001). Consequently, the advice is not to use opioids in elderly patients with headache, or to start low and increase the dose slowly (American Geriatrics Society Panel 2009). When used over a protracted period of time, opioid abuse may become a concern, especially in patients with a prior history of a substance use disorder (including tobacco use) (Ives et al. 2006; Reid et al. 2002). Although the risks are exceedingly low in older patients with no current or past history of substance abuse, it is impossible to identify every patient who will abuse prescribed opioids (Fishbain et al. 2008).

The ergot alkaloids were the first specific antimigraine therapy available. Ergotamine, previously the mainstay of acute treatment, can no longer be considered the treatment of choice in acute migraine (Goadsby and Sprenger 2010; Tfelt-Hansen et al. 2000). There are particular situations in which ergotamine is very helpful, such as in the treatment of very long attacks with headache recurrence, but dosing must be carefully monitored because ergotamine overuse can produce severe headache in addition to many vascular problems (Silberstein and McCrory 2003). Dihydroergotamine is usually better tolerated than ergotamine (less nausea and vasoconstriction), but has a poor oral bioavailability (Little et al. 1982). Dihydroergotamine administered via a nasal spray has a better bioavailability of about 40%, but the onset of action is relatively slow and it has been shown to be inferior to nasal and subcutaneous sumatriptan (Boureau et al. 2000; Touchon et al. 1996). Injectable dihydroergotamine (intravenous or intramuscular) is more effective, but produces more side effects and the mode of administration is less convenient (Goadsby and Sprenger 2010). Intermittent, chronic, and excessive use of ergotamine can lead to serious ischemic adverse events such as peripheral ischemia, arterial stenosis, myocardial infarction, and cerebral ischemia, probably due to its broad pharmacologic activity involving serotonin ($5HT_1$ and $5HT_2$), dopamine, and α-adrenoceptors (Tfelt-Hansen 2000; Wammes-van der Heijden et al. 2006). Preexisting hypertension can worsen and coronary vasoconstriction can occur, often with associated ischemic changes and anginal pain, and peripheral vasoconstriction. Ergotamine should be avoided or used with caution in elderly patients (Biondi and Saper 2000). Ergotamine overuse in patients simultaneously using cardiovascular drugs, on the contrary, increases the risk of ischemic complications almost fourfold with respect to patients using cardiovascular drugs but not using ergotamine (Wammes-van der Heijden et al. 2006).

The triptans, which are serotonin 5-HT$_{1B/1D}$ receptor agonists, are the most powerful option available to stop a migraine attack. There are seven compounds (almotriptan, eletriptan, frovatriptan, naratriptan, rizatriptan, sumatriptan, zolmitriptan), available in various formulations (tablets, nasal spray, subcutaneous injections, suppositories). Triptans, although with a less degree than ergotamine, can also cause coronary, craniovascular, and peripheral vasoconstriction possibly leading to serious complications such as myocardial infarction, ischemic stroke, and ischemic colitis, mostly in patients with cardiovascular disease or risk factors (Wammes-van der Heijden et al. 2006). Therefore, the use of triptans, like ergotamine, is contraindicated in these patients. The triptans are examples of drugs that have been thoroughly studied in clinical trials, but virtually always after excluding patients aged over 60 or 65 years. It is, however, generally thought that they may be used after the age of 60 years if, and as long as, there are no cardiac contraindications (Gladstone et al. 2004; Landy and Lobo 2005). However, especially in cases of cardiac ischemia, one should show great care with vasoconstrictive drugs such as triptans. A study of triptan use in general practice, also in elderly patients with various risk factors, has shown that there is no increased risk of stroke, myocardial infarction, cardiovascular death, ischemic heart disease, or mortality (Hall et al. 2004). When triptans are used in elderly patients, periodic cardiac screening (e.g., an electrocardiogram every 3 months) is advised. Moreover, some data referring to rizatriptan and zolmitriptan are available in the elderly. Plasma pharmacokinetics of rizatriptan appeared to be similar in the elderly and in the young (Musson et al. 2001). Zolmitriptan induced a statistically significant increase in systolic and diastolic blood pressure in the elderly compared with young adults, but this aspect was not considered to be of clinical concern (Peck et al. 1998).

CGRP is a neuropeptide thought to have a key role in the pathophysiology of migraine (Goadsby 2005). CGRP receptor antagonist telcagepant has recently been reported as effective for acute treatment of migraine with efficacy comparable to that of zolmitriptan 5 mg, but with fewer associated adverse events (Ho et al. 2008). In the trial, even if there was not an upper age limit, mean age of included patients was about 43 years and consequently results cannot be generalized to the elderly. One potential benefit of the new CGRP receptor antagonist class of acute migraine treatments is the absence of vasoconstriction, a liability of the triptans, which may allow for the safe administration of telcagepant in patients with migraine and cardiovascular disease. However, such patients were excluded from this clinical trial because of the contraindication for zolmitriptan, and further studies are necessary to determine the safety of telcagepant in patients with cardiovascular disease (Ho et al. 2008). Moreover, concerns about possible liver toxicity remain (Goadsby and Sprenger 2010). The development program of one compound, MK3207, which was undergoing phase 2 evaluation, has been discontinued because of delayed liver test abnormalities (Goadsby and Sprenger 2010).

Preventive Treatments

Preventive therapy is a crucial component of the management strategy to reduce migraine disability. Although attack frequency is usually the main impetus for prevention, sometimes intractability is the problem. Due to frequent contraindications related to acute medications, preventative drug regimens and nonpharmacologic treatments assume greater prominence when treating the elderly suffering frequent and severe headaches. Patients who typically have more than two or three migraine attacks per month might also benefit from preventive treatment, although the frequency is arbitrary and a matter of debate (Goadsby and Sprenger 2010). Preventive treatment can be divided into pharmacological and non-pharmacological therapies; one approach certainly does not exclude the use of the other, and a combination of pharmacological and non-pharmacological approaches, such as patient education, acupuncture, biofeedback, and exercise, can be useful in clinical practice. The choice of migraine preventive agent is based on effectiveness, adverse events profile, knowledge of previous efficacious or unsuccessful treatment trials, and comorbidities of the individual patient. Treatment of comorbid diseases can also be carefully chosen to improve migraine. Examples are β-blockers in cases of migraine with hypertension, antiepileptics (sodium valproate, topiramate) when the patient has migraine and epilepsy, and antidepressants to improve coexistent depression.

The use of preventive treatments in all age groups is increasing, although the efficacy of most of the prophylactic drugs is limited, and most of the available drugs are associated with many adverse effects, especially in the elderly (Lipton et al. 1993; Loder and Biondi 2005). In general, the advice in elderly is to start preventive treatment at low dosages and increase them slowly (American Geriatrics Society Panel 2009; Loder and Biondi 2005). Treatments that have proven effective in the preventive management of migraine include β-blockers, antidepressants, anticonvulsants, calcium channel blockers, serotonin antagonists, and nutraceuticals (i.e., dietary supplements with pharmacological properties). β-blockers propranolol and metoprolol, the antiepileptic drugs sodium valproate and topiramate, and the calcium channel blocker flunarizine can be considered to be first-choice drugs (Goadsby and Sprenger 2010). Flunarizine is not available in many countries and verapamil could be used as an alternative, although the evidence is much less clear for this drug with positive effects only in very small studies (Goadsby and Sprenger 2010). Relatively new drugs with some promise for the treatment of migraine include the antidepressant venlafaxine, as well as inhibitors of angiotensin-converting enzyme (ACE) and angiotensin II receptor blockers (ARBs). Anticholinergic drugs and treatment with multiple drugs must be avoided as much as possible, as they may predispose to delirium in older patients (Inouye 2006).

Migraine is clearly an inherited disposition to headache that is triggered by change: too much or too little sleep, skipping meals, weather change, change in exertion patterns, or change in stress. Thus a balanced, regular lifestyle seems desirable, although it has not been proven by evidence-based medicine that education of patients and other adjustments to lifestyle may help to reduce the frequency or severity of headaches. The same applies to the careful intake of recognized aggravating substances, such as caffeine.

Tricyclic antidepressants (including amitriptyline, desipramine, and nortriptyline), especially amitriptyline, are often used as preventive treatment for migraine and tension-type headache in adults, although without scientific evidence (Haan et al. 2006). Those same drugs can be employed also to treat postherpetic neuralgia. Caution is advised when used in the elderly (American Geriatrics Society Panel 2009; Chutka et al. 2004; Landy and Lobo 2005; Gloth 2001). Elderly patients who receive normal doses of tricyclic antidepressants usually develop higher plasma drug concentrations and metabolites than do younger patients (Chutka et al. 2004). Amitriptyline can cause anticholinergic adverse events (visual, urinary, gastrointestinal, and orthostatic hypotension), confusion, seizures, and cardiac conduction disturbances (atrioventricular blockade) (Lipton et al. 1993). Older persons rarely tolerate doses greater than 75 to 100 mg per day. Fewer adverse events are associated with nortriptyline, which may represent an appropriate alternative to amitriptyline. Tricyclic antidepressants are contraindicated in patients with cardiac dysrhythmias, closed-angle glaucoma, and urine retention (Edmeads and Wang 2006). However, the doses used for headache prevention are in general lower than those for treating depression, and adverse effects are less pronounced (Punay and Couch 2003). More recent pharmacological advances in the treatment of depression have included selective serotonin-reuptake inhibitors (SSRIs) and mixed serotonin- and norepinephrine-reuptake inhibitors (SNRIs). Those drugs have been related to a less degree of adverse events. The SNRIs (duloxetine, venlafaxine) are particularly effective in the treatment of various neuropathic pain conditions with a better adverse events profile than the tricyclic antidepressants. In contrast, SSRI drugs (sertraline, paroxetine, fluvoxamine, fluoxetine, citalopram) have not proved to be effective against pain. Caution has also been advised with the combination of triptans and SSRIs owing to the possible production of the potentially life-threatening serotonin syndrome, with symptoms such as tremor, palpitations, flushing, hypertension, and agitation (Mathew et al. 1996).

Calcium channel blockers may be used for migraine prevention. However, there are several considerations with respect to their use in the elderly. A moderate decrease in the clearance of all calcium channel blockers occurs with aging (Schwartz 1996). Older patients experience greater reductions in blood pressure and greater suppression of heart rate. Postural hypotension occurs more frequently in the elderly. When calcium channel blockers are prescribed in elderly patients, the dose must be adjusted. Caution is needed in patients with concomitant congestive heart failure (Lipton et al. 1993). In the geriatric population, verapamil has been associated with gastrointestinal bleeds caused by its antiplatelet effects (Opie 1997). Suspected gastrointestinal bleeds or bleeding points are a contraindication. Flunarizine used to be prescribed in migraine several decades ago, but its use is now very limited. Elderly patients are more susceptible to side effects, including depression and parkinsonism.

Both propranolol and timolol have been approved for migraine prophylaxis. The absolute bioavailability of propranolol doubles in the geriatric patient, thus the dose must be adjusted (McLean and Le Couteur 2004). Use may be limited because they influence congestive heart failure, conduction abnormalities, asthma, glaucoma, depressive symptoms, and diabetes (Lipton et al. 1993). β-blockers may be particularly useful in patients having also arterial hypertension or tremor.

Several antiepileptics are commonly employed to treat headache, mostly migraine and neuralgias. Sodium valproate is associated with a number of adverse events, and because of reduced hepatic mass and blood flow in the elderly these adverse events can occur more frequently in this age group. Sodium valproate can cause liver function disturbances, bone marrow suppression, decreased bone marrow density, delirium, tremor, ataxia, and, in rare cases, an extrapyramidal syndrome with dementia (Arroyo and Kramer 2001; Brodie and Kwan 2005; Chronicle and Mulleners 2004). Alopecia will not often be a problem in the elderly migraine patient. Carbamazepine is associated with multiple drug–drug interactions that may represent a relevant problem in the elderly who takes several medications. When carbamazepine is used, aspartate transaminase, alanine transaminase, complete blood count, creatinine, blood urea nitrogen, electrolytes, and serum carbamazepine levels should be monitored. Gabapentin and more recently pregabalin have been found to have beneficial effects in some forms of headache and various neuropathic pain conditions with more-benign side effect profiles than older anticonvulsant and antidepressant tricyclic drugs (Rowbotham et al. 1998; Wiffen et al. 2005). However, also gabapentin and pregabalin can be associated with sedation, ataxia, and edema. Topiramate is associated with a high risk of adverse events also in younger age groups (Chronicle and Mulleners 2004). It can cause cognitive impairment, renal stones, body weight loss, sedation, and agitation. In epilepsy, however, it seemed to be well tolerated in the elderly (Groselj et al. 2005).

The efficacy of benzodiazepines in the management of headache is limited. Current information does not support a direct analgesic effect of these drugs. The high risk profile in older adults usually obviates any potential benefit that such agents might render in terms of pain relief, although they may be justified for management of anxiety or in a trial for relief of muscle spasm, especially in common situations in which anxiety, muscle spasm, and pain coexist.

Corticosteroids can be used for the treatment of some primary headaches such as cluster headache and for secondary headache management such as giant cell arteritis. The lowest possible dose should be used to prevent steroid effects. Side effects include fluid retention and glycemic effects in short-term use and cardiovascular and bone demineralization with long-term use.

The ACE-inhibitors captopril, enalapril, and lisinopril and the ARBs candesartan, olmesartan, and telmisartan were tested mostly in non-elderly migraineurs and showed preliminary effectiveness (Bender 1995; Charles et al. 2006; Diener et al. 2009; Owada 2004; Schrader et al. 2001; Schuh-Hofer et al. 2007; Tronvik et al. 2003). Adverse events were minimal and those same compounds might be useful in elderly patients with concurrent arterial hypertension. However, it is important to remind that in the elderly, ACE-inhibitors and ARBs may cause acute renal insufficiency.

Botulinum toxin, injected into the pericranial and neck/shoulder musculature, has been studied as prophylaxis for both tension-type and migraine headache. The quality of the studies has been variable, and results often contradictory. Anyhow, some patients seem to respond to this treatment (Haan et al. 2006).

Current Research

Most of the available clinical trials referring to headache treatment excluded old subjects. To date there is no ongoing research specifically targeted to the management of headache in the elderly.

References

American Geriatrics Society Panel on the Pharmacological Management of Persistent Pain in Older Persons (2009) Pharmacological management of persistent pain in older persons. J Am Geriatr Soc 57:1331–1346

Arroyo S, Kramer G (2001) Treating epilepsy in the elderly. Drug Saf 24:991–1015

Aw TJ, Haas SJ, Liew D, Krum H (2005) Meta-analysis of cyclooxygenase-2 inhibitors and their effects on blood pressure. Arch Intern Med 165:490–496

Bender WI (1995) ACE inhibitors for prophylaxis of migraine headaches. Headache 35:470–471

Bigal ME, Liberman JN, Lipton RB (2006) Age-dependent prevalence and clinical features of migraine. Neurology 67:246–251

Biondi DM, Saper JR (2000) Geriatric headache. How to make the diagnosis and manage the pain. Geriatrics 55:40–50

Boers M, Tangelder MJ, van Ingen H, Fort JG, Goldstein JL (2007) The rate of NSAID-induced endoscopic ulcers increases linearly but not exponentially with age: a pooled analysis of 12 randomised trials. Ann Rheum Dis 66:417–418

Boureau F, Kappos L, Schoenen J, Esperanca P, Ashford E (2000) A clinical comparison of sumatriptan nasal spray and dihydroergotamine nasal spray in the acute treatment of migraine. Int J Clin Pract 54:281–286

Brennum J, Kjeldsen M, Olesen J (1992) The 5-HT1-like agonist sumatriptan has a significant effect in chronic tension-type headache. Cephalalgia 12:375–379

Brodie MJ, Kwan P (2005) Epilepsy in elderly people. BMJ 331:1317–1322

Burris JE (2004) Pharmacologic approaches to geriatric pain management. Arch Phys Med Rehabil 85 (Suppl 3):S45–S49

Castillo J, Munöz P, Guitera V, Pascual J (1999) Epidemiology of chronic daily headache in the general population. Headache 38:497–506

Charles JA, Jotkowitz S, Byrd LH (2006) Prevention of migraine with olmesartan in patients with hypertension/prehypertension. Headache 46:503–507

Christensen S, Riis A, Nørgaard M, Thomsen RW, Sørensen HT (2007) Introduction of newer selective cyclo-oxygenase-2 inhibitors and rates of hospitalization with bleeding and perforated peptic ulcer. Aliment Pharmacol Ther 25:907–912

Chronicle E, Mulleners W (2004) Anticonvulsant drugs for migraine prophylaxis. Cochrane Database Syst Rev 3:1–35

Chutka DS, Takahashi PY, Hoel RW (2004) Inappropriate medications for elderly patients. Mayo Clin Proc 79:122–139

Coleman AL (1999) Glaucoma. Lancet 354:1803–1810

Cologno D, Torelli P, Manzoni CG (1998) Migraine with aura. A review of 81 patients at 10–20 years' follow-up. Cephalalgia 18:690–696

de Abajo FJ, Garcia Rodriguez LA (2001) Risk of upper gastrointestinal bleeding and perforation associated with low-dose aspirin as plain and enteric-coated formulations. BMC Clin Pharmacol 1:1

der Heijden EA Wammes-van, Rahimtoola H, Leufkens HGM, Tijssen CC, Egberts ACG (2006) Risk of ischemic complications related to the intensity of triptan and ergotamine use. Neurology 67:1128–1134

Diener HC, Gendolla A, Feuersenger A, Evers S, Straube A, Schumacher H, Davidai G (2009) Telmisartan in migraine prophylaxis: a randomized, placebo-controlled trial. Cephalalgia 29:92–97

Dowson A, Ball K, Haworth D (2000) Comparison of a fixed combination of domperidone and paracetamol (domperamol) with sumatriptan 50 mg in moderate to severe migraine: a randomized UK primary care study. Curr Med Res Opin 16:190–197

Edmeads J (2000) Headache in the elderly. In: Olesen J, Tfelt-Hansen P, Welch KMA (eds) The headaches, 2nd edn. Lippincott Williams & Wilkins, Philadelphia, pp 947–951

Edmeads JG, Wang SJ (2006) Headaches in the elderly. In: Olesen J, Goadsby PJ, Ramadan NM, Tfelt-Hansen P, Welch KMA (eds) The headaches, 3rd edn. Lippincott Williams & Wilkins, Philadelphia, pp 1105–1110

Eriksen MK, Thomsen LL, Russell MB (2004) Prognosis of migraine with aura. Cephalalgia 24:18–22

Fishbain DA, Cole B, Lewis J, Rosomoff HL, Rosomoff RS (2008) What percentage of chronic nonmalignant pain patients exposed to chronic opioid analgesic therapy develop abuse/addiction and/or aberrant drug-related behaviors? A structured evidence-based review. Pain Med 9:444–459

Fishman SM, Wilsey B, Mahajan G, Molina P (2002) Methadone reincarnated: novel clinical applications with related concerns. Pain Med 3:339–348

Geraud G, Compagnon A, Rossi A, Cozam Study Group (2002) Zolmitriptan versus a combination of acetylsalicylic acid and metoclopramide in the acute oral treatment of migraine: a double-blind, randomised, three-attack study. Eur Neurol 47:88–89

Gladding PA, Webster MW, Farrell HB, Zeng IS, Park R, Ruijne N (2008) The antiplatelet effect of six non-steroidal anti-inflammatory drugs and their pharmacodynamic interaction with aspirin in healthy volunteers. Am J Cardiol 101:1060–1063

Gladstone JP, Eross EJ, Dodick DW (2004) Migraine in special populations. Treatment strategies for children and adolescents, pregnant women, and the elderly. Postgrad Med 115:39–50

Gloth FM (2001) Pain management in older adults: prevention and treatment. J Am Geriatr Soc 49:188–199

Goadsby PJ (2005) Calcitonin gene-related peptide antagonists as treatments of migraine and other primary headaches. Drugs 65:2557–2567

Goadsby PJ, Sprenger T (2010) Current practice and future directions in the prevention and acute management of migraine. Lancet Neurol 9:285–298

Goldstein J, Hoffman HD, Armellino JJ, Battikha JP, Hamelsky SW, Couch J, Blumenthal H, Lipton RB (1999) Treatment of severe, disabling migraine attacks in an over-the-counter population of migraine sufferers: results from three randomized placebo-controlled studies of the combination of acetaminophen, aspirin and caffeine. Cephalalgia 19:684–691

Goldstein JL, Correa P, Zhao WW, Burr AM, Hubbard RC, Verburg KM, Geis GS (2001) Reduced incidence of gastroduodenal ulcers with celecoxib, a novel cyclooxygenase-2 inhibitor, compared to naproxen in patients with arthritis. Am J Gastroenterol 96:1019–1027

Groselj J, Guerrini R, Van Oene J, Lahaye M, Schreiner A, Schwalen S (2005) Experience with topiramate monotherapy in elderly patients with recent onset epilepsy. Acta Neurol Scand 112:144–150

Haan J, Hollander J, Ferrari MD (2006) Migraine in the elderly: a review. Cephalalgia 27:97–106

Hall GC, Brown MM, Mo J, MacRae KD (2004) Triptans in migraine. The risk of stroke, cardiovascular disease, and death in practice. Neurology 62:563–568

Hawkey CJ, Jones RH, Yeomans ND, Scheiman JM, Talley NJ, Goldstein JL, Ahlbom H, Naesdal J (2007) Efficacy of esomeprazole for resolution of symptoms of heartburn and acid regurgitation in continuous users of non-steroidal anti-inflammatory drugs. Aliment Pharmacol Ther 25:813–821

Ho TW, Ferrari MD, Dodick DW, Galet V, Kost J, Fan X, Leibensperger H, Froman S, Assaid C, Lines C, Koppen H, Winner PK (2008) Efficacy and tolerability of MK-0974 (telcagepant), a new oral antagonist of calcitonin gene-related peptide receptor, compared with zolmitriptan for acute migraine: a randomised, placebo-controlled, parallel-treatment trial. Lancet 372:2115–2123

Hur C, Chan AT, Tramontano AC, Gazelle GS (2006) Coxibs versus combination NSAID and PPI therapy for chronic pain: an exploration of the risks, benefits, and costs. Ann Pharmacother 40:1052–1063

Inouye SK (2006) Delirium in older persons. N Engl J Med 354:1157–1165

Ives TJ, Chelminski PR, Hammett-Stabler CA, Malone RM, Perhac JS, Potisek NM, Shilliday BB, DeWalt DA, Pignone MP (2006) Predictors of opioid misuse in patients with chronic pain: a prospective cohort study. BMC Health Serv Res 6:46

Izhar M, Alausa T, Folker A, Hung E, Bakris GL (2004) Effects of COX inhibition on blood pressure and kidney function in ACE inhibitor-treated blacks and hispanics. Hypertension 43:573–577

Juhlin T, Björkman S, Gunnarsson B, Fyge A, Roth B, Höglund P (2004) Acute administration of diclofenac, but possibly not long term low dose aspirin, causes detrimental renal effects in heart failure patients treated with ACE-inhibitors. Eur J Heart Fail 6:909–916

Juhlin T, Björkman S, Höglund P (2005) Cyclooxygenase inhibition causes marked impairment of renal function in elderly subjects treated with diuretics and ACE-inhibitors. Eur J Heart Fail 7:1049–1056

Kalso E, Edwards JE, Moore RA, McQuay HJ (2004) Opioids in chronic non-cancer pain: systematic review of efficacy and safety. Pain 112:372–380

Kearney PM, Baigent C, Godwin J, Halls H, Emberson JR, Patrono C (2006) Do selective cyclooxygenase-2 inhibitors and traditional non-steroidal anti-inflammatory drugs increase the risk of atherothrombosis? Meta-analysis of randomised trials. BMJ 332:1302–1308

Landy SH, Lobo BL (2005) Migraine treatment throughout the lifecycle. Expert Rev Neurother 5:343–353

Limmroth V, Katsarava Z, Fritsche G, Przywara S, Diener H-C (2002) Features of medication overuse headache following overuse of different acute headache drugs. Neurology 59:1011–1014

Lipton RB, Stewart WF (1994) The epidemiology of migraine. Eur Neurol 34(suppl 2):6–11

Lipton RB, Pfeffer D, Newman LC, Solomon S (1993) Headaches in the elderly. J Pain Symptom Manage 8:87–97

Lipton RB, Stewart WF, Ryan RE, Saper J, Silberstein S, Sheftell F (1998) Efficacy and safety of acetaminophen, aspirin, and caffeine in alleviating migraine headache pain—three double-blind, randomized, placebo-controlled trials. Arch Neurol 55:210–217

Lipton RB, Stewart WF, Diamond S, Diamond ML, Reed M (2001) Prevalence and burden of migraine in the United States: data from the American Migraine Study II. Headache 41:646–657

Lisotto C, Mainardi F, Maggioni F, Dainese F, Zanchin G (2004) Headache in the elderly: a clinical study. J Headache Pain 5:36–41

Little PJ, Jennings GL, Skews H, Bobik A (1982) Bioavailability of dihydroergotamine in man. Br J Clin Pharmacol 13:785–790

Loder E, Biondi D (2005) General principles of migraine management. The changing role of prevention. Headache 45(Suppl 1):S33–S47

Lyngberg AC, Rasmussen BK, Jørgensen T, Jensen R (2005) Prognosis of migraine and tension-type headache. A population-based follow-up study. Neurology 65:580–585

MacGregor EA, Wilkinson M, Bancroft K (1993) Domperidone plus paracetamol in the treatment of migraine headache. Cephalalgia 13:124–127

Mathew NT, Tiejen GE, Lucker C (1996) Serotonin syndrome complicating migraine pharmacotherapy. Cephalalgia 16:323–327

Mattson P, Svärdsudd K, Lundberg PO, Westerberg CE (2000) The prevalence of migraine in women aged 40–70 years: a population-based study. Cephalalgia 20:893–899

McGettigan P, Henry D (2006) Cardiovascular risk and inhibition of cyclooxygenase: a systematic review of the observational studies of selective and non-selective inhibitors of cyclooxygenase 2. JAMA 296:1633–1644

McKellar G, Madhok R, Singh G (2008) Update on the use of analgesics versus nonsteroidal anti-inflammatory drugs in rheumatic disorders: risks and benefits. Curr Opin Rheumatol 20:239–245

McLean AJ, Le Couteur DG (2004) Aging biology and geriatric clinical pharmacology. Pharmacol Rev 56:163–184

Moore RA, Derry S, Makinson GT, McQuay HJ (2005) Tolerability and adverse events in clinical trials of celecoxib in osteoarthritis and rheumatoid arthritis: systematic review and meta-analysis of information from company clinical trial reports. Arthritis Res Ther 7:R644–R665

Moore RA, Derry S, Phillips CJ, McQuay HJ (2006) Nonsteroidal anti-inflammatory drugs (NSAIDs), cyxlooxygenase-2 selective inhibitors (coxibs) and gastrointestinal harm: review of clinical trials and clinical practice. BMC Musculoskelet Disord 7:79

Musson DG, Birk KL, Panebianco DL, Gagliano KD, Rogers JD, Goldberg MR (2001) Pharmacokinetics of rizatriptan in healthy elderly subjects. Int J Clin Pharmacol Ther 39:447–452

Nachit-Ouinekh F, Dartigues JF, Chrystosome V, Henry P, Sourgen C, El Hasnaoui A (2005) Evolution of migraine after a 10-year follow-up. Headache 45:1280–1287

Niccoli L, Bellino S, Cantini F (2002) Renal tolerability of three commonly employed non-steroidal anti-inflammatory drugs in elderly patients with osteoarthritis. Clin Exp Rheumatol 20:201–207

Noble M, Tregear SJ, Treadwell JR, Schoelles K (2008) Long-term opioid therapy for chronic noncancer pain: a systematic review and meta-analysis of efficacy and safety. J Pain Symptom Manage 35:214–228

Ofman JJ, MacLean CH, Straus WL, Morton SC, Berger ML, Roth EA, Shekelle PG (2002) A metaanalysis of severe upper gastrointestinal complications of nonsteroidal antiinflammatory drugs. J Rheumatol 29:804–812

Ofman JJ, MacLean CH, Straus WL, Morton SC, Berger ML, Roth EA, Shekelle PG (2003) Meta-analysis of dyspepsia and nonsteroidal antiinflammatory drugs. Arthritis Rheum 49:508–518

Opie LH (1997) Calcium channel blockers for hypertension. Dissecting the evidence for adverse events. Am J Hypertens 10:565–577

Owada K (2004) Efficacy of candesartan in the treatment of migraine in hypertensive patients. Hypertens Res 27:441–446

Pascual J, Berciano J (1994) Experience in the diagnosis of headaches that start in elderly people. J Neurol Neurosurg Psychiatry 57:1255–1257

Peck RW, Seaber EJ, Dixon RM, Layton GR, Weatherley BC, Jackson SH, Rolan PE, Posner J (1998) The pharmacodynamics and pharmacokinetics of the 5HT1B/1D-agonist zolmitriptan in healthy young and elderly men and women. Clin Pharmacol Ther 63:342–453

Prencipe M, Casini AR, Ferretti C, Santini M, Pezzella F, Scaldaferri N, Culasso F (2001) Prevalence of headache in an elderly population: attack frequency, disability, and use of medication. J Neurol Neurosurg Psychiatry 70:377–381

Punay NC, Couch JR (2003) Antidepressants in the treatment of migraine headache. Curr Pain Headache Rep 7:51–54

Rasmussen BK, Lipton RB (2006) Prognosis of migraines. In: Olesen J, Goadsby PJ, Ramadan NM, Tfelt-Hansen P, Welch KMA (eds) The headaches, 3rd edn. Lippincott Williams & Wilkins, Philadelphia, pp 429–431

Rasmussen BK, Jensen R, Schroll M, Olesen J (1991) Epidemiology of headache in a general population: a prevalence study. J Clin Epidemiol 44:1147–1157

Reid MC, Engles-Horton LL, Weber MB, Kerns RD, Rogers EL, O'Connor PG (2002) Use of opioid medications for chronic noncancer pain syndromes in primary care. J Gen Intern Med 17:173–179

Richy F, Bruyere O, Ethgen O, Rabenda V, Bouvenot G, Audran M, Herrero-Beaumont G, Moore A, Eliakim R, Haim M, Reginster JY (2004) Time dependent risk of gastrointestinal complications induced by non-steroidal anti-inflammatory drug use: a consensus statement using a meta-analytic approach. Ann Rheum Dis 63:759–766

Rosenberg JH, Silberstein SD (2005) The headache of SAH responds to sumatriptan. Headache 45:597–598

Rostom A, Dube C, Wells G, Tugwell P, Welch V, Jolicoeur E, McGowan J (2002) Prevention of NSAID-induced gastroduodenal ulcers. Cochrane Database Syst Rev CD0022960

Rowbotham M, Harden N, Stacey B, Bernstein P, Magnus-Miller L (1998) Gabapentin for the treatment of postherpetic neuralgia: a randomized controlled trial. JAMA 280:1837–1842

Santiago TV, Edelman NH (1985) Opioids and breathing. J Appl Physiol 59:1675–1685

Scher AI, Stewart WF, Ricci JA, Lipton RB (2003) Factors associated with the onset and remission of chronic daily headache in a population-based study. Pain 106:81–89

Scher AI, Stewart WF, Lipton RB (2004) Caffeine as a risk factor for chronic daily headache: a population-based study. Neurology 63:2022–2027

Schrader H, Stovner LJ, Helde G, Sand T, Bovim G (2001) Prophylactic treatment of migraine with angiotensin converting enzyme inhibitor (lisinopril): randomized, placebo controlled, crossover study. BMJ 322:1–5

Schuh-Hofer S, Flach U, Meisel A, Israel H, Reuter U, Arnold G (2007) Efficacy of lisinopril in migraine prophylaxis—an open label study. Eur J Neurol 14:701–703

Schwaiger J, Kiechl S, Seppi K, Sawires M, Stockner H, Erlacher T, Mairhofer ML, Niederkofler H, Rungger G, Gasperi A, Poewe W, Willeit J (2002) Prevalence of primary headaches and cranial neuralgias in men and women aged 55–94 years (Bruneck Study). Cephalalgia 29:179–187

Schwartz JB (1996) Calcium antagonists in the elderly. A risk–benefit analysis. Drugs Aging 9:24–36

Setakis E, Leufkens HG, van Staa TP (2008) Changes in the characteristics of patients prescribed selective cyclooxygenase-2 inhibitors after the 2004 withdrawal of rofecoxib. Arthritis Rheum 59:1105–1111

Silberstein SD, McCrory DC (2003) Ergotamine and dihydroergotamine: history, pharmacology, and efficacy. Headache 43:144–166

Silberstein S, Tepper S, Brandes J, Diamond M, Goldstein J, Winner P, Venkatraman S, Vrijens F, Malbecq W, Lines C, Visser WH, Reines S, Yuen E (2004) Randomized, placebo-controlled trial of rofecoxib in the acute treatment of migraine. Neurology 62:1552–1557

Singh G, Fort JG, Goldstein JL, Levy RA, Hanrahan PS, Bello AE, Andrade-Ortega L, Wallemark C, Agrawal NM, Eisen GM, Stenson WF, Triadafilopoulos G, SUCCESS-I Investigators (2006a) Celecoxib versus naproxen and diclofenac in osteoarthritis patients: SUCCESS-I Study. Am J Med 119:255–266

Singh G, Wu O, Langhorne P, Madhok R (2006b) Risk of acute myocardial infarction with nonselective non-steroidal anti-inflammatory drugs: a meta-analysis. Arthritis Res Ther 8:R153

Spiegel BM, Farid M, Dulai GS, Gralnek IM, Kanwal F (2006) Comparing rates of dyspepsia with Coxibs vs NSAID + PPI: a meta-analysis. Am J Med 119: 448e427–448e436

Stewart WF, Lipton RB, Celentano DD, Reed ML (1992) Prevalence of migraine headache in the United States. J Am Med Assoc 267:64–69

Tfelt-Hansen P, Olesen J, Aebelholt-Krabbe A, Melgaard B, Veilis B (1980) A double blind study of metoclopramide in the treatment of migraine attacks. J Neurol Neurosurg Psychiatry 43:369–371

Tfelt-Hansen P, Henry P, Mulder LJ, Scheldewaert RG, Schoenen J, Chazot G (1995) The effectiveness of combined oral lysine acetylsalicylate and metoclopramide compared with oral sumatriptan for migraine. Lancet 346:923–926

Tfelt-Hansen P, Saxena PR, Dahlöf C, Pascual J, Láinez M, Henry P, Diener H, Schoenen J, Ferrari MD, Goadsby PJ (2000) Ergotamine in the acute treatment of migraine. A review and European consensus. Brain 123:9–18

Touchon J, Bertin L, Pilgrim AJ, Ashford E, Bes A (1996) A comparison of subcutaneous sumatriptan and dihydroergotamine nasal spray in the acute treatment of migraine. Neurology 47:361–365

Tronvik E, Stovner LJ, Helde G, Sand T, Bovim G (2003) Prophylactic treatment of migraine with an angiotensin II receptor blocker. A randomized controlled trial. JAMA 289:65–69

Ward TM (2002) Headache disorders in the elderly. Curr Treat Options Neurol 4:403–408

Whelton A, Fort JG, Puma JA, Normandin D, Bello AE, Verburg KM, SUCCESS VI Study Group (2001) Cyclooxygenase-2–specific inhibitors and cardiorenal function: a randomized, controlled trial of celecoxib and rofecoxib in older hypertensive osteoarthritis patients. Am J Ther 8:85–95

Wiffen PJ, McQuay HJ, Edwards JE, Moore RA (2005) Gabapentin for acute and chronic pain. Cochrane Database Syst Rev CD005452

Zito G, Jull G, Story I (2006) Clinical tests of musculoskeletal dysfunction in the diagnosis of cervicogenic headache. Man Ther 11:118–129

Part 13

Medication and Headache

48 General Issues Arising from the Use of Drugs for Headache Disorders

Peer Carsten Tfelt-Hansen[1] · *Koen Paemeleire*[2]
[1]Glostrup Hospital, University of Copenhagen, Glostrup, Copenhagen, Denmark
[2]Ghent University Hospital, Ghent, Belgium

Paolo Martelletti, Timothy J. Steiner (eds.), *Handbook of Headache*, DOI 10.1007/978-88-470-1700-9_48,
© Lifting The Burden 2011

Abstract: The WHO's list of essential medicines for migraine only includes paracetamol, aspirin, ibuprofen, and propranolol at present. In the past few years, *Lifting The Burden* has been striving to include triptans as a group. It is a clinical reality indeed that patients may not respond to analgesics and NSAIDs, but may be triptan-responders. The benefit-to-tolerability ratio of triptans favors oral triptans in acute migraine treatment, but we illustrate why subcutaneous sumatriptan is the triptan of choice in acute cluster headache treatment. The individual response to prophylactic treatment is quite variable, based on individual pharmacokinetic and pharmacodynamic differences. Tailoring of drugs to patients is important in clinical practice. Barriers to optimal drug treatment of headache disorders include undertreatment and mismanagement, despite existing guidelines. Medication-overuse headache has been described in a number of headache disorders, but is most commonly encountered in migraine patients.

Established Knowledge

The treatment of headaches begins with making a diagnosis, explaining it to the patient, and developing a treatment plan taking into account the severity and frequency of the headache. Headache is most often a very painful and bothersome disorder in which drug treatment is needed acutely. In addition, when migraine, cluster headache, and tension-type headache are occurring frequently, preventive daily intake of a drug may be needed.

Acute drugs for migraine are specific drugs, such as triptans and ergot alkaloids, and nonspecific drugs such as paracetamol, aspirin, and other NSAIDs. For acute treatment of cluster headache, only quickly absorbed triptans are effective. Tension-type headaches are treated acutely with analgesics. Triptans are not effective in episodic tension-type headache (Brennum et al. 1996).

For prophylaxis of migraine several types of drugs can be used, including β-blockers, antiepileptics, and calcium channel blockers (Steiner et al. 2007). Only one drug, methysergide, was designed for migraine prophylaxis and it is rarely used because of risk of severe side effects. The prophylactic drug of first choice in cluster headache is verapamil. In frequent and chronic tension-type headache, tricyclic antidepressant drugs are used.

Worldwide, the use of drugs is heavily dependent on the WHO's list of essential drugs and this list will be discussed. Cost is still an important factor, especially with the triptans for which the patent has not expired. With all acute drugs for headache, there is the risk for overuse with resulting daily headache (see ❯ Chap. 50). Headache disorders are often chronic disorders wherefore tolerability and safety are important issues.

WHO's Essential Medicines List for Migraine

The WHO List of Essential Medicines (revised March 2010) is shown in ❯ *Table 48.1* with respect to migraine. *Lifting The Burden,* The Global Campaign to Reduce the Burden of Headache Worldwide, has in the last years argued that triptans as a group should be included in the list for migraine. WHO has, however, argued that as long as triptans have not been demonstrated to be superior to aspirin there is no need for adding the triptans to the list. Thus a meta-analysis of three randomized clinical trials (RCTs) provided evidence that effervescent aspirin 1,000 mg is as effective as sumatriptan 50 mg for the acute treatment of migraine attacks, and that both are superior to placebo (Lampl et al. 2007). This is illustrated by the

☐ Table 48.1

WHO's essential medicines list for migraine (16th edition, revised March 2010) (From http://www. who.int/medicines/publications/essentialmedicines/en/index.html)

7 Antimigraine medicines	
7.1 For treatment of acute attack	
Acetylsalicylic acid	Tablet: 300–500 mg
Ibuprofen [c]	Tablet: 200 mg; 400 mg
Paracetamol	Oral liquid: 125 mg/5 ml [c]
	Tablet 300–500 mg
7.2 For prophylaxis	
Propranolol	Tablet: 20 mg; 40 mg (hydrochloride)

[c] signifies that there is a specific indication for restricting its use to children

meta-analysis results for pain relief at 2 h, defined as a decrease in headache from moderate or severe to none or mild after 2 h, amounting to 52% (95% CI: 47–57%) for effervescent aspirin 1,000 mg, which is quite comparable to sumatriptan 50 mg (47%, 95% CI: 40–52%), and both are significantly superior to placebo (34%, 95% CI: 29–39%). These results seemingly demonstrate that the two groups of drugs, triptans and NSAIDs, are equivalent in migraine treatment (Lampl et al. 2007). Comparisons of oral triptans with other classes of acute treatments are few, and in general differences between active treatments on the primary endpoints were not dramatic (Lipton et al. 2004). Nevertheless, these data have been questioned as there is a discrepancy with experience in clinical practice (Lipton et al. 2004). We are as clinicians confronted everyday with migraine patients that do not respond to analgesics or NSAIDs. There is thus the need for more migraine-specific drugs such as triptans or ergot alkaloids. Regardless of this, a drug like effervescent aspirin should be the drug of first choice in migraine, but triptans or ergot alkaloids should be available for those patients unresponsive to aspirin. For most migraine sufferers requiring a specific antimigraine treatment, a triptan is generally a better option from both an efficacy and side-effect perspective (Tfelt-Hansen et al. 2000a).

The recommended doses of 20 mg and 40 mg for propranolol are not in agreement with the literature on migraine prophylaxis with propranolol in randomized clinical trials (RCTs) (Tfelt-Hansen and Rolan 2006). The most commonly used dose of propranolol in these RCTs is 160 mg per day and the WHO list should be changed to propranolol 40 mg and 80 mg.

Headache in general, and migraine in specific, are probably the stepchild in pain management. The use of drugs in headache and migraine should be evidence-based. "Evidence-based medicine is the conscientious, explicit, and judicious use of current best evidence in making decisions about the care of individual patients." "The practice of evidence-based medicine means integrating individual clinical expertise with the best available external clinical evidence from systematic research" (Sackett et al. 1996). Evidence-based medicine is more than just meta-analyses of drugs and procedures. WHO seemingly does not understand the second part of evidence-based medicine: the integration of individual clinical expertise into the decision. What do you do when you have a migraine patient who has unsuccessfully tried aspirin for three migraine attacks? As shown in the meta-analysis even with the optimal aspirin, effervescent aspirin 1,000 mg, 50% of the patients do not respond with headache relief and 70% are not pain free after 2 h (Lampl et al. 2007). Most patients with headache worldwide self-medicate for migraine, using aspirin and paracetamol and thus following the WHO recommendations. In some countries, a few triptans are over-the-counter drugs (Tfelt-Hansen and Steiner 2007). Triptans are currently, however, only used by 10–15% of migraine patients in Denmark and the UK (Tfelt-Hansen and Steiner 2007).

Benefit-to-Tolerability Ratio for Specific Migraine Drugs

The best available evidence comes from systematic reviews (or meta-analyses) of RCTs. In migraine there are several meta-analyses, mostly on triptans (Tfelt-Hansen et al. 2000b; Ferrari et al. 2001; McCrory and Gray 2003; Pascual 2004; Saxena and Tfelt-Hansen 2006). The efficacy is most often well described in RCTs whereas adverse events are currently reported in different ways. This makes comparison of tolerability in systematic reviews problematic. A practical example on the choice between the two administration forms of sumatriptan, oral and subcutaneous, plus the choice in cluster headache, is given in ❷ *Table 48.2*. As is shown subcutaneous sumatriptan 6 mg is both more effective and causes more adverse events than the oral form of sumatriptan 100 mg. Subcutaneous sumatriptan is also more quickly effective (relevant effect after 20 min) than oral sumatriptan (relevant effect after 60 min) (Saxena and Tfelt-Hansen 2006). Apparently, the simple benefit/tolerability is better for oral sumatriptan (32%/16% = 2) than subcutaneous sumatriptan (51%/33% = 1.5) but clinical treatment is not that simple. Most patients prefer the oral route of administration. The price of subcutaneous sumatriptan 6 mg is very high, 37 € versus 1 € for sumatriptan 50 mg (current prices in Denmark). In cluster headache the situation is different. The attack is very severe but short-lasting. So the treatment should work quickly with a high response rate. Even if intranasal sumatriptan 20 mg and zolmitriptan 5 mg are statistically superior to placebo, it is only subcutaneous sumatriptan 6 mg that has an early clinically relevant effect (❷ *Table 48.2*).

In prophylaxis of migraine, adverse events are in our experience the most frequent reasons for stopping the treatment. One should be aware of the fact that drugs result in very variable plasma levels, often five- to tenfold differences among subjects. In addition, there is a pharmacodynamic variability (Tfelt-Hansen and Edvinsson 2007). This variability is especially important in migraine prophylaxis. The dictum should be "start low, go slow." Usually we start out with ¼–½ of the dose used in RCTs and then slowly over weeks to months increase the dose depending on efficacy and tolerability. Such a tailoring of the drug to the individual patients can usually not be done in RCTs.

These examples hopefully illustrate that the benefit-to-tolerability ratio is content dependent and it is the responsibility of the physician to try optimizing the treatment of the individual patient.

Barriers to Optimal Drug Choice in the Treatment of Headache Disorders

Underdiagnosis and diagnostic delay have been well documented in a number of headache disorders, including common syndromes such as migraine and cluster headache (Lipton et al. 2001; Bahra and Goadsby 2006). Even when a correct diagnosis has been made, undertreatment and mismanagement have been observed despite the existence of guidelines for clinical practice (May et al. 2006; Steiner et al. 2007; Evers et al. 2009). Patients may receive acute treatment, but no prevention (when indicated) and vice versa. Ineffective acute drugs or prophylactic drugs

◘ Table 48.2

A practical example of the choice between two administration forms of triptans based on the benefit-to-risk ratio

Data from randomized clinical trials (RCTs)	Data not evident from RCTs and personal clinical experiences
Sumatriptan 100 mg is superior to placebo in RCTs with a therapeutic gain (TG) of 32% (Tfelt-Hansen et al. 2000a). There are 16% (95% CI: 13–19%) more adverse events after sumatriptan than after placebo. Sumatriptan 100 mg begins to have a clinically relevant effect after 60 min with a maximum after 120 min	The plasma level of sumatriptan varies considerably (four- to tenfold) after oral administration. Most patients prefer the oral route of administration. Sumatriptan 6 mg SC is very costly (37 €) versus sumatriptan tablets 50 mg (1 €)
Sumatriptan 6 mg subcutaneous (SC) has a TG of 51%. There are 33% (95% CI: 29–37%) more adverse events after sumatriptan 6 mg SC than after placebo. Sumatriptan 6 mg SC begins to have a clinically relevant effect after 20 min with a maximum effect after 60 min	
Migraine	
Efficacy-to-tolerability ratio: Both oral (TG: 32%) and SC sumatriptan (TG: 51%) are effective. Sumatriptan 6 mg SC causes more adverse events than oral sumatriptan (33% versus 16% more than placebo)	Because of the more frequent adverse events after sumatriptan 6 mg SC the oral form has clinically the best efficacy-to-tolerability ratio in migraine. The oral form is also much cheaper (1 € versus 30 €). If very quick effect is needed sumatriptan 6 mg SC is better than the oral form
Cluster headache	
Sumatriptan 6 mg SC is effective in cluster headache: within 15 min 74% of sumatriptan-treated attacks responded (no or mild headache) versus 26% of placebo-treated attacks. After nasal sumatriptan 20 mg 57% responded after 30 min versus 26% after placebo. Nasal zolmitriptan 5 mg resulted in 48% response after 30 min versus 19% response after placebo	Given the short duration and severity of attacks, rapidity of action is a crucial factor. Sumatriptan 6 mg SC has quicker onset of action and is more effective than the nasal triptans. SC sumatriptan is generally the drug of first choice

may have been proposed to patients. The proportion of IHS-defined migraineurs using only over-the-counter medications to treat their headaches was 57% in the American Migraine Study II (Lipton et al. 2001). There was a clear underuse of migraine prevention in the American Migraine Prevalence and Prevention study (Diamond et al. 2007). A significant fraction of cluster headache patients never have had access to SC sumatriptan or high-flow oxygen, both first-line acute treatments according to current recommendations (May et al. 2006; Van Alboom et al. 2009). Cluster headache patients may receive ineffective prophylactic drugs such as propranolol, carbamazepine, or amitriptyline (Van Alboom et al. 2009). Medication-overuse headache is a major public health concern and affects 0.7–1.7% of the population (Evers and Marziniak 2010). Medication-overuse headache has been described in a variety of headache disorders including tension-type headache, migraine and cluster headache (Diener and Limmroth 2004; Paemeleire et al. 2006). In principle, all acute drugs for the treatment of headache could cause MOH (Evers and Marziniak 2010).

Appropriate treatment may have been advised, but patients may lapse from care (Edmeads 2006). It is however important that resources are available to guarantee adequate follow-up of patients to ensure that optimum treatment has been established (Steiner et al. 2007). Stepped care guidelines are available in acute migraine treatment (Steiner et al. 2007), and we have made the case for triptans in nonresponders to NSAIDs in acute migraine.

References

Bahra A, Goadsby PJ (2006) Diagnostic delays and mismanagement in cluster headache. Acta Neurol Scand 109:175–179

Brennum J, Brinck T, Schriver L, Wanscher B, Soelberg Sørensen P, Tfelt-hansen P, Olesen J (1996) Sumatriptan has no clinically relevant effect in the treatment of episodic tension-type headache. Eur J Neurol 3:23–28

Diamond S, Bigal ME, Silberstein S, Loder E, Reed M, Lipton RB (2007) Patterns of diagnosis and acute and preventive treatment for migraine in the United States: results from the American migraine prevalence and prevention study. Headache 47:355–363

Diener HC, Limmroth V (2004) Medication-overuse headache: a worldwide problem. Lancet Neurol 3:475–483

Edmeads J (2006) Understanding the needs of migraine patients. Drugs 66(Suppl 3):1–8

Evers S, Marziniak M (2010) Clinical features, pathophysiology, and treatment of medication-overuse headache. Lancet Neurol 9:391–401

Evers S, Afra J, Frese A, Goadsby PJ, Linde M, May A, Sandor P (2009) EFNS guideline on the drug treatment of migraine–revised report of an EFNS task force. Eur J Neurol 16:968–981

Ferrari MD, Roon KI, Lipton RB, Goadsby PJ (2001) Oral triptans (serotonin 5-HT(1B/1D) agonists) in acute migraine treatment: a meta-analysis of 53 trials. Lancet 358:1668–1675

Lampl C, Voelker M, Diener HC (2007) Efficacy and safety of 1, 000 mg effervescent aspirin: individual patient data meta-analysis of three trials in migraine headache and migraine accompanying symptoms. J Neurol 254:705–712

Lipton RB, Diamond S, Reed M, Diamond ML, Stewart WF (2001) Migraine diagnosis and treatment: results from the American migraine study II. Headache 41:638–645

Lipton RB, Bigal ME, Goadsby PJ (2004) Double-blind clinical trials of oral triptans vs other classes of acute migraine medication – a review. Cephalalgia 24:321–332

May A, Leone M, Afra J, Linde M, Sandor PS, Evers S, Goadsby PJ (2006) EFNS guidelines on the treatment of cluster headache and other trigeminal-autonomic cephalalgias. Eur J Neurol 13:1066–1077

McCrory DC, Gray RN (2003) Oral sumatriptan for acute migraine. Cochrane Database Syst Rev (3): CD002915

Paemeleire K, Bahra A, Evers S, Matharu MS, Goadsby PJ (2006) Medication-overuse headache in patients with cluster headache. Neurology 67:109–113

Pascual J (2004) A review of rizatriptan, a quick and consistent 5-HT1B/1D agonist for the acute treatment of migraine. Expert Opin Pharmacother 5:669–677

Sackett DL, Rosenberg WM, Gray JA, Haynes RB, Richardson WS (1996) Evidence based medicine: what it is and what it isn't. Brit Med J 312:71–72

Saxena PR, Tfelt-Hansen P (2006) Triptans, 5HT1B/1D agonists in the acute treatment of migraine. In: Olesen J, Goadsby PJ, Ramadan NM, Tfelt-Hansen P, Welch KMA (eds) The Headaches, 3rd edn. Lippincott Williams & Wilkins, Philadelphia, pp 469–503

Steiner TJ, Paemeleire K, Jensen R, Valade D, Savi L, Lainez MJ, Diener HC, Martelletti P, Couturier EG (2007) European principles of management of common headache disorders in primary care. J Headache Pain 8(Suppl 1):S3–S47

Tfelt-Hansen P, Edvinsson L (2007) Pharmacokinetic and pharmacodynamic variability as possible causes for different drug responses in migraine. A comment. Cephalalgia 27:1091–1093

Tfelt-Hansen P, Rolan P (2006) Beta-adrenoceptor blocking drugs in migraine prophylaxis. In: Olesen J, Goadsby PJ, Ramadan NM, Tfelt-Hansen P, Welch KMA (eds) The Headaches, 3rd edn. Lippincott Williams & Wilkins, Philadelphia, pp 519–528

Tfelt-Hansen P, Steiner TJ (2007) Over-the-counter triptans for migraine: what are the implications? CNS Drugs 21:877–883

Tfelt-Hansen P, De Vries P, Saxena PR (2000a) Triptans in migraine: a comparative review of pharmacology, pharmacokinetics and efficacy. Drugs 60:1259–1287

Tfelt-Hansen P, Saxena PR, Dahlof C, Pascual J, Lainez M, Henry P, Diener HC, Schoenen J, Ferrari MD, Goadsby PJ (2000b) Ergotamine in the acute treatment of migraine: a review and European consensus. Brain 123(Pt 1):9–18

Van Alboom E, Louis P, Van Zandijcke M, Crevits L, Vakaet A, Paemeleire K (2009) Diagnostic and therapeutic trajectory of cluster headache patients in Flanders. Acta Neurol Belg 109:10–17

49 Hormonal Contraception and Hormone Replacement Therapy in People with Headache

E. Anne MacGregor[1] · *Astrid Gendolla*[2]
[1]The City of London Migraine Clinic, London, UK
[2]Regionales Schmerzzentrum Essen, Essen, Germany

Paolo Martelletti, Timothy J. Steiner (eds.), *Handbook of Headache*, DOI 10.1007/978-88-470-1700-9_49,
© Lifting The Burden 2011

Abstract: The International Headache Society (IHS) classifies estrogen-withdrawal headache and exogenous hormone-induced headache. These events can occur as a result of use of hormonal contraceptives and hormone replacement therapy (HRT). Hormonal contraception, particularly combined hormonal contraceptives, is a popular and effective method, with additional non-contraceptive benefits. Combined hormonal contraceptives (CHCs) typically contain synthetic ethinylestradiol. This is more potent than natural estrogen and, coupled with progestogen, inhibits ovulation, thus providing contraceptive efficacy. For many women, migraine improves or they report change in migraine frequency or severity. Migraine without aura during the hormone-free interval is often the result of estrogen "withdrawal." This can be treated with extended cycle or continuous combined hormonal contraceptives. Migraine with aura is an independent risk factor for ischemic stroke. Additional risk factors, including use of CHCs, further increase risk although the absolute risk of ischemic stroke in young women is low. Several progestogen-only and nonhormonal methods are more effective contraceptive options and are not associated with increased risk of ischemic stroke. On this basis, most authorities consider migraine with aura to be a contraindication to use of CHCs.

Hormone replacement therapy (HRT), although declining in popularity following uncertainty regarding long-term risk versus benefit, is the most effective treatment for moderate-to-severe vasomotor symptoms associated with menopause. HRT uses natural estrogens to supplement or replace ovarian estrogen at levels compatible with mean levels across the menstrual cycle. Doses are usually insufficient to suppress the natural ovarian cycle but sufficiently stabilize the perimenopausal fluctuations that are associated with vasomotor symptoms. Migraine aura is not a contraindication to use of HRT, as HRT does not appear to increase ischemic stroke risk if used for short-term treatment of vasomotor symptoms during the perimenopause. However, current use of HRT has an adverse effect on migraine frequency. Non-oral routes are recommended for women with migraine as these are less likely to have a negative effect on migraine than oral formulations. Further, continuous combined regimes appear to be better tolerated than cyclical combined HRT.

Established Knowledge

Most women require contraception at some stage during their reproductive years. Hormonal contraception, particularly combined hormonal contraceptives (CHC), is a popular and effective method, with additional non-contraceptive benefits (The American College of Obstetricians and Gynecologists 2010). Hormone replacement therapy (HRT), although declining in popularity following uncertainty regarding long-term risk versus benefit, is the most effective treatment for moderate-to-severe perimenopausal vasomotor symptoms (North American Menopause Society 2004). Both combined hormonal contraceptives and HRT contain varying proportions of estrogen and progestogens. Combined hormonal contraceptives typically use synthetic ethinylestradiol. This is more potent than natural estrogen and, coupled with progestogen, inhibits ovulation, thus providing contraceptive efficacy. Oral methods are most widely used although transdermal patches, vaginal delivery, and injectable formulations are increasing in popularity. In contrast, HRT uses natural estrogens to supplement or replace ovarian estrogen at levels compatible with mean levels across the menstrual cycle. Doses are usually insufficient to suppress the natural ovarian cycle but sufficiently stabilize the perimenopausal fluctuations that are associated with vasomotor symptoms. Unless a woman has had a hysterectomy, progestogens are necessary to provide endometrial protection.

The International Headache Society (IHS) classifies estrogen-withdrawal headache and exogenous hormone-induced headache (❯ *Tables 49.1* and ❯ *49.2*) (Headache Classification Subcommittee of the International Headache Society (IHS) 2004). These events can occur as a result of use of hormonal contraceptives and HRT. It is important that prescribers and patients are aware of the potential effects of exogenous hormones on migraine.

Effect of Combined Hormonal Contraceptives on Headache

Studies assessing headache against baseline incidence are lacking as most record incidence only after starting contraception. Hence, the effect on headache and migraine incidence of initiating hormonal contraceptives is unclear. Studies reviewing headache over time suggest that exacerbation in the early cycles of use was followed by resolution with continued use (Brill et al. 1990; Ernst et al. 2002; Sluglett and Lawson 1967). Highest incidence of headache is during the hormone-free interval (LaGuardia et al. 2005; Sulak et al. 2000, 2007).

◻ Table 49.1

Diagnostic criteria for estrogen-withdrawal headache (Adapted from Headache Classification Subcommittee of the International Headache Society [IHS] 2004)

Diagnostic criteria
A. Headache or migraine fulfilling criteria C and D
B. Daily use of exogenous estrogen for ≥3 weeks, which is interrupted
C. Headache or migraine develops within 5 days after last use of estrogen
D. Headache or migraine resolves within 3 days

Comment: Estrogen-withdrawal following cessation of a course of exogenous estrogens (such as during the pill-free interval of combined oral contraceptives or following a course of replacement or supplementary estrogen) can induce headache and/or migraine

◻ Table 49.2

Diagnostic criteria for exogenous hormone-induced headache (Adapted from Headache Classification Subcommittee of the International Headache Society [IHS] 2004)

Diagnostic criteria
A. Headache or migraine fulfilling criteria C and D
B. Daily use of exogenous hormones
C. Headache or migraine develops or markedly worsens within 3 months of commencing exogenous hormones
D. Headache or migraine resolves or reverts to its previous pattern within 3 months after total discontinuation of exogenous hormones

Comment: Regular use of exogenous hormones, typically for contraception or hormone replacement therapy, can be associated with increase in frequency or new development of headache or migraine
When a woman also experiences headache or migraine associated with exogenous estrogen-withdrawal, both codes 8.3.1 *Exogenous hormone-induced headache* and 8.4.3 *Estrogen-withdrawal headache* should be used

Although data are limited, there appears to be a dose relationship between ethinylestradiol and headache, with lower risk associated with lower doses (Fotherby 1992, 1995). There are insufficient data to assess different progestogens on headache although most studies suggest little effect (Cullberg 1972; Dunson et al. 1993; Koetsawang et al. 1995).

Effect of Hormonal Contraceptives on Migraine

Combined Hormonal Contraceptives

There are few data on the low-dose CHCs, which contain $\leq$30 mcg ethinylestradiol; most studies to date have assessed the effect of high-dose combined oral contraceptives (COCs) containing at least 50-mcg ethinylestradiol. However, evidence suggests that women with preexisting migraine experience no change or even less frequent migraine (Cupini et al. 1995; Dalton 1976; Granella et al. 1993; Kudrow 1975; Larsson-Cohn and Lundberg 1970; Machado et al. 2010; Phillips 1968; Ryan 1978; Whitty et al. 1966). Although CHCs combine ethinylestradiol and progestogens, the effects of migraine appear largely related to ethinylestradiol. There are no data on risk of non-oral CHCs.

The prevalence of headache and migraine among women using COCs was examined in a large, cross-sectional population-based study in Norway of 13,944 women (Aegidius et al. 2006). There was a significant association between use of COCs and migraine (30-mcg ethinylestradiol OR 1.4, 95% CI 1.2–1.7, $p<0.001$). This study also assessed the effect of different progestogens on migraine (Machado et al. 2010). Compared to low-dose COCs containing second-generation progestogens (levonorgestrel), there was no correlation between improvement of deterioration in migraine and use of COCs containing third-generation progestogens (desogestrel or gestodene) or contraceptives containing cyproterone acetate or chlormadinone acetate. However, women taking COCs containing drospirenone reported significantly greater improvement in migraine frequency and/severity (OR 34.9, 95% CI 1.64–707.96).

The hormone-free interval of CHCs increases risk of migraine without aura (Horowski and Runge 1986; MacGregor and Hackshaw 2002; Machado et al. 2010; Phillips 1968; Ryan 1978; Sulak et al. 2000; Whitty et al. 1966). In a retrospective study on patients on COCs with unwanted withdrawal symptoms (35% reporting headache as a symptom), almost all side effects of COCs were found to be significantly worse during the 7-day hormone-free interval compared to the 21 days of pill-taking (Sulak et al. 2002). These effects of ethinylestradiol "withdrawal" are similar to the estrogen "withdrawal" mechanism associated with menstrual migraine (see ➋ Chap. 9) (MacGregor et al. 2006).

The outcome of migraine with aura is less favorable. A clinic based case-control study reviewed 39 women with migraine with aura and 83 women with migraine without aura who had used COCs (Granella et al. 2000). Migraine with aura was worsened in 56.4% of cases compared to 25.3% of women with migraine without aura (OR 3.8, 95% CI 1.6–9.3). There was no change in 38.5% of women with migraine with aura compared to 67.5% of women with migraine without aura (OR 0.3, 95% CI 0.1–0.7). Improvement was reported by 5.1% of women with migraine with aura compared to 7.2% of women with migraine without aura (OR 0.1–4.1).

Management of Migraine in the Hormone-Free Interval

Since estrogen "withdrawal" is the most likely mechanism of migraine during the hormone-free interval, supplementing estrogen during this time should be effective. Given the association between migraine without aura and withdrawal of ethinylestradiol, treatment strategies have focused on preventing the estrogen fall. A study using 0.05-mg estradiol patches during this time suggested that this dose is suboptimal for prophylaxis although posttrial treatment with 0.1-mg doses was effective (MacGregor and Hackshaw 2002).

In a small open-label study, 11 women with menstrual migraine were treated with a 28-day cycle of 0.02-mg ethinylestradiol oral contraceptive for 21 days followed by 0.9-mg conjugated equine estrogen daily for 7 days. All women achieved at least a 50% reduction in number of headache days per cycle (mean 77.9% reduction) (Calhoun 2004).

The "tricycle" regime, i.e., taking three packets without a break, using the lowest acceptable fixed dose formulation, has been used empirically and means that the woman has only five such migraines a year instead of 13 (MacGregor and Guillebaud 1998). Randomized trials of these extended regimens using oral and transdermal CHCs show evidence of reduced headache compared to standard 21/7 regimens (LaGuardia et al. 2005; Sulak et al. 2007). There is also increasing clinical experience of the benefits of continuous, rather than just extended CHCs. A Cochrane review reported that continuous-dosing group had greater improvement of menstrual-associated symptoms (headaches, genital irritation, tiredness, bloating, and menstrual pain) compared to the cyclical regimen (Edelman et al. 2006).

A trial of 102 women taking 3 mg of drospirenone and 0.03-mg ethinylestradiol continuously showed that, compared to the usual 21/7-day regimen of combined hormonal contraceptives, a 168-day extended placebo-free regimen led to a decrease in headache severity along with improvement in work productivity and involvement in activities (Sulak et al. 2007). Similarly, an extended 84-day regimen of a transdermal contraceptive reduced the total incidence of mean headache days compared to a 21/7-day regimen (LaGuardia et al. 2005).

Continuous combined hormonal contraceptives are safe and effective method of eliminating menstrual symptoms. They are well tolerated, although unscheduled bleeding is a common reason for withdrawal from clinical trials in the first 6-months of treatment. Continued use induces amenorrhea in 80–100% of women by 10–12 months of treatment (Archer 2006). Although there are no clinical trial data regarding migraine, women who wish to have regular withdrawal bleeds may benefit from licensed low-dose COCs with shortened hormone-free intervals, such as 24/4 and 26/2-day regimens.

Progestogen-Only Contraceptives

In contrast to the effects of contraceptives containing both ethinylestradiol and progestogen, progestogen-only pills appear to have minimal effect on migraine. A population-based study of 13,944 women identified no significant association between progestogen-only pills and migraine (OR 1.3, 95% CI 0.9–1.8, $p = 0.156$) (Aegidius et al. 2006). Oral progestogen-only methods that do not inhibit ovulation are often associated with a disrupted menstrual cycle, which may increase the risk of migraine (Chumnijaraki et al. 1984). In contrast, unlicensed higher doses of oral progestogen, sufficient to inhibit ovulation, have shown benefit (Davies et al. 2003).

There are no data regarding the effect on migraine of anovulatory progestogens such as the intramuscular depot medroxyprogesterone acetate, subdermal etonogestrel, and oral desogestrel.

Effect of Hormonal Contraceptives on Migraine with Aura

A review of 36 women with migraine with aura and 86 women with migraine without aura using COCs attending a headache clinic noted 50% of women with migraine with aura reported worsening of migraine with COC use compared to 34.8% of women with migraine without aura (Cupini et al. 1995). There was no change in 27.7% of women with migraine with aura compared to 44.1% of women with migraine without aura. Improvement was reported by 0% of women with migraine with aura compared to 4.6% of women with migraine without aura. New-onset migraine was reported by 22.2% of women with migraine with aura and 16.2% of women with migraine without aura. In both groups, worsening during COC intake was more likely than improvement ($P < 0.0001$).

A study of 80 women with migraine included 13 women with migraine with aura and 67 with migraine without aura (Machado et al. 2010). More women with migraine with aura reported worsening of migraine with COC use (69.2%) compared to women with migraine without aura (25.4%) (OR 4.76, 95%CI 0.97–26.24). There was no change in 23.1% of women with migraine with aura compared to 40.3% of women with migraine without aura. Improvement was reported by 7.7% of women with migraine with aura compared to 34.3% of women with migraine without aura. New-onset migraine occurred in 12 women, including 3 cases of new-onset aura.

Progestogen-only methods appear to have little, if any, effect on migraine with aura and are a useful alternative for women whose migraine is adversely affected by combined hormonal methods (Aegidius et al. 2006). Long-acting methods are more effective than combined hormonal contraceptives (World Health Organization 2009).

As discussed below, migraine with aura is an independent risk factor for ischemic stroke. This risk is increased by use of combined hormonal contraceptives. On this basis, combined hormonal contraceptives are contraindicated for use by women with migraine with aura. Progestogen-only contraceptives are not associated with increased risk and are an alternative contraceptive option for women with migraine. Practical implications of prescribing hormonal contraceptives to migraineurs are shown in ❯ *Box 49.1*.

Box 49.1 Practical Implications of Prescribing Hormonal Contraception in Women with Migraine

- Combined hormonal contraceptives combine synthetic estrogens with progestogens in doses sufficient to inhibit ovulation.
- Combined hormonal contraceptives are available as oral, percutaneous, intravaginal, and injectable routes.
- The majority of regimes are licensed for 21 consecutive days followed by a 7-day hormone-free interval during which a withdrawal "period" occurs.
- Migraine without aura is associated with the hormone-free interval as a consequence of estrogen "withdrawal" and can be treated with licensed or unlicensed extended regimes, or continuous combined hormonal contraception.

replacement therapy (Kaiser and Meienberg 1993). All six women developed increased headache severity and accompanying visual scintillations. One patient with no previous history of migraine developed visual scintillations with no accompanying headache. Withdrawal of estrogens and additional migraine prophylaxis led to marked improvement in all women, with complete cessation of migraine in four patients.

Case reports on four women developing migraine aura following initiation of HRT showed that, in all cases, aura resolved with either a reduction in estrogen dose or change in route of delivery of estrogen (aura with conjugated equine estrogens (CEE) 1.25 mg/estradiol gel 2.25 mg daily resolved with estradiol gel 1.5 mg daily; aura with 0.625 mg CEE/2 mg oral estradiol resolved with transdermal estradiol 50 mcg; aura with transdermal estradiol 100mcg resolved when HRT was discontinued) (MacGregor 1999a).

As discussed below, perimenopausal use of HRT is not associated with increased risk of ischemic stroke. On this basis, there is no reason to contraindicate use of HRT in women with migraine with aura. Practical implications of prescribing HRT to migraineurs are shown in ❯ Box 49.2.

Box 49.2 Practical Implications of Prescribing Hormone Replacement Therapy in Women with Migraine

- HRT uses natural estrogens used continuously to provide serum estrogen levels equivalent to the average menstrual cycle.
- HRT estrogens are available in oral, percutanous, and subcutaneous preparations.
- HRT progestogens are available in oral, percutanous (combined with estrogen), and intrauterine preparations.
- Migraine with aura is a risk factor for ischemic stroke.
- Migraine aura is not a contraindication to use of HRT as HRT does not appear to increase ischemic stroke risk if used for short-term treatment of vasomotor symptoms during the perimenopause, i.e., a few years before and within 12 months of the final menstrual period.
- The lowest effective dose of non-oral estrogens necessary to control vasomotor symptoms is recommended.
- If aura starts for the first time after starting HRT, consider changing route of delivery (oral to patch, patch to gel) and/or reducing the estrogen dose.
- In women who have an intact uterus, progestogens are necessary for endometrial protection.
- Continuous progestogens are tolerated that cyclical progestogens.

Current Research

Effect of Migraine and Exogenous Hormones on Risk of Ischemic Stroke

Effect of Migraine

Case-control, cohort studies and meta-analyses indicate that migraine is an independent risk factor for ischemic stroke (Carolei et al. 1996; Etminan et al. 2005; Henrich and Horwitz 1989; Kurth et al. 2005, 2006, 2008; Lidegaard and Kreiner 2002; Nightingale and Farmer 2004; Schurks et al. 2009; Schwaag et al. 2003; Stang et al. 2005; Tzourio et al. 1993, 1995). The body of research implicates that increased risk is associated with migraine *with* aura, not migraine *without* aura (Bigal et al. 2010; Schurks et al. 2009). Risk is positively correlated with recent onset of aura and attack frequency (Donaghy et al. 2002; Kruit et al. 2004; Kurth et al. 2009; MacClellan et al. 2007).

There is some evidence that cardiovascular risk factors are more prevalent in migraineurs compared to controls, particularly high cholesterol and hypertension (Bigal et al. 2010; Scher et al. 2005). After adjusting for the presence of these risk factors, the association between migraine with aura and stroke risk remains. These findings are consistent with an increased risk of subclinical cerebellar infarcts evident on MRI (Kruit et al. 2004). Infarcts in the posterior circulation were related to the presence of aura and to attack frequency, independent of baseline risk factors.

Women aged over 45 years participating in the prospective cohort Women's Health Study were followed over 11.9 years (Kurth et al. 2006). At entry to the study, 3,577 women reported active migraine, of whom 1,418 (39.6%) reported migraine with aura. Only active migraine with aura, and not a past history, was a risk factor for ischemic cardiovascular disease. This association with ischemic stroke was significantly modified by age ($p=0.01$) with the highest association among women younger than 50 years (hazard ratio (HR) 6.16, [95% CI 2.34–16.21]).

Compared to women without migraine, women with migraine with aura in the group with the lowest Framingham risk score had a greater risk of ischemic stroke (age-adjusted HR 3.88 [95%CI 1.87–8.08]) than women with the highest Framingham risk score (HR 1.00 [95%CI 0.24–4.14]) (Kurth et al. 2008).

These findings suggest the possibility of a common genetic basis. Several studies have implicated the MTHFR genotype in migraine with aura, which is also associated with increased risk of ischemic stroke (Rubino et al. 2009; Scher et al. 2006). In women with migraine with aura who carried the TT genotype, the risk of ischemic stroke was substantially increased (multivariate adjusted RR 4.19 [95%CI 1.38–12.74] $p=0.01$) (Schurks et al. 2008).

The population-based study of 574 participants aged 55–94 years investigated the association between migraine and atherosclerosis (Schwaiger et al. 2008). Of 23 men and 88 women with a history of migraine, 36 had migraine with aura and 75 had migraine without aura. Atherosclerosis in the carotid and femoral arteries tended to be less pronounced in migraineurs compared with non-migraineurs particularly in the common carotid arteries ($p=0.009$ multivariate analysis). Migraineurs were also more likely to have a lifetime history of VTE ($p=0.02$ adjusted for age, sex, vascular risks, and HT) (Schwaiger et al. 2008). Notably, Factor V mutation affected more participants with migraine with aura compared with non-migraineurs (11.1% vs. 3.5%). Other studies have also implicated the role of coagulation abnormalities in migraine aura (Crassard et al. 2001; Moschiano et al. 2004). However, the evidence to date remains limited.

Effect of Hormonal Contraceptives

COC use is an independent risk factor for ischemic stroke with risk related to the dose of ethinylestradiol (❷ *Table 49.4*) (Carolei et al. 1996; Chang et al. 1999b; Collaborative Group for the Study of Stroke in Young Women 1975; Kemmeren et al. 2002; Lidegaard 1993, 1995; Lidegaard and Kreiner 2002; Nightingale and Farmer 2004; Petitti et al. 1996; Schwartz et al. 1998; Siritho et al. 2003; Tzourio et al. 1995; World Health Organization Collaborative Study of

◻ Table 49.4

Effect of ethinylestradiol dose on risk of ischemic stroke (Reproduced with permission from MacGregor 2007)

	Design	Sample size	Setting	Dose of ethinylestradiol (mcg)	Risk of ischemic stroke OR (95%CI)
Collaborative Group for the Study of Stroke in Young Women (1975)	Case-control	430 Cases 151 Controls	91 Hospitals in 12 US cities	≥50	4.9 (2.9–8.3)
Lidegaard (1993) and (1995)	Case-control	320 Cases 1,197 Controls	Denmark	50	2.9 (1.6–5.4)
				30–40	1.8 (1.1–2.9)
Lidegaard and Kreiner (2002)	Case-control	626 Cases 4,054 Controls	Denmark	50	4.5 (2.6–7.7)
				30–40	1.6 (1.3–2.0)
				20	1.7 (1.0–3.1)
Tzourio et al. (1995)	Case-control	72 Cases 173 Controls	France	All doses	3.1 (1.2–8.2)
				50	4.8
				30–40	2.7
				20	1.7
Carolei et al. (1996)	Case-control	308 Cases 591 Controls	Italy	All doses	1.3 (0.6–2.6)
Petitti et al. (1996)	Case-control	295 Cases 774 Controls	USA	<50	1.18 (0.54–2.59)
WHO Collaborative study (1996) (World Health Organization Collaborative Study of Cardiovascular Disease and Steroid Hormone Contraception 1996b)	Case-control	697 Cases 1,962 Controls	International	All doses (Europe)	2.24 (1.31–3.82)
				≥50	5.3 (2.56–11.0)
				<50	1.53 (0.71–3.31)
Schwartz et al. (1998)	Case-control	175 Cases 191 Controls	USA	<50	0.88 (0.44–1.76)
Chang et al. (1999) (Chang et al. 1999a)	Case-control	291 Cases 736 Controls	5 European centers	All doses	2.76 (1.01–7.55)
				≥50	7.95 (1.94–32.6)
				<50	1.19 (0.33–4.29)
Kemmeren et al. (2002)	Case-control	203 Cases 925 Controls	9 Dutch centers population based	All types	2.3 (1.6–3.3)
Siritho et al. (2003)	Case-control	234 Cases 234 Controls	4 Australian hospitals	≤50	1.76 (0.86–3.61)
Nightingale and Farmer (2004)	Case-control	190 Cases 1,129 Controls	UK General Practice Research Database	<50	2.30 (1.15–4.59)

Cardiovascular Disease and Steroid Hormone Contraception 1996b). A meta-analysis of 36 studies reported a relative risk of 2.74 (95% CI 2.24–3.35) for ischemic stroke in women using low-estrogen preparations (Chan et al. 2004). A separate meta-analysis of 16 studies reported an overall summary risk estimate for ischemic stroke among current COC users of 2.75 (95% CI 2.24–3.38) (Gillum et al. 2000). For low-dose COCs containing less than 50 mcg ethinylestradiol, the relative risk was 2.08 (95% CI 1.55–2.80). Risk remained elevated for low-estrogen preparations in population-based studies controlling for smoking and hypertension (RR 1.93, 95% CI 1.35–2.74). This would lead to an estimated 4.1 ischemic strokes per 100,000 healthy nonsmoking non-hypertensive women using COCs. Previously undiagnosed thrombophilia is a significant risk factor with risk of ischemic stroke in COC users being 13 times higher in women who are carriers of Factor V Leiden and 9 times higher in those who also have hyperhomocysteinemia (Martinelli et al. 2006).

Progestogen-only contraception is not associated with an increased risk of ischemic stroke (Heinemann et al. 1999; Lidegaard and Kreiner 2002; Poulter et al. 1999; Tzourio et al. 1995; World Health Organization Collaborative Study of Cardiovascular Disease and Steroid Hormone Contraception 1996a). The risk of ischemic stroke associated with different progestogens in COCs correlates with the dose of ethinylestradiol; there is little difference in risk associated with low-dose COCs containing second-generation progestogens (levonorgestrel and norethisterone), compared with third-generation progestogens (gestodene or desogestrel) (MacGregor 2007).

Prospective data do not support an association between migraine without aura in women of age and ischemic stroke; therefore, there is no indication to restrict use of CHCs in women with migraine without aura. In contrast, migraine with aura is an independent risk factor for ischemic stroke, although the absolute risk of ischemic stroke in young women is extremely low. The main issue is balancing risk against contraceptive efficacy. Effective contraception need not be compromised since progestogen-only and nonhormonal methods, several of which are more effective than CHCs, are not associated with increased risk (MacGregor 2007). On this basis, most authorities consider migraine with aura to be a contraindication to use of CHCs (American College of Obstetricians and Gynecologists 2006, Faculty of Sexual and Reproductive Healthcare 2009; World Health Organization 2009).

Effect of HRT

There has been much controversy regarding the risk versus benefit of HRT. The present consensus is that HRT started within 10 years of menopause to treat vasomotor symptoms does not appear to increase the risk of ischemic stroke. Risk is affected by type of estrogen and progestogen and route of delivery, with less adverse profiles associated with low-dose, non-oral routes. Limited evidence suggests that the association between migraine with aura and ischemic stroke is not statistically significantly modified by use of postmenopausal HRT. Hence migraine with aura is not a contraindication of HRT (Kurth et al. 2006). Although estrogen has favorable long-term effects on cardiovascular markers associated with reduced risk of atherosclerotic disease, it can have adverse effects on thrombotic parameters (Luyer et al. 2001; Mendelsohn 2002). The effect of HRT on migraine aura is likely to depend, at least in part, on whether any underlying mechanisms associated with aura are atherosclerotic or thrombotic. Since aura is most likely to be associated with thrombophilias rather than atherosclerotic conditions, there are benefits to non-oral estrogen replacement. Several RCTs show that transdermal estrogen has a less marked or even neutral effect on coagulation parameters compared to oral estrogen (Brosnan et al. 2007; Fait et al. 2008; Zegura et al. 2006). A dose response has also been noted (Eilertsen et al. 2006). This may account for the clinical benefits of reducing dose and route of delivery in women developing aura when starting HRT. If aura starts for the first time after starting HRT, a non-oral route should be used and the dose of estrogen should be reduced to the lowest dose necessary to control vasomotor symptoms.

Conclusions

Most women use contraception at some stage in their lives. Hormonal contraception, particularly combined hormonal contraceptives, is a popular and effective method, with additional non-contraceptive benefits. For many women, migraine improves or they report change in migraine frequency or severity. Migraine without aura during the hormone-free interval can be treated with extended cycle or continuous combined hormonal contraceptives. Migraine with aura is more likely to worsen or start de novo in association with combined hormonal contraceptive use. Of concern is that results of case-control, cohort studies and meta-analyses indicate that migraine with aura is an independent risk factor for ischemic stroke. These findings need to be viewed in the context of the low absolute risk of ischemic stroke in young women. Additional risk factors, including use of CHCs, further increase risk. On this basis, most authorities consider migraine with aura to be a contraindication to use of CHCs. Effective contraception need not be compromised since progestogen-only and nonhormonal methods, several of which are more effective than CHCs, are not associated with increased risk.

The years directly preceding menopause are marked by vasomotor symptoms and irregular menstrual cycles. Headache is a common but underreported complaint during this time. Management should be directed to treating the menopausal symptoms, which may include hormone replacement therapy. Studies suggest a significant association between migraine and current use of HRT. An understanding of the effects of different types of HRT is important as some studies suggest that a history of worsening migraine at menopause is a factor in predicting worsening migraine with HRT. However, the regime of HRT, route of estrogen, and type of progestogen may all have a significant impact on migraine. Physicians treating the menopause should be aware that non-oral routes are less likely to have a negative effect on migraine than oral formulations of estrogen replacement and continuous combined appears to be better tolerated than cyclical combined HRT. Migraine aura is not a contraindication to use of HRT, as HRT does not appear to increase ischemic stroke risk if used for short-term treatment of vasomotor symptoms during the perimenopause.

References

Aegidius K, Zwart JA, Hagen K, Schei B, Stovner LJ (2006) Oral contraceptives and increased headache prevalence: the Head-HUNT study. Neurology 66:349–353

Aegidius KL, Zwart JA, Hagen K, Schei B, Stovner LJ (2007) Hormone replacement therapy and headache prevalence in postmenopausal women. The Head-HUNT study. Eur J Neurol 14:73–78

American College of Obstetricians and Gynecologists (2006) ACOG practice bulletin. No. 73: use of hormonal contraception in women with coexisting medical conditions. Obstet Gynecol 107: 1453–1472

Archer DF (2006) Menstrual-cycle-related symptoms: a review of the rationale for continuous use of oral contraceptives. Contraception 74:359–366

Berendsen HH (2000) The role of serotonin in hot flushes. Maturitas 36:155–164

Bigal M, Kurth T, Santanello N, Buse D, Golden W, Robbins M, Lipton R (2010) Migraine and cardiovascular disease: a population-based study. Neurology 74:628–635

Brill K, Schnitker J, Albring M (1990) Long-term experience with a low-dose oral contraceptive. Gynecol Endocrinol 4:277–286

Brosnan JF, Sheppard BL, Norris LA (2007) Haemostatic activation in post-menopausal women taking low-dose hormone therapy: less effect with transdermal administration? Thromb Haemost 97:558–565

Calhoun AH (2004) A novel specific prophylaxis for menstrual-associated migraine. South Med J 97:819–822

Carolei A, Marini C, De Matteis G (1996) History of migraine and risk of cerebral ischaemia in young adults. The Italian National Research Council study group on stroke in the young. Lancet 347:1503–1506

Chan WS, Ray J, Wai EK, Ginsburg S, Hannah ME, Corey PN, Ginsberg JS (2004) Risk of stroke in women exposed to low-dose oral contraceptives: a critical evaluation of the evidence. Arch Intern Med 164:741–747

Chang C, Donaghy M, Poulter N, World Health Organisation Collaboration Study of Cardiovascular Disease and Steroid Hormone Contraception (1999a) Migraine and stroke in young women: case-control study. Br Med J 318:13–18

Chang CL, Donaghy M, Poulter N (1999b) Migraine and stroke in young women: case-control study. The World Health Organisation Collaborative Study of Cardiovascular Disease and Steroid Hormone Contraception. Br Med J 318:13–18

Chumnijaraki T, Sunyavivat S, Onthuam Y, Udomprasetgurl V (1984) Study on the factors associated with contraception discontinuation in Bangkok. Contraception 29:241–248

Collaborative Group for the Study of Stroke in Young Women (1975) Oral contraceptives and stroke in young women. Associated risk factors. JAMA 231:718–722

Crassard I, Conard J, Bousser MG (2001) Migraine and haemostasis. Cephalalgia 21:630–636

Cullberg J (1972) Mood changes and menstrual symptoms with different gestagen/estrogen combinations. A double blind comparison with a placebo. Acta Psychiatr Scand Suppl 236:1–86

Cupini LM, Matteis M, Troisi E, Calabresi P, Bernardi G, Silvestrini M (1995) Sex-hormone-related events in migrainous females. A clinical comparative study between migraine with aura and migraine without aura. Cephalalgia 15:140–144

Dalton K (1976) Migraine and oral contraceptives. Headache 15:247–251

Davies P, Fursdon-Davies C, Rees MC (2003) Progestogens for menstrual migraine. J Br Menopause Soc 9:134

Donaghy M, Chang CL, Poulter N, on behalf of the European Collaborators of the World Health Organisation Collaborative Study of Cardiovascular Disease and Steroid Hormone Contraception (2002) Duration, frequency, recency, and type of migraine and risk of ischaemic stroke in women of childbearing age. J Neurol Neurosurg Psychiat 73:747–750

Dunson TR, McLaurin VL, Israngkura B, Leelapattana B, Mukherjee R, Perez-Palacios G, Saleh AA (1993) A comparative study of two low-dose combined oral contraceptives: results from a multicenter trial. Contraception 48:109–119

Edelman A, Gallo MF, Nichols MD, Jensen JT, Schulz KF, Grimes DA (2006) Continuous versus cyclic use of combined oral contraceptives for contraception: systematic Cochrane review of randomized controlled trials. Hum Reprod 21:573–578

Eilertsen AL, Qvigstad E, Andersen TO, Sandvik L, Sandset PM (2006) Conventional-dose hormone therapy (HT) and tibolone, but not low-dose HT and raloxifene, increase markers of activated coagulation. Maturitas 55:278–287

Ernst U, Baumgartner L, Bauer U, Janssen G (2002) Improvement of quality of life in women using a low-dose desogestrel-containing contraceptive: results of an observational clinical evaluation. Eur J Contracept Reprod Health Care 7:238–243

Etminan M, Takkouche B, Isorna FC, Samii A (2005) Risk of ischaemic stroke in people with migraine: systematic review and meta-analysis of observational studies. Br Med J 330:63–65

Facchinetti F, Nappi RE, Tirelli A, Polatti F, Nappi G, Sances G (2002) Hormone supplementation differently affects migraine in postmenopausal women. Headache 42:924–929

Faculty of Sexual and Reproductive Healthcare (2009) UK Medical Eligibility Criteria for Contraceptive Use (UKMEC 2009). http://www.fsrh.org

Fait T, Vrablik M, Zizka Z, Kostirova M (2008) Changes in hemostatic variables induced by estrogen replacement therapy: comparison of transdermal and oral administration in a crossover-designed study. Gynecol Obstet Invest 65:47–51

Fotherby K (1992) Clinical experience and pharmacological effects of an oral contraceptive containing 20 micrograms oestrogen. Contraception 46:477–488

Fotherby K (1995) Twelve years of clinical experience with an oral contraceptive containing 30 micrograms ethinyloestradiol and 150 micrograms desogestrel. Contraception 51:3–12

Gillum LA, Mamidipudi SK, Johnston SC (2000) Ischemic stroke risk with oral contraceptives: a meta-analysis. JAMA 284:72–78

Granella F, Sances G, Zanferrari C, Costa A, Martignoni E, Manzoni GC (1993) Migraine without aura and reproductive life events: a clinical epidemiological study in 1,300 women. Headache 33:385–389

Granella F, Sances G, Pucci E, Nappi RE, Ghiotto N, Napp G (2000) Migraine with aura and reproductive life events: a case control study. Cephalalgia 20:701–707

Headache Classification Subcommittee of the International Headache Society (IHS) (2004) The international classification of headache disorders (2nd edn). Cephalalgia 24:1–160

Heinemann LA, Assmann A, DoMinh T, Garbe E (1999) Oral progestogen-only contraceptives and cardiovascular risk: results from the Transnational study on oral contraceptives and the health of young women. Eur J Contracept Reprod Health Care 4:67–73

Henrich JB, Horwitz LA (1989) A controlled study of ischemic stroke risk in migraine patients. J Clin Epidemiol 42:773–780

Hodson J, Thompson J, al-Azzawi F (2000) Headache at menopause and in hormone replacement therapy users. Climacteric 3:119–124

Horowski R, Runge I (1986) Possible role of gonadal hormones as triggering factors in migraine. Funct Neurol 1:405–414

Kaiser HJ, Meienberg O (1993) Deterioration of onset of migraine under oestrogen replacement therapy in the menopause. J Neurol Neurosurg Psychiatry 240:195–197

Kemmeren JM, Tanis BC, van den Bosch MA, Bollen EL, Helmerhorst FM, van der Graaf Y, Rosendaal FR, Algra A (2002) Risk of Arterial Thrombosis in Relation to Oral Contraceptives (RATIO) study: oral contraceptives and the risk of ischemic stroke. Stroke 33:1202–1208

Koetsawang S, Charoenvisal C, Banharnsupawat L, Singhakovin S, Kaewsuk O, Punnahitanont S (1995) Multicenter trial of two monophasic oral contraceptives containing 30 mcg ethinylestradiol and either desogestrel or gestodene in Thai women. Contraception 51:225–229

Kruit MC, van Buchem MA, Hofman PAM, Bakkers JTN, Terwindt GM, Ferrari MD, Launer LJ (2004) Migraine as a risk factor for subclinical brain lesions. JAMA 291:427–434

Kudrow L (1975) The relationship of headache frequency to hormone use in migraine. Headache 15:36–40

Kurth T, Slomke MA, Kase CS, Cook NR, Lee IM, Gaziano JM, Diener HC, Buring JE (2005) Migraine, headache, and the risk of stroke in women: a prospective study. Neurology 64:1020–1026

Kurth T, Gaziano JM, Cook NR, Logroscino G, Diener H-C, Buring JE (2006) Migraine and risk of cardiovascular disease in women. JAMA 296:283–291

Kurth T, Schurks M, Logroscino G, Gaziano JM, Buring JE (2008) Migraine, vascular risk, and cardiovascular events in women: prospective cohort study. Br Med J 337:a636

Kurth T, Schurks M, Logroscino G, Buring JE (2009) Migraine frequency and risk of cardiovascular disease in women. Neurology 73:581–588

LaGuardia KD, Fisher AC, Bainbridge JD, LoCoco JM, Friedman AJ (2005) Suppression of estrogen-withdrawal headache with extended transdermal contraception. Fertil Steril 83:1875–1877

Larsson-Cohn U, Lundberg PO (1970) Headache and treatment with oral contraceptives. Acta Neurol Scand 46:267–278

Lidegaard O (1993) Oral contraception and risk of a cerebral thromboembolic attack: results of a case-control study. Br Med J 306:956–963

Lidegaard Ø (1995) Oral contraceptives, pregnancy and the risk of cerebral thromboembolism: the influence of diabetes, hypertension, migraine and previous thrombotic disease. Br J Obstet Gynaecol 102:153–159

Lidegaard O, Kreiner S (2002) Contraceptives and cerebral thrombosis: a five-year national case-control study. Contraception 65:197–205

Luyer MD, Khosla S, Owen WG, Miller VM (2001) Prospective randomized study of effects of unopposed estrogen replacement therapy on markers of coagulation and inflammation in postmenopausal women. J Clin Endocrinol Metab 86:3629–3634

MacClellan LR, Giles W, Cole J, Wozniak M, Stern B, Mitchell BD, Kittner SJ (2007) Probable migraine with visual aura and risk of ischemic stroke. The stroke prevention in young women study. Stroke 38:2438–2445

MacGregor A (1999a) Estrogen replacement and migraine aura. Headache 39:674–678

MacGregor A (1999b) Effects of oral and transdermal estrogen replacement on migraine. Cephalalgia 19:124–125

MacGregor EA (2007) Migraine and use of combined hormonal contraceptives: a clinical review. J Fam Plann Reprod Health Care 33:159–169

MacGregor EA, Guillebaud J (1998) Combined oral contraceptives, migraine and ischaemic stroke. Clinical and Scientific Committee of the Faculty of Family Planning and Reproductive Health Care and the Family Planning Association. Br J Fam Plann 24:55–60

MacGregor EA, Hackshaw A (2002) Prevention of migraine in the pill-free interval of combined oral contraceptives: a double-blind, placebo-controlled pilot study using natural oestrogen supplements. J Fam Plann Reprod Health Care 28:27–31

MacGregor EA, Frith A, Ellis J, Aspinall L, Hackshaw A (2006) Incidence of migraine relative to menstrual cycle phases of rising and falling estrogen. Neurology 67:2154–2158

Machado RB, Pereira AP, Coelho GP, Neri L, Martins L, Luminoso D (2010) Epidemiological and clinical aspects of migraine in users of combined oral contraceptives. Contraception 81(3):202–208

Martinelli I, Battaglioli T, Burgo I, Di Domenico S, Mannucci PM (2006) Oral contraceptive use, thrombophilia and their interaction in young women with ischemic stroke. Haematologica 91:844–847

Mendelsohn ME (2002) Protective effects of estrogen on the cardiovascular system. Am J Cardiol 89:12E–17E, discussion 17E–18E

Misakian AL, Langer RD, Bensenor IM, Cook NR, Manson JE, Buring JE, Rexrode KM (2003) Postmenopausal hormone therapy and migraine headache. J Womens Health Larchmt 12:1027–1036

Moorhead T, Hannaford P, Warskyj M (1997) Prevalence and characteristics associated with use of hormone replacement therapy in Britain. Br J Obstet Gynaecol 104:290–297

Moschiano F, D'Amico D, Ciusani E, Erba N, Rigamonti A, Schieroni F, Bussone G (2004) Coagulation abnormalities in migraine and ischaemic cerebrovascular disease: a link between migraine and ischaemic stroke? Neurol Sci 25(suppl 3):S126–S128

Mueller L (2000) Predictability of exogenous hormone effect on subgroups of migraineurs. Headache 40:189–193

Nappi RE, Cagnacci A, Granella F, Piccinini F, Polatti F, Facchinetti F (2001) Course of primary headaches during hormone replacement therapy. Maturitas 38:157–163

Nappi RE, Sances G, Sommacal A, Detaddei S, Facchinetti F, Cristina S, Polatti F, Nappi G (2006) Different effects of tibolone and low-dose EPT in the management of postmenopausal women with primary headaches. Menopause 13:818–825

Nightingale AL, Farmer RD (2004) Ischemic stroke in young women: a nested case-control study using the UK General Practice Research Database. Stroke 35:1574–1578

North American Menopause Society (2004) Treatment of menopause-associated vasomotor symptoms: position statement of The North American Menopause Society. Menopause 11:11–33

North American Menopause Society (2010) Estrogen and progestogen use in postmenopausal women: 2010 position statement of The North American Menopause Society. Menopause 17(2):242–255

Petitti DB, Sidney S, Bernstein A, Wolf S, Quesenberry C, Ziel HK (1996) Stroke in users of low-dose oral contraceptives. N Engl J Med 335:8–15

Phillips BM (1968) Oral contraceptive drugs and migraine. Br Med J 2:99

Poulter NR, Chang CL, Farley TM, Meirik O (1999) Risk of cardiovascular diseases associated with oral progestagen preparations with therapeutic indications. Lancet 354:1610

Rodstrom K, Bengtsson C, Lissner L, Milsom I, Sundh V, Bjorkelund C (2002) A longitudinal study of the treatment of hot flushes: the population study of women in Gothenburg during a quarter of a century. Menopause 9:156–161

Rubino E, Ferrero M, Rainero I, Binello E, Vaula G, Pinessi L (2009) Association of the C677T polymorphism in the MTHFR gene with migraine: a meta-analysis. Cephalalgia 29:818–825

Ryan RE (1978) A controlled study of the effect of oral contraceptives on migraine. Headache 17:250–252

Scher AI, Terwindt GM, Picavet HS, Verschuren WM, Ferrari MD, Launer LJ (2005) Cardiovascular risk factors and migraine: the GEM population-based study. Neurology 64:614–620

Scher AI, Terwindt GM, Verschuren WM, Kruit MC, Blom HJ, Kowa H, Frants RR, van den Maagdenberg AM, van Buchem M, Ferrari MD, Launer LJ (2006) Migraine and MTHFR C677T genotype in a population-based sample. Ann Neurol 59:372–375

Schurks M, Zee RY, Buring JE, Kurth T (2008) Interrelationships among the MTHFR 677C > T polymorphism, migraine, and cardiovascular disease. Neurology 71:505–513

Schurks M, Rist PM, Bigal ME, Buring JE, Lipton RB, Kurth T (2009) Migraine and cardiovascular disease: systematic review and meta-analysis. Br Med J 339: b3914

Schwaag S, Nabavi DG, Frese A, Husstedt IW, Evers S (2003) The association between migraine and juvenile stroke: a case-control study. Headache 43:90–95

Schwaiger J, Kiechl S, Stockner H, Knoflach M, Werner P, Rungger G, Gasperi A, Willeit J (2008) Burden of atherosclerosis and risk of venous thromboembolism in patients with migraine. Neurology 71: 937–943

Schwartz SM, Petitti DB, Siscovick DS, Longstreth WT Jr, Sidney S, Raghunathan TE, Quesenberry CP Jr, Kelaghan J (1998) Stroke and use of low-dose oral contraceptives in young women. A pooled analysis of two studies. Stroke 29:2277–2284

Siritho S, Thrift AG, McNeil JJ, You RX, Davis SM, Donnan GA (2003) Risk of ischemic stroke among users of the oral contraceptive pill: The Melbourne Risk Factor Study (MERFS) Group. Stroke 34: 1575–1580

Sluglett J, Lawson JP (1967) Side-effects of oral contraceptives. Lancet 2:612

Stang PE, Carson AP, Rose KM, Mo J, Ephross SA, Shahar E, Szklo M (2005) Headache, cerebrovascular symptoms, and stroke: the atherosclerosis risk in communities study. Neurology 64:1573–1577

Sulak P, Scow R, Preece C, Riggs M, Kuehl T (2000) Hormone withdrawal symptoms in oral contraceptive users. Obstet Gynecol 95:261–266

Sulak PJ, Kuehl TJ, Ortiz M, Shull BL (2002) Acceptance of altering the standard 21-day/7-day oral contraceptive regimen to delay menses and reduce hormone withdrawal symptoms. Am J Obstet Gynecol 186:1142–1149

Sulak P, Willis S, Kuehl T, Coffee A, Clark J (2007) Headaches and oral contraceptives: impact of eliminating the standard 7-day placebo interval. Headache 47:27–37

The American College of Obstetricians and Gynecologists (2010) Noncontraceptive uses of hormonal contraception. Obstet Gynecol 115:206–218

Tzourio C, Iglesias S, Hubert JB, Visy JM, Alperovitch A, Tehindrazanarivelo A, Biousse V, Woimant F, Bousser MG (1993) Migraine and risk of ischaemic stroke: a case-control study. Br Med J 307:289–292

Tzourio C, Tehindrazanarivelo A, Iglesias S, Alperovitch A, Chedru F, d'Anglejan-Chatillon J, Bousser MG (1995) Case-control study of migraine and risk of ischaemic stroke in young women. Br Med J 310: 830–833

Warren MP, Kulak J Jr (1998) Is estrogen replacement indicated in perimenopausal women? Clin Obstet Gynecol 41:976–987

Whitty CW, Hockaday JM, Whitty MM (1966) The effect of oral contraceptives on migraine. Lancet i:856–859

World Health Organization (2009) Medical eligibility criteria for contraceptive use. WHO, Geneva

World Health Organization Collaborative Study of Cardiovascular Disease and Steroid Hormone Contraception (1996a) Ischaemic stroke and combined oral contraceptives; results of an international, multicentre, case-control study. Lancet 348:498–505

World Health Organization Collaborative Study of Cardiovascular Disease and Steroid Hormone Contraception (1996b) Haemorrhagic stroke, overall stroke risk, and combined oral contraceptives: results of an international, multicentre, case-control study. Lancet 348:505–510

Zegura B, Guzic-Salobir B, Sebestjen M, Keber I (2006) The effect of various menopausal hormone therapies on markers of inflammation, coagulation, fibrinolysis, lipids, and lipoproteins in healthy postmenopausal women. Menopause 13:643–650

50 Medication Overuse and Headache

Dimos D. Mitsikostas[1] · *Mohammed Al Jumah*[2]
[1]Athens Naval Hospital, Athens, Greece
[2]KAIMRC, King Saud Ben Abdulaziz University for Health Sciences, Riyadh, Saudi Arabia

Paolo Martelletti, Timothy J. Steiner (eds.), *Handbook of Headache*, DOI 10.1007/978-88-470-1700-9_50,
© Lifting The Burden 2011

Abstract: Medication-overuse headache (MOH) is a chronic, secondary headache disorder caused by the extensive overuse of all known symptomatic anti-headache drugs. Although its prevalence in the general population is limited to 1%, MOH has a major impact on the patient's quality of life; thus, it creates a high economic burden on society. The ICHD-II guidelines classify MOH into eight subtypes based on the overused medication. Migraine is the most common primary headache complicated by medication overuse. Typically, headaches should resolve or revert to their previous pattern within 2 months after discontinuation of the overused medication, but revised criteria have been published. MOH is often comorbid with many affective disorders; therefore, its management requires a multidisciplinary therapeutic approach, including both pharmaceutical and behavioral treatments. Withdrawal of the overused medication is necessary to improve the headaches, yet MOH frequently recurs. To treat rebound headache from withdrawal, preventive therapy can be started prior to withdrawal of the overused medication. All medications used for the prevention of the primary headache disorders involved in MOH are also effective for the prevention of MOH after withdrawal. Additional treatment of all comorbid conditions, however, is also required.

Established Knowledge

Introduction

Medication-overuse headache (MOH) is a chronic, secondary headache disorder with daily symptoms caused by the extensive overuse of symptomatic anti-headache drugs. All known anti-headache drugs can cause MOH, including specific anti-migraine agents such as ergotamines and triptans, simple analgesics, nonsteroidal anti-inflammatory drugs (NSAIDs), barbiturates, or any combination of these agents used for acute symptomatic treatment of any headache disorder (Evers and Marziniak 2010). MOH is often complicated by affective disturbances, resulting in severe damage to the patient's quality of life and a high economic burden on the society (Mitsikostas and Thomas 1999; Wiendels et al. 2006a, b). It affects not only adults but also children and adolescents (Wiendels et al. 2005). MOH does not respond to usual treatment of the primary headache disorder, and hospitalization may be necessary in certain cases. Furthermore, it is probably the most common headache disorder of patients seeking treatment in headache centers (Mitsikostas and Thomas 1999). It was not until 1951 that chronic headache was reported in patients with migraine or tension-type headache who were overusing ergotamine compounds and that withdrawal of these substances led to fewer occurrences of these chronic headaches (Peters and Horton 1951). In a second study, the authors confirmed this finding and extended it to the overuse of combinations with barbiturates and codeine (Horton and Peters 1963). In these early studies, MOH was primarily associated with the overuse of ergotamine derivatives and was therefore termed "ergotamine headache." In the 1980s, studies on MOH caused by simple analgesics and by combined analgesics were published, and MOH was recognized as a general problem of treatment for all headache subtypes (Wortz 1983; Evers and Marziniak 2010).

Classification and Diagnostic Criteria

In the first classification guidelines for headache disorders (ICHD-I 1988), MOH was termed "drug-induced headache," and a distinction was drawn only between ergotamine-induced and analgesic overuse headaches. In the ICHD-II guidelines (2004), the classification and diagnostic criteria were revised, and the disorder was termed "Medication-Overuse Headache." Soon after in 2005, a new revision was published and covered several subtypes that were missing in the ICHD-II guidelines (Silberstein et al. 2005, ❷ *Table 50.1*). This was followed by another revision in 2006 (Headache Classification Committee 2006) mainly concerning research and scientific evaluation and was termed the "appendix criteria" (❷ *Table 50.2*). There are some differences between these criteria in practice. The use of the appendix criteria has led to the identification of a greater number of patients with MOH (more sensitive), whereas the current ICHD-II revised criteria (Silberstein et al. 2005) have led to the identification of a substantial number of patients with probable, not certain, MOH (Zeeberg et al. 2009). An advantage of the appendix criteria is that they include patients from a prospective point of view (i.e., at the time of consultation) and not retrospectively (i.e., after withdrawal) (Evers and Marziniak 2010). In clinical practice, some patients are easily withdrawn and have a low risk of recurrence in contrast to patients with opioid overuse and comorbid psychiatric illness including substance dependence.

◻ **Table 50.1**

Revised ICHD-II diagnostic criteria for medication-overuse headache (Silberstein et al. 2005)

8.2 Medication-overuse headache
Diagnostic criteria
A. Headache[a] presents on ≥15 days per month fulfilling criteria C and D
B. Regular overuse[b] for ≥3 months of one or more drugs that can be taken for acute or symptomatic treatment of headache[c]
C. Headache has developed or markedly worsened during medication overuse
D. Headache resolves or reverts to its previous pattern within 2 months after discontinuation of overused medication[d]
Subtypes of medication-overuse headache
8.2.1 Ergotamine-overuse headache
Ergotamine intake on ≥10 days per month on a regular basis for >3 months
8.2.2 Triptan-overuse headache
Triptan intake (any formulation) on ≥10 days per month on a regular basis for >3 months
8.2.3 Analgesic-overuse headache
Intake of simple analgesics on ≥15 days per month on a regular basis for >3 months
8.2.4 Opioid-overuse headache
Opioid intake on ≥10 days per month on a regular basis for >3 months
8.2.5 Combination analgesic-overuse headache
Intake of combination analgesic medications[e] on ≥10 days per month on a regular basis for >3 months
8.2.6 Medication-overuse headache attributed to the combination of acute medications
Intake of any combination of ergotamine, triptans, analgesics, and/or opioids on ≥10 days per month on a regular basis for >3 months without overuse of any single class alone[f]
8.2.7 Headache attributed to other medication overuse
Regular overuse[g] for >3 months of a medication other than those described above

◻ **Table 50.1 (Continued)**

8.2.8 Probable medication-overuse headache
A. Headache fulfilling criteria A, C, and D for 8.2
B. Medication overuse fulfilling criterion B for any one of the sub forms 8.2.1–8.2.7
C. One or other of the following:
1. Overused medication has not yet been withdrawn
2. Medication overuse has ceased within the last 2 months but headache has not yet resolved or reverted to its previous pattern

[a]The headache associated with medication overuse is variable and often has a peculiar pattern with characteristics shifting, even within the same day, from migraine-like to tension-type headache

[b]Overuse is defined in terms of duration and treatment days per week. What is crucial is that treatment occurs both frequently and regularly (i.e., on 2 or more days each week). Bunching of treatment days with long periods without medication intake, practiced by some patients, is much less likely to cause medication-overuse headache and does not fulfill criterion B

[c]Medication-overuse headache can occur in patients who are headache prone when acute headache medications are taken for other indications

[d]A period of 2 months after cessation of overuse is stipulated in which improvement (resolution of headache or reversion to its previous pattern) must occur if the diagnosis is to be definite. Before cessation, or pending improvement within 2 months after cessation, the diagnosis 8.2.8 (Probable medication-overuse headache) should be applied. If such improvement does not then occur within 2 months, this diagnosis must be discarded

[e]Combinations typically implicated are those containing simple analgesics combined with opioids, butalbital, and/or caffeine

[f]The specific subform(s) 8.2.1–8.2.5 should be diagnosed if criterion B is fulfilled in respect of any one or more single class(es) of these medications

[g]The definition of overuse in terms of treatment days per week is likely to vary with the nature of the medication

◻ **Table 50.2**

Appendix criteria for medication-overuse headache (for research and clinical trial purposes only) (Headache Classification Committee 2006)

8.2 Medication-overuse headache
Diagnostic criteria
A. Headache present on $\geq$15 days per month
B. Regular overuse for >3 months of one or more acute/symptomatic treatment drugs as defined under subforms of 8.2
1. Ergotamine, triptans, opioids, or combination analgesic medications on $\geq$10 days per month on a regular basis for >3 months
2. Simple analgesics or any combination of ergotamine, triptans, analgesics, or opioids on $\geq$15 days per month on a regular basis for >3 months without overuse of any single class alone
C. Headache has developed or markedly worsened during medication overuse

Epidemiology

The 1-year prevalence of MOH is around 1% in the general population across all countries (◐ *Table 50.3*). The incidence is not known. Several studies have investigated the incidence of chronic migraine, however, and have found that within 1 year, 2.5–14% of episodic migraine

◻ Table 50.3

Prevalence of medication-overuse headache in general population studies (Modified from Evers and Marziniak 2010)

Study	Country	Period (months)	Prevalence (%)	Female (%)	Mean age (years)
Katsarava et al. (2009)	Georgia	12	0.9	NA	45.4 ± 12
Lu et al. (2001)	Taiwan	12	1.1	62	NA
Zwart et al. (2004)	Norway	NA	0.9	66	NA
Aaseth et al. (2008)	Norway	12	1.7	76	30–44
Wiendels et al. (2006a)	Netherlands	12	0.7	72	43±8
Straube et al. (2010)	Germany	6	1.0	74	53
Colas et al. (2004)	Spain	NA	1.4	92	45

NA not applicable

patients develop chronic migraine (Bigal et al., 2008a; Katsarava et al. 2004). All experts agree that medication overuse strongly predisposes to chronic migraine.

Drugs Involved

Multiple medications that are routinely used to treat headaches, migraines, or other types of pain could be the underlying cause of MOH. However, the type of overused drugs varies depending on the drugs marketed in different countries. To diagnose and subsequently manage MOH, a detailed medication history is required, including the use and dosage of over-the-counter medications. Such offending medications might include the following: acetaminophen (paracetamol), opioids, caffeine, ergotamines, NSAIDs, ASA, barbiturates, and triptans (Diener and Katsarava 2001; Limmroth et al. 2002; Goadsby 2006). The periaqueductal gray (PAG) could be a potential site of action for each of these treatments. It has been postulated that MOH may develop due to the agonist effects of these medications on the PAG. By contrast, NSAIDs are receptor antagonists (Goadsby 2006). Simple analgesics such as NSAIDs and aspirin are often included as causes of MOH (Goadsby 2006). On their own, NSAIDs seem to be weak inducers of MOH; however, if combined with caffeine, codeine, and/or barbiturates, the combination can cause MOH at a much lower dosage and after exposure for a significantly shorter period of time than simple analgesics (Katsarava and Jensen 2007). The development of MOH is both dose- and duration-dependent. Overuse of these compounds frequently leads to a state of dependency, in turn leading to MOH as the result of an interaction between a therapeutic agent used excessively and a susceptible patient (Diener 2002; Limmroth et al. 2002). The delay between first drug dose and daily headache is shortest for triptans (1–2 years), longer for ergots (3 years), and longest for analgesics (5 years) (Diener 2002).

Multiple studies have demonstrated that the most frequently overused medications are either paracetamol or combinations of paracetamol or aspirin with codeine. The second most overused drugs are triptans, followed by NSAIDs, whereas the overuse of ergotamines and opioids seems to have markedly decreased since the introduction of triptans in 1992 (Jensen and Bendtsen 2008). Still, these changes in the profile of overused drugs are despite a stable prevalence of MOH (Meskunas et al. 2006). Two retrospective, outpatient-based studies in a headache center have demonstrated that the most frequently overused drugs are combination analgesics (39–42%), followed by simple analgesics (29–38%), triptans (12–20%), opioids (6%), and ergotamines (4–11%) (Relja et al. 2004; Zeeberg et al. 2006a). In 1990, triptans were not used to treat migraine; however, 15 years later, the relative frequency of probable triptan-overuse headache has increased from 0% to 21.6%. Moreover, the relative frequency has increased for both simple analgesics (from 8.8% to 31.8%) and combinations of acute medication (from 9.8% to 22.7%). In contrast, a significant decrease in the relative frequency has been observed for ergotamine-overuse headache (from 18.6% to 0%), mostly due the overall decrease in the use of these drugs (Meskunas et al. 2006). Notably, the risk of developing MOH with the use of any of these offending medications has never been studied prospectively.

The American Migraine Prevalence and Prevention Study explored the causal relationship and the strength of association between medication overuse and migraine progression to chronic headache. This study found that the influence of medication varies according to the baseline headache frequency and drug class (Bigal and Lipton 2009). To quantify the risk of headache, users of acetaminophen were chosen as a reference group to adjust for all other factors apart from medication type. It was found that those using barbiturates (OR, 1.73; 95% CI, 1.1–2.7) or opiates (OR, 1.4; 95% CI, 1.1–2.1) were at an increased risk of incident chronic migraine (CM). Those using triptans (OR, 1.05; 95% CI, 0.8–1.6) or NSAIDs (OR, 0.97; 95% CI, 0.7–1.34), however, were not at an increased risk compared to acetaminophen users. The results were similar for women and men, except that the risk of incident CM associated with the use of opioids was higher in men (OR, 2.76) than in women (OR, 1.28) (Bigal and Lipton 2009).

Pathogenesis

It is unclear if MOH is a distinct biological identity (Goadsby 2006), and whether specific classes of medication or critical exposure doses are necessary for the development of MOH. Furthermore, the causal path is controversial: Is the overuse of symptomatic medications a cause or a consequence? It seems that not all symptomatic medications have the same significance. Bigal and Lipton (2009) summarized the evidence and drew several conclusions. (1) Opiates are associated with migraine progression with a critical dose of exposure around 8 days per month, and this effect is more pronounced in men than in women. (2) Barbiturates are also associated with migraine progression with a critical dose of exposure around 5 days per month, but this effect is more pronounced in women. (3) Triptans induce migraine progression in those with a high frequency of migraine at baseline (10–14 days per month), but not overall. (4) NSAIDs are protective in those with <10 days of headache at baseline and, similar to triptans, induce migraine progression in those with a high frequency of headaches. (5) Finally, over-the-counter agents containing caffeine increase the risk of progression (Bigal and Lipton 2009). Thus, specific classes of medications are associated with migraine progression, and a high frequency of headaches seems to be a risk factor for chronic migraine regardless of medication exposure (Bigal and Lipton 2008). According to one hypothesis, MOH is primarily a behavioral disorder. Addiction and algophobia, together with increased anxiety or depression, complete the essential psychological profile predisposing to drug overuse. Migraine often coexists with these conditions and has bidirectional influence (Merikangas and Stevens 1997; Radat and Swendsen 2005; Radat et al. 2005). On the other hand, anxiety and depression amplify pain perception (Lautenbacher and Krieg 1994). Intractable migraine is a significant reason for drug overuse, and it is likely that the combination of migraine with anxiety or depression may enhance and intensify the recurrence of migraine, resulting in drug overuse. Migraine recurrence, however, was not correlated with anxiety and depression symptoms in a survey aimed at identifying the role of affective disorders in migraine recurrence (Mitsikostas et al. 2010).

Genetic factors have also been implicated. The risk of developing MOH is much greater if there is a family history of MOH or other substance abuse, either drugs or alcohol (Cevoli et al. 2009). Recently, MOH has been associated with the Val66Met polymorphism of the brain-derived neurotrophic factor (BDNF) gene, which is also related to behavioral disorders and substance abuse (Di Lorenzo et al. 2009). Although preliminary at this stage, these findings further indicate that MOH is a biobehavioral disorder.

Several investigators have looked for a connection to different neurotransmitters and endocrine factors, including orexin A, corticotrophin releasing factor (Sarchielli et al. 2008), CSF glutamate (Vieira et al. 2007) and 5-HT2 receptors (Srikiatkhachorn and Anthony 1996; Srikiatkhachorn et al. 1994). All of these have shown significant changes in MOH patients compared to healthy controls, indicating that biological factors also contribute to the disorder. More importantly, PET imaging studies have revealed significant changes in MOH patients in the thalamus, anterior cingulate gyrus, insula/ventral striatum, inferior parietal lobe, and orbitofrontal cortex. After withdrawal therapy, all of these changes were found to be reversed, except for those in the orbitofrontal cortex, similar to other drug dependency disorders (Fumal et al. 2006).

Clinical Manifestations

Independent of the drug overused or the classification system, there are six major clinical features related to MOH:

1. It is a chronic and usually intractable headache.
2. It typically emanates from a migraine in almost 80% of cases (Diener and Dahlöf 1999; Linton-Dahlöf et al. 2000; Imai et al. 2007).
3. MOH patients often display addictive behaviors (Calabresi and Cupini 2005; Radat et al. 2008; Lundqvist et al. 2010).
4. It is very often comorbid with affective disorders (Mitsikostas and Thomas 1999; Usai et al. 2009).
5. Similar to migraine, women are two to four times more likely to suffer from MOH than men (Diener and Limmroth 2004; Aaseth et al. 2008; Bigal and Lipton 2008).
6. Triptan overuse is associated with increased migraine frequency.

The clinical features and accompanying symptoms are migraine-like in most cases, and all available symptomatic anti-migraine and analgesic substances can cause MOH. There is evidence, however, that their contributions are not equal (see pathogenesis and drugs involved). Tension-type headache, either alone or in combination with migraine, is the second more frequent primary headache involved in MOH, followed by cluster headache (Evers et al. 1996; Paemeleire et al. 2006, 2008). Other primary headaches are uncommon. Sleep disturbances such as insomnia or sleep apnea may co-occur with MOH. Both conditions require special care (e.g., diagnosis, classification, and treatment); otherwise, the outcome is likely to be very poor. A high prevalence of smokers and individuals with increased body mass index has been found among MOH patients (Straube et al. 2010), indicating that the disorder may be related to frontal lobe dysfunction (Evers and Marziniak 2010).

Management

The treatment of MOH is multidimensional and includes withdrawal of the overused substance(s), preventive pharmaceutical treatments, and behavioral therapy. All three are necessary; otherwise, the risk of recurrence is high. In order to prevent MOH, public health interventions including recommendations for the judicious use of symptomatic medications together with early use of preventative medications are essential (Rossi et al. 2009).

Withdrawal

All headache specialists agree that withdrawal therapy is necessary to improve MOH, although there is not much evidence regarding this therapy. The aims of withdrawal are several: (1) to detoxify patients from dangerous side effects caused by the overused substance(s), (2) to minimize daily headache, (3) to limit migraine progression, (4) to maximize responsiveness to new medical treatments (Zeeberg et al. 2006b), and (5) to brake the drug-induced cycle of pain-coping behavior (Rossi et al. 2009). There are several unanswered questions, however, in the withdrawal protocol that should be followed. How (abrupt or tapered), when (immediately or after preventive treatment), for how long, and in what setting (in- or outpatient) should such treatment be given, and what medications should be used? Many headache specialists are in favor of immediate and abrupt withdrawal of pain medications, whereas some believe that withdrawal may be delayed for a couple of weeks following the beginning of preventive treatment (Hagen et al. 2009). Using this approach, patients have the chance to be protected from rebound headache and to taper the overused medications more easily. In any case, opioids, benzodiazepines, and barbiturates should be discontinued gradually to avoid a withdrawal syndrome that may include severe autonomic symptoms (Evers and Marziniak 2010). Withdrawal headache occurs in most cases and seems to last for a shorter time in patients who have taken triptans (mean, 4 days) than in patients who have taken ergotamines (mean, 6.7 days) or NSAIDs (mean, 9.5 days) (Katsarava et al. 2001). Short prophylaxis for 10–20 days with high doses of naproxen (up to 1,000 mg per day) may be useful in avoiding rebound headache. In this protocol, naproxen must be given twice daily at strictly scheduled times to prevent further habituation. There is no evidence for this approach, however, other than personal experience. Much has been published and stated about the effectiveness of steroids as they do not induce abuse behaviors. Furthermore, there is evidence of altered endocrine function in chronic migraine patients with medication overuse (Rainero et al. 2006). First, Krymchantowski and Barbosa showed in a large, open-label trial that oral prednisone during the first days of drug withdrawal may be successful in detoxifying patients suffering from rebound headaches in an outpatient setting (Krymchantowski and Barbosa 2000). A subsequent Norwegian randomized controlled trial, however, which was sufficiently large and very well designed, did not confirm the findings of Krymchantowski and Barbosa. Participants were randomly assigned to receive 60 mg of prednisolone on days 1 and 2,

40 mg on days 3 and 4, and 20 mg on days 5 and 6 or placebo tablets for 6 days (Bøe et al. 2007). Another small randomized trial recently showed that prednisone might be effective in the treatment of medication withdrawal headache (Pageler et al. 2008). Thus, the use of steroids is controversial, and they should not be considered for routine treatment of rebound headache in MOH but only if other strategies have failed or are contraindicated. Some patients with severe MOH need inpatient detoxification. In this case, a 1-week admission is usually enough. Drugs for withdrawal can be given i.v. or s.c. Sumatritpan (Drucker and Tepper 1998), DHE (Silberstein et al. 1990) and NSAIDs alone or with tizanidine (Smith 2002) are suggested to treated rebound headache, together with preventive treatment. Only a few MOH patients, however, require hospitalization.

Preventive Pharmaceutical Treatment

Without a doubt, prevention in MOH should start immediately after diagnosis. The medications used depend on the primary headache disorder involved. All preventive anti-migraine drugs can be used for prevention in MOH, although evidence-based data are only available for topiramate (Diener et al. 2007; Limmroth et al. 2007). Topiramate at usual anti-migraine doses (50–150 mg) limits migraine transformation and progression and reverts chronic migraine back into episodic migraine (Mei et al. 2006). Other preventive anti-migraine medications are also suggested, including valproate, propranolol, metoprolol, and flunarizine. Although the effects of amitriptyline in migraine prophylaxis are controversial, recent data have confirmed its use in migraine patients suffering from frequent headaches (3–12 per month) (Dodick et al. 2009). Furthermore, amitriptyline might be recommended for MOH prevention for two additional reasons. Due to its antidepressive effects, it will treat possible comorbid anxiety or depressive disorders. In addition, it will also prevent tension-type headache, another comorbid disorder (Bigal et al. 2008b). Nortriptyline is another tricyclic antidepressant with potential efficacy in MOH (Domingues et al. 2009). Recent evidence has also suggested that botulinum toxin A may be effective in MOH (Mathew 2009; Silberstein et al. 2010).

Behavioral Treatment

In most cases, behavioral treatment is beneficial and includes patient education, cognitive behavioral therapy, and biobehavioral training (e.g., biofeedback, relaxation training, and stress management) (Rapoport 2008; Weeks 2009; Andrasik et al. 2009; Grazzi et al. 2009).

Outcome

Patient outcome depends on several factors, including the baseline conditions, the drug overused, the treatment followed, patient adherence, and the headache center. In a 4-year follow-up trial, almost 60% of subjects did not fulfill the MOH criteria, and their quality of life was improved. Furthermore, remission at year 1 was a significant predictor of sustained remission at year 4. Age, gender, civil status, socioeconomic situation, and type of primary headache did not influence the prognosis, but the use of ergotamines and/or opioids was significantly higher among those patients who continued to have drug overuse 4 years later

(Fontanillas et al. 2010). In another 1-year follow-up study, 53% of the treated patients remain detoxified (Hagen et al., 2009). Strategies for enhancing adherence and motivation and facilitating medical communication are necessary to improve the outcome of any case. MOH remains a therapeutic challenge for all headache specialists and includes numerous severe comorbidities that need particular and long-term attention and care.

Current Research

There has been a recent surge in the number of published and ongoing studies of MOH. These studies have dealt with many aspects of MOH such as risk factors, pathophysiology, and treatment. Although there are many questions pertaining to MOH that remain unanswered, in this section we will summarize the currently registered clinical trials of MOH treatment and recently published studies of MOH.

Risk Factors

The relationship between MOH and psychiatric disorders, especially obsessive compulsive disorder (OCD) and anxiety, is well established. A recent study evaluated the prevalence of MOH in a group of patients with psychiatric comorbidities such as anxiety and mood disorders and made comparisons between controls, patients with episodic migraine, and patients with chronic migraine. Anxiety disorders were observed with a higher prevalence of subclinical OCD in MOH patients (Cupini et al. 2009).

Pathogenesis

The mechanisms predisposing subjects to MOH or leading to disease progression remain largely unknown, but it has been postulated that particular neurobiological pathways leading to behavior and substance abuse are involved. These pathways are mediated by cognitive impulsivity. Thus, MOH may share pathophysiological mechanisms with drug addiction such as dysfunction of the frontostriatal system and central pain sensitization induced by drug overuse (Calabresi and Cupini 2005). Based on this hypothesis, BDNF seems to play a pivotal role in the pathophysiology of MOH. A single-nucleotide polymorphism in the BDNF gene, resulting in a valine to methionine substitution (Val66Met), is related to both behavioral disorders and substance abuse (Gratacòs et al. 2007). A recent study supported the idea that MOH is a substance abuse disorder by showing that the Val66Met BDNF polymorphism is a significant independent predictor of analgesic drug consumption by comparing analgesic drug use among carriers and noncarriers of this mutation (Di Lorenzo et al. 2009). Moreover, another study suggested that wolframin gene (WFS1) expression in the clinical setting of MOH might influence a patient's need for drugs, presenting as abuse behavior (Di Lorenzo et al. 2007). Wolframin is expressed in neurons involved in pain perception (Galeotti et al. 2004) and drug dependence (Bodnar and Klein 2006) through the modulation of intra-neural calcium currents. An ongoing trial is currently underway to investigate the role of the orbitofrontal cortex (OFC) in addictive behavior in patients with MOH using (18 F) FDG-PET (fluoro-deoxy-glucose positron emission tomography). The primary outcome measure of this study is basal cerebral metabolism measured using (18 F) FDG-PET before medication withdrawal, after 3 months, and after 1 year. This study is expected to be concluded in August 2011 (www. ClinicalTrials.gov).

Treatment

There has been a relatively small body of evidence guiding decisions in the management of MOH, but there are multiple ongoing trials currently registered at ClinicalTrials.gov dealing with therapeutic questions in MOH. A recent trial of prednisolone therapy showed that it is not effective in treating withdrawal headaches in patients with MOH (Bøe et al. 2007). Currently, there are no proven transitional therapies to help patients through the detoxification process. A single-center, randomized, placebo-controlled phase II trial is ongoing to assess frovatriptan as a transitional therapy in patients diagnosed with MOH. This study is comparing frovatriptan taken over a 10-day transitional period with placebo. Each participant will be enrolled for 3 months and asked to keep a detailed headache diary during this time. Before entering the study, each patient will also keep a 10-day baseline headache diary. This study is estimated to close in August 2011 (www.ClinicalTrials.gov). More recently, the New England Center for Headache has started a phase IV, double-blind, placebo-controlled detoxification study designed to assess the benefits of almotriptan and topiramate as a transitional therapies in subjects with MOH (www.ClinicalTrials.gov). The Norwegian University of Science and Technology has recently started a prospective, longitudinal, cohort follow-up study in MOH patients. The follow-up period will be 4 years after treatment withdrawal, and the study is expected to be completed in December 2010. Its design will include individuals with probable MOH who will be evaluated in a randomized, 1-year, open-label, multicenter study to determine the effects of early introduction of prophylactic treatment compared to abrupt withdrawal, including a control group (www.ClinicalTrials.gov). During follow-up, the randomized patients still living 4 years after their primary inclusion will be invited to participate in an interview evaluating their headache complaints and recurrent medication overuse.

MOH as a chronic disease shares many features with chronic pain syndromes and addictive behavior; however, it continues to represent a major challenge in headache management with many unanswered questions regarding its predisposing factors, pathophysiology, natural history, and therapy. These unanswered questions make MOH an open area for future research and study.

References

Aaseth K, Grande RB, Kvaerner KJ, Gulbrandsen P, Lundqvist C, Russell MB (2008) Prevalence of secondary chronic headaches in a population-based sample of 30–44-year-old persons. The Akershus study of chronic headache. Cephalalgia 28:705–713

Andrasik F, Buse DC, Grazzi L (2009) Behavioral medicine for migraine and medication overuse headache. Curr Pain Headache Rep 13:241–248

Bigal ME, Lipton RB (2008) Excessive acute migraine medication use and migraine progression. Neurology 71:1821–1828

Bigal ME, Lipton RB (2009) Overuse of acute migraine medications and migraine chronification. Curr Pain Headache Rep 13:301–307

Bigal ME, Serrano D, Buse D, Scher A, Stewart WF, Lipton RB (2008a) Acute migraine medications and evolution from episodic to chronic migraine: a longitudinal population-based study. Headache 48:1157–1168

Bigal ME, Rapoport AM, Hargreaves R (2008b) Advances in the pharmacologic treatment of tension-type headache. Curr Pain Headache Rep 12:442–446

Bodnar RJ, Klein GE (2006) Endogenous opiates and behavior: 2005. Peptides 27:3391–3478

Bøe MG, Mygland Å, Salvesen R (2007) Prednisolone does not reduce withdrawal headache: a randomized, double-blind study. Neurology 69:26–31

Calabresi P, Cupini LM (2005) Medication-overuse headache: similarities with drug addiction. Trends Pharmacol Sci 26:62–68

Cevoli S, Sancisi E, Grimaldi D, Pierangeli G, Zanigni S, Nicodemo M, Cortelli P, Montagna P (2009) Family history for chronic headache and drug overuse as a risk factor for headache chronification. Headache 49(3):412–418

Colas R, Muрoz P, Temprano R, Gσmez C, Pascual J (2004) Chronic daily headache with analgesic overuse: epidemiology and impact on quality of life. Neurology 62:1338–1342

Cupini LM, De Murtas M, Costa C, Mancini M, Eusebi P, Sarchielli P, Calabresi P (2009) Obsessive-compulsive disorder and migraine with medication-overuse headache. Headache 49:1005–1013

Di Lorenzo C, Sances G, Di Lorenzo G, Rengo C, Ghiotto N, Guaschino E, Perrotta A, Santorelli FM, Grieco GS, Troisi A, Siracusano A, Pierelli F, Nappi G, Casali C (2007) The wolframin His611Arg polymorphism influences medication overuse headache. Neurosci Lett 424:179–184

Di Lorenzo C, Di Lorenzo G, Sances G, Ghiotto N, Guaschino E, Grieco GS, Santorelli FM, Casali C, Troisi A, Siracusano A, Pierelli F (2009) Drug consumption in medication overuse headache is influenced by brain-derived neurotrophic factor Val66 Met polymorphism. J Headache Pain 10(5): 349–355. Epub 2009 Jun 11

Diener HC, Dahlöf CG (1999) Headache associated with chronic use of substances. In: Olesen J, Tfelt-Hansen P, Welch KMA (eds) The headaches, 2nd edn. Lippincott Williams & Wilkins, Philadelphia, pp 156–164

Diener HC, Katsarava Z (2001) Medication overuse headache. Curr Med Res Opin 17(Suppl 1):s17–21. Review

Diener HC, Limmroth V (2004) Medication-overuse headache: a worldwide problem. Lancet Neurol 3:475–483

Diener HC, Bussone G, Van Oene JC, Lahaye M, Schwalen S, Goadsby PJ, TOPMAT-MIG-201(TOP-CHROME) Study Group (2007) Topiramate reduces headache days in chronic migraine: a randomized, double-blind, placebo-controlled study. Cephalalgia 27:814–823

Dodick DW, Freitag F, Banks J, Saper J, Xiang J, Rupnow M, Biondi D, Greenberg SJ, Hulihan J, CAPSS-277 Investigator Group (2009) Topiramate versus amitriptyline in migraine prevention: a 26-week, multicenter, randomized, double-blind, double-dummy, parallel-group noninferiority trial in adult migraineurs. Clin Ther 31:542–559

Domingues RB, Silva AL, Domingues SA, Aquino CC, Kuster GW (2009) A double-blind randomized controlled trial of low doses of propranolol, nortriptyline, and the combination of propranolol and nortriptyline for the preventive treatment of migraine. Arq Neuropsiquiatr 67(4):973–977

Drucker P, Tepper S (1998) Daily sumatriptan for detoxification from rebound. Headache 38:687–690

Evers S, Marziniak M (2010) Clinical features, pathophysiology, and treatment of medication-overuse headache. Lancet Neurol 9:391–401

Evers S, Bauer B, Suhr S (1996) Ergotamine-induced headache associated with cluster headache. Neurology 46:291

Fontanillas N, Colás R, Muñoz P, Oterino A, Pascual J (2010) Long-term evolution of chronic daily headache with medication overuse in the general population. Headache 50(6):981–988

Fumal A, Laureys S, Di Clemente L et al (2006) Orbitofrontal cortex involvement in chronic analgesic-overuse headache evolving from episodic migraine. Brain 129:543–550

Galeotti N, Bartolini A, Ghelardini G (2004) Role of intracellular calcium in acute thermal pain perception. Neuropharmacology 47:935–944

Goadsby PJ (2006) Is medication-overuse headache a distinct biological entity? Nat Clin Pract Neurol 2:401

Gratacòs M, González JR, Mercader JM, de Cid R, Urretavizcaya M, Estivill X (2007) Brain-derived neurotrophic factor Val66Met and psychiatric disorders: meta-analysis of case-control studies confirm association to substance-related disorders, eating disorders, and schizophrenia. Biol Psychiatry 61:911–922

Grazzi L, Usai S, Prunesti A, Bussone G, Andrasik F (2009) Behavioral plus pharmacological treatment versus pharmacological treatment only for chronic migraine with medication overuse after day-hospital withdrawal. Neurol Sci 30(Suppl 1):S117–S119

Hagen K, Albretsen C, Vilming ST, Salvesen R, Grønning M, Helde G, Gravdahl G, Zwart JA, Stovner LJ (2009) Management of medication overuse headache: 1-year randomized multicentre open-label trial. Cephalalgia 29(2):221–232. Epub 2008 Sep 24

Headache Classification Committee (2006) New appendix criteria open for a broader concept of chronic migraine. Cephalalgia 26:742–746

Headache Classification Committee of the International Headache Society (ICHD-I) (1988) Classification and diagnostic criteria for headache disorders, cranial neuralgias and facial pain. Cephalalgia 8(suppl 7): 1–96

Headache Classification Subcommittee of the International Headache Society (ICHD-II) (2004) The international classification of headache disorders, 2nd edn. Cephalalgia 24(Suppl 1):1–160

Horton BT, Peters GA (1963) Clinical manifestations of excessive use of ergotamine preparations and management of withdrawal effect: report of 52 cases. Headache 3:214–226

Imai N, Kitamura E, Konishi T, Suzuki Y, Serizawa M, Okabe T (2007) Clinical features of probable medication-overuse headache: a retrospective study in Japan. Cephalalgia 27:1020–1023

Jensen R, Bendtsen L (2008) Medication overuse headache in Scandinavia. Cephalalgia 28:1237–1239

Katsarava Z, Jensen R (2007) Medication-overuse headache: where are we now? Curr Opin Neurol 20:326–330

Katsarava Z, Fritsche G, Muessig M, Diener HC, Limmroth V (2001) Clinical features of withdrawal headache following overuse of triptans and other headache drugs. Neurology 57:1694–1698

Katsarava Z, Schneeweiss S, Kurth T, Kroener U, Fritsche G, Eikermann A, Diener HC, Limmroth V (2004) Incidence and predictors for chronicity of headache in patients with episodic migraine. Neurology 62: 788–790

Katsarava Z, Dzagnidze A, Kukava M, Mirvelashvili E, Djibuti M, Janelidze M, Jensen R, Stovner LJ, Steiner TJ (2009) Lifting the burden: the global campaign to reduce the burden of headache worldwide and the russian linguistic subcommittee of the international headache society. Primary headache disorders in the Republic of Georgia: prevalence and risk factors. Neurology 73:1796–1803

Krymchantowski AV, Barbosa JS (2000) Prednisone as initial treatment of analgesic-induced daily headache. Cephalalgia 20:107–113

Lautenbacher S, Krieg JC (1994) Pain perception in psychiatric disorders: a review of the literature. J Psychiatr Res 28:109–122

Limmroth V, Katsarava Z, Fritsche G, Przywara S, Diener HC (2002) Features of medication overuse headache following overuse of different acute headache drugs. Neurology 59:1011–1014

Limmroth V, Biondi D, Pfeil J, Schwalen S (2007) Topiramate in patients with episodic migraine: reducing the risk for chronic forms of headache. Headache 47:13–21

Linton-Dahlöf P, Linde M, Dahlöf C (2000) Withdrawal therapy improves chronic daily headache associated with long-term misuse of headache medication: a retrospective study. Cephalalgia 20:658–662

Lu SR, Fuh JL, Chen WT, Juang KD, Wang SJ (2001) Chronic daily headache in Taipei, Taiwan: prevalence, follow-up and outcome predictors. Cephalalgia 21:980–986

Lundqvist C, Aaseth K, Grande RB, Benth JS, Russell MB (2010) The severity of dependence score correlates with medication overuse in persons with secondary chronic headaches. The Akershus study of chronic headache. Pain 148:487–491

Mathew NT (2009) Dynamic optimization of chronic migraine treatment: current and future options. Neurology 72(5 Suppl):S14–S20

Mei D, Ferraro D, Zelano G, Capuano A, Vollono C, Gabriele C, Di Trapani G (2006) Topiramate and triptans revert chronic migraine with medication overuse to episodic migraine. Clin Neuropharmacol 29:269–275

Merikangas KR, Stevens DE (1997) Comorbidity of migraine and psychiatric disorders. Neurol Clin 15:115–123

Meskunas CA, Tepper SJ, Rapoport AM, Sheftell FD, Bigal ME (2006) Medications associated with probable medication overuse headache reported in a tertiary care headache center over a 15-year period. Headache 46(5):766–772

Mitsikostas DD, Thomas AM (1999) Comorbidity of headache and depressive disorders. Cephalalgia 19:211–217

Mitsikostas DD, Vikelis M, Kodounis A, Zaglis D, Xifaras M, Doitsini S, Georgiadis G, Thomas A, Charmoussi S (2010) Migraine recurrence is not associated with depressive or anxiety symptoms. Results of a randomized controlled trial. Cephalalgia 30(6):690–695

Paemeleire K, Bahra A, Evers S, Matharu M, Goadsby PJ (2006) Medication-overuse headache in patients with cluster headache. Neurology 67:109–113

Paemeleire K, Evers S, Goadsby PJ (2008) Medication-overuse headache in patients with cluster headache. Curr Pain Headache Rep 12:122–127

Pageler L, Katsarava Z, Diener HC, Limmroth V (2008) Prednisone vs. placebo in withdrawal therapy following medication overuse headache. Cephalalgia 28:152–156

Peters GA, Horton BT (1951) Headache: with special reference to the excessive use of ergotamine preparations and withdrawal effects. Mayo Clin Proc 26:153–161

Radat F, Swendsen J (2005) Psychiatric comorbidity in migraine: a review. Cephalalgia 25:165–178

Radat F, Creac'h C, Guegan-Massardier E, Mick G, Guy N, Fabre N, Giraud P, Nachit-Ouinekh F, Lantéri-Minet M (2008) Behavioral dependence in patients with medication overuse headache: a cross-sectional study in consulting patients using the DSM-IV criteria. Headache 48:1026–1036

Radat F, Creac'h C, Swendsen JD, Lafittau M, Irachabal S, Dousset V, Henry P (2005) Psychiatric comorbidity in the evolution from migraine to medication overuse headache. Cephalalgia 25(7):519–522

Rainero I, Ferrero M, Rubino E, Valfrè W, Pellegrino M, Arvat E, Giordano R, Ghigo E, Limone P, Pinessi L (2006) Endocrine function is altered in chronic migraine patients with medication-overuse. Headache 46:597–603

Rapoport AM (2008) Medication overuse headache: awareness, detection and treatment. CNS Drugs 22:995–1004

Relja G, Granato A, Maria Antonello R, Zorzon M (2004) Headache induced by chronic substance use: analysis of medication overused and minimum dose required to induce headache. Headache 44:148–153

Rossi P, Jensen R, Nappi G, Allena M, the COMOESTAS Consortium (2009) A narrative review on the management of medication overuse headache: the steep road from experience to evidence. J Headache Pain 10:407–417

Sarchielli P, Rainero I, Coppola F et al (2008) Involvement of corticotrophin-releasing factor and orexin-A in chronic migraine and medication-overuse headache: findings from cerebrospinal fluid. Cephalalgia 28:714–722

Silberstein SD, Olesen J, Bousser MG et al; International Headache Society (2005) The international classification of headache disorders, 2nd edn (ICHD-II–revision of criteria for 8.2 Medication-overuse headache. Cephalalgia 25:460–465

Silberstein SD, Schulman EA, Hopkins MM (1990) Repetitive intravenous DHE in the treatment of refractory headache. Headache 30:334–339

Silberstein SD, Saper J, Stein M, DeGryse R, Turkel C (2010) Onabotulinumtoxin A for treatment of chronic migraine: 56-week analysis of the PREEMPT chronic migraine subgroup with baseline acute headache medication overuse. 62th AAN Annual Meeting, Toronto April 10–17, 2010.

Smith TR (2002) Low-dose tizanidine with nonsteroidal anti-inflammatory drugs for detoxification from analgesic rebound headache. Headache 42:175–177

Srikiatkhachorn A, Anthony M (1996) Serotonin receptor adaptation in patients with analgesic-induced headache. Cephalalgia 16:419–422

Srikiatkhachorn A, Govitrapong P, Limthavon C (1994) Up-regulation of 5-HT2 serotonin receptor: a possible mechanism of transformed migraine. Headache 34:8–11

Straube A, Pfaffenrath V, Ladwig KH, Meisinger C, Hoffmann W, Fendrich K, Vennemann M, Berger K (2010) Prevalence of chronic migraine and medication overuse headache in Germany-the German DMKG headache study. Cephalalgia 30(2):207–213

Usai S, Grazzi L, D'Amico D, Andrasik F, Bussone G (2009) Psychological variables in chronic migraine with medication overuse before and after inpatient withdrawal: results at 1-year follow-up. Neurol Sci 30(Suppl 1):S125–S127

Vieira DS, Naff ah-Mazzacoratti Mda G, Zukerman E, Senne Soares CA, Cavalheiro EA, Peres MF (2007) Glutamate levels in cerebrospinal fluid and triptans overuse in chronic migraine. Headache 47:842–847

Weeks RE (2009) Practical strategies for treating chronic migraine with medication overuse: case examples and role play demonstrations. Neurol Sci 30(Suppl 1):S95–S99

Wiendels NJ, van der Geest MC, Neven AK, Ferrari MD, Laan LA (2005) Chronic daily headache in children and adolescents. Headache 45:678–683

Wiendels NJ, van Haestregt A, Knuistingh Neven A, Spinhoven P, Zitman FG, Assendelft WJ, Ferrari MD (2006a) Chronic frequent headache in the general population: comorbidity and quality of life. Cephalalgia 26:1443–1450

Wiendels NJ, Knuistingh Neven A, Rosendaal FR, Spinhoven P, Zitman FG, Assendelft WJ, Ferrari MD (2006b) Chronic frequent headache in the general population: prevalence and associated factors. Cephalalgia 26:1434–1442

Worz R (1983) Effects and risks of psychotropic and analgesic combinations. Am J Med 75:139–140

Zeeberg P, Olesen J, Jensen R (2006a) Probable medication-overuse headache: the effect of a 2-month drug-free period. Neurology 66:1894–1898

Zeeberg P, Olesen J, Jensen R (2006b) Discontinuation of medication overuse in headache patients: recovery of therapeutic responsiveness. Cephalalgia 26:1192–1198

Zeeberg P, Olesen J, Jensen R (2009) Medication overuse headache and chronic migraine in a specialized headache centre: field-testing proposed new appendix criteria. Cephalalgia 29:214–220

Zwart JA, Dyb G, Hagen K, Svebak S, Stovner LJ, Holmen J (2004) Analgesic overuse among subjects with headache, neck, and low-back pain. Neurology 62:1540–1544

51 Headache as an Adverse Reaction to Medication

Anna Ferrari[1] · *Peer Carsten Tfelt-Hansen*[2]
[1]University of Modena and Reggio Emilia, Modena, Italy
[2]Glostrup Hospital, University of Copenhagen, Glostrup, Copenhagen, Denmark

Paolo Martelletti, Timothy J. Steiner (eds.), *Handbook of Headache*, DOI 10.1007/978-88-470-1700-9_51,
ⓒ Lifting The Burden 2011

Abstract: Headache is one of the most common adverse reactions induced by several drugs belonging to a wide variety of therapeutic classes, particularly cardiovascular drugs. It is probably more frequent than reported. In fact, identifying adverse reaction headache can be arduous, since headache is a non-pathognomonic symptom and a primary disorder widespread in the general population. Adverse reaction headache has no typical characteristics and can simulate a primary headache, be associated with symptoms of neurotoxicity, and be a sign of important conditions, such as pseudotumor cerebri or aseptic meningitis. Among subjects at risk are mainly the elderly. The International Classification of Headache Disorders (ICHD-II) (2004) includes headache – adverse drug reaction – in secondary forms, principally in Chap. 8, "Headaches attributed to drugs or their withdrawal," codes 8.1, 8.3, and 8.4. Among these, the most known and easily recognized is certainly nitric oxide donor–induced headache, for example, induced by glyceryl trinitrate. Headache-provoking properties of nitric oxide donors have provided a human model of primary headache to study its pathophysiology and treatment.

The stronger evidence for the diagnosis of headache as adverse reaction, i.e., a negative event with a causal link with a drug, is disappearance with suspension, and the recurrence of headache with the resumption of the drug. Temporal association between exposure to a drug and headache may instead occur by pure coincidence. In most cases, adverse reaction headache does not endanger the patient's life, it is of type A and dose-related, it occurs early in treatment (then tolerance develops), and its outcome is favorable. It can however also be very disturbing, and lead to discontinuation of the treatment. If not recognized, adverse reaction headache increases the suffering, worries the patient and the physician, and may lead to requests for investigations and the prescription of more drugs when the solution is the opposite (to reduce or stop drugs).

Established Knowledge

When one takes any medication, there is always the risk of undesirable consequences that, when harmful, are defined as adverse drug reactions (ADR) (Edwards and Aronson 2000). The adverse reaction is "a response to a drug that is noxious and unintended and occurs at doses normally used in man for the prophylaxis, diagnosis or therapy of disease, or for modification of physiological function" (WHO 1969). The essential elements of this definition are the pharmacological nature of the effect, the fact that the phenomenon is unintentional and harmful, and that it may depend on the patient, that is, there may be individual factors playing an important role. An ADR is more simply a negative event with a causal link with a medication. It is different from the adverse event that is defined as "any unwanted occurrence that may present during treatment with a pharmaceutical product, but which does not necessarily have a causal relation to the treatment" (Edwards and Aronson 2000). Here, the key element is the coincidence in time, without any suspicion of a causal association. Adverse reactions are classified into five types (❷ *Table 51.1*) and divided into serious and not-serious ones. A serious reaction is one that "results in death, requires hospital admission or prolongation of existing hospital stay, results in persistent or significant disability/incapacity, or is life-threatening." On the basis of intensity, an adverse reaction is described as: mild, when the patient is simply aware of the reaction (acceptable); moderate, when it induces a discomfort sufficient to interfere with usual activity (disturbing); and severe, if it causes incapacity to work or to do usual activity (unacceptable) (WHO 1981).

◘ Table 51.1

Types and features of adverse drug reactions

Type	Features
Type A (Augmented)	Direct extension of pharmacological action; dose-related (more frequent or more severe with higher doses); predictable on the basis of the primary pharmacological action; avoidable; most common; it is usually recognized before marketing
Type B (Bizarre)	Not dose-related (idiosyncratic); difficult to study and unpredictable on the basis of the primary pharmacological action; it only occurs in a small percentage of the population, but is often serious
Type C (Chronic)	Related to the duration of the treatment and to the doses; it can be serious and frequent
Type D (Delayed)	Related to the duration of the treatment
Type E (End of use)	Related to withdrawal after long-term therapy

The true incidence of ADRs is not known. Only a part of adverse reactions are identified and recognized as such and not attributed to the current disease. Moreover, underreporting of adverse reactions is a well-known phenomenon (Trontell 2004). It is arduous to diagnose an adverse reaction that is also a common symptom/disorder, and it is very probable that headache as adverse reaction is even more frequent than reported (Ferrari 2006). In fact, headache is both a symptom in itself not pathognomonic of any pathological condition and a primary disorder largely widespread in the general population. Only a small percentage of the population has never suffered from it, and people have often suffered from it more than once and in different occasions. The percentage of adult population with an active headache is globally 47% (Jensen and Stovner 2008). Accordingly, a person could have headache induced by a medication or simply associated with drug taking by pure coincidence. A further obstacle to the recognition comes from the information on adverse reaction headache that, with few exceptions, is still limited, although this kind of headache may be caused by many drugs (Ferrari et al. 2009). Adverse reactions that are not life-threatening, such as (usually) ADR headache, are not studied as systematically and with the same diligence as those considered serious (Michels 1999). This is unlucky, because non-serious ADRs can be very disturbing (Neidig and Koletar 2001), especially when they are chronic, compromising patients' quality of life, reducing adherence to therapy, or leading to drug discontinuation (Kaufman and Shapiro 2002; Hazel and Shakir 2006).

The social and health context raises today new problems concerning the safety of drugs: more and more people are taking more medications (Franceschi et al. 2008), there is a strong tendency to self-medication, and many drugs that needed prescription have now become over-the-counter drugs (Moen et al. 2009; Tfelt-Hansen and Steiner 2007). Biological agents that have a high potential for immunogenicity are increasing (Giezen et al. 2009), and the use of nonconventional medicine is spreading simultaneously. For example, herbal remedies are pharmacologically active and can interact dangerously with prescription drugs (Gaul et al. 2009). It is expected that the physician will be more frequently faced with iatrogenic disorders, which include headache as an adverse reaction to medication. To attempt to prevent, recognize, and manage ADR headache in clinical practice, the physician should therefore have a good knowledge of this topic.

Headache as an Adverse Drug Reaction

Drugs (❯ *Table 51.2*) that can cause headache as adverse reaction are a large legion. To provide more information, in ❯ *Table 51.2*, we have also pointed out the type of adverse reaction headache according to the criteria of the pharmacovigilance. In general, headache as an adverse reaction does not have typical characteristics. It can: (1) mimic/provoke a primary headache, most often in patients suffering from the primary headache (❯ *Table 51.3*); (2) be associated to other symptoms of neurotoxicity, as dizziness, drowsiness, fatigue, peripheral neuropathy, seizure, and encephalopathy; (3) be one of the symptoms of conditions such as pseudotumor cerebri (benign intracranial hypertension) or aseptic meningitis. In the first case, it usually concerns non-life-threatening adverse reactions, whose outcome is favorable. In the other two ones, headache may represent an early signal of a serious condition that, if recognized, can however be resolved interrupting the medication and establishing a specific treatment.

◻ Table 51.2

Drug and drug classes associated with headache as an adverse reaction and type of adverse reaction (drug-induced headaches reported in ICHD-II have not been included when there are no elements proving or suggesting the causal link between drug and headache; the codes reported in ICHD-II are in brackets) (Modified from Ferrari et al. 2009)

Drugs	Type of adverse reaction headache
Nitric oxide (NO) donors (code 8.1.1), Phosphodiesterase (PDE) inhibitors (code 8.1.2), Cocaine (code 8.1.6), Ethanol (code 8.1.4), Cannabis (code 8.1.7), Histamine (code 8.1.8), Calcium channel blockers, Antiarrhythmics, Beta-adrenergic blockers, ACE-inhibitors, Sympathomimetics (code 10.3.6), Antagonists of the at-1 receptors for angiotensin II, Statins, α_2 Adrenergic agonist (Clonidine), α_1 Adrenergic blockers (Doxazosin and Prazosin), Amiloride, Metylxanthines, β_2 Adrenergic agonists, Agents for erectile dysfunction, Nicotine (code 8.1.10), Amphetamine (code 10.3.6)	1. Headache as type A adverse drug reaction: predictable, related to the principal pharmacological action of the drugs, and dose-dependent
Amoxicillin, Carbamazepine, Diclofenac, Famotidine, Ibuprofen, Immune Globulin, Infliximab, Ketorolac, Leflunomide, Levamisole, Metronidazole, Naproxen, Ranitidine, Rofecoxib, Sulfamethoxazole, Sulfasalazine, Sulindac, Tolmetin, Trimethoprim, Valacyclovir	2. Headache as type B adverse drug reaction: idiosyncratic, unpredictable, and related to aseptic meningitis (code 7.3.2)
Amiodarone, Anabolic Steroids, Contraceptives Combination, Ciprofloxacin, Danazol, Corticosteroids, Gentamicin, Lithium Carbonate, Nalidixic Acid, Nitrofurantoin, Ofloxacin, Retinoic Acid, Tetracycline, Tyroid Hormone Replacement, Vitamin A	3. Headache as type C adverse drug reaction: after chronic medication, related to raised intracranial pressure (code 8.3 and code 7.1.2)
Caffeine-withdrawal headache (code 8.4.1), Opioid-withdrawal headache (code 8.4.2), Estrogen-withdrawal headache (code 8.4.3), Ergotamine-withdrawal headache, Cocaine-withdrawal headache, Methysergide withdrawal headache, Triptan withdrawal headache, Analgesic withdrawal headache	4. Headache as type E adverse drug reaction: related to substance withdrawal

◻ **Table 51.3**

Characteristics of headaches attributed to drugs and drug classes (Modified from Ferrari et al. 2009)

Characteristic	Drug
Migraine without aura	Cyclosporin (Steiger et al. 1994), Dipyridamole (Kruuse et al. 2006), Nitric oxide donors (Tfelt-Hansen et al. 2009), Phosphodiesterase-inhibitors (Evans and Kruuse 2004), Interferon-beta (Khromov et al. 2005), Ondansetron (Khan 2002), Tacrolimus (Ferrari et al. 2005), Sertraline (Munera and Goldstein 2001)
Migraine with aura	Nitric oxide donors (Bank 2001), Phosphodiesterase-inhibitors (Evans and Kruuse 2004), Tacrolimus (Toth et al. 2005), Fluoxetine (Larson 1993)
Typical aura without headache	Tadalafil (Dinn and Wall 2006)
Cluster headache	Nitric oxide donors (Ekbom 1968), Phosphodiesterase-inhibitors (Evans 2006)

The mechanisms of adverse reaction headache are in large measure unknown. The major ones have been considered: vasodilatation and intracranial hypertension (Asmark et al. 1989). Headache induced by most part of cardiovascular drugs seems to depend on their ability to induce vasodilatation. It is therefore a type A adverse reaction, that is, an extension of the primary pharmacological action of the drug, often dose-dependent, but occurring even at the doses normally used in therapy. Headache associated with drug-induced intracranial hypertension is instead a type B adverse reaction, unpredictable on the basis of the primary action of the drug (Ferrari 2006).

The International Classification of Headache Disorders (ICDH-II) (2004) (❷ *Table 51.4*) includes headache – adverse reaction in the secondary forms, mainly in Chap. 8, "Headaches attributed to drugs or their withdrawal," codes 8.1, 8.3, and 8.4. Among these, the most known and studied is nitric oxide donor–induced (nitroglycerin-induced) headache (code 8.1.1). This headache represents the model most used and validated for the study of the pathogenesis and therapy of migraine (Iversen et al. 1989). Nitric oxide donors (for example, isosorbide mononitrate, isosorbide dinitrate, glyceryl trinitrate, and sodium nitroprusside) can cause immediate (code 8.1.1.1) and delayed headache (code 8.1.1.2) that develops only in headache patients after a variable time, from one to several hours after administration. Delayed headache that occurs in the migraine patient after the administration of glyceryl trinitrate and has the characteristics of a migraine attack has been considered a proof of the crucial role of nitric oxide in migraine pathogenesis (Olesen et al. 1995; Tvedskov et al. 2010). In the treatment of angina or congestive heart failure with organic nitrates, headache is the most frequent adverse reaction (Tfelt-Hansen and Tfelt-Hansen 2009). Tolerance to headache usually develops in a few days; however, up to 20% of the patients do not tolerate this symptom and interrupt the drug. The frequency of nitrates-induced headache is inversely correlated with the age of the patients (Thadani and Rodgers 2006). Headache (code 8.1.2) and flushing are the more frequent adverse reactions of the phosphodiesterase-inhibitors type 5, such as sildenafil and vardenafil, employed in the therapy of erectile dysfunction (Phosphodiesterase (PDE) inhibitor–induced headache, code 8.1.2). In migraine patients, these drugs can trigger migraine attacks (Kruuse et al. 2004). Dipyridamole, a drug used in the prevention of stroke or transient ischaemic attack, causes dose-dependent headache at the beginning of the therapy

■ Table 51.4

Classification of headache as an adverse reaction to medication according to ICHD-II (2004)

Chapter 8 Headache attributed to a substance or its withdrawal	
Code	Definition
8.1	Headache induced by acute substance use or exposure
8.1.1	Nitric oxide (NO) donor–induced headache
8.1.1.1	Immediate NO donor–induced headache
8.1.1.2	Delayed NO donor–induced headache
8.1.2	Phosphodiesterase (PDE) inhibitor–induced headache
8.1.4	Alcohol-induced headache.
8.1.4.1	Immediate alcohol-induced headache
8.1.4.2	Delayed alcohol-induced headache
8.1.6	Cocaine-induced headache
8.1.7	Cannabis-induced headache
8.1.8	Histamine-induced headache
8.1.8.1	Immediate histamine-induced headache
8.1.10	Headache as an acute adverse event attributed to medication used for other indications
8.1.11	Headache attributed to other acute substance use or exposure
8.3	Headache as an adverse event attributed to chronic medication
8.3.1	Exogenous hormone-induced headache
8.4	Headache attributed to substance withdrawal
8.4.1	Caffeine-withdrawal headache
8.4.2	Opioid-withdrawal headache
8.4.3	Estrogen-withdrawal headache
Headache coded in other chapters	
7.1.2	Headache attributed to intracranial hypertension secondary to metabolic, toxic, or hormonal causes
7.3.2	Headache attributed to aseptic (non-infectious) meningitis
10.3.6	Headache attributed to acute pressor response to an exogenous agent.

in up to 70% of patients. Even if tolerance to headache develops after the first week of treatment, many patients interrupt the drug (Halkes et al. 2009; Lökk 2009). Headache caused by dipyridamole is similar to that reported in patients taking nitrates, and it is classified as phosphodiesterase inhibitor–induced headache.

Headache is a frequent adverse effect of drugs for the cardiovascular apparatus, such as ACE-inhibitors (Mangrella et al. 1998), sartans (Biswas et al. 2002), calcium channel blockers, and, above all, dihydropyridine derivates, for instance nifedipine and nisoldipine (Glasser et al. 1995; Marley and Curram 1989). With these last ones, headache already begins at the first administration, then tolerance to this effect usually develops, but up to 5 – 10% of the treated patients discontinue the medication because they do not tolerate headache (Marley and Curram 1989). Interferons-induced headache also appears immediately, within 2 h, and it persists for 24 h from the administration, together with flu-like symptoms (Pollmann et al. 2002). Non-dose-related headache is also an adverse effect of many antiviral agents. In particular, valacyclovir has been associated with cases of aseptic meningitis (Olin and Gugliotta 2003). Even 5-HT$_3$ receptor antagonists induce headache with high frequency, in up to 40% of the patients (Veneziano et al. 1995), and headache is the most common adverse effect of the proton pump inhibitors in clinical trials (Claessens et al. 2002). Among nonsteroidal anti-inflammatory drugs, indometacin induces dose-dependent headache in 15–25% of the long-term treated patients (Jacobs and Grayson 1968). Indometacin induces vasoconstriction, with reduction of the cerebral blood flow in the carotid area (Wenmalm et al. 1984). Mifepristone (Mishell et al. 1987), danazol (Asch and Greenblatt 1977), bromocriptine (Massiou et al. 2002), droloxifene (Bruning 1992), and many other hormonal agents have been reported to cause headache as an adverse effect (code 8.3.1). Hormonal contraceptives or hormone replacement therapy for menopausal subjects may worsen the severity or intensity of a preexisting headache in 18–50% of patients (Massiou and MacGregor 2000). In clinical trials with implantable contraceptives, the most frequent complaint is about headache (Brache et al. 2002). Moreover, during the period of suspension of a hormonal contraceptive or after a cycle of replacement therapy with estrogens, headache can begin, or even a migraine attack in a migraine patient, which ICHD-II (2004) classify as "oestrogen-withdrawal headache" (code 8.4.3).

Headache is the cardinal symptom of the benign intracranial hypertension (pseudotumor cerebri) (code 7.1.2) induced by drugs as glucocorticoids (Ivey and Denssesten 1969), retinoids (Visani et al. 1996), and tetracyclines (Ang et al. 2002). Other symptoms are nausea, vomiting, tinnitus, papilledema, and it can occasionally lead to paralysis of the sixth cranial nerve. The pathogenesis of benign intracranial hypertension is not known. Long-term use of glucocorticoids can cause benign intracranial hypertension more frequently in children and after a rapid decrease in glucorticoid dosage (Neville and Wilson 1970). In the majority of patients with acute promyelocitic leukemia, oral tretinoin causes increased CSF pressure and severe occipital headache. Particularly children can develop pseudotumor cerebri and papilledema (Ganguly 2005). Tetracyclines are a well-recognized cause of intracranial hypertension, above all minocycline used in young women for the therapy of acne (Mochizuki et al. 2002.) Intracranial hypertension can occur after a period of treatment with minocycline, from 2 weeks to several months. The mechanism has been attributed to decreased cerebrospinal fluid outflow at the arachnoid villi, leading to increased extracellular fluid volume and interstitial brain edema (Ang et al. 2002).

Headache caused by aseptic meningitis (code 7.3.2) is rare and not dose-related. Besides headache, fever, nuchal rigidity, confusion, nausea, and vomiting can be present. The diagnosis is difficult, and it is usually only made when infectious causes have been eliminated. The main category of causal agents is formed by nonsteroidal anti-inflammatory drugs, antibiotics, and intravenous immunoglobulin (Kepa et al. 2005). Recently, cases of aseptic meningitis have also been reported with lamotrigine (Lam et al. 2010). The most probable mechanism seems to be immunological (Kepa et al. 2005).

A clinical radiological condition defined as "reversible posterior leukoencephalopathy syndrome" is increasingly identified. This syndrome occurs in patients with a variety of tumor types, during or shortly after therapy with chemotherapeutic agents. It is manifested by headache, nausea, vomiting, altered mental status, and seizures, and it could be due to drug-induced hypertension and endothelium damage. The syndrome is reversible with treatment of concurrent hypertension or removal of the causative agent (Bhatt et al. 2009).

Diagnosis

Every time that the physician sees a patient that reports the onset of a headache he had never suffered from or a worsening or a change of preexisting headache, an adverse reaction to a medication must also be assessed in differential diagnosis. To determine the probability of a causal link between the exposure to a drug and an adverse event, four aspects must be analyzed: (1) the temporal association between the administration of the drug and the onset of the headache; (2) the pharmacological characteristics, and, in particular, if the headache is compatible with the pharmacological action of the substance, and the available knowledge of the nature and of the frequency of the adverse reactions (however, the physician must also be vigilant toward adverse reactions unexpected and never signaled before); (3) the exclusion of other causes, and (4) – the strongest proof – the response to the reduction of the dose or to the interruption of the medication (dechallenge) and the response to the readministration of the medication (rechallenge) (Rehan et al. 2009). The diagnosis of adverse reaction headache can be relatively easy for the medications for which the ability to induce headache has been broadly studied (for example, nitric oxide donors). If headache as an adverse reaction does not have particular characteristics, it can be confused with tension-type headache. This headache, which is the most common type of primary headache, lacks disease-specific features (Bendtsen and Jensen 2009). In a patient suffering from headache, headache provoked by a medication is usually similar to the preexisting one and the diagnosis may be even more complex. Migraineurs seem to be more susceptible to various endogenous or exogenous stimuli (including drug-induced headache) than individuals without migraine. Accordingly, the migraine patient can lead the physician astray reporting that the attack has been provoked by triggers such as changes of the weather, fatigue, stress, food, or menstruations (Friedman and De ver Dye 2009).

Wide interindividual differences in the response to drugs are normal, both in terms of effectiveness and of adverse effects, and certain patients are at higher risk of adverse reactions than others, because of age, genetic or environmental factors, concomitant pathologies (such as liver and kidney insufficiency), and polypharmacy (Veehof et al. 1999). The elderly population is often polymedicated and more exposed to the occurrence of adverse reactions. In the elderly, the prevalence of primary headaches decreases and the prevalence of secondary forms increases; among these, there is drug-induced headache (Reinisch et al. 2008). It will be therefore necessary to carefully assess the possibility of an adverse reaction when an old patient complains of an unusual headache, from which he has never suffered before. Another category vulnerable to adverse reactions and at risk of secondary headache is that of patients in pediatric age. Physicians are often forced to make prescriptions of drugs to children based on incomplete data of effectiveness and safety, since many drugs are only approved for use in the adult (Noah 2009).

Also when a patient with cancer suffers from a new headache, not only the possibility of a direct effect of the tumor must be considered, but also an adverse reaction to chemotherapeutic drugs or the onset of a reversible posterior leukoencephalopathy syndrome, now reported with increasing frequency (Vaughn et al. 2008).

Headache is also one of the most frequent side effects after placebo. More specifically, this headache is a nocebo (from Latin: I will harm) response, which is an unpleasant symptom which emerges after the administration of placebo. The nocebo phenomenon is caused by negative expectations or by doubts about treatments. Females, elderly people, and patients who are anxious or depressed are more likely to experience nocebo effect (Barsky et al. 2002).

Headache is one of the most common symptoms among those who determine physician's consultation. The fact that drug administration or discontinuation is temporally associated with a headache does not prove that the drug has a causal role and in no way excludes the need to evaluate other causes.

Treatment

An accurate diagnosis and the evaluation of the severity of adverse reaction headache and of its impact on the normal daily activities are key elements to decide how to behave. If the physician recognizes the headache as drug-induced, judges this reaction as not-serious, and fully informs the patient of this, the patient removes the fear of a disease and may agree to continue the drug (especially when essential to its health) despite the headache. The majority of headaches as adverse drug reactions are dose-dependent (type A). The treatment can therefore be easy: decreasing the dose of the drug till the disappearance of the adverse effect and the least effective dose. If on reducing the dose, the therapeutic effect also disappears, it is obviously necessary to change the kind of drug. Since the frequency of adverse effects is not identical for all the agents of a class, another drug of the same class could not cause the same problem. When the headache is associated with other symptoms or signs of neurotoxicity, such as visual disturbances, the physician should be alarmed and the drug should be immediately discontinued.

Published studies on treatment of drug-induced headaches are very limited. In two studies including patients with chronic migraine with medication overuse, topiramate was superior to placebo for migraine days (Diener et al. 2009). The few indications available suggest that topiramate and gabapentin are effective in children with headache caused by serotonin receptor antagonists (Veneziano et al. 1995) and that acetazolamide is useful to counteract the development of pseudotumor cerebri by retinoids in children treated with vitamin A for the therapy of acute promyelocytic leukemia (Ganguly 2005). Specific medications, such as triptans, may be indicated for acute treatment only if the drug worsens a preexisting primary headache, such as migraine. These drugs should not however be prescribed to patients with pathologies that contraindicate their employment: for example, patients suffering from cardiovascular disease in treatment with nitrates or calcium channel antagonists. Headaches developing after the abrupt withdrawal of a drug readily respond to the restart of the same drug, which may be then reduced more gradually. These headaches tend however to end naturally usually within days to 1 week.

Prevention remains the best therapy even in the case of headache caused by drugs. In patients already suffering from primary headache (especially migraine), the use of drugs that can cause headache or migraine attacks should be avoided. If the drug is vital and irreplaceable (which is rare), it is necessary to warn the patient that it could cause headache.

Conclusion

It is impossible to completely avoid adverse reactions, among which is adverse reaction headache. Simple approaches (❂ Table 51.5), such as prudent and appropriate use of drugs, familiarity with side effects and drug interactions, and telling the patient to adhere to the prescribed dose, are certainly helpful in reducing adverse reactions to a minimum (Aronson 2009). Today, a lot of information about drugs is directly addressed to patients in inserts, so

■ Table 51.5

Key messages for physicians and patients

Physicians	Patients
Before prescribing a drug able to frequently induce headache as adverse effect, investigate on a possible preexisting headache	If you suffer from headache, report it to your doctor before he prescribes you drugs
In the differential diagnosis of a new headache, keep in mind the possibility of an adverse drug reaction	When you go to the doctor, bring with you a list of the medications you are taking
Be aware of confounding by the high prevalence of primary headache	Ask your doctor of the possible adverse effects that you can expect from the drugs that he prescribes you
Note that the temporal link between a drug and a headache may just be by chance; search other explanations	Always refer to your doctor if you use nonconventional therapies, such as herbal remedies
Be prepared for unpredictable, unexpected adverse drug reactions	Always tell your doctor if you are allergic to certain drugs, if you are nursing, pregnant, or if you plan to be
Identify patients at risk	Read the package insert of the drug that has been prescribed to you
Give the patient information and clear instructions on drugs and how to take them	Follow the dosage that the doctor has prescribed
Periodically evaluate the therapy that you have prescribed	Inform your doctor immediately if you think the drug produces strange effects or adverse reactions
Do not prescribe drugs of doubtful effectiveness	Do not take medications recommended by friends or relatives or because you have heard or read of them on Internet

they should also take an active and responsible role in the process of care, which includes the reporting of adverse effects. Recognizing and documenting adverse events may help to prevent the recurrence of the reaction. Even if an adverse reaction headache does not endanger the life of the patient, its nonrecognition can cause instead pain, unnecessary anxiety, and social costs: requests of investigations, consultations, and prescription of additional drugs when the solution is the opposite, that is, to reduce or discontinue drugs (Gautier et al. 2003).

References

Ang ER, Zimmerman JC, Malkin E (2002) Pseudotumor cerebri secondary to minocycline intake. J Am Board Fam Pract 15:229–233

Aronson JK (2009) Medication errors: what they are, how they happen, and how to avoid them. QJM 102: 513–521

Asch RH, Greenblatt RB (1977) The use of impeded androgen-danazol- in the management of benign breast disorders. Am J Obstet Gynecol 127:130

Asmark H, Lundberg PO, Olsson S (1989) Drug-related headache. Headache 29:441–444

Bank J (2001) Migraine with aura after administration of sublingual nitroglycerin tablets. Headache 41:84–87

Barsky AJ, Saintfort R, Rogers MP, Borus JF (2002) Nonspecific medication side effects and the nocebo phenomenon. J Am Med Assoc 287:622–627

Bendtsen L, Jensen R (2009) Tension-type headache. Neurol Clin 27:525–535

Bhatt A, Farooq MU, Majid A, Kassab M (2009) Chemotherapy-related posterior reversible leukoencephalopathy syndrome. Nat Clin Pract Neurol 5:163–169

Biswas PN, Wilton LV, Shakir SW (2002) The safety of valsartan: results of a postmarketing surveillance study on 12881 patients in England. J Hum Hypertens 16:795–803

Brache V, Faundes A, Alvarez F, Cochon L (2002) Nonmenstrual adverse events during use of implantable contraceptives for women: data from clinical trials. Contraception 65:63–74

Bruning PF (1992) Droloxifene, a new anti-oestrogen in postmenopausal advanced breast cancer: preliminary results of a double-blind dose-finding phase II trial. Eur J Cancer 28:1404–1407

Claessens AA, Heerdink ER, van Eijk JT, Lamers CB, Leufkens HG (2002) Determinants of headache in lansoprazole users in the Netherlands: results from a nested case-control study. Drug Saf 25:287–295

Diener HC, Dodick DW, Goadsby PJ, Bigal ME, Bussone G, Silberstein SD (2009) Utility of topiramate for the treatment of patients with chronic migraine in the presence or absence of acute medication overuse. Cephalalgia 29:1021–1027

Dinn RB, Wall M (2006) Tadalafil associated with typical migraine aura without headache. Cephalalgia 26: 1344–1346

Edwards IR, Aronson JK (2000) Adverse drug reactions: definitions, diagnosis, and management. Lancet 356:1255–1259

Ekbom K (1968) Nitrolglycerin as a provocative agent in cluster headache. Arch Neurol 19:487–493

Evans RW (2006) Sildenafil can trigger cluster headaches. Headache 46:173–174

Evans RW, Kruuse C (2004) Phosphodiesterase-5 inhibitors and migraine. Headache 44:925–926

Ferrari A (2006) Headache: one of the most common and troublesome adverse reactions to drugs. Curr Drug Saf 1:43–58

Ferrari U, Empl M, Kim KS, Sostak P, Forderreuther S, Starube A (2005) Calcineurin inhibitor-induced headache: clinical characteristics and possible mechanisms. Headache 45:211–214

Ferrari A, Spaccapelo L, Gallesi D, Sternieri E (2009) Focus on headache as an adverse reaction to drugs. J Headache Pain 10:235–239

Franceschi M, Scarcelli C, Niro V, Seripa D, Pazienza AM, Pepe G, Colusso AM, Pacilli L, Pilotto A (2008) Prevalence, clinical features and avoidability of adverse drug reactions as cause of admission to a geriatric unit: a prospective study of 1756 patients. Drug Saf 31:545–556

Friedman DI, De ver Dye T (2009) Migraine and the environment. Headache 49:941–952

Ganguly S (2005) All-trans retinoic acid related headache in patients with acute promyelocytic leukemia: prophylaxis and treatment with acetazolamide. Leu Res 29:721

Gaul C, Eismann R, Schmidt T, May A, Leinisch E, Wieser T, Evers S, Henkel K, Franz G, Zierz S (2009) Use of complementary and alternative medicine in patients suffering from primary headache disorders. Cephalalgia 29:1069–1078

Gautier S, Bachelet H, Bordet R, Caron J (2003) The cost of adverse drug reactions. Expert Opin Pharmacother 4:319–326

Giezen TJ, Mantel-Teeuwisse LHG (2009) Pharmacovigilance of biopharmaceuticals: challenges remain. Drug Saf 32:811–817

Glasser SP, Ripa S, Garland WT, Weiss R, Nademanee K, Singh S, Bittar N (1995) Antianginal and antiischemic efficacy of monotherapy extended-release nisoldipine (Coat Core) in chronic stable angina. J Clin Pharmacol 35:780–784

Halkes PH, van Gijn J, Kappelle LJ, Koudstaal PJ, Algra A, European/Australasian Stroke Prevention in Reversible Ischaemia Trial Study Group (2009) Risk indicators for development of headache during dipyridamole treatment after cerebral ischaemia of arterial origin. J Neurol Neurosurg Psychiatry 80:437–439

Hazell L, Shakir SA (2006) Under-reporting of adverse drug reactions: a systematic review. Drug Saf 29: 385–396

Headache Classification Subcommittee of the International Headache Society (2004) The international classification of headache disorders, 2nd edn. Cephalalgia 24(Suppl 1):1–160

Iversen HK, Olesen J, Tfelt-Hansen P (1989) Intravenous nitroglycerin as an experimental model of vascular headache. Basic characteristics. Pain 38:17–24

Ivey KJ, Denssesten L (1969) Pseudotumor cerebri associated with corticosteroid therapy in an adult. J Am Med Assoc 208:1698–1700

Jacobs JH, Grayson MF (1968) Trial of an anti-inflammatory agent (indomethacin) in low back pain with and without radicular involvement. Br Med J 3:158–160

Jensen R, Stovner LJ (2008) Epidemiology and comorbidity of headache. Lancet Neurol 7:354–361

Kaufman DW, Shapiro S (2002) Epidemiological assessment of drug-induced disease. Lancet 356: 1339–1343

Kepa L, Oczko-Grzesik B, Stolarz W, Sobala-Szczygiel B (2005) Drug-induced aseptic meningitis in suspected central nervous system infections. J Clin Neurosci 12:562–574

Khan RB (2002) Migraine-type headaches in children receiving chemotherapy and ondansetron. J Child Neurol 17:857–858

Khromov A, Segal M, Nissinoff J, Fast A (2005) Migraines linked to interferon-beta treatment of multiple sclerosis. Am J Phys Med Rehabil 84:644–647

Kruuse C, Frandsen E, Schifter S, Thomsen LL, Birk S, Olesen J (2004) Plasma levels of cAMP, cGMP and CGRP in sildenafil-induced headache. Cephalalgia 24:547–553

Kruuse C, Lassen LH, Iversen HK, Oestergaard S, Olesen J (2006) Dipyridamole may induce migraine in patients with migraine without aura. Cephalalgia 26:925–933

Lam GM, Edelson DP, Whelan CT (2010) Lamotrigine: an unusual etiology for aseptic meningitis. Neurologist 16:35–36

Larson EW (1993) Migraine with typical aura associated with fluoxetine therapy: case report. J Clin Psychiatry 54:235–236

Lökk J (2009) Dipyridamole-associated headache in stroke patients–interindividual differences? Eur Neurol 62:109–113

Mangrella M, Motola G, Russo F, Mazzeo F, Giassa T, Falcone G, Rossi F, D'Alessio O, Rossi F (1998) Hospital intensive monitoring of adverse reactions of ACE inhibitors. Minerva Med 89:91–97

Marley JE, Curram JB (1989) General practice data derived tolerability assessment of antihypertensive drugs. J Int Med Res 17:473–478

Massiou U, MacGregor EA (2000) Evolution and treatment of migraine with oral contraceptives. Cephalalgia 20:170–174

Massiou H, Launay JM, Levy C, El-Amrani M, Emperauger B, Bousser MG (2002) SUNCT syndrome in two patients with prolactinomas and bromocriptine-induced attacks. Neurology 58:1698–1699

Michels KB (1999) Problems assessing non serious adverse drug reactions: antidepressant drug therapy and sexual dysfunction. Pharmacotherapy 19:424–429

Mishell DR, Shoupe D, Brenner PF, Lacarra M, Horenstein J, Lahteenmaki P, Spitz IM (1987) Termination of early gestation with the anti-progestin steroid RU 486: medium versus low dose. Contraception 35:307–321

Mochizuki K, Takahashi T, Kano M, Terajima K, Hori N (2002) Pseudotumor cerebri induced by minocycline therapy for acne vulgaris. Jpn J Ophthalmol 46:668–672

Moen J, Antonov K, Larsson CA, Lindblad U, Nilsson JL, Råstam L, Ring L (2009) Factors associated with multiple medication use in different age groups. Ann Pharmacother 43:1978–1985

Munera PA, Goldstein A (2001) Migraine and sertraline. J Am Acad Child Adolesc Psychiatry 40:1125–1126

Neidig JL, Koletar SL (2001) Safety reporting in clinical trials. J Am Med Assoc 285:2077–2078

Neville BGR, Wilson J (1970) Benign intracranial hypertension following corticosteroid withdrawal in childhood. Br Med J 3:554–556

Noah BA (2009) Just a spoonful of sugar: drug safety for pediatric population. J Law Med Ethics 37:280–291

Olesen J, Thomsen LL, Lassen LH, Olesen IJ (1995) The nitric oxide hypothesis of migraine and other vascular headaches. Cephalalgia 15:94–100

Olin JL, Gugliotta JL (2003) Possible valacyclovir-related neurotoxicity and aseptic meningitis. Ann Pharmacother 37:1814–1817

Pollmann W, Erasmus LP, Feneberg W, Then Bergh F, Straube A (2002) Interferon beta but not glatiramer acetate therapy aggravates headaches in MS. Neurology 59:636–639

Rehan HS, Chopra D, Kakkar AK (2009) Physician's guide to pharmacovigilance: terminology and causality assessment. Eur J Intern Med 20:3–8

Reinisch VM, Sostak P, Straube A (2008) Headache in the elderly. MMW Fortschr Med 7:42–44

Steiger MJ, Farrah T, Rolles K, Harvey P, Burroughs AK (1994) Cyclosporin associated headache. J Neurol Neurosurg Psychiatry 57:1258–1259

Tfelt-Hansen P, Steiner TJ (2007) Over-the-counter triptans for migraine: what are the implications? CNS Drugs 21:877–883

Tfelt-Hansen PC, Tfelt-Hansen J (2009) Nitroglycerin headache and nitroglycerin-induced primary headaches from 1846 and onwards: a historical overview and an update. Headache 49:445–456

Tfelt-Hansen P, Daugaard D, Lassen LH, Iversen HK, Olesen J (2009) Prednisolone reduces nitric oxide-induced migraine. Eur J Neurol 16:1106–1111

Thadani U, Rodgers T (2006) Side effects of using nitrates to treat angina. Expert Opin Drug Saf 5:667–674

Toth CC, Burak K, Becker W (2005) Recurrence of migraine with aura due to tacrolimus therapy in a liver transplant recipient successfully treated with sirolimus substitution. Headache 45:245–246

Trontell A (2004) Expecting the unexpected - drug safety, pharmacovigilance, and prepared mind. N Engl J Med 351:1385–1387

Tvedskov JF, Iversen HK, Olesen J, Tfelt-Hansen P (2010) Nitroglycerin provocation in normal subjects is not a useful human migraine model? Cephalalgia 30:928–932

Vaughn C, Zhang L, Schiff D (2008) Reversible posterior leukoencephalopathy syndrome in cancer. Curr Oncol Rep 10:86–91

Veehof LJ, Stewart RE, Meyboom-de Jong B et al (1999) Adverse drug reactions and polypharmacy in the elderly in general practice. Eur J Clin Pharmacol 55:533–536

Veneziano M, Framarino Dei Malatesta M, Bandiera AF, Fiorelli C, Galati M, Paolucci A (1995) Ondansetron-induced headache. Our experience in gynecological cancer. Eur J Gynaecol Oncol 16: 203–207

Visani G, Bontempo G, Manfroi S, Pazzaglia A, D'Alessandro R, Tura S (1996) All-trans-retinoic acid and pseudotumor cerebri in a young adult with acute promyelocytic leukemia: a possible disease association. Haematologica 81:152–154

Wenmalm A, Carlsson F, Edlund A, Eriksson S, Kaijser L, Nowak J (1984) Central and peripheral haemodynamic effects of non-steroidal anti-inflammatory drugs in man. Arch Toxicol Suppl 7: 350–359

World Health Organization (1969) International drug monitoring: the role of the hospital. WHO Tech Rep Ser 425:5–25

World Health Organization (1981) Cancer treatment: WHO recommendations for grading of acute and subacute toxicity. Cancer 47:207–214

Part 14

Complementary and Alternative Care in Headache

52 Biobehavioral, Complementary and Alternative Treatments for Headache

Tom Whitmarsh[1] · *Dawn C. Buse*[2,3]
[1]Glasgow Homeopathic Hospital, Glasgow, Scotland, UK
[2]Albert Einstein College of Medicine of Yeshiva University, Bronx, NY, USA
[3]Montefiore Headache Center, Bronx, NY, USA

Paolo Martelletti, Timothy J. Steiner (eds.), *Handbook of Headache*, DOI 10.1007/978-88-470-1700-9_52,
© Lifting The Burden 2011

Abstract: Headache management and research into headache in the Western World is largely based on drugs and pharmacology. This chapter is concerned with the nondrug management of headache. Biobehavioral techniques, such as biofeedback, cognitive-behavioral therapy, and relaxation, have much evidence of efficacy in headache either alone or in combination with pharmacotherapy, and have become standard components of treatment programs at many specialty headache centers, especially in USA. Their use and applicability in the rest of the world is much less studied. Complementary and alternative treatments (CAM) are very widely used by the general population and by headache sufferers. There is good evidence from clinical trials that acupuncture can help people with migraine and with tension-type headache (TTH), in fact, it has become more or less mainstream in some countries. Chiropractic and other spinal manipulative therapies for headache are not well-supported in their effectiveness in headache by well-performed trials even though it may seem reasonable to patients that there is a role for neck-manipulation in headache. There is a plethora of uncontrolled studies and case reports in the literature. Similar comments can be made about other therapies and headache, like homeopathy, reflexology, and yoga, where there are many case reports and only a few well-performed trials, usually with small numbers and done by enthusiasts. Vagus nerve stimulation has been suggested as a possible therapy for intractable headache.

Introduction

Management of headache and research into headache treatment in the developed Western World at the moment is overwhelmingly drug- and pharmacology-based. Other strategies that are potentially effective need to be helped to come to the fore either alone or in combination with more conventional therapies. This chapter aims to review treatments for headache that have demonstrated empirical efficacy and/or are popular and widely used.

Widely used in some countries and well-established, biobehavioral techniques, such as biofeedback, cognitive-behavioral therapy, and relaxation training, are often lumped into the category of "complementary and alternative" medicine (CAM). Experienced practitioners of these therapies do not regard what they do in this light and would not put their therapies in this category. Accordingly, this chapter will review evidence on biobehavioral therapies as well as CAM therapies commonly used in headache management – such as acupuncture, chiropractic, osteopathy, homeopathy, and nutrition.

Biobehavioral Therapies

While there are a range of relatively safe and effective pharmacological treatments for migraine, non-pharmacologic treatments play an important role in comprehensive and effective headache management. Meta-analyses comparing certain biobehavioral with pharmacological treatments have shown similar efficacy between some approaches, and demonstrated that benefits following the biobehavioral interventions were maintained over time at increased rates comparing to outcomes following medication discontinuation (Mathew 1981; Holroyd et al. 1988; Holroyd and Penzien 1990; Penzien et al. 1990).

There are several empirically validated, biobehavioral interventions with demonstrated efficacy in headache management. These therapies may be offered individually or in conjunction with pharmacotherapy (Goslin et al. 1999). In fact, some combinations of pharmacological and non-pharmacological approaches are even more effective than either approach individually (Holroyd et al. 1995, 2001). In addition, combined treatment can help maintain positive outcomes (Grazzi et al. 2002) and improve treatment compliance (Rains et al. 2006a, b). Non-pharmacological interventions offer the benefits of being relatively safe and cost-effective without the potential for drug interactions or side effects. They are useful for patients who need or want to avoid medication use, such as women who are pregnant, lactating, or trying to become pregnant (Scharff et al. 1996), and may augment the effectiveness of other treatments or minimize the need for their use (Penzien et al. 2002).

There is a large and constantly growing body of published evidence examining the use of biobehavioral therapies for headache and migraine including meta-analytic studies and evidence-based reviews (Andrasik 2007; Nestoriuc and Martin 2007; Nestoriuc et al. 2008a, b). As a result, biobehavioral treatments with demonstrated empirical efficacy for headache management have become standard components of specialty headache centers and multidisciplinary pain-management programs and are endorsed by the American Medical Association, the World Health Organization, and the National Institutes of Health as well as many other professional organizations (Goslin et al. 1999). Published consensus-based reviews have been conducted including the US Headache Consortium (an expert panel composed of representative of the American Academy of Family Physicians, American Academy of Neurology, American Headache Society, American College of Emergency Physicians, American College of Physicians-American Society of Internal Medicine, American Osteopathic Association, and National Headache Foundation) (Campbell et al. 2000), the Cochrane collaboration (Nicholson et al. 2004), the Division 12 Task Force of the American Psychological Association (Task Force on Promotion and Dissemination of Psychological Procedures 1995), the Canadian Headache Society (Pryse-Phillips et al. 1998), and the Association for Applied Psychophysiology and Biofeedback (Yucha and Gilbert 2004).

The US Headache Consortium published "scientifically sound, clinically relevant practice guidelines" (Campbell et al. 2000) for the treatment and management of migraine headache based on an extensive review of the medical literature and compilation of expert consensus (Goslin et al. 1999). The guidelines include data and recommendations on the utility of non-pharmacological (behavioral and physical) treatments (Campbell et al. 2000), in which they opine that non-pharmacological treatments are particularly well suited for patients who:

(a) Have a preference for non-pharmacological interventions
(b) Display a poor tolerance for specific pharmacological treatments
(c) Exhibit medical contraindications for specific pharmacological treatments
(d) Have insufficient or no response to pharmacological treatment
(e) Are pregnant, are planning to become pregnant, or are nursing
(f) Have a history of long-term, frequent, or excessive use of analgesic or acute medications that can aggravate headache problems (or lead to decreased responsiveness to other pharmacotherapies)
(g) Exhibit significant stress or deficient stress-coping skills

Biobehavioral treatments for headache can be divided into the categories of cognitive-behavioral therapy (CBT), biobehavioral training (i.e., biofeedback, relaxation training, and stress management), education, and lifestyle modification. The US Headache Consortium assigned the following treatments "Grade A" evidence (meaning that there were multiple well-designed randomized clinical trials, directly relevant to the recommendation, which yielded a consistent pattern of findings) for their use: relaxation training, thermal biofeedback combined with relaxation training, electromyographic biofeedback, and cognitive-behavioral therapy (for prevention of migraine). "Grade B" evidence (meaning that some evidence from randomized clinical trials supported the recommendation, but the scientific support was not optimal) was given for behavioral therapy combined with preventive drug therapy to achieve added clinical improvement for migraine.

Cognitive-Behavioral Therapy (Established Knowledge)

The US Headache Consortium found "Grade A" evidence for cognitive-behavioral therapy (CBT) for the preventive treatment of migraine (Campbell et al. 2000). CBT is an empirically validated, psychotherapeutic treatment comprised of cognitive and behavioral theories and strategies. Cognitive strategies focus on identifying and challenging maladaptive or dysfunctional thoughts, beliefs, and responses to stress (Beck et al. 1979). Cognitive foci of CBT for headache management include enhancing self-efficacy (i.e., the patient's belief in his or her ability to succeed or accomplish a certain task) (Bandura 1977), encouraging patients to adopt an internal locus of control (i.e., a belief that the mechanism for change lies within oneself as opposed to an external locus of control or the belief that only the health-care provider (HCP), medication, or medical procedures have the power for change) (Heath et al. 2008), and eliminating catastrophizing (a hopeless and overwhelming way of thinking). Research has demonstrated that low self-efficacy and external locus of control, and catastrophizing predict poor outcomes to treatment and reduced quality of life in headache sufferers (Holroyd et al. 2007). Other targets of cognitive interventions include assertiveness training, increasing coping skills, and cognitive reappraisal and restructuring (Holroyd and Andrasik 1982).

Behavioral strategies in headache management include modifying behaviors that may maintain or exacerbate headaches and replacing them with healthy behaviors (Nicholson et al. 2005). Behavioral interventions for headache include education, the use of headache diaries, identification and avoidance of triggers, and lifestyle modification. To avoid and manage headache exacerbations, migraineurs should maintain a regular and healthy lifestyle, especially during times when they are most vulnerable to an attack (e.g., premenstrually, during times of increased stress). This includes practicing proper sleep hygiene and maintaining a regular sleep–wake schedule, maintaining a regular and healthy diet, getting regular exercise, avoidance of excessive caffeine or alcohol consumption, smoking cessation, and regular practice of stress management, relaxation techniques, and self-care.

Cognitive-behavioral interventions may be employed in headache management in several ways. With CBT, the patient may be able to directly manage and relieve symptoms, avoid headache-eliciting episodes or occurrences, and improve overall coping. CBT strategies may also help the headache sufferer manage comorbid symptoms, such as depression and anxiety, which have been demonstrated to increase the negative effects of migraine on a sufferer's life including HRQoL and headache-related disability. Additionally, CBT strategies can target and eliminate potential risk factors for headache progression (from episodic to chronic migraine or daily headache). Several modifiable risk factors for transformation have been identified including frequency of migraine attacks, obesity, acute medication overuse, caffeine overuse, stressful life events, depression, and sleep disorders (Bigal and Lipton 2006). These risk factors provide targets for CBT interventions.

Biofeedback (Established Knowledge)

Biofeedback is a technique that involves monitoring physiological processes of which the patient may not be consciously aware and/or does not believe that he or she has voluntary control. Through various equipment and methods, biological or physiological information is converted into a signal that is then "fed back" to the patient. Through biofeedback training, the patient develops increased awareness of physiological functions and learns to control their physiologic state (Sovak et al. 1981; Penzien and Holroyd 1994; Schwartz and Andrasik 2003). While monitoring physiological responses, patients are taught relaxation skills such as diagrammatic breathing or visualization to induce the "relaxation response" (Benson 1975), which is comprised of calming of the sympathetic nervous system and the complimentary activation of the parasympathetic nervous system (Schwartz and Andrasik 2003; Andrasik and Flor 2008).

Many modalities may be monitored through biofeedback including peripheral skin temperature (TEMP-FB), blood-volume-pulse (BVP-FB), electromyographic (EMG-FB), electroencephalographic (EEG-FB), and galvanic skin response (GSR-FB) feedback. The strongest evidence for biofeedback for tension-type headache involves using EMG-FB with the goal of teaching patients to reduce pericranial muscle activity (Goslin et al. 1999). The strongest evidence for migraine management is for thermal, EMG, and BVP biofeedback and relaxation training (Campbell et al. 2000). Thermal biofeedback, also known as "hand warming biofeedback" or "autogenic feedback" (when combined with components of autogenic therapy), involves monitoring finger temperature (a measure of circulation) with a sensitive thermometer. Patients are taught that higher finger temperature corresponds to a more relaxed state and their goal is to raise their finger temperature. During or preceding a headache the body may enter the "fight or flight" state (activation of the sympathetic nervous system). As sympathetic activity increases, circulation to the extremities decreases and finger temperature decreases. Conversely, as parasympathetic activity increases and the relaxation response is activated, circulation and extremity temperature increases.

The US Consortium Guidelines assigned "Grade A" level evidence to thermal biofeedback with relaxation training for statistically significant improvement in headache management (Blanchard et al. 1980; Campbell et al. 2000). Additionally, Nestoriuc et al. (2008a) conducted a comprehensive efficacy review of biofeedback for headache management in adults. They examined data from two recently published meta-analyses, which included 150 outcome studies, of which 94 met inclusion criteria. The authors reported medium-to-large mean effect sizes for biofeedback for the treatment of headache, and found that treatment effects were maintained over an average follow-up period of 14 months, both in completer and intention-to-treat analyses. In addition to the reduction of attack frequency, significant effects were also found for improvements in self-efficacy, symptoms of depression and anxiety, and medication use.

Relaxation Training (Established Knowledge)

Relaxation techniques help patients minimize physiological responses to stress and decrease sympathetic arousal. The US Headache Consortium gave "Grade A" status to relaxation training for prevention of migraine (Campbell et al. 2000). Relaxation training may include a variety of techniques (Penzien and Holroyd 1994). The classic procedure "Progressive Muscle

Relaxation Training" (PMRT), which was first published in 1938, involves tensing and relaxing various muscle groups while attending to the resulting contrasting sensations (Jacobson 1938). Other relaxation techniques include visual or guided imagery, cue-controlled relaxation, diaphragmatic breathing, hypnosis, and self-hypnosis (Bernstein et al. 2000; Rime and Andrasik 2007).

To achieve the benefits from relaxation, patients may use any techniques or tools that quiet the mind and calm the body including meditation, prayer, yoga, listening to pleasant music, listening to guided relaxation sessions, or any other method that a patient finds effective. Although techniques can be quickly learned, they require regular practice in order to become effective, automatic responses especially, during pain/headache attacks or stressful situations.

Complementary and Alternative (CAM) Therapies and Other Nonconventional Treatments

CAM refers to "those forms of treatment which are not widely in use by orthodox healthcare professionals" (British Medical Association 1993). Another definition of Complementary Medicine is "diagnosis, treatment and/or prevention which complements mainstream medicine by contributing to a common whole, by satisfying a demand not met by orthodoxy, or by diversifying the conceptual frameworks of medicine" (Ernst et al. 1995). There might be an unfortunate tendency to lump all nonconventional practices together as "alternative" and label them all as either "good" or "bad," depending on one's preference. Viewed more holistically, there are approaches on both sides of a notional dividing line which bring health benefits to particular individuals. There is little to guide us in knowing in advance which sufferers will benefit from which therapy. It is perhaps one of the tasks of medicine over the next few decades to integrate nonconventional therapies into treatment pathways, the prime goal being to alleviate suffering and promote health. This is beginning to happen in therapy of headache with such treatments as acupuncture or butterbur and riboflavin. Nonconventional treatments of headache have been reviewed in the past (Whitmarsh 1999; Mauskop 2001) and to a certain extent, this chapter represents an improvement and update.

Three studies from the group led by Eisenberg have documented the rise through the 1990s, then stability of usage and status of CAM therapies in general from 1990 to 2002 (Eisenberg et al. 1993; Eisenberg et al. 1998; Tindle et al. 2005), and show that these therapies are very popular, but a major concern is the relatively low likelihood of users telling their HCPs that they are indeed using other therapies. For example, in the first paper, 34% of a national US sample by phone interview of over 18-year-olds ($n = 1,539$) had used at least one of 16 listed CAM therapies in the past year and 72% of the users had not told their health-care provider (HCP) about their CAM use. The authors estimated that in 1990, Americans made 425 million visits to providers of unconventional therapy. The second paper surveyed use in 1997 and found that there had been an increase of total visits of 47.3% to 629 million, with little change in the proportion of nondisclosure of use that remained very high. The third study, based on a much bigger sample size, found little change from 1997 to 2002 in the proportion of Americans reporting use of at least one CAM therapy (about 35%) in the preceding year. HCPs could potentially inadvertently put patients at risk of interactions with other treatments (e.g., with some herbal remedies), or misattribute changes in the clinical state of patients to their suggested interventions when in reality it had to do with the therapy not revealed, which the patient was using at the same time.

Some studies have looked specifically at CAM use in specialized headache clinics and found it to be common. For example, in 110 chronic tension-type headache patients attending a specialist headache clinic in Italy, past use of a CAM therapy was 22.7% and 40% in the past year; 41.1% of the patients felt it had been beneficial for their headache. The most frequently used therapies were chiropractic (21.9%), acupuncture (17.8%), and massage (17.8%) (Rossi et al. 2006). Sixty percent of users had not informed their HCPs. The same group looked at 481 patients with migraine (Rossi et al. 2005) and found that 31.3% reported CAM use in the past, with 17.1% using CAM in the last year. The CAM therapy was perceived as beneficial by 39.5% of the patients who had used them, but 61% of users had not informed their HCPs of use. A general survey of 73 patients with headache syndromes attending a head and neck clinic (von Peter et al. 2002) found that 85% of them were using at least one form of CAM for their pain and 60% of them felt it was beneficial. Some have found the beginnings of a suggestion of benefit in these figures (Whitmarsh 2002a). The rising tide of concern amongst patients in the Western World about the side effects of conventional pharmaceuticals has been considered one reason for the rapid rise in popularity of many forms of unconventional medicine (Whorton 1999).

Some have felt that conventional trial design can never be fully applied to therapies that are by their nature individualized like complementary therapies and have put forward the claims of uncontrolled, outcome studies (Walach and Jonas 2002; Spence et al. 2005). These tend to rely on very large numbers or magnitude of effect to provide power, or are just ignored. There is suspicion of the over-reliance on statistical rather than clinical significance of interventions (Ziliak and McCloskey 2008). The CAM field reports a lot of case experiences thinking along these lines and it must be remembered that most of these therapies cannot be patented and there are not well-developed research networks in place in CAM; so for these reasons amongst others, there is not a lot of money available in CAM and not a huge amount of research done. Others feel that conventional trial methodologies can be used and adapted to investigate almost any intervention (Diener 2008).

Physical Treatments: Acupuncture, Chiropractic, Physical and Occupational Therapies, and Massage

Data on the efficacy of physical treatments for migraine are limited by small sample size, poor study design, and weak results (Biondi 2005). Physicians and patients are advised to make cautious and individualized judgments about the utility of physical treatments for migraine treatment and management. In some cases these modalities may provide valuable addition to first-line pharmacological and biobehavioral treatments; however, cost, time, and potential adverse effects should be weighed carefully.

Acupuncture (Established Knowledge)

Data on the efficacy of acupuncture for migraine treatment and management are mixed. The National Institutes of Health (NIH) Consensus Development Program issued the following statement in 1997: "Acupuncture as a therapeutic intervention is widely practiced in the United States. There have been many studies of its potential usefulness. However, many of these studies provide equivocal results because of design, sample size, and other factors. The issue is further complicated by inherent difficulties in the use of appropriate controls, such as placebo and sham acupuncture groups" (NIH Consensus Conference 1998). More recent meta-analyses and systematic reviews echo the same sentiments that while some research shows positive efficacy, the quality of research and, therefore, the ability to draw conclusions remains a little unclear at this time.

For many years a large number of case reports and RCTs have been published suggesting benefit of acupuncture in various kinds of headache. A problem has been widespread applicability and availability "in the real world" of methods and whether this treatment could be shown to be cost-effective. Concerns here have been successfully addressed in two papers reporting a very well-designed study and its effect on cost (Vickers et al. 2004; Wonderling et al. 2004). The authors randomized 401 patients with "chronic headache" (mostly migraine) to receive either acupuncture (provided by "qualified, experienced acupuncturists," mostly physiotherapists working within the national health service) or usual care. Patients completed a daily diary of headache and medication use for a 4-week baseline period and then 3 months and 1 year after randomization. Severity of headache was recorded four times per day and the total summed to give a "headache score." The SF-36 health status questionnaire was completed at baseline, 3 months and 1 year. Scores for headache severity fell by 34% in the acupuncture group compared with 16% in controls at 12-month follow-up ($p = 0.0002$), which is equivalent to 22 fewer days of headache/year. Medication use was lower in the acupuncture group and SF-36 data favored acupuncture, reaching significance for the health domains of physical role functioning, energy, and change in health. Data on the use of resources showed that patients in the acupuncture group made fewer visits to general practitioners and complementary practitioners and took fewer days off sick. The authors conclude by saying that "a policy of using a local acupuncture service in addition to standard care results in persisting, clinically relevant benefits for primary care patients with chronic headache, particularly migraine. Expansion of NHS acupuncture services for headache should be considered." The subsequent cost-effectiveness analysis allied to this trial concurs with this view, finding the cost of acupuncture per quality-adjusted life year (QALY) gained to be £9,180. On this analysis, acupuncture does not result in an overall cost saving, but is probably better value for money than several interventions currently recommended. This kind of cost analysis has been rarely done with headache treatments, but, for example, the cost per QALY of sumatriptan compared with oral caffeine and ergotamine is £16,000 (Evans et al. 1997).

Acupuncture would appear to have become nearly mainstream, to be thought of as one of the options in the management of headache with the publication of updates of Cochrane reviews of acupuncture in migraine (Linde et al. 2009a) and TTH (Linde et al. 2009b). An earlier Cochrane review concluded that evidence for acupuncture in the prophylaxis of migraine and of tension-type headache was "promising but not sufficient" (see ❷ Chap. 54). The revised, updated advice is now split into two reviews. The authors were able to consider 12 additional trials in migraine and six additional trials in TTH and conclude that acupuncture is a valuable non-pharmacological tool in headache management (see ❷ Chap. 21).

An editorial in the journal *Cephalalgia* (Diener 2008) supported the use of acupuncture in headache, and highlighted two large trials in Germany one of which was an RCT of 302 patients with migraine (Linde et al. 2005). They were randomized into three groups – one received acupuncture, one received "sham" acupuncture (where needles are used, but their placement is not based on the "philosophical" concepts underlying classical acupuncture), and one was a waiting list control. Results did not differ between real and sham acupuncture, with a response rate in these groups of about 50%. The waiting list control response rate was only

15%. It seems that the effect in many trials is to do with needling in itself and not so much on the ideas of classical acupuncture. The other trial is on a very large scale in TTH (Jena et al. 2008). 11,874 patients were treated in an open fashion with acupuncture in addition to standard care. The percentage reduction of headache days over 6 months was 45%. The authors also randomized 1,613 patients to receive acupuncture with 1,569 in a usual care control group. Over 3 months, the acupuncture group had a decrease in number of headache days from 8.4 to 4.7 compared to the control group who only saw a reduction from 8.1 to 7.5.

Spinal Manipulative Therapies (SMT) (Current Research)

Spinal manipulative therapies include such treatments as chiropractic, osteopathy, and physiotherapy. A cervicogenic origin, or at least a contribution from neck dysfunction in various types of headache, has been debated for many years. To patients, who often suffer neck pain or tender muscle-point activation in the neck with different types of headache, it can frequently seem obvious that some sort of physical treatment needs to be given to help their pain. The chiropractic literature is particularly rich in discussion of the role of the neck in headache and is replete with single cases, case series, and uncontrolled studies, which suggest beneficial effects of cervical spine manipulation in various forms of headache. Data from controlled trials are limited by small sample size, with at least one well-planned trial having to be stopped because of low recruitment (Vernon et al. 2009). Few trials have appeared in the last two decades and those that have are small, with typically 20–30 patients included. In the USA, where the vast majority of chiropractic is carried out, there are an estimated 18–38 million manipulations of the cervical spine for headache each year (Shekelle and Coulter 1997). This literature discusses frustration at the relative lack of attention paid by conventional HCPs at the role of the cervical spine in the generation and maintenance of headache, with comments such as "this coherent paradigm is largely disregarded in orthodox circles" (Vernon 1995). In particular, it is felt that the current model of cervicogenic headache by IHS criteria is too restrictive. Quite obviously, chiropractors only use manipulation when there is something to treat, which will almost always be changes in the cervical spine not detectable by conventional diagnostic techniques.

There have been at least two reviews of spinal manipulative treatment (Bronfort et al. 2001) and physical treatments for headache (Biondi 2005) published in predominantly "chiropractic" and "conventional" journals, respectively. The "conventional" study reviewed literature related to chiropractic, osteopathy, physiotherapy, and massage in headache and the "chiropractic" study reviewed with similar criteria. Both reported a lack of evidence in controlled trials to firmly establish SMT as a first-line treatment option in any kind of primary headache and both found that there was not enough research to fully comment on and make clear recommendations of the place of SMT in the treatment of headache. The "conventional" study concludes that on trial evidence, physiotherapy is more effective than acupuncture or massage in the treatment of TTH and appears to be most beneficial in patients with a high frequency of headache episodes, especially when combined with other treatments like thermal biofeedback, relaxation training, and exercise; chiropractic manipulation demonstrates a trend toward benefit in TTH and the evidence for an effect here is better than chiropractic in migraine. The "chiropractic" study concludes that there is moderate evidence that SMT has short-term efficacy similar to amitriptyline in the prophylaxis of chronic TTH and migraine; there is moderate evidence that SMT is more efficacious than massage for cervicogenic headache and that SMT has an effect comparable to commonly used first-line prophylactic prescription drugs for TTH and migraine.

The best trials in chiropractic treatment of headache diagnosed by IHS criteria are in chronic TTH (Boline et al. 1995) and in migraine (Tuchin et al. 2000). In the TTH study, 126 patients were randomized to either chiropractic manipulation or to standard drug therapy with low-dose amitriptyline. The chiropractic group ($n = 70$) received 20 min of treatment twice a week for 6 weeks and the amitriptyline group ($n = 56$) received 10–30 mg of amitriptyline daily for 6 weeks. Both groups improved during the treatment period in all outcome measures (headache frequency, headache intensity, over-the-counter medication usage, functional health status assessed by SF-36). However, once the treatment was stopped, the benefits did not persist in the amitriptyline group and all these measures quickly returned to baseline. The SMT group, though, showed persisting benefits 4 weeks after the treatment stopped, with 32% reduction in headache intensity, 42% reduction in frequency, 30% reduction in over-the-counter medication usage, and 16% improvement in functional health status. In the migraine study, 127 Australian volunteers were recruited by media advertising. The mean duration of headache was 18.1 years. They were randomized to receive either 2 months of chiropractic treatment, or 2 months of sham neck interferential therapy (in which electrodes are applied to the neck, but the current is turned off). All subjects kept detailed headache diaries and follow-up was quite long for these sorts of studies, being 6 months. The treatment group showed an improvement in migraine frequency ($p < 0.005$), duration ($p < 0.01$), disability ($p < 0.01$), and medication use ($p < 0.001$) compared to the control group.

There is evidence from a pilot study, in 24 adults with cervicogenic headache and associated neck pain, of a dose–response relationship in the benefit of chiropractic manipulation (Haas et al. 2004). Patients were given one, three, or four treatments per week for 3 weeks. Patients improved more in their pain with a higher number of chiropractic treatments.

Research in osteopathy is even less well-developed. A small study compares osteopathic manipulation of the head and neck (including cranial osteopathic techniques involving treatment to the bones of the skull, conventionally regarded as "fixed" in position) with progressive muscular relaxation (PMR) (Anderson and Seniscal 2006) in TTH. Twenty-nine patients were recruited and randomized. All practiced PMR at home while the experimental group also received three osteopathic treatments. After 6 weeks, the osteopathy group had a significant improvement in the number of headache days per week ($p = 0.16$).

An osteopathic physician may provide the same outcomes as a conventional physician for less cost. One study retrospectively reviewed the case records of two residency clinics of patients treated for migraine over 5 years (Schabert and Crow 2009). One clinic was osteopathic and offered SMT in addition to standard treatment. The other was entirely conventional and did not offer SMT. Costs were tabulated for both clinics and pain ratings at each visit were tabulated. Electronic records from 631 patients were analyzed (1,427 migraine-related visits). Average cost per patient visit was approximately 50% less at the osteopathic vs. conventional clinic ($159.63 vs. $363.84), the difference due to a lower number of prescription drugs being prescribed. There was no difference between the two clinics in the patient's ratings of pain severity. The authors conclude that the inclusion of osteopathic techniques in a treatment regime for patients with migraine may lower the cost of the treatment regime.

Cervical manipulation has been implicated as causing some forms of stroke. This is taken very seriously amongst the chiropractic community (Blum 2008), even if the risk is probably not high, especially in those without preexisting risk factors. One review (Hurwitz et al. 1996) identified 136 references to complications of cervical spine manipulation from 1966 to 1996.

Twenty-three of these occurred when headache was the presenting complaint, but the authors concluded that serious complications of cervical spine manipulation have a very low incidence of between ten and 20 per 10 million manipulations. Even so, some HCPs feel that patients undergoing SMT should be consented for risk of stroke or vascular injury from the procedure (Smith et al. 2003). The authors of this study reviewed all patients under age 60 with cervical artery dissection ($n = 151$) and ischemic stroke or TIA from between 1995 and 2000 at two academic stroke centers. Three hundred and six age- and sex-matched control participants were selected; 51 patients were studied with their matched controls, by questionnaire and interview. In univariate analysis, patients with dissection were more likely to have had SMT within 30 days (14% vs. 3%, $p = 0.032$) and to have had head or neck pain preceding stroke or TIA (76% vs. 40%, $p = 0.001$). Multivariate analysis suggests that vertebral artery dissection is independently associated with SMT within 30 days (OR 6.62, 95% CI 1.4–30) and pain before stroke (OR 3.76, 95% CI 1.3–11). Chiropractors make the point that the signs that can presage a stroke or TIA are often the same signs that lead a person to seek chiropractic care 3 (Blum 2008), so maybe the safe position comes down to clinical awareness.

How is the nonspecialized manipulator to decide when referral for physical therapy to the neck is appropriate? Hurwitz et al. (1996) attempted to list criteria for referral. The review lists clinical characteristics of patients who are most likely to benefit or it is uncertain that they will benefit from SMT, which look like a first step toward guidelines for referral. In all lists, the presence of cervical signs and symptoms and normal neurological examination are emphasized. A summary of the review was sent to nine experts in the field of cervical manipulation and headache (an orthopedic surgeon, a neurosurgeon, two neurologists, a primary care physician, and four chiropractors). The panel members used a risk-benefit scale to rate the appropriateness of cervical manipulation in a wide-ranging list of 736 clinically detailed scenarios. Their opinions were collated and a conference was held with discussion of contentious points. After discussion, the panel re-rated all the scenarios, judging 82 as appropriate, 230 as uncertain, and 424 as inappropriate for cervical spine manipulation. While this review is over a decade old, it still seems to be the best guide (Shekelle and Coulter 1997).

Physical Therapy, Occupational Therapy, and Exercise (Established Knowledge)

The impact of chronic pain including migraine headache on daily life can be severe, even during the interictal periods (i.e., time between attacks) (Buse et al. 2007). Patients with chronic diseases with episodic manifestations such as migraine may remain in bed or do very little on days when pain is particularly severe, then compensate with intense over activity on days when they are pain free. This pattern of overexertion leads to a sense of frustration on the part of the patient and makes it difficult to participate reliably in work, social and vocational or educational activities.

Exercise improves physical functioning, may reduce BMI, and may reduce the somatic and cognitive experience of pain. Exercise can also have a beneficial impact on depression, anxiety, and quality of life, and help regulate sleep–wake cycles and appetite. A supervised physical therapy program of reconditioning and therapeutic exercise can provide benefit on many levels for patients who may not have the knowledge or motivation or who may not be physically capable of engaging in regular physical exercise on their own. A structured review of data on physical treatments for headache reported that physical therapy is more effective than massage therapy or acupuncture for the treatment of headache and is most effective when combined with other treatments such as biofeedback, relaxation training, and exercise (Biondi 2005).

Occupational therapists can help patients incorporate effective pain-management strategies into activities of everyday life. Specific strategies can include goal setting, group programs, pacing techniques, assertive communication, and the use of appropriate body mechanics during everyday activities and assistive devices or environmental modifications to support independent function. Both physical and occupational therapies are aimed at increasing patients' use of independent pain-management modalities and reducing disability and dependence on medication.

Massage (Current Research)

Little data exists on the efficacy of massage as a treatment for migraine. However, one study found that massage led to reduction in migraine frequency and improvement in sleep quality when compared to control participants (Lawler and Cameron 2006). The authors also observed beneficial effects on perceived stress and coping efficacy and noted that during sessions, massage induced decreases in state anxiety, heart rate, and cortisol.

Yoga (Current Research)

Yoga is an ancient Indian, nonreligious practice that includes breathing techniques, mindfulness, meditation, and building of strength, flexibility, and stamina through physical postures and routines. Many varieties exist. Hatha yoga, which focuses on breathing and postures, is one of the most commonly practiced forms of yoga. Yoga has been demonstrated to produce positive effects on such physiological measures as on heart rate, blood pressure, galvanic skin response, respiratory rate, fasting blood glucose, breath holding time, auditory and visual reaction times, and intraocular pressure (Ospina et al. 2007). Benefit has been demonstrated with a combined pharmacologic and yoga approach among chronic tension-type headache (Bhatia et al. 2007) and in a randomized trial among migraine sufferers (John et al. 2007). In fact, John et al. (2007) demonstrated that migraine sufferers enrolled in a 3-month yoga program demonstrated improvement in headache frequency, severity of migraine, pain factors, anxiety, and depression when compared with a self-care control group.

Other Therapies

Homeopathy (Current Research)

Four RCTs have been published of homeopathy in headache, mostly in migraine. They have been reviewed as a whole and the results felt to be saying that homeopathy is ineffective in headache (Ernst 1999). One out of four is very positive for homeopathy in headache (in this case migraine) in a conventional sense (Brigo and Serpelloni 1991). The authors randomized

60 patients to receive either homeopathy or placebo for 3 months. They demonstrated highly significant and clinically relevant reductions in frequency ($p = 0.0001$) and severity of headache and reduction in analgesic use. Three trials are negative, two in migraine (Straumsheim et al. 2000; Whitmarsh et al. 1997) and one in "chronic headache" (Walach et al. 1997) according to International Headache Society (IHS) trial criteria, which became available only after the first study was published. The view that they are entirely "negative" has been extensively criticized as too simple (see, e.g., Whitmarsh 2002b). When patient well-being outcomes are taken into account, rather than crude numbers of attacks per month (the main IHS criterion of effect of a treatment), three out of four trials show a positive result for homeopathy, including all the trials in migraine.

Outside the rarefied world of clinical trials, does homeopathy perform well in the real world? It would appear so. This question was addressed by an observational study of the quality of life in patients with headache receiving homeopathic treatment (Muscari-Tomaioli et al. 2001). The authors studied 53 patients with "chronic headache," a mix of migraine with and without aura and TTH. SF-36 health status questionnaires were filled in prospectively before treatment was commenced with classical homeopathy and again after 4–6 months. Results were compared and showed that all health dimensions statistically significantly improved, with marked improvements in pain and the strongest results being in the "bodily pain" and "vitality" parameters ($p < 0.0001$).

Another observational study has been performed from the headache clinic in Athens (Kivellos et al. 2009). Seventy-two migraineurs with a mean age of 32 years opted for homeopathy treatment. Thirty-one of them had previously had conventional treatment with tricyclic antidepressants or anti-epileptics and were regarded as "resistant." Headache Impact Test 6 (HIT-6) scores were 62 ± 4 (mean $\pm$ SD) at baseline and improved at 6 months to 47 ± 8 ($p < 0.0009$ Wilcoxon signed ranks test), which improvement persisted at 12-months (HIT-6 41 ± 7, $p < 0.0009$ vs. 6 months). Migraine severity (VAS) decreased by 71% and frequency by 80% at 12 months ($p < 0.0001$ for both comparisons vs. baseline). Mood too, was consistently better at 12 months according to patient self-report.

A larger prospective observational study in primary care (Witt et al. 2009) enrolled 230 adults and 74 children with "chronic headache," who were consecutive patients beginning homeopathic treatment and treated by 73 different physicians. They were followed for 2 years and kept records of complaint severity, quality of life (QoL), and medication use. The mean duration of headache in the adults was 9.3 years and in the children 2.44 years. Severity of complaints showed marked improvement in the first 3 months of treatment, continuing on to the end of the study. For headache, standardized effects (mean change divided by standard deviation at baseline) in adults was 1.63 (95% CI 1.78–1.49), 2.27 (2.45–2.09), and 2.44 (2.63–2.25) at 3, 12, and 24 months, respectively. In children, the standardized effects at these times were 1.67 (1.91–1.44), 2.55 (2.82–2.28), and 2.74 (3.03–2.46). The QoL among adults improved over time, but this improvement was not observed in the children. Use of conventional treatment and health service use decreased markedly. The authors comment that while this observational but uncontrolled study shows a consistent improvement in patients seeking homeopathic treatment because of headache (the vast majority already treated, usually conventionally) over 24 months, conclusions about the relationship between treatment and observed effect should not be drawn because of the trial design. Investigation of homeopathy in headache treatment perhaps is a good example of conventional methods not being necessarily always the best way to show the benefits to patients of nonconventional treatments.

Nutrition (Current Research)

Many foods have been reported idiosyncratically to trigger migraine (Peatfield et al. 1984) and most physicians routinely search for possible trigger factors of migraine, including dietary ones and counsel avoidance (Sun-Edelstein and Mauskop 2009). Foods often said to trigger attacks of migraine, such as cheese, chocolate, alcohol, and citrus fruit, have not generally been found in well-performed trials to in fact do so (Crawford and Simmons 2006). The idea of migraine as a food-allergic disorder has often been raised (Grant 1979). Evidence for this comes from notable improvements in headache frequency and/or severity after exclusion of various foods from the diet, followed by double-blind placebo controlled reintroductions of specific food triggers in pediatric (Egger et al. 1983) and adult (Cornwell and Clarke 1991) migraine. In the pediatric study, 85% of 98 migraine sufferers became headache-free following an elimination diet for 4 weeks. Sixty responders were then challenged in a double-blind trial with the offending foods and only redeveloped migraine with true foods, not with "sham" foods. Correlations of food-induced migraine with specific immunoglobulin E to foods implicated by dietary exclusion (by radioallergosorbent testing) (Munro et al. 1980) and with skin testing to dietary allergens (Mansfield et al. 1985) have been noted, along with a protective effect of sodium chromoglycate (Munro et al. 1984). Little has been published recently about research into dietary or food-allergic research in migraine, but it does seem to be an area that warrants further investigation.

A specific concern in headache management has been the role played by caffeine. This substance is frequently avoided by headache sufferers in one report of children and adolescents with chronic daily headache; overuse of caffeine in the form of cola drinks was held to be responsible for the headaches (Hering-Hanit and Gadoth 2003). Over a 5-year period in a tertiary headache clinic in a general hospital in Israel, the authors encountered 36 children and adolescents with daily or near-daily headache who were heavy consumers of cola drinks. The mean age of the subjects was 9.2 years (range 6–18) and the mean headache duration was 1.8 years (range 0.6–5). All were heavy cola-users and used at least 1.5 L of cola drinks per day (192.88 mg caffeine) and a mean of 11 L (range 10.5–21) of cola drinks per week, which is equivalent to 1414.5 mg caffeine (range 1350.1–2700.3). The patients were encouraged to withdraw gradually from the cola drinks, which resulted in complete cessation of headache in 33 subjects. The other three subjects continued to suffer from occasional migraine without aura attacks. The authors comment that withdrawal from these drinks can be achieved gradually without withdrawal headache and with the complete disappearance of the chronic daily headache. The authors very much implicate the caffeine in the drinks as the cause of the headache, but fizzy drinks contain many other ingredients and the headache might conceivably be due to other constituents. In this light, it is interesting to consider the report that a popular no-calorie sweetener, sucralose, can be responsible for triggering migraine (Patel et al. 2006).

Other Therapies

Reflexology (Current Research)

This therapy relies on the theoretical notion that all parts of the body and any dysfunction in them, including the head, are in some way reflected in "reflex zones" in the feet. The reflexologist examines the feet (especially the soles) and assesses the state of the tissues there.

Any changes in a reflex zone's state are held to reflect dysfunction in the organ represented, and the reflexologist attempts to change the organ's state with forms of pressure to the feet and relieve the dysfunction in the associated organ. In one study from Denmark, 220 patients with chronic headache were diagnosed by IHS criteria by a consultant physician (Launso et al. 1999): 76 (35%) had TTH, 41 (18%) had migraine, 42 (19%) had a mixture of both, and 61 (28%) were "undetermined." By their final treatment of a course of reflexology, 78% of the patients reported that they were "cured" with no more headaches (23%) or had experienced relief (55%). There was a concomitant reduction in use of conventional drugs.

Vagus Nerve Stimulation (Current Research)

Another therapy that has been tried in chronic, refractory migraine is vagus nerve stimulation (VNS). This does not come under the CAM banner, but is certainly not conventional! VNS is an effective treatment for drug-resistant epilepsy and possibly depression. There is one very small report of implanting VNS in four men and two women with disabling chronic cluster headache and migraine (Mauskop 2005). In one man and one woman with chronic migraine, VNS produced dramatic improvement with restoration of the ability to work. Two patients with chronic cluster had significant improvement of their headaches. So four out of six patients with otherwise intractable headache had a clinically very useful response and the author comments that VNS may be a useful option for chronic headache.

Conclusion

Biobehavioral and CAM therapies play an important role in the comprehensive care of the headache or migraine sufferer. Biobehavioral techniques such as CBT, biofeedback, and relaxation training have empirical evidence for their efficacy in headache management. Other CAM therapies have varying levels of empirical support, but may be popular with sufferers. It is incumbent upon people caring for those with headache to understand something of these therapies to be able to guide persons with migraine appropriately and also to help encourage trust so that interactions can be avoided. Decisions about their use should be made by HCPs and patients jointly taking into consideration potential benefits, risks, and costs.

Biobehavioral and CAM therapies may be used individually or in conjunction with mainstream pharmacological interventions. And in fact they may augment the effectiveness of other treatments, or minimize the need for their use. A combination of pharmacological approaches with certain non-pharmacological approaches has been demonstrated to be superior to either approach on its own, to help maintain positive outcomes and to improve treatment adherence.

Biobehavioral tools should be used prophylactically and practiced on a regular basis in order to maintain homeostasis and manage stress so that the patient does not trigger a headache attack in the first place. Patients can be taught ways to modify thoughts, feelings, and behaviors with CBT. They can be taught to manage the physiological effects of stress with biofeedback and relaxation training.

Some behavioral techniques can be incorporated by HCPs during an appointment (e.g., education, diaphragmatic breathing, and guided imagery), some can be self-taught and practiced by the patient (e.g., relaxation practice and stress management), and some require a referral to an appropriately trained professional (e.g., biofeedback training, CBT). In any case, educating and encouraging patients to train their physiology through biofeedback and relaxation, adopt healthy lifestyle habits, and recognize and mediate the effects of stress in their lives provides patients with a set of tools for headache management that will benefit them throughout their lifetime.

In daily practice, seeing headache sufferers, it is very helpful to have as wide a range of therapeutic options available as possible, both conventional and those less widely known and used, that have demonstrated efficacy and are safe and appropriate for the patient.

References

Anderson RE, Seniscal C (2006) A comparison of selected osteopathic treatment and relaxation for tension-type headaches. Headache 46(8):1273–1280

Andrasik F (2007) What does the evidence show? Efficacy of behavioural treatments for recurrent headaches in adults. Neurol Sci 28:S70–S77

Andrasik F, Flor H (2008) Biofeedback. In: Breivik H, Campbell WI, Nicholas MK (eds) Clinical pain management: practice and procedures, 2nd edn. Hodder & Stoughton, London, pp 153–166

Bandura A (1977) Self-efficacy: toward a unifying theory of behavioral change. Psychol Rev 84:191–215

Beck AT, Rush AJ, Shaw BF, Emery G (1979) Cognitive therapy of depression. Guilford, New York

Benson H (1975) The relaxation response. William Morrow, New York

Bernstein DA, Borkovec TD, Hazlett-Stevens H (2000) New directions in progressive relaxation training: a guidebook for helping professions. Praeger, Westport

Bhatia R, Dureja GP, Tripathi M, Bhattacharjee M, Bijlani RL, Mathur R (2007) Role of temporalis muscle over activity in chronic tension type headache: effect of yoga based management. Indian J Physiol Pharmacol 51(4):333–344

Bigal ME, Lipton RB (2006) Modifiable risk factors for migraine progression. Headache 46:1334–1343

Biondi DM (2005) Physical treatments for headache: a structured review. Headache 45(6):738–746

Blanchard EB, Andrasik F, Ahles TA et al (1980) Migraine and tension headache: a meta-analytic review. Behav Ther 14:613–631

Blum CL (2008) Chiropractic and stroke: what are our responsibilities? J Vertebr Subluxat Res 15 Jul 2008: 1–4

Boline PD, Kassack K, Bronfort G, Nelson C, Anderson AV (1995) Spinal manipulation vs. amitriptyline for the treatment of chronic tension-type headaches: a randomized clinical trial. J Manipulative Physiol Ther 18(3):148–154

Brigo B, Serpelloni G (1991) Homeopathic treatment of migraines: a randomized double-blind controlled study of sixty cases (homeopathic remedy versus placebo). Berlin J Res Homoeopath 1(2):98–106

British Medical Association (1993) Complementary medicine new approaches to good practice. Oxford University Press, Oxford

Bronfort G, Assendelft WJ, Evans R, Haas M, Bouter L (2001) Efficacy of spinal manipulation for chronic headache: a systematic review. J Manipulative Physiol Ther 24(7):457–466

Buse DC, Bigal ME, Rupnow MFT, Reed ML, Serrano D, Biondi DM, Hulihan JF, Lipton RB (2007) The migraine interictal burden scale (MIBS): results of a population-based validation study headache. Headache 47(5):778

Campbell JK, Penzien DB, Wall EM (25 Apr 2000) Evidence-based guidelines for migraine headache: behavioral and physical treatments. http://www.aan.com/professionals/practice/pdfs/g10089.pdf. Accessed Apr 2010

Cornwell N, Clarke L (1991) Dietary modification in patients with migraine and tension-type headache. Cephalalgia 11(Suppl 11):143–144

Crawford P, Simmons M (2006) What dietary modifications are indicated for migraines? J Fam Pract 55(1): 62–66

Diener HC (2008) Acupuncture for the treatment of headaches: more than sticking needles into humans? Cephalalgia 28:911–913

Egger J, Wilson J, Carter CM, Turner MW, Soothill JF (1983) Is migraine food allergy? A double-blind controlled trial of oligoantigenic diet treatment. Lancet 2:865–869

Eisenberg DM, Kessler RC, Foster C et al (1993) Unconventional medicine in the United States: prevalence, costs, and patterns of use. N Engl J Med 328(4):246–252

Eisenberg DM, Davis RB, Ettner SL et al (1998) Trends in alternative medicine use in the United States, 1990–1997. J Am Med Assoc 280:1569–1574

Ernst E (1999) Homeopathic prophylaxis of headaches and migraine? A systematic review. J Pain Symptom Manage 18(5):353–357

Ernst E, Mills S et al (1995) Complementary medicine – a definition (letter). Br J Gen Pract 48:506

Evans KW, Boan JA, Evans JL, Suaib A (1997) Economic evaluation of oral sumatriptan compared with oral caffeine ergotamine for migraine. Pharacoeconomics 12:565–577

Goslin RE, Gray RN, McCrory DC et al (1999) Behavioral and physical treatments for migraine headache. Technical review 2.2 (Prepared for the Agency for Health Care Policy and Research under Contract No 290-94-2025). http://wwwclinpolmcdue.edu. Accessed Apr 2010

Grant ECG (1979) Food allergies and migraine. Lancet 2:966–968

Grazzi L, Andrasik F, D'Amico D et al (2002) Behavioral and pharmacologic treatment of transformed migraine with analgesic overuse: outcome at three years. Headache 42:483–490

Haas M, Groupp E, Aickin M, Fairweather A, Ganger B, Attwood M et al (2004) Dose response for chiropractic care of chronic cervicogenic headache and associated neck pain: a randomized pilot study. J Manipulative Physiol Ther 27(9):547–553

Heath RL, Saliba M, Mahmassani O, Major SC, Khoury BA (2008) Locus of control moderates the relationship between headache pain and depression. J Headache Pain 9:301–308

Hering-Hanit R, Gadoth N (2003) Caffeine-induced headache in children and adolescents. Cephalalgia 23(5):332–335

Holroyd KA, Andrasik F (1982) A cognitive-behavioral approach to recurrent tension and migraine headache. In: Kendall PC (ed) Advances in cognitive-behavioral research and therapy, vol 1. Academic, New York, pp 275–320

Holroyd KA, Penzien DB (1990) Pharmacological versus non-pharmacological prophylaxis of recurrent migraine headache: a meta-analytic review of clinical trials. Pain 42:1–13

Holroyd KA, Holm JE, Hursey KG et al (1988) Recurrent vascular headache: home-based behavioral treatment versus abortive pharmacological treatment. J Consult Clin Psychol 56:218–223

Holroyd KA, France JL, Cordingley GE et al (1995) Enhancing the effectiveness of relaxation-thermal biofeedback training with propranolol hydrochloride. J Consult Clin Psychol 63:327–330

Holroyd KA, O'Donnell FJ, Stensland M, Lipchik GL, Cordingley GE, Carlson BW (2001) Management of chronic tension-type headache with tricyclic antidepressant medication stress management therapy and their combination: a randomized controlled trial. J Am Med Assoc 285:2208–2215

Holroyd KA, Drew JB, Cottrell CK, Romanek KM, Heh V (2007) Impaired functioning and quality of life in severe migraine: the role of catastrophizing and associated symptoms. Cephalalgia 27:1156–1165

Hurwitz EL, Aker PD, Adams AH, Meeker WD, Shekelle PG (1996) Manipulation of the cervical spine. A systematic review of the literature. Spine 21:1746–1760

Jacobson E (1938) Progressive relaxation. University of Chicago Press, Chicago

Jena S, Witt CM, Brinkhaus B, Wegscheider K, Willich SN (2008) Acupuncture in patients with headache. Cephalalgia 28(9):969–979

John PJ, Sharma N, Sharma CM, Kankane A (2007) Effectiveness of yoga therapy in the treatment of migraine without aura: a randomized controlled trial. Headache 47(5):654–661

Kivellos S, Papilas K, Karageorgiou K, Vithoulkas G (2009) Observational prospective study of homeopathic treatment in patients with migraine. Cephalalgia 29:107

Launso L, Brendstrup E, Arnberg S (1999) An exploratory study of reflexological treatment for headache. Altern Ther Health Med 5(3):57–65

Lawler SP, Cameron LD (2006) A randomized controlled trial of massage therapy as a treatment for migraine. Ann Behav Med 32(1):50–59

Linde K, Streng A, Jurgens S, Hoppe A, Brinkhaus B, Witt C, Wagenpfeil S, Pfaffenrath V, Hammes MG, Weidenhammer W, Willich S, Melchart D (2005) Acupuncture for patients with migraine: a randomized controlled trial. J Am Med Assoc 293(17):2118–2125

Linde K, Allais G, Brinkhaus B, Manheimer E, Vickers A, White AR (2009a) Acupuncture for migraine prophylaxis. Cochrane Database Syst Rev 21 Jan 2009(1):CD001218

Linde K, Allais G, Brinkhaus B, Manheimer E, Vickers A, White AR (2009b) Acupuncture for tension-type headache. Cochrane Database Syst Rev 21 Jan 2009(1):CD007587

Mansfield LE, Vaughan TR, Waller SF, Haverly RW, Ting S (1985) Food allergy and migraine, double-blind and mediator confirmation of an allergic aetiology. Ann Allergy 55:126–129

Mathew NT (1981) Prophylaxis of migraine and mixed headache: a randomized controlled study. Headache 21:105–109

Mauskop A (2001) Alternative therapies in headache. Is there a role? Med Clin North Am 85(4):1077–1084

Mauskop A (2005) Vagus nerve stimulation relieves chronic refractory migraine and cluster headaches. Cephalalgia 25(2):82–86

Munro J, Carini C, Brostoff J, Zilkha K (1980) Food allergy in migraine. Study of dietary exclusion and RAST. Lancet 2:1–4

Munro J, Carini C, Brostoff J (1984) Migraine is a food-allergic disease. Lancet 2:719–721

Muscari-Tomaioli G, Allegri F, Miali E, Pomposelli R, Tubai P, Targhetta A et al (2001) Observational study of quality of life in patients with headache, receiving homeopathic treatment. Br Homeopathic J 90(4):189–197

Nestoriuc Y, Martin A (2007) Efficacy of biofeedback for migraine: a meta-analysis. Pain 128:111–127

Nestoriuc Y, Martin A, Rief W, Andrasik F (2008a) Biofeedback treatment for headache disorders: a comprehensive efficacy review. Appl Psychophysiol Biofeedback 33:125–140

Nestoriuc Y, Rief W, Martin A (2008b) Meta-analysis of biofeedback for tension-type headache: efficacy specificity and treatment moderators. J Consult Clin Psychol 76:379–396

Nicholson RA, Penzien D, McCrory DC et al (2004) Behavioral therapies for migraine (protocol). Cochrane Database Syst Rev (1):CD004601. doi:101002/14651858CD004601

Nicholson RA, Nash JM, Andrasik F (2005) A self-administered behavioral intervention using tailored messages for migraine. Headache 45:1124–1139

NIH Consensus Conference (1998) Acupuncture. J Am Med Assoc 280(17):1518–1524

Ospina MB, Bond K, Karkhaneh M et al (2007) Meditation practices for health: state of the research (AHRQ). Evid Rep Technol Assess Jun 2007(155):1–263

Patel RM, Sarma R, Grimsley E (2006) Popular sweetener sucralose as a migraine trigger. Headache 46(8):1303–1304

Peatfield RC, Glover V, Littlewood JT, Sandler M, Clifford-Rose F (1984) The prevalence of diet-induced migraine. Cephalalgia 4:179–183

Penzien DB, Holroyd KA (1994) Psychosocial interventions in the management of recurrent headache disorders – II: description of treatment techniques. Behav Med 20:64–73

Penzien DB, Johnson CA, Carpenter DE, Holroyd KA (1990) Drug vs behavioral treatment of migraine: long-acting propranolol vs home-based self-management training. Headache 30:300

Penzien DB, Rains JC, Andrasik F (2002) Behavioral management of recurrent headache: three decades of experience and empiricism. Appl Psychophysiol Biofeedback 27:163–181

Pryse-Phillips WE, Dodick DW, Edmeads JG, Gawel MJ, Nelson RF, Purdy RA, Robinson G, Stirling D, Worthington I (1998) Guidelines for the nonpharmacologic management of migraine in clinical practice. Can Med Assoc J 159:47–54

Rains JC, Lipchik GL, Penzien DB (2006a) Behavioral facilitation of medical treatment for headache – part I: review of headache treatment compliance. Headache 46:1387–1394

Rains JC, Penzien DB, Lipchik GL (2006b) Behavioral facilitation of medical treatment for headache – part II: theoretical models and behavioral strategies for improving adherence. Headache 46:1395–1403

Rime C, Andrasik F (2007) Relaxation techniques and guided imagery. In: Waldman SD (ed) Pain management, vol 2. Saunders/Elsevier, Philadelphia, pp 1025–1032

Rossi P, Di Lorenzo G, Malpezzi MG, Faroni J, Cesarino F, Di Lorenzo C et al (2005) Prevalence, pattern and predictors of use of complementary and alternative medicine (CAM) in migraine patients attending a headache clinic in Italy. Cephalalgia 25(7):493–506

Rossi P, Di Lorenzo G, Faroni J, Malpezzi MG, Cesarino F, Nappi G (2006) Use of complementary and alternative medicine by patients with chronic tension-type headache: results of a headache clinic survey. Headache 46(4):622–631

Schabert E, Crow WT (2009) Impact of osteopathic manipulative treatment on cost of care for patients with migraine headache: a retrospective review of patient records. J Am Osteopath Assoc 109(8):403–407

Scharff L, Marcus DA, Turk DC (1996) Maintenance of effects in the nonmedical treatment of headaches during pregnancy. Headache 36:285–290

Schwartz MS, Andrasik F (2003) Biofeedback: a practitioner's guide, 3rd edn. Guilford, New York

Shekelle PG, Coulter I (1997) Cervical spine manipulation: summary report of a systematic review of the literature and a multidisciplinary expert panel. J Spinal Dis 10:223–228

Smith WS, Johnston SC, Skalabrin EJ, Weaver M, Azari P, Albers GW et al (2003) Spinal manipulative therapy is an independent risk factor for vertebral artery dissection. Neurology 60(9):1424–1428

Sovak M, Kunzel M, Sternbach RA, Dalessio DJ (1981) Mechanism of the biofeedback therapy of migraine: volitional manipulation of the psychophysiological background. Headache 21:89–92

Spence DS, Thompson EA, Barron SJ (2005) Homeopathic treatment for chronic disease: a 6-year, university-hospital outpatient observational study. J Altern Complement Med 11(5):793–798

Straumsheim P, Borchgrevink C, Mowinckel P, Kierulf H, Hafslund O (2000) Homeopathic treatment of migraine: a double blind, placebo controlled trial of 68 patients. Br Homeopathic J 89(1):4–7

Sun-Edelstein C, Mauskop A (2009) Foods and supplements in the management of migraine headaches. Clin J Pain 25(5):446–452

Task Force on Promotion and Dissemination of Psychological Procedures (1995) Training in and dissemination of empirically-validated psychological treatments: report and recommendations. Clin Psychol 48:3–23

Tindle HA, Davis RB, Phillips RS, Eisenberg DM (2005) Trends in use of complementary and alternative medicine by US adults: 1997–2002. Altern Ther Health Med 11(1):42–49

Tuchin PJ, Pollard H, Bonello R (2000) A randomized controlled trial of chiropractic spinal manipulative therapy for migraine. J Manipulative Physiol Ther 23(2):91–95

Vernon HT (1995) The effectiveness of chiropractic manipulation in the treatment of headache: an exploration of the literature. J Manipulative Physiol Ther 18:611–617

Vernon H, Jansz G, Goldsmith CH, McDermai C (2009) A randomized, placebo-controlled clinical trial of chiropractic and medical prophylactic treatment of adults with tension-type headache: results from a stopped trial. J Manipulative Physiol Ther 32(5):344–351

Vickers AJ, Rees RW, Zollman CE, McCarney R, Smith CM, Ellis N, Fisher P, Van Haselen R (2004) Acupuncture for chronic headache in primary care: large, pragmatic, randomized trial. Br Med J 328:744

von Peter S, Ting W, Scrivani S, Korkin E, Okvat H, Gross M, Oz C, Balmaceda C (2002) Survey on the use of complementary and alternative medicine among patients with headache syndromes. Cephalalgia 22(5):395–400

Walach H, Jonas WB (2002) Homeopathy. In: Lewith G, Jonas WB, Walach H (eds) Clinical research in complementary therapies. Principles, problems and solutions. Churchill Livingstone, Edinburgh, pp 793–798

Walach H, Haeusler W, Lowes T, Mussbach D, Schamell U, Springer W et al (1997) Classical homeopathic treatment of chronic headaches. Cephalalgia 17(2):119–126

Whitmarsh TE (1999) The role of complementary therapies in headache treatment. In: Goadsby G, Dowson AJ, Miles A (eds) The effective management of headache. Aesculapius Medical Press, London

Whitmarsh TE (2002a) The nature of evidence in complementary and alternative medicine: ideas from trials of homeopathy in headache. In: Callahan D (ed) The role of complementary and alternative medicine. Georgetown University Press, Washington, DC

Whitmarsh T (2002b) Survey on the use of complementary and alternative medicine among patients with headache syndromes (editorial). Cephalalgia 22(5): 331–332

Whitmarsh TE, Coleston-Shields DM, Steiner TJ (1997) Double-blind randomized placebo-controlled study of homoeopathic prophylaxis of migraine. Cephalalgia 17(5):600–604

Whorton JC (1999) The history of complementary and alternative medicine. In: Jonas WB, Levin JS (eds) Essentials of complementary and alternative medicine. Lippincott, Williams & Wilkins, Philadelphia

Witt CM, Ludtke R, Willich SN (2009) Homeopathic treatment of chronic headache (ICD-9: 784.0) – a prospective observational study with 2-year follow-up. Forsch Komplementärmed 16(4):227–235

Wonderling D, Vickers AJ, Grieve R, McCarney R (2004) Cost effectiveness analysis of a randomized trial of acupuncture for chronic headache in primary care. Br Med J 328:747

Yucha C, Gilbert C (2004) Evidence-based practice in biofeedback and neurotherapy. Association for Applied Psychophysiology and Biofeedback, Wheat Ridge

Ziliak ST, McCloskey DN (2008) The cult of statistical significance. How the standard error cost us jobs, justice and lives. The University of Michigan Press, Ann Arbor

53 Magnesium, Vitamins and Herbal Preparations

Alexander Mauskop[1] · *Christina Sun-Edelstein*[2]
[1]New York Headache Center, New York, NY, USA
[2]Centre for Clinical Neurosciences and Neurological Research,
St Vincent's Hospital, Melbourne, Australia

Paolo Martelletti, Timothy J. Steiner (eds.), *Handbook of Headache*, DOI 10.1007/978-88-470-1700-9_53,
© Lifting The Burden 2011

Abstract: Headache patients frequently seek alternatives to traditional acute and preventative treatments, given the side effects often associated with conventional medications. In this chapter, the available evidence for the use of magnesium, coenzyme Q_{10} (CoQ_{10}), riboflavin, butterbur, feverfew, and alpha lipoic acid in migraine prevention are reviewed. Areas of ongoing research, particularly in pharmacogenetics, are also discussed. Although further research with large-scale randomized controlled trials (RCTs) is necessary to better clarify the efficacy of these vitamins, supplements, and herbal preparations, we recommend the consideration of oral magnesium supplementation in migraineurs in whom there is clinical suspicion of magnesium deficiency, given its safety and tolerability. Butterbur is also recommended for migraine prophylaxis given the positive results from two randomized controlled trials. Though the clinical efficacy data for feverfew, CoQ_{10}, riboflavin, and alpha lipoic acid are equivocal, these substances may also be considered in patients who express an interest in alternative treatments.

Established Knowledge

Introduction

In recent years, there has been a surge in interest in alternative treatment options for common disorders such as headache. Traditional medications are often expensive or associated with side effects, and are not always effective. As a result, patients frequently seek safe, efficacious, and inexpensive alternatives, either to augment or replace their conventional medications. Vitamins, supplements, and herbal preparations are appealing in that they appear more "natural" and therefore less toxic than traditional medications. Furthermore, they are often perceived to be more helpful than conventional care for the treatment of headache and neck and back conditions (Eisenberg et al. 2001). Many users of alternative treatments do not disclose their use of these treatments, believing that their physicians would not understand or incorporate nontraditional therapies into their medical treatment plan (Rossi et al. 2005; Eisenberg et al. 2001). An understanding and awareness of complementary and alternative options has therefore become an important aspect of headache management for physicians.

In this chapter, the existing evidence for the use of magnesium, CoQ_{10}, riboflavin, butterbur (*Petasites hybridus*), feverfew, and alpha lipoic acid in migraine prophylaxis are reviewed. Areas of ongoing research, particularly in pharmacogenetics, are also discussed.

Magnesium

Magnesium and Migraine Pathophysiology

Magnesium, an essential cation that plays a vital role in multiple physiological processes, may be involved in several different aspects of migraine pathogenesis. Magnesium deficiency has been associated with cortical spreading depression (Mody et al. 1987), neurotransmitter release (Coan and Collingridge 1985), platelet aggregation (Baudouin-Legros et al. 1986), and vasoconstriction (Altura and Altura 1982, 1989), all of which are important elements of our current understanding of migraine pathophysiology. Its concentration influences serotonin receptors, nitric oxide synthesis and release, inflammatory mediators, and various other migraine-related receptors and neurotransmitters (Bianchi et al. 2004). Magnesium also plays a role in the control of vascular tone and reactivity to endogenous hormones and neurotransmitters, via its relationship with the NMDA receptor (Turlapaty and Altura 1980; Altura et al. 1987). Deficiency in magnesium also facilitates the generation and release of substance P (Weglicki and Phillips 1992), which subsequently acts on sensory fibers and produces headache pain (Moskowitz 1984).

Magnesium Deficiency

In addition to its role in migraine pathogenesis, magnesium deficiency can be seen in any chronic medical illness, including cardiovascular disease, diabetes, pre-eclampsia, eclampsia, sickle cell disease, and chronic alcoholism. Symptoms of low magnesium include premenstrual syndrome, leg muscle cramps, coldness of extremities, weakness, anorexia, nausea, digestive disorders, lack of coordination, and confusion.

Although a relationship between magnesium deficiency and migraine had been speculated for years, the lack of simple and reliable ways of measuring magnesium content in soft tissues made it difficult to clarify the association. Inconsistent results were attributed to the use of total magnesium levels, since it is the ionized form of magnesium (IMg^{2+}) which truly reflects disturbed magnesium metabolism (Altura et al. 1992). However, the development of a specific ion-selective electrode for magnesium has allowed the accurate and rapid measurement of serum ionized magnesium levels (Altura et al. 1992, 1994).

A pilot study of 40 patients with an acute migraine attack found that 50% of the patients had low levels of ionized magnesium (Mauskop et al. 1995). In these patients, basal serum IMg^{2+} level correlated with the efficacy of 1 g of intravenous magnesium in treating an attack (Mauskop et al. 1995; Mauskop et al. 1996). Of the patients in whom pain relief was sustained over 24 h, 89% had a low serum IMg^{2+} level; only 16% of patients who had no relief had a low IMg^{2+} level. However, total magnesium levels in all subjects were within normal limits.

Migraine has been associated with a systemic magnesium deficiency, as inferred from a study (Trauninger et al. 2002) showing that increased magnesium retention occurred in migraineurs when compared to normal controls after oral loading with 3,000 mg of magnesium lactate (the magnesium load test) during a 24 h interictal period. Low levels of magnesium in the brain (Ramadan et al. 1989) and cerebrospinal fluid (Jain et al. 1985) have also been reported, but interictal studies on serum (Gallai et al. 1992; Sarchielli et al. 1992; Schoenen et al. 1991; Thomas et al. 1992; Mauskop et al. 1993), plasma (Facchinetti et al. 1991; Smeets et al. 1994), and intracellular (Gallai et al. 1993, 1994; Schoenen et al. 1991; Thomas et al. 1992; Facchinetti et al. 1991; Smeets et al. 1994) magnesium levels in migraineurs and patients with tension-type headache have yielded inconsistent results. However, interictal levels of red blood cell (RBC) magnesium have been shown to be decreased in migraineurs with (Gallai et al. 1993) and without aura (Schoenen et al. 1991; Facchinetti et al. 1991), as well as in juvenile migraine patients with and without aura (Soriani et al. 1995). These results were corroborated by a study (Thomas et al. 2000) which showed low total magnesium in erythrocytes and low ionized magnesium in lymphocytes in migraine patients, both of which increased significantly after a 2-week trial of drinking mineral water containing 110 mg/l magnesium. Given its commercial availability, the RBC magnesium assay may therefore be a better way of assessing for deficiency, since serum magnesium levels are unreliable, except when low.

Treatment with Oral Magnesium

Three double-blind RCTs have shown therapeutic efficacy of Mg^{2+} supplementation in headache patients. In the first, oral magnesium supplementation in 24 women with menstrual migraine yielded positive results (Facchinetti et al. 1991). Subjects in the treatment group received 360 mg of magnesium pyrrolidone carboxylic acid in three divided doses. Women received 2 cycles of study medication, taken daily from ovulation to the first day of flow. Results showed a significant reduction in the number of days with headache ($p < 0.1$) and the total pain index ($p > 0.03$), as well as an improvement of the Menstrual Distress Questionnaire score in the treatment group compared to placebo.

A larger study of 81 patients with migraine headaches also showed a significant improvement in patients on active therapy (Peikert et al. 1996). Attack frequency was reduced by 41.6% in the magnesium group and by 15.8% in the placebo group. The active treatment group received 600 mg of trimagnesium dicitrate in a water-soluble granular powder taken every morning. Most recently, Koseoglu et al. (2008) studied the prophylactic effects of 600 mg/day of oral magnesium citrate supplementation in patients with migraine without aura and found that active treatment resulted in a significant decrease in migraine attack frequency and severity. A fourth RCT showed no effect of oral magnesium on migraine (Pfaffenrath et al. 1996). This negative result has been attributed to the use of a poorly absorbed magnesium salt, since diarrhea occurred in almost half of patients in the treatment group.

The most common adverse effect associated with oral magnesium supplementation is diarrhea, and patients should be cautioned about this possibility. Magnesium toxicity is rare in patients with normal renal function. It is marked by the loss of deep tendon reflexes followed by muscle weakness. Severe toxicity can lead to cardiac muscle weakness, respiratory paralysis, and death (Mauskop and Altura 1998).

Magnesium and Menstrually Related Migraine

Magnesium deficiency may be especially common in women with menstrually related migraine. A clinical study by Facchinetti et al. (1991) showed that women with menstrual migraine reported a significant decrease in headache days, and an improvement in the Menstrual Distress Questionnaire Score, after receiving treatment with oral magnesium. A prospective study (Mauskop et al. 2002) with 270 women, 61 of whom had menstrually related migraine, showed that the incidence of IMg^{2+} deficiency was 45% during menstrual attacks, 15% during nonmenstrual attacks, 14% during menstruation without a migraine, and 15% between menstruations and between migraine attacks.

Treatment with Intravenous Magnesium

Intravenous magnesium has been used in the treatment of acute migraine with inconsistent results. In the pilot study (Mauskop et al. 1995) described under "*Magnesium Deficiency*" a strong correlation between the clinical response and the levels of serum IMg^{2+} was found ($p < 0.01$). Though the study was not double-blinded or placebo-controlled, both the researchers and subjects were blinded to the IMg^{2+} levels. A subsequent study (Mauskop et al. 1996) showed that 1 g of magnesium sulfate resulted in rapid headache relief in patients with low serum IMg^{2+} levels.

In a single-blind RCT involving 30 patients with moderate to severe migraine attacks (Demirkaya et al. 2001), treatment with 1 g intravenous magnesium sulfate was superior to placebo in terms of both response rate (100% for magnesium sulfate vs. 7% for placebo) and pain-free rate (87% for magnesium sulfate and 0% for placebo). Mild side effects including flushing and a burning sensation in the face and neck were common, but did not require discontinuation of treatment. Furthermore, none of the subjects reported headache recurrence during the 24 h after treatment. Bigal et al. (2002), in a double-blind RCT, showed that 1 g of magnesium sulfate resulted in a statistically significant improvement in pain and associated symptoms compared with controls in subjects with migraine with aura. Though migraine without aura patients did not show a significant difference in pain relief compared to those receiving placebo, they did have a significantly lower intensity of photophobia and phonophobia.

Two RCTs have been conducted in emergency room settings, neither of which showed that magnesium was more effective than placebo in aborting attacks (Corbo et al. 2001; Cete et al. 2005).

Supplements and Mitochondrial Dysfunction

Mitochondrial dysfunction, which leads to impaired oxygen metabolism, has been speculated to play a role in migraine pathophysiology (Koo et al. 1993; Lanteri-Minet and Desnuelle 1996), as migraineurs have been shown to have reduced mitochondrial phosphorylation potential in between headaches (Bresolin et al. 1991; Montagna et al. 1994a). This is the basis for the use of supplements that enhance mitochondrial function in the treatment of migraine, such as riboflavin, coenzyme Q_{10}, and alpha lipoic acid.

Riboflavin

Riboflavin, also known as vitamin B2, is a precursor for flavin mononucleotides that are cofactors in the electron transport chain of the Krebs cycle. It plays an essential role in membrane stability and the maintenance of energy-related cellular functions. One well-designed RCT evaluating the use of riboflavin in migraine prophylaxis was positive, showing that daily use of 400 mg riboflavin for 3 months resulted in a 50% reduction in attacks in 59% of patients, compared to 15% for placebo. Two minor adverse reactions, diarrhea and polyuria, were reported in the treatment group (Schoenen et al. 1998).

Coenzyme Q_{10}

Coenzyme Q_{10} (CoQ_{10}) is an endogenous enzyme cofactor made by all cells in the body. It is a component of the mitochondrial electron transport chain, and generates energy via its involvement in aerobic cellular respiration. Two small studies have demonstrated some benefit effects in the treatment of migraine. The first, an open-label study (Rozen et al. 2002) in which 31 patients with migraine used 150 mg daily of CoQ_{10} for 3 months, found that 61% had at least a 50% reduction in migraine days without significant adverse events. Supplementation was effective within the first month of therapy. Later, a small RCT (Sandor et al. 2005) evaluating the efficacy of 100 mg of CoQ_{10} three times daily in 42 subjects showed that CoQ_{10} significantly decreased attack frequency, headache days, and days with nausea. Gastro-intestinal disturbances and "cutaneous allergy" were reported at a low rate.

Although there are no RCTs on CoQ_{10} in children, supplementation may be especially effective in the treatment of pediatric migraine. CoQ_{10} levels were measured in a study (Hershey et al. 2007) of 1,550 patients (mean age 13.3 ± 3.5 years) with frequent headaches, and found that nearly a third of subjects were below the reference range. Supplementation with 1–3 mg/kg per day of CoQ_{10} in liquid gel capsule formulation resulted in a significant improvement in total CoQ_{10} levels, headache frequency, and degree of headache disability.

Alpha Lipoic Acid

Alpha lipoic acid (also known as thioctic acid) is another compound that enhances mitochondrial oxygen metabolism and ATP production (Matalon et al. 1984). It has been evaluated as a migraine preventative treatment in one open pilot study (unpublished data, discussed in Magis et al. 2007) and one small RCT (Magis et al. 2007) thus far. In the RCT, 54 subjects received either 600 mg alpha lipoic acid or placebo daily for 3 months. The nonsignificant results were attributed to the underpowered nature of the study. However, there was a clear trend for reduction of migraine frequency after treatment with alpha lipoic acid. Within-group analyses also showed a significant reduction in attack frequency, headache days, and headache severity in the treatment group.

Herbal Preparations

Butterbur

Over the past decade, *Petasites hybridus* root extract, also known as butterbur, has emerged as a promising new treatment in migraine prevention. The butterbur plant is a perennial shrub found throughout Europe and parts of Asia, and was used in ancient times for its medicinal properties. Though its mechanism of action is not fully understood, *Petasites* likely acts through calcium channel regulation and inhibition of peptide-leukotriene biosynthesis, thereby influencing the inflammatory cascade associated with migraine (Eaton 1998; Sheftell et al. 2000; Pearlman and Fisher 2001). While the butterbur plant itself contains pyrrolizidine alkaloids which are hepatotoxic and carcinogenic, these compounds are removed in the commercially available preparations, such as Petadolex®.

Several studies have been conducted to evaluate the efficacy of *Petasites hybridus* in the prevention of migraine. In the first RCT (Grossman and Schmidrams 2000), 50 mg of Petadolex twice daily showed a significantly reduced number of migraine attacks and migraine days per month compared to placebo. However, due to flawed statistical analyses, an independent re-analysis of efficacy criteria (Diener et al. 2004) was undertaken, which confirmed the superiority of the butterbur extract over placebo for all primary variables of efficacy. Subsequently, a three-arm, parallel-group, RCT of 245 patients comparing *Petasites* extract 75 mg twice daily, *Petasites* extract 50 mg twice daily, and placebo twice daily (Lipton et al. 2004) showed that the higher dose of *Petasites* extract was more effective than placebo in decreasing the number of monthly migraine attacks.

A multicenter prospective open-label study (Pothmann and Danesch 2005) of Petodolex in 109 children and adolescents with migraine resulted in 77% of all patients reporting a reduction in migraine frequency of at least 50%. Ninety-one percent of participants felt substantially or at least slightly improved after four months of treatment. More recently, a prospective, partly double-blind, RCT assessing the efficacy of Petadolex and music therapy in primary school children with migraine (Oelkers-Ax et al. 2008) showed that at 6-month follow-up, both music therapy and butterbur root extract were superior to placebo ($p = 0.018$ and $p = 0.044$, respectively) in reducing headache frequency, but only among those that completed the study. In the analysis including all treated patients, treatment groups did not differ significantly during follow-up.

Petadolex was well tolerated in all of the above studies, and no serious adverse events occurred. The most frequently reported adverse reactions were mild gastrointestinal events, especially eructation (burping).

Feverfew

Feverfew is a herbal preparation that was used in Europe for centuries in the treatment of fevers, headache, inflammation, and arthritis. It is currently available as the dried leaves of the weed plant *tanacetum pathenium*, and may act in migraine prophylaxis by inhibiting both platelet aggregation as well as the release of serotonin from platelets and white blood cells. Feverfew may also have anti-inflammatory action via the inhibition of prostaglandin synthesis and phospholipase A (Heptinstall et al. 1985, 1987; Pugh and Sambo 1988; Makheja and Bailey 1982). Anti-migraine activity is likely to be related to the parthenolides within the leaves.

Several RCTs have been conducted over the past decades with conflicting results (Johnson et al. 1985; Murphy et al. 1988; Kuritzky et al. 1994; De Weerdt et al. 1996; Palevitch et al. 1997; Vogler et al. 1998). Furthermore, a 2004 Cochrane review (Pittler and Ernst 2004) of double-blind RCTs assessing the clinical efficacy and safety of feverfew in migraine prevention concluded that there was insufficient evidence to suggest that feverfew is more effective than placebo in migraine prophylaxis. No major safety or tolerability issues were identified.

However, given that inconsistencies in study results were thought to be related to wide variations in the strength of the active ingredient (parthenolide) (Draves and Walker 2003) and differences in the stability of feverfew preparations (Willigmann and Freudenstein 1998), a new, more stable feverfew extract (MIG-99) was evaluated in a RCT involving 147 patients (Pfaffenrath et al. 2002). Although none of the doses were significant for the primary endpoint, a subset of patients with a high frequency of migraine attacks did seem to benefit. In a follow-up multicenter RCT with 170 subjects (Diener et al. 2005), randomized to 6.25 mg TID of MIG-99 or placebo, a statistically significant and clinically relevant reduction in migraine frequency in the MIG-99 group compared to placebo was reported.

Side effects reported in the RCTs include gastrointestinal disturbances, mouth ulcers, and a "post-feverfew syndrome" of joint aches.

Treatment Summary

Further research with large-scale RCTs is needed to better clarify the efficacy of vitamins and supplements in the treatment of migraine. However, based on the available information, our recommendations are as follows:

- Oral magnesium supplementation should be considered in migraineurs in whom there is clinical suspicion of magnesium deficiency, given its safety and tolerability. Daily treatment with 400 mg of chelated magnesium, magnesium oxide, or slow-release magnesium is recommended in patients with premenstrual syndrome, cold extremities, and leg or foot muscle cramps. Higher doses of up to 1,000 may be required and tolerated in some cases, although diarrhea may limit increased dosing.

- We use intravenous magnesium for acute treatment of migraine, where it has been effective in up to 50% of patients in our experience. Intravenous treatment is also an option for patients who cannot tolerate or absorb oral magnesium supplementation. Monthly (often premenstrual) prophylactic infusions of 1 g of magnesium sulfate offer substantial benefit to some patients as well.

- *Petasites hybridus*, or butterbur, is recommended for migraine prophylaxis given the positive results from 2 RCTs. The dosage is 75 mg twice daily.

- Coenzyme Q_{10} 300 mg or riboflavin 400 mg daily may be a good option for some patients, having shown benefit in 1 RCT.

- Though the clinical efficacy data pertaining to feverfew, and alpha lipoic acid are equivocal, these substances may be considered in patients who express an interest in alternative treatments.

Current Research

Current research on the use of vitamins and supplements appears to be moving forward in the field of pharmacogenetics. Drawing from reports of mitochondrial DNA mutations in migraineurs with stroke episodes (Majamaa et al. 1997; Ojaimi et al. 1998), previous 31P magnetic resonance spectroscopy studies showing an interictal impairment of mitochondrial oxidative phosphorylation in migraineurs (Welch et al. 1989; Barbiroli et al. 1992, Montagna et al. 1994b), and other studies showing that enhancers of oxidative phosphorylation such as riboflavin have preventative efficacy in migraine (Schoenen et al. 1998; Boehnke et al. 2004), a recent pharmacogenetic study (DiLorenzo et al. 2009) demonstrated that riboflavin may be more effective in the treatment of migraine patients with non-H mitochondrial DNA haplotypes. Given that riboflavin is effective in deficiencies of the electron transport chain complex I (Penn et al. 1992; Bernsen et al. 1993), the authors hypothesized that mitochondrial haplogroups differentially influence the activity of the various complexes. They further hypothesized that these results may have ethnic implications, since haplogroup H is predominantly found in the European population.

Supplementation with B vitamins, especially folate (vitamin B9), may have a future role in migraine prevention. Decreased folate and elevated homocysteine (folate is a cofactor in homocysteine metabolism) have been associated with some forms of ischemic vascular disease, endothelial dysfunction, and congenital abnormalities of the heart and neural tube (De Bree et al. 2002; Hobbs et al. 2005). Taking into account the comorbidity of migraine and stroke (Tzourio et al. 1993; Merikangas et al. 1997; Kurth 2007) and the presumed role of homocysteine in the disruption of vascular endothelial function, it has been speculated that elevated homocysteine may be involved in the pathophysiology underlying migraine and stroke. Homocysteine is metabolized via a B12- dependent enzyme methylenetretrahydrofolate reductase (MTHFR) or a B6-dependent pathway (Wang et al. 2007) and therefore elevated levels can be decreased by vitamin supplementation with folate, vitamin B12, and vitamin B6. Supplementation with these vitamins has already been shown to reduce the risk of stroke, and of the three vitamins, folate is thought to play the primary role (Wang et al. 2007). In addition, a polymorphism in the MTHFR gene (MTHFRC677T), specifically the TT genotype, has been associated with an increased risk of migraine with aura (Rubino et al. 2009; Scher et al. 2006).

Recently, a RCT assessing daily vitamin supplementation with 2 mg folic acid, 25 mg vitamin B6, and 400 µg of vitamin B12 for 6 months was undertaken to ascertain the effects on homocysteine levels and migraine disability, frequency, and severity in 52 patients with migraine with aura. The relationship between MTHFRC677T genotype and treatment response was also assessed (Lea et al. 2009). Vitamin supplementation resulted in a reduction of homocysteine levels by 39%, as well as a marked decrease in severe migraine disability, headache frequency, and pain severity. The treatment effect on both homocysteine levels and migraine disability was associated with the MTHFRC677T genotype in that carriers of the C allele showed a greater response when compared to those of TT genotypes. Treatment was well tolerated with no adverse events reported. DiRosa et al. (2007), in a small, open-labeled study of children with migraine, found that 6 months of daily treatment with 5 mg of folic acid resulted in a complete resolution of migraine attacks in 60% of patients and a reduction of headaches in the remaining subjects.

Gingkolide B, a herbal constituent extract from ginkgo biloba tree leaves, was recently shown to be effective in reducing both aura frequency and duration in a multicenter, open, preliminary trial (D'Andrea et al. 2009). Fifty women with migraine with aura or migraine aura without headache received Migrasoll®, a combination of 60 mg ginkgo biloba terpenes phytosome and very low concentrations of CoQ_{10} and vitamin B2. In addition to a significant decrease in attack frequency and duration, 42.2% of subjects experienced a total disappearance of aura by the end of the treatment period (4 months). Its mechanism of action in migraine therapy may relate to its modulation of gluamate's excitatory effect on the central nervous system (CNS), thus inhibiting cortical spreading depression (Bryn et al. 2004), its inhibition of platelet activating factor (Nogami et al. 1997), or its activity against the formation and deposition of free radicals in the CNS (Droy-Lefaix and Doly 1992).

Conclusions

Alternative treatments for migraine, including vitamins, supplements, and herbal preparations, have gained increased attention in recent years as more and more patients seek options outside the realm of conventional medications. While some of these therapies have demonstrated benefit in relatively small RCTs, the implementation of large-scale studies is necessary in order to better establish their efficacy and gain wider acceptance among physicians accustomed to using traditional treatments. Other future goals include the identification and investigation of other potential alternative treatments for headache management and the establishment of biomarkers that can assist in the development of these therapies.

References

Altura BT, Altura BM (1982) The role of magnesium in etiology of strokes and cerebrovasospasm. Magnesium 1:277–291

Altura BT, Altura BM (1989) Withdrawal of magnesium causes vasospasm while elevated magnesium produced relaxation of tone in cerebral arteries. Neurosci Lett 20:323–327

Altura BM, Altura BT, Carella A, Gebrewold A, Murakawa T, Nishio A (1987) Mg^{2+}- Ca^{2+} interaction in contractility of vascular smooth muscle: Mg^{2+}

versus organic calcium channel blockers on myogenic tone and agonist-induced responsiveness of blood vessels. Can J Physiol Pharmacol 65:729–745

Altura BT, Shirley T, Young CC, Dell'Ofrano K, Handwerker SM, Altura BM (1992) A new method for the rapid determination of ionized Mg^{2+} in whole blood, serum and plasma. Meth Find Exp Clin Pharmacol 14:297–304

Altura BT, Shirley TL, Young CC, Dell'Ofrano K, Hiti J, Welsh R, Yeh Q, Barbour RL, Altura BM (1994) Characterization of a new ion selective electrode for ionized magnesium in whole blood, plasma, serum and aqueous samples. Scand J Clin Lab Invest Suppl 54(217):21–36

Barbiroli B, Montagna P, Cortelli P et al (1992) Abnormal brain and muscle energy metabolism shown by 31P magnetic resonance spectroscopy in patients affected by migraine with aura. Neurology 42: 1209–1214

Baudouin-Legros M, Dard B, Guichency P (1986) Hyperreactivity of platelets from spontaneously hypertensive rats role of external magnesium. Hypertension 8:694–699

Bernsen PL, Gabreels FJ, Ruitenbeek W, Hamburger HL (1993) Treatment of complex I deficiency with riboflavin. J Neurol Sci 118:181–187

Bianchi A, Salomone S, Caraci F et al (2004) Role of magnesium, coenzyme Q10, riboflavin, and vitamin B12 in migraine prophylaxis. Vitam Horm 69:297–312

Bigal ME, Bordini Ca, Tepper SJ, Speciali JG (2002) Intravenous magnesium sulphate in the acute treatment of migraine without aura and migraine with aura. A randomized, double-blind, placebo-controlled study. Cephalalgia 22:345–353

Boehnke C, Reuter U, Flach U et al (2004) High-dose riboflavin treatment is efficacious in migraine prophylaxis- an open study in a tertiary care centre. Eur J Neurol 11:475–477

Bresolin N, Martinelli P, Barbiroli B et al (1991) Muscle mitochondrial DNA deletion and 31P-NMR spectroscopy alterations in a migraine patient. J Neurol 104:182–189

Bryn W, Coran MH, Schultz PG, Rimbach G, Krucker T (2004) Age-related effect of ginkgo biloba on synaptic plasticity and excitability. Neurobiol Aging 25:955–962

Cete Y, Dora B, Ertan C, Ozdemir C, Oktay C (2005) A randomized prospective placebo-controlled study of intravenous magnesium sulphate vs. metoclopramide in the management of acute migraine attacks in the emergency department. Cephalalgia 25:199–204

Coan EJ, Collingridge GL (1985) Magnesium ions block an N-methyl D-aspartate receptor-mediated component of synaptic transmission in rat hippocampus. Neurosci Lett 53:21–26

Corbo J, Esses D, Bijur PE, Iannaccone R, Gallagher EJ (2001) Randomized clinical trial of intravenous magnesium sulfate as an adjunctive medication for emergency department treatment of migraine headache. Ann Emerg Med 38:621–627

D'Andrea G, Bussone G, Allais G et al (2009) Efficacy of ginkgolide B in the prophylaxis of migraine with aura. Neurol Sci 30(Suppl 1):S121–S124

De Bree A, Verschuren WM, Kromhout D et al (2002) Homocysteine determinants and the evidence to what extent homocysteine determines the risk of coronary heart disease. Pharmacol Rev 54:599–618

De Weerdt CJ, Bootsma HPR, Hendricks H (1996) Herbal medicines in migraine prevention: randomized double-blind placebo-controlled crossover trial of feverfew preparation. Phytomedicine 3:225–230

Demirkaya S, Vural O, Dora B, Topcuoglu MA (2001) Efficacy of intravenous magnesium sulfate in the treatment of acute migraine attacks. Headache 41:171–177

Di Rosa G, Attina S, Spano M et al (2007) Efficacy of folic acid in children with migraine, hyperhomocysteinemia and MTHFR polymorphisms. Headache 47:1342–1344

Diener HC, Rahlfs VW, Danesch U (2004) The first placebo-controlled trial of a special butterbur root extract for the prevention of migraine: reanalysis of efficacy criteria. Eur Neurol 51:89–97

Diener HC, Pfaffenrath V, Schnitker J, Friede M, Henneicke-von Zepelin HH (2005) Efficacy and safety of 6.25 mg t.i.d. feverfew CO2-extract (MIG-99) in migraine prevention- a randomized, double-blind, multicentre, placebo-controlled study. Cephalalgia 25(11):1031–1041

DiLorenzo C, Pierelli F, Coppola G et al (2009) Mitochondrial DNA haplogroups influence the therapeutic response to riboflavin in migraineurs. Neurology 72:1588–1594

Draves AH, Walker SE (2003) Parthenolide content of Canadian commercial feverfew preparations: label claims are misleading in most cases. Can Pharm J RPC 136:23–30

Droy-Lefaix MT, Doly M (1992) EGb 761, a retinal free-radical scavenger. In: Christen Y, Constantin J, Lacour M (eds) Effect of ginkgo biloba extract (EGb 761) and central nervous system. Elsevier, Paris

Eaton J (1998) Butterbur, herbal help for migraine. Nat Pharm 2:23–24

Eisenberg DM, Kessler RC, Van Rompay MI, Kaptchuk TJ, Wilkey SA, Appel S, Davis RB (2001) Perceptions about complementary therapies relative to conventional therapies among adults who use both: results from a national survey. Ann Intern Med 135:344–351

Facchinetti F, Sances G, Borella P, Genazzani AR, Nappi G (1991) Magnesium prophylaxis of menstrual migraine: effects on intracellular magnesium. Headache 31:298–301

Gallai V, Sarchielli P, Costa G et al (1992) Serium and salivary magnesium levels in migraine results in a group of juvenile patients. Headache 32:132–135

Gallai V, Sarchielli P, Morucci P, Abbritti G (1993) Red blood cell magnesium levels in migraine patients. Cephalalgia 13:94–98

Gallai V, Sarchielli P, Morucci P, Abbritti G (1994) Magnesium content of monomuclear blood cells in migraine patients. Headache 34:160

Grossman M, Schmidrams H (2000) An extract of Petasites hybridus is effective in the prophylaxis of migraine. Int J Clin Pharmacol Ther 38:430–435

Heptinstall S, White A, Williamson L, Mitchell JRA (1985) Extracts of feverfew inhibit granule secretion in blood platelets and polymorphonuclear leukocytes. Lancet 1:1071–1074

Heptinstall S, Goenewegen WA, Spangenberg P, Loesche W (1987) Extracts of feverfew may inhibit platelet behaviour via neutralisation of suphydryl groups. J Pharm Pharmacol 39:459–465

Hershey AD, Powers SW, Vockell AB et al (2007) Coenzyme Q10 deficiency and response to supplementation in pediatric and adolescent migraine. Headache 47:73–80

Hobbs CA, Cleves MA, Melnyk S et al (2005) Congenital heart defects and abnormal maternal biomarkers of methionine and homocysteine metabolism. Am J Clin Nutr 81:147–153

Jain AC, Sethi NC, Balbar PK (1985) A clinical electroencephalographic and trace element study with special reference to zinc, copper and magnesium in serum and cerebrospinal fluid (CSF) in cases of migraine. J Neurol Suppl 232:161

Johnson ES, Kadam NP, Hylands DM, Hylands PJ (1985) Efficacy of feverfew as prophylactic treatment of migraine. Br Med J 291:569–573

Koo B, Becker LE, Chuang S et al (1993) Mitochondrial encephalomyopathy, lactic acidosis, stroke-like episodes (MELAS): clinical, radiological, pathological, and genetic observations. Ann Neurol 34:25–32

Koseoglu E, Talashoglu A, Gonul AS, Kula M (2008) The effects of magnesium prophylaxis in migraine without aura. Magnes Res 21:101–108

Kuritzky A, Elhacham Y, Yerushalmi Z, Hering R (1994) Feverfew in the treatment of migraine: its effect on serotonin uptake and platelet activity. Neurology 44(Suppl 2):293 P

Kurth T (2007) Migraine and ischaemic vascular events. Cephalalgia 27:965–975

Lanteri-Minet M, Desnuelle C (1996) Migraine and mitochondrial dysfunction. Rev Neurol 152: 234–238

Lea R, Colson N, Quinlan S, Macmillan J, Griffiths L (2009) The effects of vitamin supplementation and MTHFR (C677T) genotype on homocysteine-lowering and migraine disability. Pharmacogenet Genomics 19:422–428

Lipton RB, Gobel H, Einhaupl KM, Wilks K, Mauskop A (2004) Petsites hybridus root (butterbur) is an effective preventive treatment for migraine. Neurology 63:2240–2244

Magis D, Ambrosini A, Sandor P et al (2007) A randomized double-blind placebo-controlled trial of thioctic acid in migraine prophylaxis. Headache 47:52–57

Majamaa K, Turkka J, Karppa M, Winqvist S, Hassinen IE (1997) The common MELAS mutation A3243G in mitochondrial DNA among young patients with an occipital brain infarct. Neurology 49:1331–1334

Makheja AM, Bailey JM (1982) A platelet phospholipase inhibitor from the medicinal herb feverfew (Tanacetum parthenium). Prostaglandins Leukot Med 8:653–660

Matalon R, Tumpf DA, Kimberlee M et al (1984) Lipoamide dehydrogenase deficiency with primary lactic acidosis: favorable response to treatment with oral lipoic acid. J Pediatr 104:65–69

Mauskop M, Altura BM (1998) Magnesium for migraine: rationale for use and theapeutic potential. CNS Drugs 9:185–190

Mauskop A, Altura BT, Cracco RQ, Altura BM (1993) Deficiency in serum in ionized magnesium but not total magnesium in patients with migraines. Possible role of ICa^{2+}/IMg^{2+} ratio. Headache 33:135–138

Mauskop A, Altura BT, Cracco RQ et al (1995) Intravenous magnesium sulfate relieves migraine attacks in patients with low serum ionized magnesium levels: a pilot study. Clin Sci 89:633–636

Mauskop A, Altura BT, Cracco RQ, Altura BM (1996) Intravenous magnesium sulfate rapidly alleviates headaches of various types. Headache 36:154–160

Mauskop A, Altura BT, Altura BM (2002) Serum ionized magnesium levels and serum ionized calcium/ionized magnesium ratios in women with menstrual migraine. Headache 42:242–248

Merikangas KR, Fenton BT, Cheng SH, Stolar MJ, Risch N (1997) Association between migraine and stroke in a large-scale epidemiological study of the United States. Arch Neurol 54:362–368

Mody I, Lambert JD, Heinemann U (1987) Low extracellular magnesium induces epileptiform activity and spreading depression in rat hippocampal slices. J Neurophysiol 57:869–888

Montagna P, Cortell P, Barbiroli B (1994a) Magnetic resonance spectroscopy studies in migraine. Cephalalgia 14:184–193

Montagna P, Cortelli P, Monari L et al (1994b) 31P magnetic resonance spectroscopy in migraine without aura. Neurology 44:666–669

Moskowitz MA (1984) The neurobiology of vascular head pain. Ann Neurol 16:157–168

Murphy JJ, Heptinstall S, Mitchell JR (1988) Randomised double-blind placebo-controlled trial of feverfew in migraine prevention. Lancet 2:189–192

Nogami K, Hirashima Y, Endo S, Takaku A (1997) Involvement of platelet-activating factor (PAF) in glutamate neurotoxicity in rat neuronal cultures. Brain Res 754:72–78

Oelkers-Ax R, Leins A, Parzer P, Hillecke T, Bolay HV, Fischer J, Bender S, Hermanns U, Resch F (2008) Butterbur root extract and music therapy in the prevention of childhood migraine: an explorative study. Eur J Pain 12:301–313

Ojaimi J, Katsabanis S, Bower S et al (1998) Mitochondrial DNA in stroke and migraine with aura. Cerebrovasc Dis 8:102–106

Palevitch D, Earon G, Carasso R (1997) Feverfew (Tanacetum parthenium) as a prophylactic treatment for migraine: a placebo-controlled doulbe-blind study. Phytother Res 11:508–511

Pearlman EM, Fisher S (2001) Preventive treatment for childhood and adolescent headache: role of once-daily montelukast sodium. Cephalalgia 21:461

Peikert A, Wilimzig C, Kohne-Volland R (1996) Prophylaxis of migraine with oral magnesium: results from a prospective, multi-center, placebo-controlled and double-blind randomized study. Cephalalgia 16:257–263

Penn AMW, Lee JWK, Thuillier P et al (1992) MELAS syndrome with mitochondrial tRNALeu (UUR) mutation: correlation of clinical state, nerve conduction, and muscle 31P magnetic resonance spectroscopy during treatment with nicotinamide and riboflavin. Neurology 42:2147–2152

Pfaffenrath V, Wessely P, Meyer C et al (1996) Magnesium in the prophylaxis of migraine-A double-blind, placebo-controlled study. Cephalalgia 16:436–440

Pfaffenrath V, Diener HC, Fisher M, Friede M, Henneicke-von Zepelin HH (2002) The efficacy and safety of Tanacetum parthenium (feverfew) in migraine prophylaxis- a double-blind, multicentre, randomized placebo-controlled dose-response study. Cephalalgia 22:523–532

Pittler MH, Ernst E (2004) Feverfew for preventing migraine. Cochrane Database Syst Rev 1:CD002286

Pothmann R, Danesch U (2005) Migraine prevention in children and adolescents: results of an open study with a special butterbur root extract. Headache 45:196–203

Pugh WH, Sambo K (1988) Prostaglandin synthetase inhibitors in feverfew. J Pharm Pharmacol 40:743–745

Ramadan NM, Halvorson H, Vande-Linde A et al (1989) Low brain magnesium in migraine. Headache 29:590–593

Rossi P, Di Lorenzo G, Malpezzi MG et al (2005) Prevalence, pattern and predictors of use of complementary and alternative medicine (CAM) in migraine patients attending a headache clinic in Italy. Cephalalgia 25:493–506

Rozen TD, Oshinsky ML, Gebeline CA, Bradley KC, Young WB, Schechter AL, Silberstein SD (2002) Open label trial of Coenzyme Q10 as a migraine preventive. Cephalalgia 22:137–141

Rubino E, Ferrero M, Rainero I et al (2009) Association of the C677T polymorphism in the MTHFR gene with migraine: a meta-analysis. Cephalalgia 29:818–825

Sandor PS, DiClemente L, Coppola G, Saenger U, Fumal A, Magis D, Seidel L, Agosti RM, Schoenen J (2005) Efficacy of coenzyme Q10 in migraine prophylaxis: a randomized controlled trial. Neurology 64:713–715

Sarchielli P, Coata G, Firenze C, Morucci P, Abbritti G, Gallai V (1992) Serum and salivary magnesium levels in migraine and tension-type headache. Results in a group of adult patients. Cephalalgia 12:21–27, 42

Scher AI, Terwindt GM, Verschuren WMM et al (2006) Migraine and MTHFRC677T genotype in a population-based sample. Ann Neurol 59:372–375

Schoenen J, Sianard-Gainko J, Lenaerts M (1991) Blood magnesium levels in migraine. Cephalalgia 11:97–99

Schoenen J, Jacquy J, Lanaerts M (1998) Effectiveness of high-dose riboflavin in migraine prophylaxis. Neurology 50:466–470

Sheftell F, Rapoport A, Weeks R, Walker B, Gammerman I, Baskin S (2000) Montelukast in the prophylaxis of migraine: a potential role for leukotriene modifiers. Headache 40:158–163

Smeets MC, Vernooy CB, Souverjin JHM, Ferrari MD (1994) Intracellular and plasma magnesium in familial hemiplegic migraine and migraine with and without aura. Cephalalgia 14:29–32

Soriani S, Arnaldi C, De Carlo L et al (1995) Serum and red blood cell magnesium levels in juvenile migraine patients. Headache 35:14–16

Thomas J, Thomas E, Tomb E (1992) Serum and erythrocyte magnesium concentrations and migraine. Magnes Res 5:127–130

Thomas J, Millot JM, Sebille S, Delabroise AM et al (2000) Free and total magnesium in lymphocytes of migraine patients- effect of magnesium-rich mineral water intake. Clin Chim Acta 295:64–75

Trauninger A, Pfund Z, Koszegi T, Czopf J (2002) Oral magnesium load test in patients with migraine. Headache 42:114–119

Turlapaty PDMV, Altura BM (1980) Magnesium deficiency produces spasms of coronary arteries: relationship to etiology of sudden death ischemic heart disease. Science 208:198–200

Tzourio C, Iglesias S, Hubert JB et al (1993) Migraine and risk of ischaemic stroke: a case-control study. BMJ 307:289–292

Vogler BK, Pittler BK, Ernst E (1998) Feverfew as a preventive treatment for migraine: a systematic review. Cephalalgia 18:704–708

Wang X, Qin X, Demirtas H et al (2007) Efficacy of folic acid supplementation in stroke prevention: a meta-analysis. Lancet 369:1876–1882

Weglicki WB, Phillips TM (1992) Pathobiology of magnesium deficiency: a cytokine/neurogenic inflammation hypothesis. Am J Physiol 263(pt 2): R734–R737

Welch KM, Levine SR, D'Andrea G, Schultz LR, Helpern JA (1989) Preliminary observations on brain energy metabolism in migraine studied by in vivo phosphorus 31 NMR spectroscopy. Neurology 39:538–541

Willigmann I, Freudenstein J (1998) Production of a stable feverfew (Tanadetum parthenium) extract as an active substance for a pharmaceutical product. In: Poster symposium. Society for Medicinal Plant Research, Vienna

54 Traditional Treatments for Headache

Redda Tekle Haimanot[1] · *Sheng–Yuan Yu*[2] · *K. Ravishankar*[3] ·
Mario Fernando Prieto Peres[4] · *Luiz Paulo Queiroz*[5]
[1]Addis Ababa University, Addis Ababa, Ethiopia
[2]Chinese PLA General Hospital, Beijing, People's Republic of China
[3]The Headache and Migraine Clinic, Joslok Hospital and Research Center,
Lilavati Hospital and Research Center, Mumbai, India
[4]Universidade Federal de São Paulo, São Paulo, Brazil
[5]Universidade Federal de Santa Catarina, Florianópolis, Brazil

Paolo Martelletti, Timothy J. Steiner (eds.), *Handbook of Headache*, DOI 10.1007/978-88-470-1700-9_54,
© Lifting The Burden 2011

Abstract: Traditional remedies for headache are widely practiced throughout the world. They appear to be more popular in Africa, Asia, and South America. In this chapter, the different methods used traditionally to manage headache in these parts of the world are described by experienced experts in the field. In China, acupuncture and herbs constitute the main approaches while in India Ayurveda, homeopathy, yoga, head massage, herbs, and dietary remedies are commonly used. In Africa and Ethiopia in particular, herbal medication, cauterization, and cupping with or without bloodletting are often employed to traditionally treat different type of headaches. In South America, medicinal plants appear to dominate although spiritual therapy is also getting more and more popular. The increasing use of secretion from frog has also been reported in Brazil. The chapter has also interesting descriptions of the traditional beliefs and hypotheses on the causation of headache as perceived by various cultures in different countries.

What comes out of the various experiences is the wide use of traditional remedies in headache treatment worldwide. In terms of herbal medication, it is evident that different ingredients and dosage are prescribed to different patients. Dosages are often not standardized and therefore have the potential risks of harmful side effects. In addition, the use of traditional methods to treat any symptom of headache could delay the diagnosis and management of serious conditions such as meningitis and other intracranial pathologies.

The popularity of traditional medicine is so significant that some countries particularly in Africa are working toward integrating effective and safe traditional remedies into their national health-care systems. The World Health Organization (WHO) is coordinating such efforts so that safety is not compromised when traditional remedies are popularized.

Introduction

Headache is a very common and universally recognized medical condition. The approach to its treatment reflects cultural diversity. The socioeconomic development and literacy level of a community influences on how headache is perceived and medical treatment sought. In rural societies, the symptoms of headache may be ignored or suppressed. In these communities, traditional treatment may be the only option. Moreover, despite the availability of modern medicine, many people may rely more on traditional medical practice because of its cultural acceptability, easy accessibility, and affordability.

According to World Health Organization (WHO) in some Asian and African countries, 80% of the population depends on traditional medicine for primary health care. Herbal medicines are the commonest in use and the most lucrative. Traditional medicine can treat various infections and conditions. For instance, the new antimalarial drug, artemisinin was developed from *Artemisia annua* L., a plant used in China for almost 2,000 years. Unfortunately, counterfeit, poor quality, or adulterated herbal products in international markets present serious safety threats to patients (WHO 2000). Traditional African medical practice involving herbalists, diviners, and midwives is culturally deep rooted and popular. However, within this extensive practice there are misdiagnosis of diseases and the dangers of toxic side effects. As a result, attempts are being made in some African countries to regulate and integrate traditional medicine into the national health delivery system and WHO has formulated a strategy to address the issue (WHO 2002).

This chapter deals with the different types of traditional treatments employed for headache in different parts of the world. Traditional Chinese and Indian (Ayurveda) medicines are the most ancient and still the most widely used. A great deal of scientific research and evidence-based investigation has been carried out on Chinese traditional medicine. Indian Ayurveda needs more work in this scientific field while very little research has been published on African and South American traditional medicine for headache. The five authors' chapter will present overviews of Chinese, Indian, African, and South American traditional treatments employed for headache. The Chinese approach of using acupuncture and herbs is described together with some insight into our modern understanding of their mechanism of action.

Chinese Traditional Treatments

Although medications remain the mainstay therapy for headache, the patients also continue to suffer discomfort and interference with activities of daily life. Moreover, adverse effects of medications may lead to limitations of drug therapy. Acupuncture and Chinese herbs are Chinese traditional medicine for treating headaches that have been widely used in clinical practice for over 3,000 years. This chapter focuses on the history and traditional Chinese theory, modern mechanism, and clinical practice of acupuncture and Chinese herbs, providing some information about their state and challenge.

Acupuncture

History and Traditional Chinese Theory of Acupuncture

Acupuncture and Chinese herbal medicine comprise a system of health care that originated in China more than 3,000 years ago. Traditional Chinese medicine is based on the Chinese concept of energy balancing where there are two forces within the body that require balance in order to achieve health. The two forces are commonly referred to as *Yin* (negative) and *Yang* (positive). The aim of treatment with acupuncture is to restore the body systems to balance between *Yin* and *Yang* via inserting acupuncture needles to influence the flow of *QI* (pronounced "chee"), which circulates and flow through 12 organs and 12 meridians of the body. The 359 classic acupoints are distributed along these meridians (Ernst 2006). The *QI* circulates within the deeper organs and connects to the superficial skin via acupoints. Therefore, the stimulation of specific acupoints can influence flow of *QI* in the meridians and in the organs. In the state of a normal healthy body, a balance exists between these organs. When injury, disease, emotional trauma, or infection occurs, the natural flow of *QI* may be affected and altered. If *QI* is blocked, it would result in pain and inflammation. The stimulation of relevant acupoints is supposed to dissolve *QI* blockage.

Modern Views on the Mechanism of Acupuncture

Modern medical research suggests that the mechanism of acupuncture treatment of headache is multifaceted and multi-leveled and includes the following. (1) Acupuncture has a good analgesic effect. It may increase pain thresholds by regulating the secretion of endogenous opioids that play a role in analgesic effects. It has been determined that endogenous opioids, such as endorphins, enkephalin, and dynorphin, can bind to opiate receptors in brain and nerve endings to cause analgesic effects and regulate human emotions (Takeshige et al. 1992; Guyton and Hall 2001). Some studies have shown that acupuncture could increase the level of enkephalin and dynorphin in plasma (Yu et al. 1997) and the central nervous system (Chen et al. 1996; Fu 2000). The enhanced enkephalin was correlated with increased pain threshold and the block of pain transmission. It has been observed that the increased enkephalin in the reticular paragigantocellularis (RPGC) during acupuncture could bind to opiate receptors at the endings of nociceptive primary afferents, suppress the release of substance P (SP) from these terminals, and result in a block of pain transmission (Yu et al. 1985; Raj 1986). Besides stimulation of RPGC in rats by acupuncture, there is also an increase in beta endorphin and leucine encephalin secretion, which play an important role in acupuncture analgesia (Zhao 1995). (2) Acupuncture can improve oxygen metabolism and blood flow in the brain. Single photon emission computed tomography scan (SPECT), brain perfusion imaging, and magnetoencephalography have shown that during stimulation of some acupoints, blood flow in the contralateral cerebral cortex and thalamus, ipsilateral basal ganglia, bilateral cerebellum, and also local activities of brain function have a trend of increase. This suggests that acupuncture can have a good effect on regulation of blood flow in the cerebral cortex (Wang and Jia 1996; Dhond et al. 2007). Migraine often causes cerebral vasomotor dysfunction. Acupuncture can improve cerebral blood flow and change the blood supply to brain tissue, which may be the role of acupuncture in helping to alleviate migraine. (3) Acupuncture can improve metabolic disorder. It has been observed that acupuncture application causes changes in the concentrations of K^+, Na^+, Mg^{2+}, and Ca^{2+} in the neurons (Deng 1995; Demirkaya et al. 2001). The recent studies showed that the biochemical changes are associated with the pathogenesis of migraine. Mg^{2+} deficiency has been implicated in the pathogenesis of migraine and tension-type headache (Altura and Altura 2001; Demirkaya et al. 2001; Zhao and Stillman 2003). During treatment of migraine attacks with 1 g intravenous magnesium sulfate, the pain disappeared in 13 patients (86.6%), diminished in 2 patients (13.4%), and accompanying symptoms disappeared in all 15 patients (100%) (Demirkaya et al. 2001). (4) Acupuncture has a good anti-inflammatory effect (Yu et al. 1995; Yu et al. 1996). A study has shown that acupuncture could play a role in modulation of neurogenic inflammation by release of endorphins, which exert an anti-inflammatory effect and analgesia (Ceccherelli et al. 2002). (5) Affecting the immune system. It has been determined that the levels of interleucin-2, interferon gamma, and the activity of natural killer cells of the spleen are increased by applied acupuncture (Yu et al. 1997; Yu et al. 1998).

Clinical Practice of Acupuncture

Acupuncture has been widely used in treating headaches around the world, but its effectiveness is still controversial. Many trials and numerous systematic reviews of acupuncture have recently become available. A systematic review (Melchart et al. 2002) by the Cochrane Collaborative published in 2002 identified 16 randomized studies on true acupuncture and migraine. In 11 of 16 migraine studies, the effectiveness of true acupuncture was compared with sham acupuncture, including number of days with headache, frequency of attacks, and attack intensity. Most studies reported differences in favor of acupuncture for at least one outcome. In five studies, the effects of acupuncture were significantly better than placebo. Three studies showed trends in favor of acupuncture, while two studies found no significant difference between true and sham acupuncture. The remaining one study was inconclusive due to the high dropout rate during the study. The author's overall conclusion about that the majority of the migraine studies showed at least a trend in favor of true acupuncture. This review suggests the effectiveness of acupuncture for treating headaches needed further study. A recent systematic review, less available and accessible in the West (Sun and Gan 2008), demonstrated that acupuncture is an effective treatment for headache. Specifically, acupuncture is superior to sham with a significantly higher response rate in patients with migraine and tension-type headache, and a significantly reduced headache intensity at late follow-up. Interestingly, subgroup analysis found that acupuncture is more effective in reducing headache intensity than sham in tension-type headache, but it did not provide the same positive result for migraine. When compared with pharmacological and waiting list options, acupuncture was also more effective for reducing headache intensity and frequency. Moreover, the Cochrane review of 22 trials in 2009 (Linde et al. 2009) showed acupuncture is effective in the prophylaxis of migraine. Six trials compared acupuncture to no prophylactic treatment or routine care only. After 3–4 months, patients receiving acupuncture had higher response rates and fewer headaches. Four trials compared acupuncture to proven prophylactic drug treatment. The authors conclude that acupuncture is at least as effective as, or possibly more effective than, prophylactic drug treatment, and has fewer adverse effects and that acupuncture should be considered a treatment option for patients willing to undergo this treatment. However, there are also some opposite opinions. For example, a review of 57 trials in Japanese from 1978 to 2006 showed that there is limited evidence that acupuncture is more effective than no treatment, and inconclusive evidence that trigger point acupuncture is more effective than placebo, sham acupuncture, or standard care (Itoh et al. 2007). Furthermore, a recent systematic review with meta-analysis of randomized, controlled trials suggested that acupuncture compared with sham for tension-type headache has limited efficacy for the reduction of headache frequency (Davis et al. 2008). Researchers have noted that the results of investigations of acupuncture as a treatment for migraine are difficult to interpret. Many researchers have pointed out that some aspects of the studies need to be further improved, including complete understanding of the physiological effects of acupuncture, identification of suitable sham or placebo treatments, standardization of acupoint selection and treatment course among randomized, clear adequacy of acupuncture "dose," the effective blinding of participants, more scientific researches and international cooperation, and so on (Davis et al. 2008; Kelly 2009).

Chinese Herbs

Basics of Traditional Chinese Medicine

Traditional Chinese medicine has been a frequent therapy for headache for thousands of years. The treatment of Chinese medicine is based on *Yin-Yang* and *Zang-Fu* theories. Chinese herbs are used to balance the body. For instance, when the cause of headache is disharmony of the liver system (diagnosed according to Chinese medicine), the principle of treatment is to balance the flow of liver *QI*. The Chinese herbs *Chuan gong, Tian Ma, Gou Teng, Du Li* in combination with other herbs are commonly used (Song and Hao 2001). The prescription is based on specific symptoms of each patient as well as the experience of each practitioner. The duration of Chinese herbal treatment is usually 1–2 months and also depends on individual patient's condition. Chinese herbal medicine is a traditional Chinese therapy for headache and is very powerful in balancing the body. It has been observed that Chinese herbs can significantly reduce the pain intensity, shorten the time of headache attacks, reduce the frequency of the headache, and prevent the attack of headache.

The Mechanism of Traditional Chinese Herbs

The mechanism of action of traditional Chinese herbs on headache has not been worked out, although limited studies show it perhaps includes the following.

Regulating Neurotransmitters

Tou Feng capsule can block the decreased concentration of 5-HT, norepinephrine (NE), and dopamine (DA) in the brain of a rat migraine model, to keep the level of neurotransmitters up, and improve blood flow in the brain (Yao et al. 2002). Some studies showed that *Xue Fu Zhu Yu Tang* (Li 2006), *Headache Power* (Song and Hao 2001), and *oral compound Gastrodia* (Lu et al. 2004) can prolong blood clotting time, increase pain threshold, and result in relieving migraine symptoms.

Regulating Neuropeptide

It has been observed that in a rat model of migraine using nitroglycerin, *Tong Xin Luo Capsule* can downregulate expression of calcitonin gene-related peptide (CGRP) mRNA in brainstem and trigeminal ganglion (Yang et al. 2006) and *Tou Feng capsule* decreases CGRP and histamine in rat serum (Yao et al. 2001). CGRP is known to correlate with headache.

Regulating Expression of C-Fos and C-Jun

Several recent trails show that *Tong Feng Yin* inhibits the increased expression of c-fos and c-jun (Ren et al. 2000), and *Xiao Yao Di Bi Liquid* blocks the increased expression of c-fos in rat brainstem and hypothalamus in a model of migraine using nitroglycerin (Hu et al. 2004).

Regulating Function of Blood Vessel

Da Chuan Gong Wan, which is commonly used to treat headache in China, can inhibit excessive dilation of cerebral blood vessels caused by nitrous oxide (NO) (Yang et al. 2005).

Clinical Practice of Traditional Chinese Herbs

The traditional Chinese herbal medicine for headache treatment can be divided into oral drug (i.e., single herb and many herbs together) and topical drug (e.g., herbal fumigation and injecting to acupoints), but many herbs together have been mainly used in clinical practice. For example, it is reported that 32 cases of migraine were treated with the mixture *Yang Xue Chu Feng Tong Luo Tang* (Huang et al. 2003), which consists of: *Dang Gui* and *Ge Gen*, 15 g each, *Bai Shao, Chuan Xiong, Qiang Huo*, and *Tu Yuan*, 30 g each, *Sheng Di*, 20 g, *Jing Jie, Fang Feng, Bai Zhi, Tao Ren, Hong Hua*, and *Di Long*, 10 g each, and *Xi Xin*, 6 g. If there was accompanying nausea and vomiting, *Ban Xia* and *Wu Zhu Yu* were added. If there were heart palpitations and insomnia, *Shi Chang Pu* and stir-fried *Suan Zao Ren* were added. If there was scanty *QI*, bodily vacuity, and lack of strength, *Huang Qi* and *Dang Shen* were added. One packet of these medicinals was decocted in water and administered per day in two divided doses, morning and evening. Ten days equaled one course of treatment, and outcomes were analyzed after three successive courses (i.e., *at* 30 days). Cure was defined as complete disappearance of the headaches and all accompanying symptoms with no recurrence within half a year. Marked effect was defined as basic disappearance of headaches and accompanying symptoms with one to two recurrences. Improvement was defined as a decrease in the severity of the headaches and three to five recurrences. No effect meant that there was no improvement in the headache. Based on these criteria, 24 cases were judged cured, 6 cases showed a marked effect and the duration of the headache recurrences was short, and 2 cases improved. Therefore, the author concluded that those herbs can effectively treat migraine.

Many traditional Chinese medicine products have now been made from the traditional Chinese herbs as raw materials, in order that they can be easily taken. The commonly used products are *Zhen Tian capsule, Tian Shu capsule, Tou Tong Ning capsule, Yang Xue Qing Nao granules, Tong Tian oral liquid,* and so on. One study randomly divided 100 patients with tension-type headache into a treatment group (50 cases) treated with *Eprisome and Tian Shu capsule,* and a control group (50 cases) treated with *Tian Shu capsule,* for 2 weeks. Cure was defined as no recurrence of headache and disappearance of accompanying symptoms of headache. Marked effect was defined as frequency of headache reduced more than 70% and the duration of time was markedly shorted. Effect was defined as frequency of headache reduced to 35% $\sim$ 69% and the duration of time was shortened. NO effect was defined as frequency of headache reduced less than 35%. A total effectiveness rate included cure rate, marked effect rate, and effect rate. Based on these criteria, the total effectiveness rate of the treatment group was 91.67% and the control group 76.60%. There was significant difference ($P < 0.05$) between treatment group and control group (Zhang et al. 2008). It has also been observed that *Tou Tong Ning* capsule significantly decreases the frequency and the duration of time of migraine attacks, comparing with placebo (Ren et al. 2009). Moreover, there have been a lot of clinical observations on traditional Chinese medicine products treating headaches, most of which showed they are effective.

There has not been enough evidence to confirm the efficiency of traditional Chinese herbs in headache, because the present clinical trials have often been done (1) lacking uniform criteria of diagnosis and clinical evaluation; (2) lacking standard dosage; (3) lacking scientific research design and systematic prospective study; (4) with insufficient samples. Most of the trials used the diagnostic system of traditional Chinese medicine, which is very different from the classification and diagnostic criteria by IHS. Traditional Chinese medicine focuses on individuation of treatment, i.e., the different ingredients and their dosages for different patients.

Indian Traditional Treatment

Traditional treatments are often used along with conventional treatment in the treatment of migraine and tension-type headache. Pharmacological treatment of migraine is complex, and there is no ideal treatment or universally agreed upon guideline. Not all patients respond to the same medications, many develop unacceptable side effects and some are reluctant to take medications. Overuse of acute medications can lead to "medication overuse headache" (MOH) further complicating management strategies. These concerns force patients who have tried out conventional headache therapies to explore complementary or alternative or traditional therapies (Rossi et al. 2005; Evans and Taylor 2006).

The term "Traditional Medicine" or "Alternative Medicine" means any form of medicine that is outside the mainstream of Western medicine or allopathy or orthodox medicine and refers to a broad set of health-care practices that are not integrated into the dominant health-care system. (WHO 2000) The World Health Organization (WHO) defines traditional medicine as "the health practices, approaches, knowledge and beliefs incorporating plant, animal and mineral-based medicines, spiritual therapies, manual techniques and exercises, applied singularly or in combination to treat, diagnose and prevent illnesses or maintain well-being" (WHO 2000). Practices of traditional medicine vary greatly from country to country, and from region to region and are influenced by factors such as history, culture, and attitudes.

Traditional medicine has not been officially recognized in many countries. Consequently, education, training, and research in this area have not received due attention and support. Further scientific research is needed to provide additional evidence of its safety and efficacy. The lack of research data is mainly due to the absence of research methodology for evaluating traditional medicine. Efficacy assessment of traditional medicine may be quite different from conventional medicine.

Traditional treatment looks at most problems as the result of complex mind–body disharmonies. A common traditional treatment method utilized is Herbal. Medicinal herbs have been used as "nutritional supplements" with special properties. Practitioners of traditional treatment also use a range of physical approaches that range from acupuncture to massage or soft tissue manipulation. Each traditional healer has ethnically based sets of treatment for enhancing the outcome and for reestablishing proper nerve function, proper blood flow, and proper structural function. Traditional healers also use psychotherapeutic approaches.

Complementary and alternative medicine (CAM) is often perceived by the public to be more helpful than conventional care for the treatment of headache. In many regions, there is a notion that allopathic medicines taken on a long-term basis are harmful and have side effects. As a result many patients resort to complementary and alternative therapies like acupuncture, biofeedback therapy, relaxation therapy, herbal remedies, and vitamin or mineral supplementation. Plants have been employed as a herbal remedy for migraine treatment and prophylaxis; examples include Feverfew (*Tanacetum parthenium*) and Butterbur (*Petasites hybridus*). Recent studies have demonstrated the effectiveness of acupuncture and yoga in the reduction of migraine headache (Mauskop 2008; Gaul et al. 2009).

Headache patients in India are exposed to the following traditional treatments: Ayurveda, Homeopathy, Yoga, Herbs, Diets, and Massage. They are detailed below (Ravishankar 2004).

Ayurveda

Ayurveda is a traditional medical system used by many in India. Ayurveda is the complete balance of the body, mind, and spirit, including emotions and psychology. Ayurveda includes in its considerations longevity, rejuvenation, and self-realization therapies through herbs, diet, exercise, yoga, aromas, tantras, mantras, and meditation. The hypothesis is that headache usually arises from a stomach disturbance. A better acid–alkali balance in the body may be responsible for reducing the frequency of migraine. There is a close correlation between the symptoms of migraine with those of Amla-pitta of Ayurveda (state of acid–alkali imbalance in the body) causing symptoms such as: brahma (confusion), moorcha (fainting), aruchi (anorexia), aalasya (fatigue), chardi (vomiting), prasek (nausea), mukhmadhurya (sweetness in the mouth), and shiroruja (headache). So the correlation between the cause and symptoms of Amla-pitta of Ayurveda match the current diagnostic criteria of migraine.

Prakash et al. (2006) carried out a study with a uniform ayurvedic treatment protocol (AyTP) comprising five ayurvedic medicines. A uniform treatment protocol was first designed and the same was offered to all migraine patients. Generally, the patients who visited the clinics for AyTP were not satisfied with conventional therapy. Out of 406 patients who were offered this protocol, 204 patients completed 90 days of this treatment. Complete disappearance of headache and associated symptoms at completion of AyTP was seen in 72 (35.2%). In 144 (70.5%) of patients, the marked reduction of migraine frequency and pain intensity observed maybe because of AyTP.

A combination of these five Ayurvedic medicines can markedly reduce the migraine frequency in some migraine patients. The combination of Narikel Lavan, Sootashekhara Rasa, Sitopaladi Churna, Rason Vati, and Godanti Mishran in conjunction with regulated lifestyle and diet may have restored the acid–alkali balance, and restored the functioning of the gastrointestinal system. The herbo-mineral ayurvedic medicines used for migraine treatment contained bhasma of silver, copper, and mercury and many immunomodulatory medicinal herbs, namely, *Allium sativum, Eclipta alba, Cinnmomum zeylanica, Zingiber officinalis, Piper longum, Piper nigrum, Bambusa arumdinaceae, Ellettaria cardamomum* and *Cinnamomum cassia, Ferula northrax, Citrus acida,* etc. Some ingredients used for medicine preparations are moderate to severely toxic in the raw form (ashodhit). However, intricate processing (shodhan) converts these toxic materials to complex mineral forms that are nontoxic but improper processing/manufacturing of ayurvedic medicines may result in severe toxicity. Hence, the safety profile of the combined formulations was first established in animal models (Prakash et al. 2006).

Though this was an open-labeled study, it does allow a conclusion to be drawn about the efficacy of Ayurvedic treatment in migraine. However, to ascertain the real effectiveness of Ayurvedic treatment protocols, a properly controlled clinical trial with a larger patient population is required. Recent studies have indicated that Ayurvedic medicines can be effective in treatment of tension-type headache also.

Homeopathy

For some people who find that prescription treatment for headaches is not effective enough or that the side effects are too uncomfortable to allow for treatment to continue, homeopathic medicine may be one option. It is considered an alternative treatment to conventional drugs and medications. It is thought to be less likely to cause side effects in comparison with prescription strength medications (Ravishankar 2004).

Homeopathy is based on the concept of using extremely small amounts of substances, which in large amounts can induce the same symptoms that are being treated. Homeopathy is meant to enhance the body's natural healing and encourages your body's own ability to heal itself. Homeopathic treatment aims to address each person uniquely, rather than simply recommending one specific treatment for everyone who suffers from headaches, for example. Homeopathy also abides by the ethos that a person should be treated as a whole and treatments are therefore likely to be multifaceted (Headache Homeopathy website).

Homeopathic treatment uses diluted quantities of various plant, mineral, or animal substances to focus on the root cause of an illness. Treatment is thought to increase the production of endorphins, which are the body's natural painkillers. Treatment may be aimed at various areas such as stress or allergies as well as symptoms occurring during an attack. Homeopathic medicines are available over the counter but it is preferable to receive guidance from a homeopathic practitioner. Dosage and frequency of the preparations will vary and you may use only one medicine or a combination. Medications may be used early on when headache pain initially begins, and also daily for long-term prevention.

Homeopathy is rarely a cure or quick fix although some people believe headaches can stop completely after appropriate use of homeopathy. There are approximately 250 remedies to choose from for migraine headache in homeopathy. Medicines may require some time to take effect and are intended to manage and relieve headache pain. Homeopathic medications can also have contraindications with prescription medications, so it is crucial to discuss this after you combine different treatments, to ensure you do not compromise your health. Although homeopathic preparations are considered quite safe, reactions such as a skin rash can occur and so caution should still be used.

Yoga

Through various yogic techniques, a person can avoid and control headaches. Yoga postures and pranayama can help alleviate the pain of headache by releasing tension and stress. A regular routine of Yoga exercise, breathing techniques, and meditation can help to prevent chronic headache or reduce their severity.

Yoga is a complete science of life that originated in India many thousands of years ago. Yoga is one of the six orthodox systems of Indian Philosophy. Yoga means "union" in Sanskrit, the classical language of India. Yoga is an ancient practice that helps create a sense of union in body, mind, and spirit. Yoga provides a holistic approach to lifestyle.

The exercises (action) of Yoga are designed to put pressure on the glandular systems of the body, thereby increasing its efficiency and total health. It strengthens the spinal cord, energizes the inner cells, and activates the whole nervous system. "Bhramri Pranayam" is the most efficient Yoga practice to reduce headache. Some of the Yoga poses that are greatly suggested in such cases include suryanamaskar, bhujanga asana, pawan muktasana, sirsasana, kapalabhati, shitali pranayama, savasana, jalandhar banha, and kunjal jal neti. Inverted postures increase oxygen to the brain and can also reduce headache. Neck exercises play a vital role in curing headache. Yoga practice helps to ease tension, increase flexibility, and tone the muscles. Anuloma Viloma is the special breathing technique that cures headache to a great extent. Tension headaches, also categorized as muscle contraction, often can be alleviated through deep breathing and relaxation asanas, especially while lying down in a quiet place. Exercises that stretch the muscles can release the tension that often causes headaches (John et al. 2007).

There are many ways in which yoga benefits the body. It improves muscle tone, flexibility, strength and stamina, improves circulation, and stimulates the immune system. Yoga decreases the metabolic rate, lowers heart rate, and reduces the workload of the heart. Yoga lowers levels of chemicals associated with stress. It decreases high blood pressure, reduces stress and tension, anxiety, depression, irritability, and improves concentration. Yoga also helps to increase self-awareness, enabling you to address physical symptoms before they become severe.

John et al. (2007) conducted a randomized controlled trial that evaluated the effectiveness of yoga on migraine headache and found that yoga had beneficial effects on various migraine parameters. They arrived at the preliminary conclusion that integrated yoga therapy could be an additional treatment for migraine.

Herbs

The following herbs are found easily in India and are used for headache relief:

1. Betel (*Piper betle*): Betel leaves have analgesic and cooling properties.
2. Clove (*Syzygium aromaticum*): The aroma of the clove has a headache-allaying effect. It can soothe the nerves and bring it back to a pacified state.
3. Garlic (*Allium sativum*): Garlic has almost miraculous properties in relieving headaches, of whatever type they are. Their juice slowly permeates the head region and acts as a painkiller.
4. Ginger (*Zingiber officinale*): Ginger has painkilling properties. Due to this property, it is used as an external application on the affected head region. This gives relief from the headache.

Dietary Treatments

When there is a headache, consuming a sweet preparation or even a spoonful of sugar helps. In many places in India, "Jalebi" and milk are given to prevent morning headaches. Milk and ghee are also beneficial in headaches. Preferably, the milk of a cow should be warmed and had when there is a headache. Rice is the preferred carbohydrate to be taken in times of headache. The water left after cooking the rice should be had when it is warm, with a dash of ghee added in it. Spicy and fried foods are to be avoided when there is a headache.

Head Massage

Head massage is one of the traditional methods in India of using oils to massage your neck, shoulders, scalp, and face to get rid of headache. The Indian head massage headache treatment takes care of the mind, body, and the spirit. In addition to soothing your condition of acute pain in the head, Indian massage therapy is said to help by reinstalling or repairing the movements of your joints, by enhancing the supply of oxygen and glucose to your brain, by improving the circulation of cerebrospinal fluid, by relieving muscle tension, and by stimulating the process of blood circulation in the body. If you use oil as part of the massage, it helps to calm your nervous system too. Indian head massage headache treatment is done following particular massage methods like squeezing, rubbing, gently tapping, and prodding (Massage Therapy for Headache website).

If you are suffering from sinus headache, then the Indian head massage headache treatment will work upon your acupressure points to allay the sinus pressure, stimulate blood circulation, and enhance your vigilance. Indian head massage treatment for headache is suitable for people of all age and sex. Only those who have complaints of degenerative spinal disorders, osteoporosis, and arthritis should not be allowed to go through head massage treatment for headache. If the steps of Indian massage treatment for headache are rightly followed, the outcome is sure to be effective.

Conclusion

Comprehensive headache management should ideally include both conventional medicine and complementary or alternative or traditional medicine (CAM) – see ❍ Chap. 52. Traditional treatments have been tried out mostly in migraine patients. CAM is used widely in tertiary headache care as adjectives or alternatives. The goal is to find effective means to reduce, by at least 50%, the number of headaches, their intensity or their duration, while improving the functional quality of life (Rossi et al. 2005; Evans and Taylor 2006).

The use of CAM is based on patient preference or in those who respond poorly to conventional drugs or who have contraindications to drugs. CAM or "Herbal remedies" are considered as natural and safe but some have potentially harmful side effects. It is best for pregnant women to avoid all traditional treatments except magnesium. Most traditional treatments however are not scientifically studied.

Data about CAM use in different countries show different patterns (WHO 2000). There are five commonly utilized CAM medications for headache prevention. The following traditional treatment options used in other countries, are not commonly used in India – biofeedback, aromatherapy, chiropractic manipulation, hypnosis, craniosacral manipulation, Feverfew, Petasites, magnesium, CoQ10. Factors such as age, gender, education, headache severity, disability, chronicity of headache, and attitude can all influence CAM treatment. Regional differences in income and health-care systems, especially the willingness of health insurance to reimburse the cost of such treatment influence the use of CAM therapies. In difficult or refractory headache situations, one should take advantage of all resources. CAM therapies should be incorporated into medical education. Good trials are needed. Ideally one should combine both conventional treatment and traditional treatment.

Traditional Treatments in Africa with Emphasis on Ethiopia

Traditional or ethnomedical practice is widespread in African countries. For instance, in South Africa between 70% and 80% of the population use the traditional medical sector as their first contact for advice and for treatment of health concern (Kasilo 2000).

A survey in Ethiopia has shown that 80% of Ethiopians use traditional remedies as a primary source of health care (Kassaye et al. 2006). Traditional beliefs are so culturally entrenched that 14% of Ethiopian Jewish migrants visiting a mental health center in Israel attributed their psychiatric and other physical problems to a type of spirit possession (Arieli and Aycheks 1994). There are also evidences that Ethiopian immigrants in Israel continue to perform traditional bloodletting in their new country of residency. Their common reason for the procedure was that the blood was too dark or impure due to diseases such as headache, "feeling of pressure in the blood," fainting, weakness, or nausea (Tandeter et al. 2001).

The majority of African populations live in rural areas where health-care coverage is low. The recourse of rural people to traditional treatment is because it is culturally accepted, easily accessible, and affordable. The lack of knowledge and exposure to modern treatment methods contributes to the popularity of traditional medical practice.

Traditional treatment is influenced by the way the causation of illness is perceived in the cultural and social context of the country or the society. In Ethiopia, it is believed that health is a state of equilibrium within the body and between the body and the outside. Excess heat, cold, drink, worms, and sun can disrupt this equilibrium and cause disease. For instance, excess sun is thought to cause headache, eye disease, earache, and other conditions (Hodes 1997). Vecchiato has identified two broad etiological domains: naturalistic and magico-religious. The naturalistic illness results from external factors, contagion, interpersonal conflict, or personal excesses while the magico-religious domain illness is attributed to God (Allah), nature, demonic spirits, ancestral ghosts, magical forces (evil eye, sorcery, and curses), and breech of social taboos or personal vows (Vecchiato 1993). As a consequence, two types of traditional healers are easily identified. These are the diviner and the herbalist. There is often an overlap whereby an herbalist may prescribe his/her recipe combined with spiritual mysticism.

African traditional medical skills and practitioners or healers are very diverse in their skills and therapeutic approaches, which range from the use of herbal medication to that of spirituality with magical religious orientation. The healers learn their trade from a family member (parents, uncle, etc.), or through apprenticeship under a well-known practitioner in the community. There are also those that claim to have become healers through a spiritual calling. The mean age of a traditional healer in Central Ethiopia was 53.7 years and the majority practiced their trade on a part-time basis (Teferi and Hahn 2002).

Ethnomedical practice in Ethiopia takes different forms depending on the type of the sickness and how the problem is perceived. The specialization of the healers is also quite diverse. They include tooth extractors, uvula cutters, cuppers, amulet writers, those that perform cauterization, exorcists, and seers (Hodes 1997).

Modalities of Traditional Treatment

In Africa, different methods are used in traditional treatment. The modalities of ethnomedical approaches differ from country to country and even within the same country the practices may vary depending on geography, ethnicity, and other sociocultural environmental factors.

Besides traditional bonesetters and birth attendants, the commonest modality of traditional medical practice is ethnobotanical remedies using medicinal plants. In Africa, the rural people and urban poor very much rely on the use of herbal medicine. These are prescribed and provided by herbalists but may be self-administered. The predominant dosage forms are liquid preparations. The deep-rooted cultural belief in the ethnomedical practice is so strong that in many places the traditional healers and the remedies they offer may be preferred over modern medicines and procedures. The herbalist that collects and administers the medicinal plants is treated with respect by the community. He or she in turn preserves his/her special status in the community through secrecy of his/her art and the creation of an environment of mysticism.

Mental illness traditionally is attributed to supernatural forces such as evil spirits that enter a person's body or the shadow cast by an evil eye (Alem and Argaw 1993). Most patients go to priests, magicians, sorcerers, and traditional healers/diviners (Giel and Van Luij 1968; Alem and Argaw 1993). Holy spring water is used extensively to treat patients with psychosocial or psychiatric problem. Drinking and bathing in holy waters together with prayers by priests is often used for a constellation of illness both physical and mental.

Children with throat and respiratory infection or simple febrile illness may undergo uvulectomy performed by a traditional healer in unsterile conditions. This approach has often been complicated by sepsis or tetanus.

Amulets, made of strips of parchment on which biblical or koranic verses are written in ink and rolled up in leather bags are used both prophylactically and therapeutically against evil spirits, bearers of the evil eye, and sorcerers. Epilepsy is commonly believed by rural people to be caused by evil spirit or contagion while touching a seizing person (Tekle-Haimanot et al. 1991). Hence, the wearing of amulets by persons with epilepsy is quite common.

Cauterization is employed with the belief that intense heat destroys the disease-causing substance. It is employed to treat different painful conditions including chest or back pain, headache, and abdominal cramps.

Cupping with or without bloodletting is also practiced with the belief that the procedure will extract "bad unhealthy blood." The procedure is again used in painful conditions as in cauterization.

Bloodletting is commonly practiced in some parts of Ethiopia to treat headache, fever, stiff neck, or abdominal pain. The bloodletting is carried out with an incision on the forearm. In rural areas, cuts and bleeding from the eyelids is used as the treatment of choice for eye diseases like conjunctivitis.

Role of Ethnomedical Practice in the Treatment of Headache

In the rural setting, traditional remedies are commonly used in the treatment of headaches in Africa in general and in Ethiopia in particular. The simplistic traditional approach of treating headache is the application of a tight cotton scarf around the head. Among people living in "enset" (false banana) growing areas in Ethiopia, the cotton scarf is replaced by strong "enset" fibers. The application of butter over the scalp and the consumption of coffee are other forms of self-medications that are applied to treat headache.

Herbalists use the leaves of different plants to treat headaches. The common method of administration of the remedy is in the form of sniffing of a liquid extract via the respiratory system. In South Africa, the tea of the dried leaves of Lion tail (Leonotis and Leonuris) is taken to treat headache. Some of the herbs used to treat headache in Ethiopia include *Mentha pipertia*, *Nigella sativa* (Black seed), *Ocimum basilicum* (Basil), and *Rata chalepensis*.

The approach to treat headache of the migraine character is more dramatic and involves experts. One practice is the use of cautery over the site of the throbbing headache. It is carried out with red-hot charcoal, hot iron, or a burning stick.

Cupping is also used in persistent chronic headache and migraine in particular. In the rural area, bleeding is usually made on the temple and cupping is performed using a cow horn with a hole at the end where the suction is applied by the practitioner (Pankhurst 1965). When it is combined with bloodletting ("bleed-cupping"), in some African cultures herbal ointment is applied with follow-up herbal drugs. Some cultures also rub hot herbal ointment across the patient's eyelids to cure the headache.

Conclusion

The traditional treatment of headache in the African culture is quite varied. It may be as simple as drinking coffee or the tying a tight scarf around the head or as invasive as cauterization, bleed-cupping or bloodletting. The use of these traditional methods of treatment could delay the diagnosis and management of serious conditions such as meningitis and other intracranial pathologies. Moreover there are studies to show that traditional medicines carry the risk of dangerous toxicity. A study in South Africa demonstrated that 18% of all acute poisonings were due to traditional medicines, most (86.6%) of all death from acute poisoning were as a result of poisoning with traditional medicines and the traditional healer is the main source (Joubert and Sabeta 1982). However, the position that traditional medical practitioners occupy in African societies is so influential and important that efforts are being made to involve them in the national health-care system through training and evaluation of effective remedies.

Traditional Treatments for Headaches in South America

Headache treatment can be preventive and acute; also pharmacological and non-pharmacological (Lipton et al. 2007). A non-pharmacological approach is frequently used by patients (Dodick and Silberstein 2007), not always prescribed or initiated by their physicians. Self-initiated treatment or coping strategies depend mainly on the patients' cultural background.

Evidence-based medicine is biased toward available randomized clinical trials (RCTs) and generally focuses on medication. Less evidence is available in medicine for non-pharmacological approaches.

In South America, many coping strategies and natural, cultural-based treatments are available. Some of them are linked to spiritual practices and/or religious activities.

South America is a predominantly catholic continent. In 2007, the Brazilian population was surveyed regarding religious affiliation. 64% were catholics, 17% pentecostals, 5% non-pentecostals, and 3% spiritist. Most of them believe in God (97%), in miracles (87%), in life after death (60%), and many in reincarnation (44%) (Serafim 2007).

Limited data are available regarding traditional treatments used in Latin America; we describe in this chapter the most common practices seen in our environment.

Carod-Artal and Vázquez-Cabrera (2008) have studied headache and migraine treatments in native cultures in Central and South America. Three different tribes were studied. An anthropological field study was conducted with Tzeltal Maya (Mexico), Kamayurá (Brazil), and Uru-Chipaya (Bolivia) American Indians. Migraine is called *yaxti-wanjol chawaj* by Tzeltal shamans. They wash the head of the patient with an herbal solution to treat headache. The boiled leaves of a shrub called *payté wamal* (*Tagetes nelsonii*) were used to relieve migraine. Migraine is called "monkey's disease" by Kamayurá natives. The disease is supposed to be originated by the revenge of the killed monkey's spirit, striking to Kamayurá hunter on his head. It is treated with an herbal infusion (*Serjania* sp.) applied in the eyes of the patient. Migraine is called *eskeclamix* by Uru-Chipaya people; and is treated by drinking the *cañahua* plant (*Chenopodium pallidicaule*) boiled with water. The patient's head may also be washed with shaman's fermented urine.

In Brazil, specially common and typical in the North-Northeast culture, a treatment called "garrafada" is used for several disorders, including headaches and migraine. Herbs are prepared with diverse (and not very well known) tree barks syrup.

Regarding use of homemade remedies, Santos et al. carried out a study evaluating 105 teachers of primary schools on the outskirts of Belo Horizonte, Brazil. Interestingly, 69 (65.7%) thought that certain diseases could be treated with homemade remedies and 54 (78.3%) were able to associate a particular disease with a particular medicinal plant. Lemon balm (*Melissa officinalis*) and Macela flower (*Achyrocline satureioides*) were pointed as healing plants for headaches (Santos et al. 1995). Another study conducted in 2009 surveyed medicinal plants used by academics of a health school in Paraná, Brazil. Results showed that 73% of respondents use medicinal plants. From these, 49% stated they use it for digestive disorders and 24.3% for nervous system disorders (including headache, stress, and anxiety). Macela flower (*Achyrocline satureioides*), Chamomile (*Matricaria chamomilla*), Lemon balm (*Melissa officinalis*), and Espinheira-santa (*Maytenus ilicifolia*) were used for headaches (Aquino Rutkanskis and Cruz-Silva 2009).

In 2006, 100 patients from two public health units in Espírito Santo, Brazil were interviewed concerning medicinal plants. Headache treatments were provided by the following plants: Rosemary oil (*Rosmarinus officinalis*), Orange seed (*Citrus sinensis*), Lemon balm (*Melissa officinalis*), and Margaridinha (*Leucanthemum parthenium*) (Taufner et al. 2006).

However, several concerns can be highlighted by this kind of therapy. In 2003, Amaral evaluated medicinal plants available in the informal commerce of São Luís, Maranhão, Brazil, and found that most herbs were not passed for consumption and 81.5% had bacterial contamination. (Amaral et al. 2003).

The use of the hallucinogenic brew *ayahuasca*, obtained from infusing the shredded stalk of the *malpighiaceous* plant *Banisteriopsis caapi* with the leaves of other plants such as *Psychotria viridis* is found in a religious community called Santo Daime and "União dos vegetais." This religion is also called "forest religion" due to its connection with Amazon region. According to Lang, this tradition is a "spiritual mission that conduct their followers to cure and regeneration processes, through the use of *ayahuasca* (Lang 2008).

Another substance used in Brazil is the frog secretion *Phyllomedusa bicolor*, also known as Kambô. According to a recent publication, (Lima and Labate 2007) the use of this kind of substance is increasing in Brazil, especially in urban cities. Its users vary from tappers to health professionals and the cure for conditions such as, diabetes, heart disease, headache, and migraine are mentioned.

Concerning religious and spiritual treatments, we should mention two different groups: the Pentecostal evangelic churches and the Spiritists.

In Pentecostal evangelic churches, worship services are performed in order to bless individuals and in some cases take away demoniac spirits causing the disorder. According to Nascimento Cunha et al. (2008) some unpleasant events, interpreted as punishment by God, are cured depending on the performance of duties and obligations. There are several television programs regarding these therapies stating cures for lots of medical conditions, including headaches. This can be clearly seen in an excerpt from an article published in 2007. A young man stated: "I remember one day that I had a very severe headache. The Evangelical minister prayed and the pain went away" (Pacheco et al. 2007).

Spiritism is a Christian popular religion in Latin America. Its perspective on mental disorders exerts a great influence in Brazil (Moreira-Almeida and Neto 2005; Moreira-Almeida et al. 2005). Spiritist theory supports the survival of the spirit after death with an exchange of knowledge between the incarnated and disincarnated spirits. A model of spiritual etiology without rejecting the biological, psychological, and social causes of mental disorders is used. The Spiritist etiologic model for mental disorders includes the negative influences of discarnated spirits (termed "obsession") and trauma experienced in previous lives. Several therapeutic approaches are recommended in a variety of conditions including headaches such as the use of "fluidified" (magnetized) water, reading religious texts, prayers, energy healing using hands ("passes"), disobsession (treatment for "obsession"), efforts to live according to ethical principles, and spiritual surgery.

Conclusion

As reported above, there are several traditional treatments for headaches in Latin America, in which two groups are well defined, medicinal plants and spiritual therapy. Most of them are used frequently; however, studies showing their results are lacking in the literature.

References

Alem A, J.L., Argaw M. (1993) Traditional perceptions and treatment of mental disorders in central Ethiopia. Year book of cross-cultural medicine and psychopathology. pp 105–119

Altura BM, Altura BT (2001) Tension headaches and muscle tension: is there a role for magnesium? Med Hypotheses 57:705–713

Amaral F, Coutinho D, Ribeiro M, Oliveira M (2003) Avaliação da qualidade de drogas vegetais comercializadas em São Luís/Maranhão. Rev Bras Farmacognosia 13:27–30

Aquino Rutkanskis A, Cruz-Silva C (2009) Use of medicinal plants by academics of area health of Assis Gurgacz School in the Cascavel city – PR. Cultivando o saber 2(4):69–85

Arieli A, Aycheks S (1994) Mental disease related to belief in being possessed by the "Zar" spirit. Harefuah 126:636–642

Carod-Artal F, Vázquez-Cabrera C (2008) An anthropological study about headache and migraine in native cultures from Central and South America. Headache J Head Face Pain 47(6):834–841

Ceccherelli F, Gagliardi G, Ruzzante L, Giron G (Jun 2002) Acupuncture modulation of capsaicin-induced inflammation: effect of intraperitoneal and local administration of naloxone in rats A blinded controlled study. J Altern Complement Med 8(3):341–349

Chen Z, Hendner J, Hedner T (1996) Substance P induced respiratory excitation is blunted by delta-receptor specific opioids in the rat medulla oblongata. Acta Physiol Scand 157(2):165–173

Davis MA, Kononowech RW, Rolin SA, Spierings EL (2008) Acupuncture for tension-type headache: a meta-analysis of randomized, controlled trials. J Pain 9(8):667–677

Demirkaya S, Vural O, Dora B (2001) Efficacy of intravenous magnesium sulfate in the treatment of acute migraine attacks. Headache 41:171–177

Deng QS (1995) Ionic mechanism of acupuncture on improvement of learning and memory in age mammals. Am J Chin Med 23(1):1–9

Dhond RP, Kettner N, Napadow V (Jul-Aug 2007) Neuroimaging acupuncture effects in the human brain. J Altern Complement Med 13(6):603–616

Dodick D, Silberstein S (2007) Migraine prevention. Pract Neurol 7(6):383

Ernst E (2006) Acupuncture-a critical analysis. J Intern Med 259(2):125–137

Evans RW, Taylor FR (Jun 2006) "Natural" or alternative medications for migraine prevention. Headache 46(6):1012–1018

Fu H (2000) What is the material base of acupuncture? The nerves! Med Hypotheses 54(3):358–359

Gaul C, Eismann R, Schmidt T, May A et al (Oct 2009) Use of complementary and alternative medicine in patients suffering from primary headache disorders. Cephalalgia 29(10):1069–1078

Gedif T, Hahn HJ (2002) Herbalists in Addis Ababa and Butajira, central Ethiopia: Mode of service delivery and traditional pharmaceutical practice. Ethiop J Health Dev 16(2):191–197

Giel R, Van Luij KJN (1968) Faith healing and spirit possession in Ghion, Ethiopia. Soc Sci Med 2:63–79

Guyton AC, Hall JE (2001) Textbook of medical physiology. WB Saunders, Philadelphia

Headache Homeopathy. http://www.headacheexpert.co.uk/HeadacheHomeopathy.html

Herbs in the Treatment of headache. http://www.ayushveda.com/ayurveda-articles/headache.htm

Hodes RM (1997) Cross-cultural medicine and diverse health beliefs-Ethiopian abroad. Isr West J Med 166:29–36

Hu HQ, Wang XL, Zhou YH, Fu XJ, Liu W, Wang DX, Fu Q (2004) The effect of Xiao Yao Di Bi Liquid on the expression of c-fos gene in rat of migraine. Chin J Clin Pharmacol Ther 9(7):774–777

Huang QZ, Shan X, Zhong Y (2003) The treatment of 32 cases of migraine headache by Yang Xue Chu Feng Tong Luo Tang Shanxi. Chin Med 5:19–20

Itoh K, Katsumi Y, Hirota S, Kitakoji H (2007) Randomised trial of trigger point acupuncture compared with other acupuncture for treatment of chronic neck pain. Complement Ther Med 15(3):172–179

John PJ, Sharma N, Sharma CM, Kankane A (2007) Effectiveness of yoga therapy in the treatment of migraine without aura: A randomized controlled trial. Headache 47:654–661

Joubert P, Sebata B (1982) The role of prospective epidemiology in the establishment of a toxicology service for a developing community. S Afr Med J 62:853–854

Kasilo O (2000) Traditional African Medicine. In: WHOs Traditional Medicine, better science, policy and services for health development: Proceedings of a WHO international symposium, Awaji Island, Hyogo Prefecture, Japan, pp 86–94

Kassaye KD, Amberbir A, Getachew B, Mussema Y (2006) A historical overview of traditional medicine practices and policy in Ethiopia. Ethiop J Health Dev 20:127–134

Kelly RB (2009) Acupuncture for pain. Am Fam Physician 80(5):481–484

Lang A (2008) Espiritismo no Brasil. Cad CERU 19:171–185

Li CM (2006) The study on effect of Xue Hu ZHu Yu Tang on rat of migraine. Shan Xi Zhong Yi Xue Yuan Xue Bao 7(2):13–14

Lima E, Labate B (2007) "Remédio da Ciência" e "Remédio da Alma": os usos da secreção do kambô (Phyllomedusa bicolor) nas cidades. Campos-Revista de Antropologia Social 8(1):71–90

Linde K, Streng A, Jürgens S, Hoppe A, Brinkhaus B, Witt C, Wagenpfeil S, Pfaffenrath V, Hammes MG, Weidenhammer W, Willich SN, Melchart D (2005) Acupuncture for patients with migraine: a randomized controlled trial. JAMA 293(17):2118–2125

Linde K, Allais G, Brinkhaus B, Manheimer E, Vickers A, White AR (2009) Acupuncture for migraine prophylaxis. Cochrane Database Syst Rev 21(1):CD001218

Lipton R, Bigal M, Diamond M, Freitag F, Reed M, Stewart W (2007) Migraine prevalence, disease burden, and the need for preventive therapy. Neurology 68(5):343

Liu JP (2009) Observation on the effects of Feng Xue Ning Tong for treatment migraine. Hen Nan Tradit Chin Med 29(1):59

Lu JS, Gao QJ, Feng YY (2004) The role of oral compound Gastrodia on rat of migraine. Yi Yao Tao Bao 23(3):137–139

Massage Therapy for Headache. http://www.ehow.com/how_1964_massage-away-headache.html

Mauskop A (2008) Complementary and alternative treatments for migraine. Drug Dev Res 68:424–427

Melchart D, Linde K, Fischer P, Berman B, White A, Vickers A, Allais G (2002) Acupuncture for idiopathic headache. Cochrane Database SystRev 3: CD001218

Moreira-Almeida A, Neto F (2005) Spiritist views of mental disorders in Brazil. Transcult Psychiatry 42(4):570

Moreira-Almeida A, Almeida A, Neto F (2005) History of "Spiritist madness" in Brazil. Hist Psychiatry 16(1):5

Nascimento Cunha M, Gomes Z, Maia F, Nascimento T (2008) Discurso religioso, hegemonia pentecostal e mídia no Brasil. Rev Caminhando 13(21):87–96

Pacheco E, Ribeiro R, Silva S (2007) "Eu era do mundo": transformações do auto-conceito na conversão pentecostal. Psic: Teor e Pesq 23(1):53–62

Pankhurst R (1965) An historical examination of traditional Ethiopia medicine and surgery. Ethiop Med J 3:157–172

Prakash VB, Pareek A, Narayan JP (2006) Observational study of ayurvedic treatment on migraine without aura. Int J Head 26:1317

Raj PP (1986) Acupuncture. In: Raj PP (ed) Practical management of pain. Year Book, Chicago, pp 799–820

Ravishankar K (2004) Barriers to headache care in India and effort to improve the situation. Lancet Neurol 3:564–567

Ren YX, Peng C, Yao G (2000) The effect of Tuo Yin on the expression of c-fos and c-jun genes in rat of migraine. Cheng Du Zhong Yi Yao Univ Xue Bao 23(3):34–36

Ren D, Wang KH, Huang LJ (2009) Observation on the effects of Tou Tong Ning capsule on migraine. Guangxi Tradit Chin Med 32(5):23–25

Rossi P, Di Lorenzo G, Malpezzi MG, Faroni J, Cesarino F, Di Lorenzo C et al (2005) Prevalence, pattern and predictors of use of complementary and alternative medicine (CAM) in migraine patients attending a headache clinic in Italy. Cephalalgia 25:493–506

Santos M Dias A, Martins M (1995) Knowledge and use of alternative medicine by elementary school children and teachers. Rev Saúde Pública 29(3):221–227

Serafim M. (2007) Recortes da pesquisa Datafolha sobre religião no Brasil. http://mauricioserafim.net/2007/05/08/recortesda-pesquisa-datafolha-sobre-religiao-no-brasil/

Song LG, Hao J (2001) The document analysis of Chinese medicine for treatment migraine from 1995 to 1999. Shan Dong Yi Yao Univ Xue Bao 25(3):195–197

Sun YX, Gan TJ (2008) Acupuncture for the management of chronic headache: a systematic review. Anesth Analg 107(6):2038–2047

Takeshige C, Nakamura A, Asamoto S, Arai T (1992) Positive feed-back action of pituitary beta endorphin on acupuncture analgesia afferent pathway. Brain Res Bull 27(1):37–44

Tandeter H, Grynbaum M, Borkan J (2001) A qualitative study on cultural bloodletting among Ethiopian immigrants. Isr Med Assoc J 3:937–939

Taufner C, Ferraço E, Ribeiro L (2006) The use of medicinal plants as an alternative herbal therapy in public health units at Santa Teresa and at Marilandia, ES. Natureza line 4(1):30–39

Tekle-Haimanot R, Abebe M, Forsgren L et al (1991) Attitudes of rural people in central Ethiopia toward epilepsy. Soc Sci Med 32:203–209

Traditional Medicine, Health System Governance and Service Delivery WHO/Geneva. http://whqlibdoc.who.int/hq/2000/WHO_EDM_TRM_2000.1.pdf

Vecchiato N (1993) Traditional medicine. In: Koos H, Zein ZA (eds) The ecology of health and disease in Ethiopia. West view, Boulder, pp 157–178

Wang F, Jia SW (1996) Effect of acupuncture on regional cerebral blood flow and cerebral functional activity evaluated with single-photon emission computed tomography]. Zhong guo Zhong Xi Yi Jie He Za Zhi 16(6):340–343

WHO (2000) General guidelines for methodologies on research and evaluation of traditional medicine WHO/EDM/TRM/2000. WHO, Geneva

WHO (2002) Traditional Medicine strategy 2002-2005. WHO/EDM/TRM/2002. WHO, Geneva

Yang HJ, Li G, Bian BL (2005) The protective effect of Da Chun Gong Wan on low serotonin-mediated hypersensitivity state of NO. China J Exp Tradit Med Formulae 11(1):28–30

Yang XS, Chen XY, Hu YM, Gu F (2006) The effect of Tong Xin Luo Capsule on expression of CGRP and α-2CGRP genes in rat of migraine. J Int Neurol Neurosurg 33(4):299–232

Yao G, Chen ML, Ren YX (2001) The effect of Tuo Feng Capsule on the level of CGRP, ET and His genes in serum of rat of migraine. Cheng Du Zhong Yi Yao Univ Xue Bao 24(4):38–41

Yao G, Hu Y, Chen ML, Peng C, Wang YT (2002) Effect of Tou Feng capsule on the level of Monoamine neurotransmitters in rat of migraine. Chin Patent Med 24(1):43–45

Yoga for headache. http://www.indianetzone.com/42/yoga_headache.htm

Yu Y, Zhou S, Liu LG (1985) Distribution of metenkephalin and its changes in cervical spinal cord and medulla oblongata of dog during operation under acupuncture anesthesia. Zhen Ci Yan Jiu 10:289–294

Yu SY, Kuang PG, Pu CQ, Zhang FY, Liu JX (1995a) Inhibiting effects of Tianrong acupoint therapy on mast cells on dura mater. Acupunct Res 20(4):34–38

Yu SY, Kuang PG, Zhang FY, Liu JX (1995b) Anti-inflammatory effects of Tianrong acupoint therapy on blood vessels of dura mater. J Tradit Chin Med 15(3):1–5

Yu SY, Kuang PG, Zhang FY, Liu JX (1996) Plasma extravasation in different tissues innervated by trigeminal nerve following electrical stimulation of the unilateral trigeminal ganglion. Chin J Pain Med 2(2):109–113

Yu SY, Kuang PG, Wang ZJ, Chen HN (1997a) Effects of Tianrong acupoint therapy on concentrations of β-endophin in plasma of the patients with migraine. Chin J Pain Med 3(2s):28

Yu SY, Kuang PG, Zhang FY, Liu JX (1997b) Effects of Tianrong acupoint therapy on concentrations of dynorphin A1-13 in CSF and plasma of the patients with migraine. Acupunct Res 22(4):216–218

Yu Y, Kasahara T, Sato T, Guo S, Liu Y, Asano K, Hisamitsu T (1997c) Enhancement of splenic interferon-gamma, interleukin-2, NK cytotoxicity by S36 acupoint acupuncture in F344 rats. Jpn J Physiol 47(2):173–178

Yu Y, Kasahara T, Sato T, Asano K, Yu G, Fang J (1998) Role of endogenous interferon-gama on the enhancement of splenic NK cell activity by electroacupuncture stimulation in mice. J Neuroimmunol 90(2):176–186

Zhang CY, Mao CJ, Wen ZM (2008) Observation on the effects of Eprisome and Tian shu capsule for the patients of tension headache. Chin J Pract Nerv Dis 11(4):42–43

Zhao L (1995) Role of opioid peptides of rat's nucleus reticulari paragigantocellularis lateralis (RPGL) in acupuncture analgesia. Acupunct Electrother Res 20(1):89–100

Zhao C, Stillman C (2003) New developments in the pharmacotherapy of tension-type headaches. Expert Opin Pharmacother 4:2229–2237

Part 15

Non-Governmental Organizations in Headache

55 The Role of Lay Organizations in Relieving the Burden of Headache: South American Perspective

Lorenzo Gardella
Sanatorio Parque, Rosario, Santa Fe, Argentina

Paolo Martelletti, Timothy J. Steiner (eds.), *Handbook of Headache*, DOI 10.1007/978-88-470-1700-9_55,

Abstract: Headache is a high prevailing disorder among general population.

Millions of people suffer from headaches all over the world. Most of them are bad diagnosed and are not given a correct treatment, being affected their individual, social, and working life; headaches affect their quality of life. People who suffer from headaches do not function at their best not only during the attacks but also during asymptomatic periods.

The public health significance of headaches is often overlooked probably because of their episodic nature and the fact that most of the times there is no death risk involved.

It is essential to work toward a better understanding of migraine at all levels, including recognition by health insurers, government departments, and nongovernmental organizations (NGOs) in order to improve health services and provide better patient care.

That is the reason why we insist on the importance of founding nongovernmental organizations since they keep a good relationship among doctors, patients, and other interested sectors and they work supervising Self Assistance Groups.

These institutions provide information to headache sufferers in remote areas of the country and they set a formal relationship with the World Headache Alliance (WHA), the International Headache Society (IHS), and the World Health Organization (WHO) to start an efficient global campaign using the mass media available to spread all these objectives.

Background

Headaches affect people in the years of greater productivity (Linet and Stewart 1987; Rasmussen et al. 1991; Breslau and Davis 1992; Stewart et al. 1992; Lainez et al. 1996). Migraine is one of the 20 causes of "years of life lost with disability (YLD-DALY)" (Osterhaus and Townsend 1991; Stewart et al. 1996). This index is duplicated when considering all types of headaches (Headache Classification Committee of the International Headache Society 1988). So it should be very important to establish an efficient and effective approach to the diagnosis and cure of headache disorders. And it is necessary to have a new outlook on the overall care of these patients and guarantee them a better quality of life (Osterhaus and Townsend 1991; Edmeads et al. 1993).

There are lots of treatments that professional neurologists have to treat headache disorders nowadays. New drugs have excellent results for patients during their crisis (Celentano et al. 1992). Besides, preventive medication and non-pharmacological opportunities (physical activities, diet, sleeping control, oriental alternative treatments, biofeedback, Transcutaneous Electric Nerve Stimulation, Production of a diary, etc.) (Russell et al. 1992) give our patients more chances to relieve their pain episodes. But, besides our medical and professional intervention, we need to aware the population; we must inform them about these new possibilities. Headache ought to be a public health concern. In many countries, headaches are given a low priority in the assignment of health-care resources (Cull et al. 1992; de Lissovoy and Lazarus 1994). Many governments, seeking to constrain health-care costs, do not acknowledge the substantial burden of headache on society (Osterhaus et al. 1992).

It is in this sense that we emphasize the role of nongovernmental organizations (NGOs). An NGO is a private entity with humanitarian and social purposes and objectives defined by its members. It is created independent of local, regional, and national governments, as well as international organizations. Its membership is made up of voluntary lay people. In order to be economically able to carry out their activities, the NGOs rely on the support of beneficial foundations, the pharmaceutical industry, and different companies for donations. They also organize different events to raise funds.

In the cases in which NGOs are funded totally or partially by governments, the NGO maintains its nongovernmental status and excludes government representatives from membership in the organization. The number of international operating NGOs is estimated at 40,000. National numbers are even higher: Russia has 277,000 NGOs, India is estimated to have between one million and two million NGOs.

By 1800, nearly 200 "friendly societies" were founded in England to deal with the burden of headache, and many self-improvement associations were brought to North America by immigrant groups (Osterhaus 1993). The British Migraine Association was formed in 1958, the Swedish in 1960; the National Headache Foundation (EEUU) was formed in 1970 and the Canadian in 1974. Recently, there has been an explosion in the interest and development of headache groups in many more countries and in most continents. This growth may be the resultant need to provide patients with new information and optimism for a brighter, pain-free future.

The Role of Lay Organizations

Headache organizations are able to provide their audiences with credible, accurate, and up-to-date information on headache. They do this via broadcast, and print-media, newsletters, pamphlets, books, video and audio tapes, seminars, fax, Internet, and most recently the Web. They bring patients together through literature, personal contact, events, educational forums, and in some cases, through self-help or support groups.

Headache disorders not only affect headache sufferers, they also afflict the life of those who live with them. It is for this reason that the information supplied to the sufferer must be passed on to spouses, partners, family members, friends, bosses, and coworkers. People that live with headache sufferers should comprehend them, help them, and learn to live with them since their role is really important in the treatment of the sufferer. Headache patients almost universally report a lack of understanding among many people close to them. There are myths surrounding headache disorders, but the reality is of course, that headache is a valid, medical, neurobiological disorder (Von Korff et al. 1992). It is misunderstood within families, workplaces, and social circles. In a recent study, 51% of patients reported that their doctor does not take headache seriously enough (Stang and Osterhaus 1993; Wells 1993; Lipton et al. 1995).

Headache nongovernmental organizations make a broader public, which may not be directly touched by headache sufferers, aware of the serious nature of headache disorders and society's consciousness becomes appropriately sympathetic to the needs of headache patients.

Advocacy is a possible major role that all headache organizations could play. All countries could benefit from the development of their own organization reflecting local culture, practice, and social norms. The World Headache Alliance is formed to foster the development and continuance of such organizations. It is the Alliance's vision to see global participation in worldwide awareness events and educational projects aimed at efficiently making the world a better place for headache patients.

Even though nongovernmental organizations are directed or coordinated by specialized doctors, the active participation is performed by lay people who are not professionals, but in general suffer or have been victims of important headaches. For many of them headaches are still a burden to be relieved and others have remarkably improved and are grateful or want their experience to be known regarding their quality of life and how it has changed for better. These people participate in an active way and their collaboration is really important since their testimonies are of great significance.

The role of headache groups from countries affiliated to the World Headache Alliance (WHA) consists in the organization of talks in different places as schools, gymnasiums, beauty centers, for the community and neighbor population. These talks should be addressed to nonmedical professionals such as psychologists, pharmaceuticals, dentists, opticians, chiropractors, and physiotherapists among others, because these professionals are in permanent contact with headache sufferers. It is the purpose of these meetings to aware the population on the lack of attention given to headache by health care, to awake health authorities to make the best use of our human and technological resources, to encourage research for the diagnosis and treatment of headaches, to develop "public education programs," to inform by mass communication media that headaches are treatable medical illnesses, to promote "screening programs" to help identify headache sufferers, to establish which are each one's responsibilities and priorities, and build public consciousness regarding the impact of headaches on people´s quality of life.

It is also nongovernmental organizations' aim to do their best to widen and activate collaboration with colleagues abroad. Cooperation between scientists of different countries could be helpful in many ways. It could include methodological workshops, short visits of scientists to experienced laboratories, and training of young doctors and technicians in these laboratories.

References

Breslau N, Davis GC (1992) Migraine, physical health and psyquiatric disorders: a prospective epidemiologic study of young adults. J Psychiatr Res 27:211–221

Celentano DD, Stewart WF, Lipton RB (1992) Medication use and disability among migraniers. A national probability sample survey. Headache 32:223–228

Cull RE, Wells NEJ, Miocevich ML (1992) The economic cost of migraine. Brit J Econ 2:103–115

de Lissovoy G, Lazarus SS (1994) The economic cost of migraine: the present state of knowledge. Neurology 44:856–862

Edmeads J, Findly H, Tugwell P et al (1993) Impact of migraine and tension type headaches on life-style, consulting behaviour and medication use: a Canadian population survey. Can J Neurol Sci 20:131–137

Headache Classification Committee of the International Headache Society (1988) Classification and diagnostic criteria for headache disorders, cranial neuralgias and facial pain. Cephalalgia 8(Suppl 7):1–96

Lainez JM, Titus F, Cobaleda S et al (1996) Socioeconomic impact of migraine. Funct Neurol 11:133

Linet MS, Stewart WF (1987) The epidemiology of migraine. In: Blau JN (ed) Migraine clinical,

therapeutic, conceptual and research aspects. Chapman & Hall, London, pp 451–477

Lipton RB, Stewart WF, VonKorff M (1995) Migraine impact and functional disability. Cephalalgia 15(suppl 15):4–9

Osterhaus JT (1993) The burden of migraine. Can J Neurol Sci 20(Suppl 4):35

Osterhaus JT, Townsend RJ (1991) The quality of life of migranieurs: a cross-sectional profile. Cephalalgia 11(Suppl 11):103–104

Osterhaus JT, Gutterman DG, Plachetka JR (1992) Healthcare resource and lost labor costs of migraine headache in the United States. Pharmacoeconomics 2:67–76

Rasmussen BK, Jensen R, Schroll M et al (1991) Epidemiology of headache in a general population: a prevalence study. J Clin Epidemiol 44:1147–1157

Russell MB, Rasmussen BK, Brennum J et al (1992) Presentation of a new instrument: the diagnostic Headache diary. Cephalalgia 12:369–374

Stang PE, Osterhaus JT (1993) Impact of migraine in the United States: data from the national health interview survey. Headache 33:29–35

Stewart WF, Lipton RB, Celentano DD et al (1992) Prevalence of migraine headache in the United States. J Am Med Assoc 267:64–69

Stewart WF, Lipton RB, Simon D (1996) Work related disability: results from the American Migraine Study. Cephalalgia 16:231–238, OSLO

Von Korff M, Ormelk J, Keefe F et al (1992) Grading the severity of chronic pain. Pain 50:133149

Wells NEJ (1993) The cost of migraine to society. Poster presented at the 7th World congress of pain, Paris

56 The Role of Lay Organizations in Relieving the Burden of Headache: African Perspective

Regina N. M. Kamoga
Community Health And Information Network (CHAIN), Kampala, Uganda

Paolo Martelletti, Timothy J. Steiner (eds.), *Handbook of Headache*, DOI 10.1007/978-88-470-1700-9_56,
© Lifting The Burden 2011

Abstract: "For anyone who has suffered from a headache knows that it's not just a headache. A headache prevents you from doing the things you are passionate about; it denies you the freedom to enjoy life thus compromising the quality of life."

Although headaches are among the most common medical problem, they are also given the least attention, mainly because they are not considered to be life threatening.

In Uganda, like elsewhere in the world, a headache is not regarded as a serious problem. There is hardly any information on headaches and its management. There is lack of specialists to handle headache patients. The physicians do not have adequate diagnostic skills and facilities, which result in wrong diagnosis and treatment. This is mainly due to inadequate capacity of the country to train health workers and ability to provide adequate health facilities.

Evidence available to WHO shows that, at primary health-care level in Africa, Asia, and Latin America Regions, only about 40% of all patients were treated in accordance with clinical guidelines for many common conditions and there has been no improvement over the past 15 years.

A low level of awareness is yet another barrier to reducing the burden of headache. The lay organizations have a key role to play by raising public awareness about the headache and its management. This involves mobilizing and educating the public about the headache problem, so as to provide an understanding as to what a headache is, the different types of headaches, symptoms, how to manage it, the headache treatment available, and its proper use. A number of approaches have been used including, among others, advocacy that involves all stakeholders including decision makers, political and community leaders, the media, and the public; as well as lobbying government to develop and implement professional development programs to update knowledge and skills in order to respond to new and rapidly evolving challenges of health care.

The Role of Lay Organizations

Normally when people suffer from a headache, they consider self-treatment as the first option. If it persists, they will go to private units or clinics that are informal with limited infrastructure and uncertain quality of services. Visiting a major hospital will be the last option as it is normally preferred for more serious conditions and for hospitalization.

Traditional healers also play a big role in Uganda especially in treatment of headaches.

This is because of the misinformation and beliefs people have, many people especially in the rural areas associate headache with ancestral spirits or witchcraft and mental problem. They believe that one has annoyed his ancestral spirits and therefore needs to reconcile with them. Others think they have been bewitched by an enemy. Because of these beliefs, people seek traditional/herbal remedies to treat the headaches. This has resulted into people being subjected to crude methods and practices that are not only unsafe but also dangerous to their lives. Such practices include among others cutting of the vein on the side of the head where the throbbing pain is , this is meant to drive away "spirits," looking up at the morning sun, putting herbal concoctions in the nose, and many others. It is therefore the responsibility of lay organisations together with the Ministry of Health to protect the public against such practices.

The role of lay organizations in Uganda is significant but not without challenges. The biggest challenge is how to effectively disseminate information to a public with low literacy levels. This calls for innovative ways of disseminating information. The lay organizations develop strategies that enable them reach the wider community. It is believed that when people receive and share information in an appropriate way, they are able to understand their condition and are able to seek treatment early and adhere to their medication.

To bridge the gap, organizations such as the International Institute of Alternative and Complementary Medicine in Uganda have helped reduce headache burden by bringing a whole new approach to diagnosing headache.

"When a patient comes he/she is given a full diagnosis and depending on the nature of the headache, a genetical health predispositions test is performed to establish the underlying problem within the system and then appropriate treatment is given," says Dr Juuko Ndawula, Director of the International Institute of Alternative and Complementary Medicine in Uganda (personal communication in 2010).

Lay organizations have also used methods such as media both electronic and newsprint; however, the challenge is the literacy levels, coupled with the poor reading culture makes it difficult for people to access information. The Television as well does not reach many people especially in the rural areas due to poor infrastructure and poverty.

Oral transmission of information has been used since time immemorial and serves as an effective way of transmitting headache information that is through stories, music and drama, community meetings, and debates, to reach out to the rural community.

Public awareness campaigns are aimed at talking to crowds of people in the community. The campaigns are organized by involving traditional leaders, community leaders, and community volunteers; the local leaders command a lot of respect in the community. Other occasions include village meetings and market days.

Posters, brochures, and pamphlets are used to deliver appropriate messages, this need to be translated in different local languages.

Community-to-community collaboration is another strategy that is used to disseminate information at the community level. This is where different communities come together to share knowledge and experiences on an issue. It is usually through exchange visits that can be conducted between individual/community/organizations.

Community support groups, where people with the same health condition meet and share knowledge and experiences on how to manage their condition is yet another way of helping lifting the burden of headache.

It is however important to note that all the methods above need to take into consideration the target group, appropriate message and its relevance to the local conditions. This is mainly because every society has its unique way of doing things in terms of societal norms, beliefs, taboos, and practices. A lot of resources both human resource and financial resources is also required by lay organisations to effectively do their work, yet many organisations are constrained and not able to provide the needed services. All stakeholders, public and private need to work together to help lift the headache burden.

References

Ministry of Health (2009) Uganda human resources for health report. Kampala, Uganda

Ministry of Health (2009) Uganda national communication strategy for promoting rational use of medicines. Kampala, Uganda, pp 9–11

Tripartite Training Programme (DENIVA/URDT/ACFODE) (1999) Management training for civil society organisation, promoting change. Kampala

Woytek R, Shroff-Mehta P, Mohan PC (eds) (2004) Indigenous knowledge. Local pathways to global development. Knowledge and Learning Group, African Region/The World Bank

57 The Role of Lay Organizations in Relieving the Burden of Headache: European Perspective

Valerie Hobbs
OUCH (UK) Organisation for the Understanding of Cluster Headache, Tenby, Pembrokeshire, UK

Paolo Martelletti, Timothy J. Steiner (eds.), *Handbook of Headache*, DOI 10.1007/978-88-470-1700-9_57,
© Lifting The Burden 2011

Abstract: "They're unique, they're expert and they're crucial." So says Professor Peter Goadsby of UCSF and The National Hospital for Neurology and Neurosurgery, referring to one particular lay support organization for headache sufferers.

Much underestimated and sometimes dismissed as being ill-informed timewasters, the medical profession is now beginning to recognize the increasingly important role that is filled by lay organizations, particularly in supporting sufferers.

The general public's view is that headache is a minor health problem, but given that approximately 10 million people in the UK suffer headache in one form or another and the cost to the economy is approximately £7 billion per annum, this is not a minor health problem.

Most headache sufferers will self-diagnose and self-treat with over-the-counter remedies, but in the UK for the estimated 12% with severe and/or rare headache conditions access to a correct diagnosis and treatment can take anything from 2 to 25 years.

Lay patient organizations have an important part to play in raising awareness of the various conditions, promoting a better understanding of them, providing information and support to sufferers and their families, promoting better liaison between sufferers and the medical profession, and by supporting research into headache conditions.

Established Knowledge

The International Headache Society headache classification has 14 different groups of headache, encompassing around 600 different headache types. In the UK, there are four main support groups for headache sufferers: Migraine Action, Migraine Trust, OUCH (UK) (Organisation for the Understanding of Cluster Headache), and the Trigeminal Neuralgia Association. Each organization has members who suffer not only from the eponymous condition, but from other less well known but severe headache types, some even suffering from multiple headache types. All four organizations speak as one voice through Headache UK, an alliance of all four organizations with two professional organizations, BASH and MIPCA. Headache UK is able to speak at governmental and national level regarding headache and together with the All Party Parliamentary Group on Headache Disorders has launched two early day motions in the Commons regarding diagnosis and treatment of headache disorders.

The individual organizations provide vital support to sufferers of the rarer conditions, who can feel very isolated and who suffer at levels stated by Professor Goadsby as being the most severe suffered by mankind, in fact one condition, cluster headache is referred to as "suicide headache" as it is so painful.

Very often, sufferers are unable to find support even from their own family members; their constant suffering renders them exhausted through lack of sleep, and working and existing on a day-to-day level is difficult in the extreme. Loss of employment, the concomitant financial loss, and lack of understanding can lead to deep depression and total loss of self-esteem. Support organizations provide information that is not provided by the medical professions, such as information on employment issues, state benefits, how supporters can help sufferers, basic information on use of medications and explaining treatments.

All of the major headache charities have help lines, which are a vital means of contact to the newly diagnosed and a useful reference point for health professionals. They all provide printed information and have detailed Web sites and members' fora. They all strive for liaison with the medical profession and very often provide a useful patient cohort for research purposes, as well as some financial resources.

Current Research

There is very little in the literature regarding not only the role of the lay organizations, but also the huge impact that headache has on the lives not only of the sufferer but also their supporters. There is of course the Headache Impact Test, but that does not deal with the question in full detail. No account is taken of the embarrassment factor of having an attack in public; how a child feels seeing a much loved parent in the extremes of a headache attack; the lack of understanding and awareness of those observing an attack, and of the life-changing effects of suffering a severe headache condition. Many lose their jobs altogether, or have to change their type of employment as there may be a headache-triggering element in their existing employment environment. Relationships can break up under the pressure of living with someone with a long-term chronic pain condition, adding to the depression and loss of self-esteem. Lay patient organizations provide very valuable support in these areas, but this needs to be backed up by a better understanding from the medical profession.

Being able to speak to other sufferers has, anecdotally, been shown to be one of the most important factors for the sufferers themselves. Similarly, supporter talking to supporter encourages the view that "you are not alone" with whatever headache condition is involved. All the headache charities organize meetings at various venues all over the country, thus aiding public awareness and, by inviting health professionals to participate, encourages good liaison between the patients and the primary and secondary carers.

More research needs to be done in the areas of the benefits of lay support organizations and also the impact that severe headache can have on a patient's life, leading to better diagnosis, treatment, and outcomes, and inclusion of better neurological training for all doctors, to enable correct diagnosis and treatment.

Conclusion

Lay organizations will continue to relieve the headache burden, by provision of nonmedical support, advice and guidance, both to sufferers and to the medical profession. A symbiotic relationship between the organizations and the medical profession should engender mutual respect and understanding and an acceptance of the vital part that lay organizations have to play in relieving the burden of headache.

In the twenty-first century, the doctor–patient relationship is undergoing a gradual change, with the patient taking a more proactive role. This proactivity can only be accomplished by the patient learning more about their condition from information and advice supplied by patient lay organizations.

References

Goadsby PJ (2007) Cluster headache (DVD). DMA Video, London

Headache UK Manifesto (2009) Migraine action, migraine trust. BASH, MIPCA, OUCH (UK), London

http://ihs-classification.org ICHD II; various, Mar 2010

http://www.headacheexpert.co.uk/facts-figures-about-headaches.html. Accessed Apr 2010

58 *Lifting The Burden*: The Global Campaign Against Headache

Timothy J. Steiner[1,2] · Lars Jacob Stovner[8] · Zaza Katsarava[3] ·
Rigmor Jensen[4] · Gretchen L. Birbeck[5,6] · Paolo Martelletti[7]
[1]Norwegian University of Science and Technology, Trondheim, Norway
[2]Faculty of Medicine, Imperial College London, London, UK
[3]University of Essen, Essen, Germany
[4]Glostrup Hospital, University of Copenhagen, Glostrup, Copenhagen, Denmark
[5]Michigan State University, East Lansing, MI, USA
[6]Chikankata Health Services, Mazabuka, Zambia
[7]School of Health Sciences, Sapienza University of Rome, Rome, Italy
[8]Norwegian University of Science and Technology and St. Olavs Hospital, Trondheim, Norway

Parts of this contribution have also been published as part of a Springer Open Choice article which is freely available at springerlink.com – DOI 10.1007/s10194-007-0428-1

Paolo Martelletti, Timothy J. Steiner (eds.), *Handbook of Headache*, DOI 10.1007/978-88-470-1700-9_58,
© Lifting The Burden 2011

Abstract: Headache disorders are highly prevalent, ubiquitous, often lifelong and disabling. They are largely treatable, but everywhere are under-recognized, underdiagnosed, and undertreated. In many countries, they are simply not acknowledged as illnesses requiring health care, and in all countries they have low priority. The Global Campaign against Headache (GC), launched in collaboration with the World Health Organization, is a response to this public-health disaster.

This chapter briefly describes the origins of the Global Campaign, its vision and purpose, its structure and three stages, and its activities and achievements during the 7 years since its launch.

Introduction

People who are affected by headache disorders, and professionals working in the field of headache, know that these disorders are real and often lifelong illnesses. They are not only highly prevalent, affecting men, women, and children, they are also disabling.

And they are ubiquitous. Headache disorders are not complaints only of rich countries. While huge lost-productivity costs resulting from headache disorders focus the attention in high-income countries, the humanitarian burdens of headache – pain and suffering, lifestyle compromises, damaged relationships, and lost opportunities – weigh no less heavily elsewhere. Poverty and its consequences of poor sanitation and infectious diseases may seem to be of overwhelming priority in many low-income countries, but why should headache and the burdens it imposes be any less disagreeable in the presence of hunger and other illness?

It is an irony that effective treatments that could alleviate these burdens are within reach. Research into disease mechanisms and the discoveries of the last 15 years have hugely benefited a few while failing to touch most of the world's headache-blighted lives. Yet the reality is that, for the vast majority of those whose quality of life is spoiled by headache, effective treatment requires no expensive equipment, tests, or specialists. The essential components of effective medical management are awareness of the problem, correct recognition and diagnosis, avoidance of mismanagement, appropriate lifestyle modifications, and informed use of cost-effective pharmaceutical remedies. The principal reason why the burdens attributable to headache persist, and indirect costs remain so high, is failure of health-care systems to provide these simple measures. Instead, there are artificial barriers throughout the world to access to care.

The key factor underlying this public-health disaster is education failure at every level. Lack of awareness and understanding of headache disorders among the general public allows myths to persist that they are not real and not worthy of medical attention. Lack of inclusion of diagnosis and management of headache disorders in the training curricula of health-care providers leaves them unskilled and therefore unwilling to offer health care in this field. Lack of recognition of the humanitarian burden and socioeconomic cost attributable to headache disorders leads health-policy makers grossly to misjudge the priority due to them. Headache disorders in many countries are simply not acknowledged as illnesses requiring health care, and everywhere they have low priority.

Lifting The Burden: A Response

In September 2003, the World Health Organization (WHO) signed a Memorandum of Understanding that brought into being the Global Campaign against Headache (GC), known as *Lifting The Burden*.

This truly important event for people worldwide affected by headache signaled WHO's recognition of headache disorders as a global public-health priority. It did not come about easily: there are many competing claims upon WHO's limited resources, and WHO accords priority only where it is manifestly due. Headache disorders in fact fulfill all of the criteria against which WHO assesses priority: they are highly prevalent, ubiquitous, disabling, and to a large extent treatable. While we all knew this, WHO required proof of it. This was quite right, and proof was provided, first at a technical consensus meeting on headache disorders hosted at WHO headquarters in Geneva in April 2000 (World Health Organization 2000) and then, crucially, by assimilating the evidence on migraine for WHO's *Global Burden of Disease Survey 2000* (GBD2000) (migraine had not featured in the earlier GBD1990). The outcome was conclusive: Migraine, on its own, was shown to be among the top 20 causes in the world of years of life lost to disability (World Health Organization 2001). Headache disorders came in from the cold.

Initially the GC was a partnership between WHO, International Headache Society (IHS), European Headache Federation (EHF), and World Headache Alliance (WHA), all of whom were cosignatories to the Memorandum of Understanding. It has moved on since. *Lifting The Burden* is now a legal entity in its own right, incorporated and registered as a charity in the United Kingdom, and admitted into Official Relations with WHO, markers of considerable success in its formative years. More broadly based now, the GC is better described as a collaboration between WHO, international nongovernmental organizations, academic institutions, and many willing individuals around the world. Its academic base has moved from Imperial College London to the Norwegian University of Science and Technology (NTNU), where it is better supported; the interests and research priorities of the Department of Clinical Neuroscience at NTNU enthusiastically embrace headache and global public health.

The originally conceived three stages of the GC have been described in detail before (Steiner 2004). In summary, first is to know the nature, scope, and scale of the problem – that is, the burden of headache – everywhere in the world ("knowledge for action"). It is perhaps extraordinary that, in 2003, very little was known of the prevalence or burden of any headache disorder for more than half the people of the world (Stovner et al. 2007): those living in most of the Western Pacific including China, all of South East Asia including India, all of Eastern Europe including Russia, most of Eastern Mediterranean, and most of Africa. Second is to exploit this knowledge, as it is gathered, to persuade governments, health-care providers and the public that, on clear evidence, headache *must* have higher health-care priority ("awareness for action"). Third, and the ultimate purpose of the GC, is to work with local policy makers and principal stakeholders to plan and implement health-care services for headache, ensuring these are appropriate to local systems, resources, and needs ("action for beneficial change").

Changing the world is a challenging task. Rather than suffer Descartes' paralysis from uncertainty (Descartes 1901), *Lifting The Burden* adopted the indomitable spirit invoked by American poetess, Marianne Moore (❯ *Box 58.1*), and set about the task with an aspirational vision (❯ *Box 58.2*). It took the three stages of the task apart into multiple steps, all with achievable objectives that, when reassembled at some time in the future, would lead to that vision (*A journey of a thousand miles begins with a single step* (attributed to Confucius)).

Box 58.1: I May, I Might, I Must

If you will tell me why the fen
appears impassable, I then
will tell you why I think that I
can get across it if I try.

Marianne Moore (1887–1972)

Box 58.2: The Global Campaign's Vision

Lifting The Burden envisions a future world in which headache disorders are recognized every-where as real, disabling, and deserving of medical care. In this future world, all who need care have access to it without artificial barriers.

The First Seven Years

Filling the very large gaps in knowledge for action has been the first priority. No standard methodology existed for population-based burden-of-headache studies, so *Lifting The Burden* developed its own. The model calls for a representative mix of urban and rural population samples, encountered by door-to-door "cold-calling" at randomly selected households; from each household, one adult, also randomly selected, is interviewed; the structured diagnostic questionnaire, based on ICHD-II, is validated in a pilot study within the population to be surveyed.

Applying this model, studies have been completed in Georgia (Kukava et al. 2007; Katsarava et al. 2009a, b) and Moldova (Moldovanu et al. 2007) and have reached the analysis stage in Russia (Ayzenberg et al. 2010), China (Yu et al.), and India; others are underway in Zambia and Pakistan, and more are planned in Saudi Arabia, Ethiopia and, possibly, Morocco, Abu Dhabi, Guatemala, Belize, Serbia, and Brazil. So far, these have revealed an extraordinarily high prevalence of daily headache in countries of Eastern Europe, highly prevalent migraine in Russia and, especially, in India (as represented by Karnataka State), and a prevalence of migraine in China, where it had been thought to be low, that is not very dissimilar from the global average of 11% (Stovner et al. 2007).

Lifting The Burden is a partner in *Eurolight*, a project supported by the European Com-mission Public Health Executive Agency to survey the impact of headache throughout Europe. This has harvested information from people with headache in Austria, France, Germany, Ireland, Italy, Lithuania, Luxembourg, the Netherlands, Spain, and the United Kingdom (Andrée et al. 2010). All of this will soon be published.

As for awareness, at the International Headache Congress in Kyoto in October 2005, the *Kyoto Declaration on Headache* was drafted with the guidance and signed in the presence not only of WHO's Regional Director for the Western Pacific Region but also of representatives of the Japanese Ministry of Health, Labour and Welfare. *Lifting The Burden* secured the inclusion of headache disorders in the *Atlas of Neurological Disorders* (World Health Organization, World Federation of Neurology 2004), produced in 2005 jointly by WHO and the World Federation of Neurology (WFN), and as a major chapter in WHO's later publication, *Neurological disorders: public health challenges* (World Health Organization 2007). All of these, not only because they have the imprimatur of WHO but also because their content is compelling, enter the consciousness of politicians, bringing awareness to them of headache as a substantial cause of public ill-health (Martelletti et al. 2007). So, too, does *Lifting The Burden*'s joint review with WHO showing the paucity of headache research in low- and middle-income countries (Mateen et al. 2008), and even more so will the joint global survey for WHO's *Atlas of Headache Disorders*, due to be published in 2011. The *Atlas of Headache Disorders*, one in the continuing series of Atlases published by WHO, will include data on headache and headache services gathered from more than 100 countries.

Politically more telling than all of these will be the inclusion of migraine and, for the first time, tension-type headache and medication-overuse headache in the new *Global Burden of Disease Study 2010* (GBD 2010). GBD2010 is a major revision of GBD2000, the importance of which, for the cause of headache, is highlighted above: it is essential for the future that GBD2010 accords due weight to the worldwide burden of headache, and *Lifting The Burden* has put much into assimilating, analyzing, and presenting the evidence on which this depends.

As *Lifting The Burden* considers models of headache service delivery and organization, and endeavors to make evidence-driven recommendations for change (Antonaci et al. 2008; Steiner et al. 2011), one clear principle is that most headache management belongs in primary care. The numbers of people who need it make this so (Steiner et al. 2011), but it is anyway the case that *most* headache management does not benefit from involvement of specialists. Nonexperts in primary care can do it perfectly well, although they do need some training.

Education is a central pillar of beneficial change (Steiner 2004, 2005). Training doctors to be better at managing headache is a huge undertaking on its own, but completely necessary: the current deficiencies in training, themselves engendered by the low priority given to headache, are at the heart (though not the whole cause) of the universal health-care failures for headache. Education is required at all levels, and therefore an undertaking to be shared – with IHS, EHF, and similar organizations, of course, but also with the universities. Within the GC is the Master's Degree in Headache Medicine at Sapienza University, Rome. This annual theoretical and practical course, now in its eighth year, is delivered by an international faculty (Martelletti et al. 2005). It is a training-the-trainers program, directed at specialists but with the hope of reaching primary care, the intended target, as the trainees return as trainers to their home countries.

Management by nonexperts in primary care can be made better also by the provision of practical clinical management supports, upon which *Lifting The Burden* embarked by assembling a writing and review group from all world regions in order to ensure multicultural relevance – a cardinal requirement of everything the GC is engaged in. Already produced, or in development, are diagnostic aids applying the criteria of ICHD-II, but simplified; regional management guidelines developed, where these exist, by harmonizing national guidelines (Steiner et al. 2007); information sheets for patients to aid understanding and promote compliance with treatment (Steiner 2007a); and universally acceptable indices of impact and treatment outcome (Steiner 2007b). The last was developed at a technical consensus meeting on headache outcome measures at WHO headquarters in April 2006, and follow-up validation and evaluation studies are being conducted in six countries.

This *Handbook of Headache*, written by authors from all over the world, is also aimed at nonspecialists. It is a supplement to these aids, providing detail when this is required.

Because good translation is crucial to multicultural relevance, *Lifting The Burden* has developed translation standards and protocols for GC materials (Peters 2007).

Lifting The Burden is working with, and supporting, the Cochrane collaboration, fostering systematic reviews of treatments for headache. One of the purposes is to be able to advise WHO on revisions to its essential medicines list, which, in time, will encourage availability worldwide of the drugs most needed to treat headache effectively.

As for actual intervention, *Lifting The Burden* has developed a headache-service model, to be tested soon in Georgia and later, if plans go forward, in Serbia, Bulgaria, and Abu Dhabi. The model is adaptable, but involves first assessing local need, together with willingness to pay, upon which sustainability will depend. The next steps in Georgia are to establish three clinics, provide free care and drugs to geographically defined populations and show the benefits of treatment to people and of the service to population health. Only once these benefits are apparent, the service will charge according to willingness to pay in order to become self-sustaining.

Ultimately, *Lifting The Burden* must evaluate what it helps to create, and amend it, in an iterative process if necessary, to achieve what is best possible. This raises a fundamental question: What is a good headache service? Surprisingly, or perhaps not, "quality" in the context of headache services has no accepted definition. Indeed it is not easily defined, although in part it must lie in the attainment of good outcomes, which can be measured. In preparing its proposals for headache-service quality evaluation, soon to be published, *Lifting The Burden* has undertaken a worldwide consultation.

Conclusion

This is a summary of what has happened. Not everything has been included. We believe *Lifting The Burden* can be pleased with and proud of its first 7 years. The activities represent many more than a single step (*A journey of a thousand miles begins with a single step* (attributed to Confucius)); more importantly, the steps are all in one and the right direction – each part of a cohesive, managed project directed toward a clear purpose. They involve actions in 28 countries, a seventh of the world's total.

Acknowledgments

The collaborations underpinning these activities include WHO of course, its headquarters in Geneva and the Regional Offices for South East Asia and Western Pacific; they include IHS and, notably, its Russian Linguistic Subcommittee, EHF, WHA, WFN, and the Pain, Palliative and Supportive Care (PaPaS) group of the Cochrane Collaboration. At national level they include: in Austria: Konventhospital Barmherzige Brüder, Linz; in Belgium: University of Ghent; in Brazil: the Federal University of Santa Catarina, Florianopolis, and Botucatu Medical School; in China: the Ministry of Health, the PLA General Hospital, Beijing, the Fourth Military Medical University, Xian, Xiaya Hospital of Centre-south University, Changsha, Affiliated Huashan Hospital of Fudan University, Shanghai, the First Affiliated Hospital of Sun Yat-sen

University, Guangzhou, and the First Hospital of Jilin University, Changchun; in Denmark: the Danish Headache Centre, Glostrup, and the University of Copenhagen; in Ethiopia: the University of Addis Ababa; in France: Hôpital Pasteur, Nice, and Hôpital Lariboisière, Paris; in Georgia: Tbilisi Medical University; in Germany: the University of Essen and the Institute for Health and Rehabilitation Sciences, Ludwig Maximilians University, Munich; in India: the National Institute for Mental Health and Neurosciences, Bangalore; in Italy: the National Neurological Institute C Mondino, Pavia, Sapienza University, Rome, Department of Neurology Policlinic of Monza, the University of Turin and the Neurological Institute Carlo Besta, Milan; in Japan: the Ministry of Health, Labour and Welfare and the International Headache Center, Kawasaki, Kanagawa; in Luxembourg: Centre de Recherche Public de la Santé; in Moldova: Chisinau State Medical and Pharmaceutical University; in the Netherlands: Medisch Centrum Boerhaave, Amsterdam; in Norway: the Norwegian National Headache Centre and the Norwegian University of Science and Technology, Trondheim; in Pakistan: DOW University of Health Sciences, Karachi; in Portugal: Hospital da Luz, Lisbon; in Russia: Setchenov Moscow Medical Academy and the Institute of Sociology, Russian Academy of Sciences, Moscow; in Saudi Arabia: King Abdullah International Medical Research Center, Riyadh, and the Saudi Arabia National Guard; in Serbia: the Ministry of Health and the Institute of Neurology and School of Medicine, Belgrade; in Spain: University Clinic Hospital, Valencia University; in Sri Lanka: the University of Colombo; in United Arab Emirates: the Health Authority – Abu Dhabi (HAAD); in the United Kingdom: Imperial College London, the City of London Migraine Clinic, the University of Oxford, and Isis Medical Media Ltd, Tonbridge; in the United States of America: Albert Einstein College of Medicine, Bronx NY, Brigham and Women's Hospital, Boston MA, Duke University, Durham NC, Geisinger Clinic, Center for Health Research, Danville PA, Michigan State University, East Lansing MI, the New England Center for Headache, Stamford CT, Park Nicollet Headache Clinic & Research Center, Minneapolis MN, Roosevelt Hospital, New York NY, Uniformed Services University, Bethesda MD, and the University of North Carolina, Chapel Hill NC; in Zambia: Chainama Hills College Hospital, Lusaka. And at individual level, they include many people, far too numerous to list.

All of these, and the many sponsors, we warmly thank.

This chapter is based on two editorials published in *Journal of Headache and Pain* (Steiner 2005; Steiner et al. 2010).

References

Andrée C, Vaillant M, Barre J, Katsarava Z, Lainez JM, Lair M-L, Lanteri-Minet M, Lampl C, Steiner TJ, Stovner LJ, Tassorelli C, Sándor PS (2010) Development and validation of the EUROLIGHT questionnaire to evaluate the burden of primary headache disorders in Europe. Cephalalgia 30:1082–1100

Antonaci F, Valade D, Lanteri-Minet M, Láinez JM, Jensen J, Steiner TJ (2008) Proposals for the organisation of headache services in Europe. Intern Emerg Med 3:S25–S28

Ayzenberg I, Katsarava Z, Mathalikov R, Chernysh M, Osipova V, Tabeeva G, Steiner TJ on behalf of *Lifting The Burden*: the Global Campaign to Reduce Burden of Headache Worldwide and the Russian Linguistic Subcommittee of the International Headache Society (2010) The burden of headache in Russia: validation of the diagnostic questionnaire in a population-based sample. Eur J Neurol. doi: 10.1111/j.1468-1331.2010.03177.x [Epub ahead of print]

Descartes R (1901) Principles of human knowledge. In Veitch J (trans, 1901, reprinted 1988) The meditations and selections from the principles. Open Court, Illinois, p 130

Katsarava Z, Dzagnidze A, Kukava M, Mirvelashvili E, Djibuti M, Janelidze M, Jensen R, Stovner LJ, Steiner TJ (2009a) Prevalence of cluster headache in the Republic of Georgia: results of a population-based study and methodological considerations. Cephalalgia 29:949–952

Katsarava Z, Dzagnidze A, Kukava M, Mirvelashvili E, Djibuti M, Janelidze M, Jensen R, Stovner LJ, Steiner TJ (2009b) Primary headache disorders in the Republic of Georgia: prevalence and risk factors. Neurology 73:1796–1803

Kukava M, Dzagnidze A, Mirvelashvili E, Djibuti M, Fritsche G, Jensen R, Stovner LJ, Steiner TJ, Katsarava Z (2007) Validation of a Georgian language headache questionnaire in a population-based sample. J Headache Pain 8:321–324

Martelletti P, Haimanot RT, Lainez MJA, Rapoport AM, Ravishankar K, Sakai F, Silberstein SD, Vincent M, Steiner TJ (2005) The global campaign to reduce the burden of headache worldwide. The International Team for Specialist Education (ITSE). J Headache Pain 6:261–263

Martelletti P, Steiner TJ, Bertolote JM, Dua T, Saraceno B (2007) The definitive position of headache among the major public health challenges. An end to the slippery slope of disregard [editorial]. J Headache Pain 8:149–151

Mateen F, Dua T, Steiner T, Saxena S (2008) Headache disorders in developing countries: research over the past decade. Cephalalgia 28:1107–1114

Moldovanu I, Pavlic G, Odobescu S, Rotaru L, Craciun C, Ciobanu L, Corcea G, Steiner T, Katsarava Z (2007) The prevalence of headache disorders in the Republic of Moldova: a population-based study. Cephalalgia 27:673

Peters M (2007) Translation protocols. J Headache Pain 8(suppl 1):S40–S47

Steiner TJ (2004) Lifting the burden: the global campaign against headache. Lancet Neurol 3:204–205

Steiner TJ (2005) *Lifting The Burden*: the global campaign to reduce the burden of headache worldwide. J Headache Pain 6:373–377

Steiner TJ (2007a) Information for patients. J Headache Pain 8(suppl 1):S26–S39

Steiner TJ (2007b) The HALT and HART indices. J Headache Pain 8(suppl 1):S22–S25

Steiner TJ, Paemeleire K, Jensen R, Valade D, Savi L, Lainez MJA, Diener H-C, Martelletti P, Couturier EGM (2007) European principles of management of common headache disorders in primary care. J Headache Pain 8(suppl 1):S3–S21

Steiner TJ, Birbeck GL, Jensen R, Katsarava Z, Martelletti P, Stovner LJ (2010) *Lifting The burden*: the first 7 years. J Headache Pain 11:451–455

Steiner TJ, Antonaci F, Jensen R, Lainez MJA, Lanteri-Minet M, Valade D on behalf of the European Headache Federation and *Lifting The Burden*: The Global Campaign against Headache (2011a) Recommendations for headache service organisation and delivery in Europe. J Headache Pain. doi: 10.1007/s10194-011-0320-x

Stovner LJ, Hagen K, Jensen R, Katsarava Z, Lipton RB, Scher AI, Steiner TJ, Zwart J-A (2007) The global burden of headache: a documentation of headache prevalence and disability worldwide. Cephalalgia 27:193–210

World Health Organization (2000) Headache disorders and public health: education and management implications. WHO, Geneva

World Health Organization (2001) World health report 2001. WHO, Geneva

World Health Organization (2007) Neurological disorders: public health challenges. WHO, Geneva

World Health Organization, World Federation of Neurology (2004) Atlas: country resources for neurological disorders. WHO, Geneva

Yu S-Y, Cao X-T, Zhao G, Yang X-S, Qiao X-Y, Fang Y-N, Feng J-C, Liu R-Z, Steiner TJ (2011) The burden of headache in China: validation of diagnostic questionnaire for a population-based survey. J Headache Pain 12:141–146

Resources and Links

Global Resources

World Health Organization
www.who.int
www.who.int/mental_health/neurology/headache/en

Action to promote global public health is among the missions of the World Health Organization (WHO). Campaigns committed to global public-health priorities, planned and conducted in collaboration with non-governmental organizations, are a means of accomplishing strategic goals. Since 2004, the year in which the Global Campaign against Headache was launched, WHO has given its formal support to activities aimed at reducing the burden of headache worldwide.

Lifting The Burden: The Global Campaign Against Headache
www.l-t-b.org; www.liftingtheburden.org

Lifting The Burden is a UK-registered charitable company. Its purpose is to direct and implement the Global Campaign against Headache in collaboration with WHO and in partnership with other non-governmental organisations, academic institutions, and individuals worldwide, with the ultimate objective of reducing the global burden of headache. Central to the Campaign, and essential for its purposes, are educational initiatives at various levels: aimed at health-care providers, health policy-makers, employers, schools, people affected by headache, and the general public.

Professional Organizations

International Headache Society
www.ihs-headache.org
Founded 1981

European Headache Federation
www.ehf-org.org
Founded 1992

American Headache Society
www.americanheadachesociety.org
Founded 1959

Post-Graduate Education

Sapienza University of Rome
Department of Clinical and Molecular Sciences

Master in Headache Medicine
http://w3.uniroma1.it/headache
   The Master Degree in Headache Medicine is a central pillar of *Lifting The Burden*'s educational activity. The annual part-time 1-year course is delivered by a faculty of international experts and comprises didactic lectures and practical clinical demonstrations, supported by distance learning. In the academic year 2010–2011, the course is offered for the eighth time.

University of Central Lancashire, Preston
School of Public Health & Clinical Sciences
PG CERT Management of Headache in Primary Care
www.uclan.ac.uk/information/courses/pgcert_management_of_headache_primary_care.php

   This postgraduate part-time modular course, completed within 1 academic year, focuses on the management of headache in primary care.

Scientific Journals

Cephalalgia
http://cep.sagepub.com
The Official Journal of the International Headache Society, first published in 1981.

Headache
www.headachejournal.org
The Official Journal of the American Headache Society, first published in 1961.

The Journal of Headache and Pain
www.springer.com/10194
The Official Journal of *Lifting The Burden* and of the European Headache Federation, first published in 2000.

Guidelines

Headache Classification Subcommittee of the International Headache Society (2004) The International Classification of Headache Disorders. 2nd ed. *Cephalalgia* 24 (Suppl 1): 9–160
   Since the first edition of 1988, and the second of 2004, the international classification of headache disorders has provided a common language for scientific, clinical and educational endeavour in the field of headache.

   Steiner TJ, Martelletti P (eds) (2007) WHO/LTB/EHF Aids for Management of Common Headache Disorders in Primary Care. *J Headache Pain* 8:S1–S47
   This compendium of aids for headache management in primary care includes guides for diagnosis and management of headache disorders, as well as information that may be given to patients.

Lay Organizations

World Headache Alliance
www.w-h-a.org

European Headache Alliance
www.e-h-a.eu

American Headache Society – Committee for Headache Education
www.achenet.org

Index

Lightning Source UK Ltd.
Milton Keynes UK
UKOW04n1900090514

231420UK00006B/192/P